HEALTH
for the
WHOLE
PERSON

The Complete Guide to Holistic Medicine

HEALTH *for the* WHOLE PERSON

edited by
Arthur C. Hastings, Ph.D. • James Fadiman, Ph.D. • James S. Gordon, M.D.

Westview Press • Boulder, Colorado

Based on a report for the U.S. government prepared by the Institute of Noetic Sciences, San Francisco, California, for the National Institute of Mental Health.

Published in 1980 in the United States of America by
  Westview Press, Inc.
  5500 Central Avenue
  Boulder, Colorado 80301
  Frederick A. Praeger, Publisher

Library of Congress Cataloging in Publication Data
Main entry under title:
Health for the whole person.
  Based on a report prepared by the Institute of Noetic Sciences for the National Institute of Mental Health.
  Includes bibliographies and indexes.
  1. Holistic medicine. I. Hastings, Arthur. II. Fadiman, James, 1939- III. Gordon, James Samuel.
IV. Institute of Noetic Sciences.
R733.H4   613   79-25285
ISBN 0-89158-883-3
ISBN 0-89158-884-1 pbk.

Printed and bound in the United States of America

CONTENTS

Foreword, *Senator Edward M. Kennedy* ix
Preface xi
Acknowledgments xiii
The Contributors xv

PART ONE
HOLISTIC MEDICINE

1   The Paradigm of Holistic Medicine, *James S. Gordon, M.D.* 3

    Annotated Bibliography 28

PART TWO
THE CONTEXT OF HEALTH

2   The Social Context of Health, *Leonard J. Duhl, M.D.* 39

    Annotated Bibliography 49

3   Family Therapy and Physical Illness, *Richard Rabkin, M.D.* 53

  Annotated Bibliography 61

4   Ecological Factors in Health, *Stephen Lerner, Michael Lerner, Ph.D.,*
and Jane Borchers, M.A. 65

  Annotated Bibliography 70

5   Medical Self-Care: Self-Responsibility for Health,
Tom Ferguson, M.D. 87

  Annotated Bibliography 100

PART THREE
MODALITIES FOR HEALTH
AND MENTAL HEALTH

THE ROLE OF THE MIND

6   The Mind in Health and Disease, *Kenneth R. Pelletier, Ph.D.* 107

  Annotated Bibliography 110

7   Biofeedback, *Joe Kamiya, Ph.D., and*
Joanne Gardner Kamiya, M.A. 115

  Annotated Bibliography 125

8   Autogenic Therapy, *Erik Peper, Ph.D., and*
Elizabeth Ann Williams 131

  Annotated Bibliography 136

9   Hypnosis, *David B. Cheek, M.D.* 139

  Annotated Bibliography 153

10   Meditation and Holistic Medicine,
Deane H. Shapiro, Jr., Ph.D. 159

  Annotated Bibliography 166

11   Psychic Healing, *Stanley Krippner, Ph.D.* 169

  Annotated Bibliography 172

12   The Placebo Effect: A Neglected Asset in the Care of Patients,
Herbert Benson, M.D., and Mark D. Epstein 179

  Annotated Bibliography, *David Zeiger and*
Arthur Hastings, Ph.D. 186

THE ROLE OF THE BODY

13 The Physical Disciplines and Health,
    Donald B. Ardell, Ph.D. 191

        Annotated Bibliography 204

14 Touch: Working with the Body, *Robert Frager, Ph.D.* 209

        Annotated Bibliography 218

15 Chiropractic, *Victoria Simons, D.C.* 227

        Annotated Bibliography 236

16 Eastern Spiritual and Physical Disciplines and Health:
    Annotated Bibliography, *Arthur Hastings, Ph.D.,*
    James Fadiman, Ph.D., and James S. Gordon, M.D. 241

HEALING INPUTS

17 Food and Nutrition, *James Fadiman, Ph.D.* 247

        Annotated Bibliography 256

18 The Therapeutic Use of Plants, *Leslie J. Kaslof* 263

        Annotated Bibliography 270

19 Music and Sound in Health, *Helen L. Bonny, Ph.D.* 277

        Annotated Bibliography 282

20 The Use of Light and Color in Health,
    Philip C. Hughes, Ph.D. 285

        Annotated Bibliography 296

PART FOUR
APPLICATIONS
THROUGHOUT THE LIFE CYCLE

21 Alternatives in Childbirth, *James S. Gordon, M.D., and*
    Doris B. Haire 303

        Annotated Bibliography 318

22 Holistic Approaches to Oral Health and Dentistry,
    Leo Wollman, M.D., Erwin DiCyan, Ph.D.,
    George Goldberg, D.D.S., and Arthur Hastings, Ph.D. 333

Annotated Bibliography, *Leo Wollman, M.D., and
Arthur Hastings, Ph.D.* 341

23 Stress: The New Etiology, *Thomas H. Holmes, M.D.* 345

Annotated Bibliography 357

24 Holistic Approaches to Healthy Aging and Programs for
the Elderly, *Ken Dychtwald, Ph.D.* 363

Annotated Bibliography 373

25 Dying and Death, *Charles A. Garfield, Ph.D.* 379

Annotated Bibliography 389

PART FIVE
ALTERNATIVE MEDICAL PERSPECTIVES

26 Homoeopathic Medicine, *Harris L. Coulter, Ph.D.* 395

Annotated Bibliography 401

27 Chinese Medicine and Holistic Health,
David E. Bresler, Ph.D., C.A. 407

Annotated Bibliography 420

28 Indigenous and Traditional Systems of Healing,
Arthur Kleinman, M.D. 427

Annotated Bibliography 436

29 Alternative Forms of Diagnosis, *Arthur Hastings, Ph.D.* 443

Annotated Bibliography 458

PART SIX
SOCIAL AND POLITICAL IMPLICATIONS

30 Holistic Health Centers, *James S. Gordon, M.D.* 467

Annotated Bibliography 479

31 The Future of Health Care in the United States,
Rick J. Carlson, J.D. 483

Annotated Bibliography 496

Name and Title Index 503
Subject Index 523

FOREWORD

Senator Edward M. Kennedy

The benefits of our present health care system are unequally distributed and its costs prohibitive even to those who can take advantage of them. Statistics tell us that the children of poor and minority women are far more likely than middle class infants to die at birth or in the weeks thereafter, that people who live in inner city and poor rural areas are more likely to become mentally and physically ill than those who live in our affluent suburbs, that a single major illness may bankrupt even a well-to-do middle-class family. It is clear that we need some kind of national health-care program to extend the benefits of medical care to all Americans, to ensure that health will not be bought at the price of economic security.

In recent years we have begun to realize that we need to make changes in the kind of health care we provide to Americans as well as in its distribution and cost. We know a good deal about helping people when they are acutely ill, about responding to and treating catastrophic illness and massive trauma. We know and are able to do far less about the chronic diseases – hypertension and insomnia, diabetes, arthritis, alcoholism, and mental illness – that afflict and will increasingly afflict our aging population. And we are only at the beginning of our efforts to prevent illness and promote health.

Health for the Whole Person, encyclopedic in scope, modest in tone, tells us a good deal about why our present health care system is not adequate to meet the needs of the American people, and better yet, it tells us some of the directions we might pursue to improve our health. It shows us that we have lost sight of the capacity of the family, the culture, and the society to produce and relieve individual illness. It brings to our attention techniques – diet and exercise, touch, and introspection – that we have ignored or neglected, and perhaps most importantly it shows us that these techniques can be used to help people to help themselves. . . . I hope it will be only one of many attempts to bridge the gap between physical and mental illness, to promote a more holistic approach to the health of our nation.

PREFACE

This book presents attitudes, information, and tools for a holistic approach to medicine, health, and mental health. In our discussions among ourselves and with the contributing authors we defined three aspects of a holistic approach. First, such an approach involves expanding our focus to include the many personal, familial, social, and environmental factors that promote health, prevent illness, and encourage healing. Second, a holistic approach views the patient as an individual person, not as a symptom-bearing organism. This attitude emphasizes the self-responsibility of the person for his or her health and the importance of mobilizing the person's own health capacities, rather than treating illness only from the outside. Third, the holistic approach tries to make wise use of the many diagnostic, treatment, and health modalities that are available in addition to the standard materia medica – including alternative medical and healing systems as well as psychological techniques and physical modalities. Some of these methods of treatment and health practices are already accepted, others are accepted but not applied in practice, and still others need further research to explore the range of their uses.

This volume presents information about these varied aspects and practices of holistic medicine. Each chapter surveys a specific topic and is followed by an extensive bibliography containing critical annotations on the most important theoretical and practical references for that area. The discussions and bibliographies have been written for the health care professional and for the layman who wishes to become more knowledgeable in his or her own health practices.

But do remember that as yet there is no specific holistic medicine orthodoxy. There is no holistic therapy regime for arthritis or leukemia nor is there a holistic treatment of choice for schizophrenia. Rather, the holistic approach in medicine is a context and a set of principles to guide our attitudes toward health, our therapeutic practices, and our relationships with body and mind, patients, the environment, and health care. We ourselves must provide the integration.

Arthur Hastings
James Fadiman
James S. Gordon

ACKNOWLEDGMENTS

This book is based on a report prepared by the Institute of Noetic Sciences for the National Institute of Mental Health and was partially supported with federal funds provided under contract no. 278-77-0040 (SM): "A Comprehensive Critical Bibliography on 'Holistic Medicine and Its Relevance to Current Health and Mental Health Theory and Practice.'" The original report is planned to be made available from the Superintendent of Documents, Washington, D.C., under the title *Holistic Medicine,* published by the National Institute of Mental Health. For the present volume the report was re-edited, and new and additional material was added.

The Institute of Noetic Sciences, located in San Francisco, is a nonprofit educational and research organization founded by former astronaut Edgar D. Mitchell. Its purpose is to sponsor the growth and development of the tools, techniques, and applications of science to the study of mind, brain, and body relationships and their applications to health, education, and medicine.

The staff that prepared the report for the Institute of Noetic Sciences consisted of Arthur Hastings and James Fadiman, codirectors, and Susan Swanson, administrator. Editorial responsibilities for the book were divided among the codirectors and James S. Gordon of the National Institute of Mental Health. Janette Harrington was responsible for manuscript preparation.

Staff reviewers included David Zeiger, Phyllis Mattson, Susan Emigh,

Valeria Dumitru, David Hall, and Felicity Hall. We also wish to thank the following colleagues and associates for their assistance and suggestions: Frank Barr, James Beal, Diane Brown, Emmanuel Cheraskin, Osmond Crosby, Sharon Curtin, Lawrence Dickey, George Engel, Karen Fitzgerald, Jerome Frank, Don Gerrard, Gloria Goldsmith, Jules D. Gordon, Elmer Green, Willis Harman, Robert C. Heffron, Richard Hicks, Rick Ingrasci, Lori Kaplan, Alan Levy, Salvador Minuchin, Dawa Norbu, Brendan O'Regan, John Ott, James Polidora, Tarthang Tulku, and T. J. Tsarong. In addition, our appreciation goes to the California Institute of Transpersonal Psychology and its staff, Menlo Park, for their help.

The contents of this publication are the opinions of the authors and the editors and do not necessarily reflect the views or policies of the National Institute of Mental Health of the Department of Health, Education, and Welfare, nor does mention of trade names, commercial products, or organizations imply endorsement by the U.S. government.

A. H.
J. F.
J.S.G.

THE CONTRIBUTORS

Donald B. Ardell, Ph.D., M.C.P. President, Planning for Wellness, Mill Valley, California. Author of *High Level Wellness: An Alternative to Doctors, Drugs and Disease* and *High Level Wellness for Young People or Anyone Under the Influence of an Adult.*

Herbert Benson, M.D. Associate professor of medicine, Harvard University Medical School, Boston, Massachusetts, and Department of Behavioral Medicine, Beth Israel Hospital, Boston, Massachusetts. Author of *The Mind-Body Effect* and *The Relaxation Response.*

Helen Lindquist Bonny, Ph.D., R.M.T. Director, Department of Music Therapy, The Catholic University of America, Washington, D.C., and director, Institute for Consciousness and Music Training Seminars, Baltimore, Maryland. Author of *The Role of Taped Music Programs in the Guided Imagery and Music Process, Facilitating GIM Sessions,* coauthor (with L. M. Savary) of *Music and Your Mind: Listening with a New Consciousness,* contributor of "Music Therapy/Guided Imagery" in *Wholistic Dimensions in Healing,* edited by Leslie J. Kaslof.

Jane Borchers, M.A. Research associate, Commonweal, Inc., Bolinas, California. Coauthor of *Common Knowledge.*

David E. Bresler, Ph.D., C.A. Director, Pain Control Unit, University of California, Los Angeles, California; adjunct assistant professor of anesthesiology, gnathology, and occlusion and of psychology, UCLA School of Medicine, School of Dentistry, and the College of Letters and Sciences; executive director, Center for Integral Medicine, Pacific Palisades, California. Author of *Free Yourself from Pain*, coeditor and contributor of *Mind, Body and Health: Toward an Integral Medicine* (in press).

Rick J. Carlson, J.D. Health policy specialist, Commonweal, Inc., Bolinas, California; Health Resource Group, Mill Valley, California; Health Resources and Communication, Inc., San Francisco, California. Editor of *The Frontiers of Science and Medicine;* author of *The End of Medicine, The Dilemmas of Punishment*, and *Future Directions in Health Care.*

David B. Cheek, M.D., F.A.C.O.G. Gynecology and obstetrics, San Francisco, California. Attending staff, Children's Hospital and Pacific Medical Center, San Francisco; contract faculty, California School of Professional Psychology, Berkeley, California. Coauthor of *Clinical Hypnotherapy.*

Harris Livermore Coulter, Ph.D. Washington, D.C. Author of *Homoeopathic Medicine; Divided Legacy: A History of the Schism in Medical Thought*, vol. 1, *The Patterns Emerge: Hippocrates to Paracelsus;* vol. 2, *Progress and Regress: Van Helmont to Claude Bernard;* vol. 3, *Science and Ethics in American Medicine, 1800–1920.*

Erwin DiCyan, Ph.D. Pharmacology. Author of *Without Prescription, Vitamins in Your Life, Vitamin E and Aging*, and *Creativity—Road to Self Discovery.*

Leonard J. Duhl, M.D. Professor of public health and urban social policy, Department of City and Regional Planning, University of California, Berkeley, California. Author of *The Urban Condition: People and Policy in the Metropolis*, coauthor of *Making Whole: Health for a New Epoch* (in press).

Ken Dychtwald, Ph.D. Psychologist, Berkeley, California. President, Association for Humanistic Gerontology. Author of *Bodymind*, editor (with A. Villoldo) of *Human Potential: Glimpses into the 21st Century* (in press) and author of *Lifelong Health and Well-being* (forthcoming).

Mark D. Epstein. Harvard University Medical School, Boston, Massachusetts.

James Fadiman, Ph.D. Lecturer, Stanford University, Palo Alto, California; professor, California Institute of Transpersonal Psychology, Menlo Park, California. Coauthor (with Robert Frager) of *Personality and Personal Growth;* editor of *Exploring Madness, The Proper Study of Man;* and coeditor of *Relax.*

Tom Ferguson, M.D. Editor of *Medical Self-Care*, Inverness, California.

Robert Frager, Ph.D. Director, California Institute of Transpersonal Psychology, Menlo Park, California. Author (with James Fadiman) of *Personality and Personal Growth.*

Charles A. Garfield, Ph.D. Assistant clinical professor of medical psychology, Cancer Research Institute, University of California Medical Center, San Francisco, California; founder and chairman, Shanti Project, Berkeley, California. Author of *Stress and Survival: The Emotional Realities of Life-Threatening Illness* and *Psychosocial Care of the Dying Patient.*

George Goldberg, D.D.S. Price-Pottenger Nutritional Foundation, Santa

Monica, California; Southern Academy of Clinical Nutrition, Florida.

James S. Gordon, M.D. Research psychiatrist and consultant on alternative forms of service, Center for Studies of Child and Family Mental Health, National Institute of Mental Health, Rockville, Maryland. Author of *Special Study of Alternative Services: Report to the President's Commission on Mental Health* and *Caring for Youth: Essays on Alternative Services;* coeditor and contributor to *Mind, Body and Health: Toward an Integral Medicine* (in press).

Doris B. Haire. President, American Foundation for Maternal and Child Health, New York City; former president, International Childbirth Association, Milwaukee, Wisconsin. Author of *The Cultural Warping of Childbirth;* contributing author to *Prevention of Embryonic Fetal and Perinatal Disease.*

Arthur Hastings, Ph.D. Research associate, Institute of Noetic Sciences, San Francisco, California; professor, California Institute of Transpersonal Psychology, Menlo Park, California; adjunct professor, John F. Kennedy University, Orinda, California. Coauthor of *Argumentation and Advocacy, Group Communication Through Computers,* vol. 2, and *Changing Images of Man.*

Thomas H. Holmes, M.D. Professor of psychiatry and behavioral sciences, University of Washington School of Medicine, Seattle, Washington. Coauthor of "Life Change and Illness Susceptibility," in *Separation and Depression: Clinical and Research Aspects,* edited by J. P. Scott and E. C. Senay; *The Nose: An Experimental Study of Reactions Within the Nose in Human Subjects During Varying Life Experiences.*

Philip C. Hughes, Ph.D. Director of environmental photobiology, Duro-Test Corporation, North Bergen, New Jersey.

Joanne Gardner Kamiya, M.A. Research associate, Langley Porter Institute, University of California Medical School, San Francisco, California.

Joe Kamiya, Ph.D. Professor of medical research in residence, Langley Porter Institute, University of California Medical School, San Francisco, California. Coeditor and contributor to *Biofeedback and Self-Control.*

Leslie J. Kaslof. Founder, International Institute for Biological and Botanical Research and the National Council on Wholistic Therapeutics and Medicine, Brooklyn, New York. Author of *Herb and Ailment Cross-Reference Chart;* editor of *Wholistic Dimensions in Healing.*

Arthur Kleinman, M.D., M.A. Associate professor and head, Division of Cross-Cultural Psychiatry, Department of Psychiatry and Behavioral Sciences, University of Washington, Seattle, Washington. Author of *Patients and Healers in the Context of Culture: An Exploration of the Borderland between Anthropology, Medicine, and Psychiatry* (in press); coeditor of *Renewal in Psychiatry.*

Stanley Krippner, Ph.D. Humanistic Psychology Institute, San Francisco, California. Author of *Song of the Siren;* coauthor of *Dream Telepathy;* author of *The Realms of Healing;* editor of *Advances in Parapsychological Research,* vols. 1 and 2.

Michael Lerner, Ph.D. Executive director, Commonweal, Inc., Bolinas, California. Coauthor of *Common Knowledge.*

Stephen Lerner. Research director, Commonweal, Inc., Bolinas, California. Coauthor of *Common Knowledge;* editor of *Working Papers.*

Kenneth R. Pelletier, Ph.D. Assistant clinical professor, Department of Psychiatry and the Langley Porter Neuropsychiatric Institute, University of California School of Medicine, San Francisco, California; assistant professor, Department of Public Health, University of California, Berkeley; director of the Psychosomatic Medicine Clinic, Berkeley, California. Author of *Mind as Healer, Mind as Slayer: A Holistic Approach to Preventing Stress Disorders, Toward a Science of Consciousness,* and *Holistic Medicine: From Stress to Optimum Health;* coauthor of *Consciousness: East and West.*

Erik Peper, Ph.D. Director, Biofeedback and Family Therapy Institute, Berkeley, California; faculty, Center for Interdisciplinary Science, San Francisco State University, San Francisco, California. Coauthor of *Mind/Body Integration: Essential Readings in Biofeedback;* author of *Relaxation: A Bibliography* and *From the Inside-out: A Self-teaching and Laboratory Manual for Biofeedback and Self Regulation.*

Richard Rabkin, M.D. Associate clinical professor, New York University School of Medicine, New York. Author of *Inner and Other Space* and *Strategic Psychotherapy.*

Deane H. Shapiro, Jr., Ph.D. President, Institute for the Advancement of Human Behavior, Portola Valley, California; dean of academic affairs, Pacific Graduate School of Psychology, Palo Alto, California; clinical instructor, Department of Psychiatry and Behavioral Sciences, Stanford University Medical School, Stanford, California. Author of *Precision Nirvana;* coeditor of *Meditation: Self-regulation Strategy and Altered State of Consciousness.*

Victoria Simons, D.C. Private chiropractic practice, Falls Church, Virginia.

Elizabeth Ann Williams. Institute for Interdisciplinary Science, San Francisco State University, San Francisco, California.

Leo Wollman, M.D. Psychiatrist, Brooklyn, New York. Editor of *The Journal of the American Society of Psychosomatic Dentistry and Medicine;* author of *Write Yourself Slim* and *Hypnosis in Marriage and Divorce.*

David J. Zeiger, Stanford Sleep Research Center, Stanford University Medical School, Stanford, California.

Part One

HOLISTIC MEDICINE

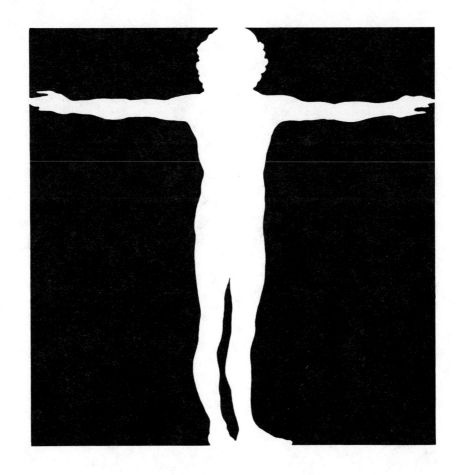

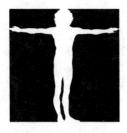

THE PARADIGM OF HOLISTIC MEDICINE

James S. Gordon, M.D.

The concept of "holism" was first introduced by the South African philosopher Jan Christian Smuts in 1926. To Smuts holism was an antidote to the analytic reductionism of the prevailing sciences. It was a way of comprehending whole organisms and systems as entities greater than and different from the sum of their parts (Smuts, 1926).

In the last several years holistic (sometimes spelled wholistic) medicine has come to denote both an approach to the whole person in his or her total environment and a variety of healing and health-promoting practices. This approach, which encompasses and is at times indistinguishable from humanistic, behavioral, and integral medicine, includes an appreciation of patients as mental and emotional, social and spiritual, as well as physical beings. It respects their capacity for healing themselves and regards them as active partners in, rather than passive recipients of, health care. Such an approach has always been an integral part of the healer's heritage. It is named and emphasized now to correct our tendencies to equate medicine and health care with the treatment of disease entities; to ignore the shaping force of familial, social, and economic contexts on health and disease; and to confuse (in Osler's words) the patient with his illness.

Through a series of chapters specifically written for it, this volume attempts to describe the familial, social, cultural, and ecological contexts that modify and shape both our health and our medical practice; to summarize our current knowledge of many healing modalities that have, until recently, been neglected by most Western allopathic physicians; and to demonstrate how these modalities are currently being applied in settings that address a variety of bio-psychosocial problems. Each of the chapters is supplemented by a critical anno-tated bibliography.

It is important to realize that individual techniques practiced by thousands of physicians and nurses, mental health professionals, and lay people are not neces-sarily holistic, even when they claim to address themselves to "the whole person." Acupuncture is, for example, one aspect of Chinese medicine, and that elegant and useful system is still only a part of the larger whole that healing can and should be. It has little to offer the victim of an automobile accident and does not teach a physician how to alter the interpersonal dynamics that may maintain and encourage chronic illness. Holistic practitioners use all the techniques that are helpful to their patients: biofeedback, meditation, and modern fluid replacement as well as ancient energy balance, surgery, and acupuncture. Holistic medicine is a model or paradigm, not just the techniques that are used within its practice.

This chapter describes the paradigm or model of holistic medicine. It ex-plores the forces that have created the need for a more holistic approach to medicine and outlines some of the principles that are or ought to be part of the theory and practice of any form of health and medical care that presumes to call itself holistic.

The Biomedical Background

In the last several centuries Western civilization has been shaped by a system of thought and a world view we variously call rational, scientific, or mechanistic. Emphasizing analysis, action, and achievement, it has helped to create a technol-ogy that has brought enormous material advances to a significant sector of the developed world. This technology has made it possible for people in any part of the world to be in instantaneous communication with one another, it has enabled us to move for considerable periods of time beyond the gravitational pull of the earth, and it has helped us to resolve matter into particles so small that even our most sophisticated instruments can observe them only indirectly. It has pro-duced telephones and televisions, satellites and space programs, nuclear medi-cine and nuclear weapons.

The medicine we practice reflects this method of thought and relies on the technology it has produced. Since the philosopher Descartes separated a tran-scendent nonmaterial mind from the material and mechanical operations of the body, science has been concerned with ever more accurately resolving that body into its component parts. From Harvey's physiological observations to modern biochemistry, from Vesalius's gross anatomy through Leeuwenhoek's micro-scopic researches to the ultrastructural anatomy revealed by the electron micro-scope, science has honed in ever more finely on the irreducible forms and func-tions that sustain our physical being.

In the mid-nineteenth century this mechanistic model was informed by two important sets of observations: (1) that particular organic entities—bacteria— were instrumental in producing particular disease states and characteristic pathological lesions; and (2) that certain substances—antitoxins and vaccines— could improve the individual's ability to ward off the effects of these and other pathogens. Koch's observations as well as Von Behring's and Jenner's innoculations paved the way for Ehrlich's discovery of a "magic bullet" that could destroy the spirochetes of syphillis and trypanosomiasis while sparing their human host.

Investigators and clinicians began to move like an advancing army on disease. Fleming discovered the antibiotic penicillin and Florey tested it clinically; insulin was isolated and used in the treatment of diabetics. The increasing sophistication of the technology brought ever more dramatic results. Kidneys were transplanted to patients who lacked them; a machine pumped blood through the body while surgeons repaired its diseased heart.

No longer viewed as a God-sent affliction, an imbalance between the individual and the environment, or a sign of moral insufficiency, disease became explicable in particular bacteriological, biochemical, and pathophysiological terms. Biomedical scientists believed that once they found the offending pathogen or uncovered the basic metabolic error they would be able to synthesize the appropriate antibiotic, to repair the damaged organ, or to replace the missing chemical. Optimistic researchers and clinicians came to expect that every disease, including the deviant behaviors and the contorted interpersonal relationships that they began to call "mental illness," would some day be traced to particular pathogens or resolved into particular biochemical abnormalities. The congealed heart and the twisted mind would, on appropriate examination, reveal the malfunctioning cell and the twisted molecule.

The explanatory power and the very real achievements of this biomedical model tended over time to narrow the perspective of those who adopted it, to prevent them from fully appreciating the importance of the social, economic, and environmental determinants of health and illness. Their conviction and the power and prestige they accumulated cast a shadow over the work of other less "scientific" healers. Rival healing professions and perspectives gradually disappeared (Thomsonian medicine), were relegated to "fringe" status (homoeopathy, chiropractic, naturopathy), or were absorbed into mainstream biomedicine (osteopathy and midwifery).

In the early part of this century the biomedical model extended its domain beyond the bounds of physical and even mental disease. Birth and death, those most inevitable of human processes, were taken from the familiar home context in which they had always taken place to the hospital. Armed with analgesics, anesthetics, forceps, and scalpels, obstetricians urged newborns out into the bright light of delivery rooms. Physicians and nurses, determined to use all their knowledge and skill to prolong life, usurped the roles of family members in the care of the terminally ill.

Later, conditions that had been viewed in religious, moral, economic, or political terms acquired medical metaphors and demanded medical intervention. Juvenile delinquency, social protest, the struggles of Blacks and women to obtain their rights, and the activities of our children were variously diagnosed and, where occasion permitted, treated as illnesses. Young people who could not sit still in school rooms, prisoners who protested jail conditions, and, occasionally, civil rights workers who wanted to vote were all given pills to treat the mental illnesses that presumably caused them to behave in this fashion.

Meanwhile, other health care professionals contributed to a model that was both less imperialistic and more comprehensive. Nevertheless, researchers in psychosomatic medicine insisted on the connection between their patients' emotional and physical condition, schools of public health continued to be concerned with the poverty and exploitative working conditions that fostered mental defects and physical illness, and anthropologists reported on the efficacy of "primitive" healers' techniques and the cures that faith alone seemed able to effect. But these disciplines were regarded as extramedical specialties, not dimensions of medicine itself. Modern medicine meant biomedicine, highly refined and technologically based diagnostic procedures and surgical and pharmacological intervention, with a focus on the individual patient and his or her disease.

The Challenge to Biomedicine

Approximately twenty years ago faith in the efficacy and exclusivity of the biomedical model and in the institutions and attitudes that were reinforced and sustained by it began to erode. In 1959 René Dubos, a research microbiologist, suggested in *Mirage of Health* that the advances he and others had made in the development of antibiotics and other remedies had far less to do with the improved health of the population of industrialized nations than a variety of economic, social, nutritional, and behavioral advances. Five years later the U.S. Surgeon General's report (1964) clearly revealed the association between one behavior, smoking, and such serious and often fatal illnesses as emphysema, chronic bronchitis, hypertension, and lung cancer. At the same time, in the wake of the civil rights movement Blacks and others began to declare that good health and respectful health care were, like the vote, a right; women questioned the medical treatment they received at the hands of mostly male physicians; mine workers challenged the working conditions that produced so much death and debility; and all Americans began to wonder when "magic bullets" would be discovered to attack the chronic conditions—arthritis, hypertension, cancer, and cardiovascular and cerebrovascular disease—which had replaced infectious disease as major killers and cripplers.

Meanwhile the most prestigious scientific journals were publishing reports on the side effects and inadequacies of the medicines that physicians daily prescribed for their patients. New strains of bacteria developed resistance to the wondrous antibiotics that had destroyed their ancestors and then to the antibiotics that were synthesized to replace them. Aspirin, long thought to be benign, turned out to be responsible for a virtual epidemic of gastrointestinal bleeding. Chloramphenicol was implicated in the sudden deaths of children whose infections were successfully treated. And a tranquilizer, thalidomide, normally prescribed for pregnant women, was found to cross through placentas to produce babies with tiny flipperlike arms and legs.

The cost of medical care mounted even more rapidly than concern about the equity of its distribution or its effectiveness. Even after the passage of Medicare and Medicaid legislation, families in the half of our population that were neither poor enough nor old enough to qualify for government assistance, nor rich enough to afford comprehensive insurance, could be pauperized by a single major illness (Knowles, 1977). Hospital charges swelled with the costs of exhaustive batteries of laboratory tests and the purchase and maintenance of such expensive technological innovations as radiation therapy units and ultrasound scanners, and physicians' fees increased almost as precipitously. From 1950 to 1965 the cost of medical care increased from $10 to $40 billion, from 4 percent to almost 6 percent of the gross national product. Five years later it was almost $70 billion and over 7 percent of the GNP.

In the last decade the acceleration of medical costs and the increasingly apparent limitations of medical care have provided both background and motive force for an ever broader and more articulate critique of modern biomedicine and its theoretical underpinnings. This critique, whose dimensions I will outline in the next section of this chapter, is in turn creating the context for a new way of looking at ourselves and our bodies, for a new model of health and illness care that enriches and enlarges modern biomedicine.

The Critique

Historical Reevaluation

Even some of those who contributed most to the underpinnings of the biomedical view of health and illness believed that it was dangerously narrow. The "father of modern pathology," Rudolph Virchow, was as concerned with public health as he was with microscopic diagnosis. He once remarked that "medicine is a social science and politics nothing but medicine on a grand scale." Pasteur himself is said to have declared on his deathbed that "Bernard is right. The pathogen is nothing, the terrain is everything." Nonetheless, many medical historians persisted in emphasizing the overwhelming importance of biomedical discoveries in combatting illness and improving health (Marti-Ibanez, 1952). In the last several years, however, Thomas McKeown (1976) has substantially revised conventional opinion about the effects of medical progress on our health. He has marshalled a wealth of data that substantiates Dubos's pioneering effort to put the achievements of biomedicine in a historical perspective.

Drawing on public health statistics from England and Wales in the last three centuries, McKeown has demonstrated that medical advances generally coincided with, rather than caused, improvements in the health of the population. His meticulous researches show that only 10 percent of the improvement in mortality from infectious disease can be traced to individual medical intervention — including the dramatic and sometimes lifesaving use of antibiotics. According to McKeown, our better health can largely be attributed to factors unrelated to medicine. These include improvements in nutrition (secondary to better food sources and methods of cultivation), in the environment (especially the treatment and regulation of food and water), and in our behavior (particularly the change in reproductive patterns that limited the size of the population).

When McKeown applies the lessons of his revisionist history to our current situation, he concludes that the remedies for the chronic diseases that afflict our aging, sedentary, overfed, and ecologically besieged population must once again come from changes in diet, behavior, and the environment.

The Discovery of Our National Ill Health

It was clear to epidemiologists, even before Dubos and McKeown drove the point home, that the burden of mortality and morbidity in developed nations was shifting from acute infections to chronic stress-related disorders. During the last ten years, however, we have become acutely aware of the prevalence and destructiveness of these disorders.

An authoritative collection of essays edited by the late president of the Rockefeller Foundation (Knowles, 1977) informs us that by 1974 some 50 percent of our deaths resulted from cardiovascular and cerebrovascular disease and another 19 percent could be attributed to cancer. Twenty-four million Americans currently have hypertension (a major predisposing cause of both cardiovascular and cerebrovascular disease), and a like number are afflicted with sleep-onset insomnia. Twice as many have regular headaches and three times that number are more than twenty pounds above their optimal weight. A recent report by the President's Commission on Mental Health (1978) tells us that 9 million Americans are alcoholic and that "15 percent of our population needs some form of mental health services."

Limitations and Dangers of the Current Medical System

This prevalence of chronic disease and discomfort, the generally unsatisfactory progress of our multibillion dollar "war on cancer" (Schneiderman, 1979), together with our mixed record of improving our survival at either end of the life cycle — the United States still ranks fifteenth in the world in overall infant mortality and has since 1900 only extended the life span of 45-year-olds by four and one half years (Bureau of the Census, 1977) – has caused many within and outside the health professions to wonder if the range of modern medicine's effectiveness is far more limited than it initially seemed.

This skepticism has been augmented by an increasing number of studies that demonstrate unnecessary, counterproductive, and dangerous practices in our medical system. Some, like Mather's (1971) randomized examination of home versus hospital treatment of acute myocardial infarction, raise pointed questions about high-technology, hospital-based medicine. In that study mortality rates were comparable for heart attack patients treated in intensive care units and at home. Others highlight our physicians' and our society's promiscuous use of pharmacological agents that are addictive, potentially dangerous, and often unnecessary – 5 to 7 billion Valium and Librium each year and 20,000 tons or 225 aspirin per person per year (Brecher, 1973). Still others indict our surgical practice. Surveys of the prevalence, cost, and lethality of unnecessary surgery (U.S. House of Representatives, 1976) have revealed that 2.4 million unnecessary operations costing $3.9 billion and 11,900 lives were performed in 1974 alone. A follow-up study several years later (U.S. House of Representatives, 1978) painted almost the same picture.

Several writers, including particularly Carlson (1975) and Illich (1976), have assembled an impressive and frightening array of statistics on iatrogenic (physician- and hospital-caused) illness and inadequate and misdirected treatment. Together these studies, which are largely drawn from refereed medical journals, indict the quality of our best care, the thoroughness with which it is delivered, and the environment in which it takes place. Carlson describes one study of emergency room patients undertaken at Baltimore City Hospital (and repeated with essentially identical results at the prestigious Johns Hopkins Hospital) by Robert Brook and colleagues (1973). Brook demonstrated that only 94 of 141 emergency room patients completed diagnostic studies ordered for them, that only 37 of the 98 who received X-rays were informed of the results, and that only 14 of 38 who had abnormal X-rays received adequate therapy for the conditions that were diagnosed. Illich cites figures to show that 1 out of 5 patients admitted to a typical research hospital acquires an iatrogenic disease. He adds, quoting a 1973 U.S. Department of Health, Education, and Welfare report, that 7 percent of all patients suffer compensable injuries while hospitalized.

The Psychosomatic Critique

Exemplary clinicians and researchers from Hippocrates to Osler, from Walter B. Cannon to Hans Selye, have emphasized the inextricability of mind and body, of physical and emotional health. However, many of their contemporary heirs have forgotten that an illness affects both body and mind, that it is their job to help their patients regain emotional as well as biochemical balance. In practice most conditions are regarded as either physical or mental and are assigned to the specialist—psychiatrist or internist—into whose domain they fall. Even those that are called psychosomatic—peptic ulcers, hypertension, thyrotoxicosis, ulcerative colitis, asthma, and others—are often treated pharmacologically, as if they were exclusively somatic, while in common speech "It's just psychosomatic" has come to mean "It's imaginary."

In the last several years a growing understanding that many chronic diseases are related to high levels of tension and anxiety has revived interest in the view that all illness is psychosomatic. A number of recent works (Pelletier, 1977) have explored the implications of Selye's (1956) decades-old research into the psychophysiology of stress and have provided evidence to substantiate and extend the clinical descriptions of such psychosomatic pioneers as Franz Alexander, Helen Flanders Dunbar, Wilhelm Reich, and George Engel. Research evidence indicates that people who have recently experienced significant loss (LeShan and Worthington, 1956; Holmes and Masuda, 1973) and particularly those who are not close to their parents (Thomas and Duszynski, 1974) are more likely to develop a variety of chronic diseases than matched controls. Also, hard-driving, time-obsessed "type A personalities" are far more likely to become hypertensive than more relaxed people of the same age, race, and class (Friedman and Rosenman, 1974).

Some researchers have begun to trace the complex and perhaps hypothalamically medicated pathways by which these and other emotional factors are translated into altered neurophysiological and immune states and ultimately into chronic illnesses (Stein, Schiavi, and Camerino, 1976). Others, among them Engel (1977), Frank (1978), and Eisenberg (1977), are using this information to help them build the base for a new, less narrow medical model of health and illness.

The Contextual Critique

During the last twenty years researchers making use of techniques derived from family therapy, sociology, and anthropology have begun to demonstrate what astute clinicians have always known or suspected—that the incidence, manifestation, and course of a variety of physical as well as "emotional" illnesses are intimately connected with the economic and cultural, social and familial context in which the afflicted individual lives and works. For example, the elegant work with diabetic children of Minuchin and his coworkers (1978), has shown a clear relationship between their free fatty-acid levels and their parents' interactions; Gajdusek and Gibbs's (1975) studies of the slow virus, kuru, have implicated specific cultural practices in its transmission; and Brenner's (1975) epidemiological work has demonstrated a clear relationship between fluctuations in our national economy and the incidence of a variety of disease conditions.

Similarly, it has become increasingly clear that successful treatment of even the most discrete clinical entity can be frustrated by ignorance of the familial and cultural context in which it occurs (Kleinman et al., 1978).

The Insights of Modern Physics

The behavioral and social sciences have challenged the context of biomedical observation and the scope of its treatment, but post-Einsteinian physics has begun to call its accuracy – and indeed the very scientific method on which biomedicine is based – into question. Years ago Heisenberg (1958) noted that in atomic physics the observer's perspective and the instruments he used modified the object being observed. Today health care professionals whose scientific education has been shaped by the implications of relativity theory and quantum mechanics are emphasizing the inherent subjectivity of all diagnostic judgments, including those based on the most advanced of our technologies. They are suggesting that we may, simply by observing and defining it, shape the nature, course, and outcome of our patients' health and illness.

The Spiritual Critique

Modern physics has also contributed to the construction of the spiritual critique of biomedicine. We have learned in recent years that at subatomic levels, high-enough speeds, and great-enough distances matter and energy are interconvertible and time and space are continuous; that some phenomena are by their very nature inaccessible to direct observation; and that, at any rate, all observations are shaped by and in turn shape the observer. Increasingly the scientists' vision of the universe and the language they use have come to resemble those of the mystics. All things do appear to be seamlessly and wondrously interconnected, and all attempts to describe them are inadequate and, although heroic, are still somehow beside the point.

In widely read books, the physicist Capra (1975) and the psychologist LeShan (1974) have elucidated the commonalities of modern scientific observation and mystical experience. Their work helps to humble the proud objectivity of medical scientists, to remind us that through most of our history medicine itself has been a sacred art. Healing was God's work and the healer – priest or shaman – was a catalyst to, or vessel for, a power variously labeled as God or nature. In recent years this scientific sanction has encouraged clerics, physicians, and lay people who are dissatisfied with the aridity of both contemporary religion and medicine to try to forge a new synthesis of healing practice, scientific research, and spirit.

Anecdotes about "faith healing," "miracle" cures, and unexplained recoveries from usually fatal illnesses have prompted investigators to measure – and to find – significant biochemical changes in plants and animals subjected to a "healing" touch (Grad, 1965; Smith, 1972), to document spontaneous remissions and miracle cures (Everson and Cole, 1966; Frank, 1973), to examine rather than to factor out the nonspecific healing interactions that have been called the placebo effect (Benson and Epstein, 1975; Benson, 1979; Shapiro, 1970), and to encourage and to mobilize the healing powers of faith and hope, intention and touch

(Krieger, 1975; LeShan, 1974; Simonton, Matthews-Simonton, and Creighton, 1978).

Though this work has not been sufficiently replicated it does suggest that forces lying outside the domain of biomedical observations—including attitudes and expectations we have traditionally thought of as religious—can have effects on health and illness.

The Political Critique

During the 1960s the political critique of U.S. medicine focused on the inequities of health care distribution, the persistent folly of keeping soldiers healthy so they could die in Vietnam, the excess profits made by some providers of health care, and the unmet needs of those who suffered from such specific diseases as black and brown lung (Ehrenreich and Ehrenreich, 1970). In the late 1960s the rallying cry of the Medical Committee for Human Rights was "Health care is a right, not a privilege."

In the 1970s the clinical approach itself came under fire. Its leftist critics saw it as a reflection of a capitalist system and an individualist ideology manipulated by powerful multinational corporations bent on improving their financial status at the expense of people's health. In this view our medical system diverts attention from the political and social origins of illness by focusing on the proximate causes in the bodies of those who become ill (Turshen, 1977). Congruently, Knowles (1977) notes that only 0.5 percent of our health budget is spent on prevention and 2.5 percent on health promotion and education.

The Ecological Critique

More recently this anticapitalist critique has been enlarged still further by an ecological perspective that emphasizes the increasing counterproductivity of the technologies we have used to subdue the nature around and within us. Its advocates insist that we must change our approach—in agriculture, energy development, and transportation as well as in medicine—from conquest and expansion to coexistence and adaptation.

This point of view, first suggested two hundred years ago by Rousseau, has been articulated most clearly in the context of modern medicine by René Dubos (1968). Dubos and others note that our urban living space is in many cases so polluted, overcrowded, and crime ridden that it makes a decent life difficult; that the factories and offices we have created to help relieve us of the stress of surviving are promoting an unprecedented number of stress-related illnesses; that the technologies we have created to cure disease and prolong life are causing new diseases and perpetuating lives that lack vitality.

Without denying the achievements of our technology—some argue that the limits of these achievements almost had to be reached before the urge to do more could be tempered—the ecological critique insists that we must conserve our resources and restrain our appetites, that we must adapt to the limits of the natural world and of our own nature rather than try to coerce them into accommodating to our desires.

The Consumer Critique

During the last ten years broadly based national movements for political and social justice have yielded to specific kinds of consumer activism and to more local struggles – on behalf of homeless young people or battered women, against proposed nuclear power plants, and for greater control over local energy development or social services (Gordon, 1978). Attempts to gain more control over the health care system (and over the minds and bodies that we submit to it) have flourished in this climate. A number of the activists of the 1960s, who by now are experiencing some of the vulnerability that attends their own aging process, have turned their energies to analyzing the social and economic forces that produce ill health and poor health care, creating alternatives that are more democratic as well as more efficient, and learning how to take care of themselves in the process (Gordon, 1978; Ferguson, 1979).

Although a variety of individuals of all ages have been active in the movement for self-care, patients' rights, and institutional reform, women have consistently led efforts for change. Ten or fifteen years ago many women were ignorant about their own bodies, angrily ashamed of the anxieties that overtook them in the offices of condescending male physicians (Boston Women's Health Book Collective, 1976). Today women in increasing numbers feel confident and knowledgeable enough to question their physicians' findings and the safety and necessity of the medications and procedures that they prescribe. Some have turned for aid in childbirth from male doctors to female midwives (Gordon and Haire, in press), from the medication and isolation of hospital delivery to the familiarity and warmth of undrugged childbirth in their own homes and birthing centers. Others have begun to experiment with nonpharmacological home remedies for "female" problems and to organize clinics and self-help groups (Gordon, 1978). The articles and books they have written to inform other women (Boston Women's Health Book Collective, 1976; Arms, 1977) have provided a catalyst and a model for health care consumers of both sexes and of all ages.

The Humanistic Critique

Many health professionals have become impatient with the bureaucratization and specialization of medical treatment and are as dissatisfied with offering impersonal and fragmented care as their patients are with receiving it. In recent years young physicians have, in increasing numbers, forsaken the lucrative and prestigious specialties for the comprehensiveness and sustained personal contact of family practice. In 1974, 821 of them entered family practice internships and residencies and in 1978 that number more than doubled to 1,756 (Graettinger,

1978a, 1978b). Far larger numbers of health care professionals—nurses and social workers, educators and physical therapists, as well as physicians in all specialties—have tried to find ways to "humanize" a practice that appears to take an enormous psychological toll on its members. (Physicians, for example, have extremely high rates of suicide, drug addiction, and alcoholism.) Many have become involved in personal psychotherapy and the human potential movement. Several health care professionals organized the Institute for the Study of Humanistic Medicine (Miller et al., 1975), an educational and research group designed to help its staff, their colleagues, and their students become more aware of their own needs and more sensitive to their patients.

The Cross-Cultural Critique

The efforts of critics to point out the failures of the U.S. medical system, of physicians trying to humanize themselves and their relationships with their patients, and of consumers trying to reclaim control over their own bodies and take an active role in their own care have been catalyzed by the discovery of the health care systems and practices of other countries and other cultures. New or newly translated information on several indigenous systems (Kleinman, Eisenberg, and Good, 1978)—including the Tibetan, the Indian, and particularly the Native American (Boyd, 1974)—suggests that there are other ways of conceptualizing and, indeed, of curing illness.

In recent years, however, the richest and most suggestive possibilities have been raised by developments in the People's Republic of China (Horn, 1971; Sidel and Sidel, 1974). Since the 1949 revolution the Chinese have mobilized their energies to provide effective models of public health (the elimination of venereal disease and the virtual eradication of schistosomiasis), of health service delivery (a well-organized and decentralized system), and consumer participation (the use of barefoot doctors and the inclusion of patients in ward care and decision making). They have revived interest in their traditional systems of medicine and have made considerable strides in using them in conjunction with the most modern Western methods.

Some Americans have continued to feel that the Chinese model is largely irrelevant to our practice, that the efficacy of such techniques as acupuncture depends on the Chinese people's docility or their cultural attitudes, that their public health measures are suitable only for underdeveloped countries and attainable only at the price of individual freedom.

Many unmoved by the Chinese model have been impressed by the viewpoint of a country more similar to our own. In *A New Perspective on the Health of Canadians* (LaLonde, 1975), the Canadian minister of health questioned not only the success but also the utility of individual medical care and the biomedical model on which it is based. Although it did not ignore the role and training of physicians, the importance of research, or the biomedical causes and pharmacological remedies of illness, this influential report placed its greatest emphasis on the behavioral, social, and environmental context of health and illness. According to the LaLonde Report (as it came to be known) further advances in the health of Canadians (who already receive medical care as a right) would come only when they changed the behaviors—alcohol and tobacco abuse, poor nutrition, and sedentary living—that made them vulnerable to disease, only when the people of that nation undertook individual efforts as well as a national strategy for health promotion.

The Financial Imperative

All the critiques listed above have their adherents within and outside of the medical profession, and all are helping to shape an emerging holistic model of medicine and health care that includes but is not limited to biomedical science. However, none of them—nor all of them together—is exerting as much pressure for change in our current medical and health care systems as the ever-increasing cost of caring for our aging and chronically ill population. Last year the total expenses for health care were $162.6 billion, or 8.8 percent of the gross national product. Each year the cost of health care has been rising at a rate twice that of all other costs (U.S. Department of Health, Education, and Welfare, 1978). The search for more comprehensive and effective ways of conceptualizing and organizing health care, for alternative therapies, for a more holistic approach to health and illness will continue—not only because the evidence suggests it is valid and moral but also because we simply cannot afford to continue as we have been.

The remainder of this chapter will discuss the holistic paradigm that is beginning to emerge in the theory and practice of medicine and health care.

The Paradigm of Holistic Medicine

The paradigm or model of holistic medicine has evolved in tandem with the critique of modern biomedicine. Each informs, stimulates, enlarges, and tempers the other. This model is, at least potentially, a corrective to the excesses of biomedicine, a supplement to its deficiencies, and an affirmation of its deepest and most enduring strengths. It sets our contemporary concern with the cure of diseases in the larger frame of health care, enlarges and enriches the roles of both health care providers and patients, and provides a framework within which many techniques—old and new, Western and non-Western—may be used.

The outline of characteristics that follows is my own synthesis. It is probably both larger and less distinct than any individual practice and undoubtedly omits features that some practitioners would consider essential. It does, I think, provide some sense of the form, content, and spirit of the holistic medicine that is evolving as well as a framework for the remainder of this volume.

1. *Holistic medicine addresses itself to the physical, mental, and spiritual aspects of those who come for care.* The practitioners of holistic medicine are concerned with helping their patients heal the split that has stripped the mind of its power to experience and control the body, that has stripped the body of its wisdom and intentionality, and that has ruptured the bond between these two and the spirit that gives them both meaning. In the language of science, human beings are "open systems" (Brody and Sobel, 1979) and may be addressed at a variety of levels, the psychosocial and spiritual as well as the biochemical and physiological.

Holistic practitioners are as interested in the coloring of the mood that preceded an attack of chest pain and the meaning it had for the patient as in the dimensions of the electrocardiographic changes that followed it. Their therapeutic approach may include a meditative technique (Benson, 1975); dietary changes and exercise to improve cardiovascular functioning; psychotherapy to mitigate the depression and rage that predispose a person to myocardial infarction (Parkes et al., 1969); or pastoral counseling to help someone confront the despair that can be as lethal as any anatomic pathology (Schmale, 1972).

On a professional level holistic medicine recalls the healer's physical, psychological, and spiritual functions from the specialists – internists, mental health professionals, and clerics – to whom they have been parceled out, reuniting them in each practitioner as well as in the teams of health care workers – physicians and nurses, psychotherapists, ministers, acupuncturists, chiropractors, nutritionists, health educators, and others – who jointly staff and run holistic health centers and clinics.

2. *Although it appreciates the predictive value of data based on statistical studies, holistic medicine emphasizes each patient's genetic, biological, and psychosocial uniqueness as well as the importance of tailoring treatment to meet each individual's needs.* Medical schools today recognize that the majority of their graduates' future patients will suffer from a small number of chronic debilitating psychophysiological conditions. Nonetheless they emphasize – in their grand rounds and in the readings they assign – the exotic disease, the rare tumor, the vital importance of the single finding that distinguishes one slightly different pathological condition from another. Holistic medicine, by contrast, emphasizes the uniqueness of each *person,* the complex socioeconomic and psychological factors that in addition to biochemical and physiological factors characterize each person's health or illness. It encourages students and practitioners to spend considerable time with their patients, to explore and appreciate the minute particularity of the new world that each patient brings to them, to become sensitive to the complex psychology and uncommon life of people with common diseases.

Each person will require a different approach – different forms of exercise, a different diet, a different pharmacological treatment, and different kinds of psychotherapeutic intervention. One asthmatic adolescent may best be treated in a group that runs several miles a day. Another may be seen in the context of a systems-oriented family therapy (Minuchin et al., 1978). The first may work out her anger and improve her vital capacity through daily running. The second may diminish her anxieties and increase her self-confidence through biofeedback techniques. One may be able to discontinue antiasthmatic medication almost immediately, the other may have to continue occasionally to use it.

3. *A holistic approach to medicine and health care includes understanding and treating people in the context of their culture, their family, and their community.* A holistic perspective respects the ways culture shapes pathophysiology and distinguishes between the anatomical lesions that constitute a "disease" state or diagnostic category and the individual's experience of "illness" (Kleinman et al., 1978). This kind of perspective leads to a respect for culturally sanctioned views of illness and its treatment and to the incorporation of indigenous healers where their services are appropriate. It also provides a theoretical basis for including families and communities in the therapeutic process, for working to change as well as to understand their dynamics.

Some practitioners have discovered (Minuchin et al., 1978) that they can alter the biochemistry and physiology of some asthmatic, diabetic, and anorectic children by helping their families change the patterns of relating that precipitate acute attacks and maintain chronic illness. Others have learned to augment their individual treatment by mobilizing the family's capacity for emotional support. This approach has been used with chronic pain patients (Bresler and Trubo, 1979; Shealy, 1976), hypertensives (Hoebel, 1977), and cancer patients (Simonton, Matthews-Simonton, and Creighton, 1978). Still others have assembled an extended network of family and friends to help individuals deal with chronic disease by reintegrating them into an effective cultural and social support system (Speck and Atteneave, 1973).

4. *Holistic medicine views health as a positive state, not as the absence of disease.* Holistic practitioners tend to measure well-being on a continuum that ascends from clinical disease through the absence of disease to the World Health Organization's definition of "complete physical and mental well-being" to a state of extraordinary vigor, joy, and creativity that some are beginning to call "super health" (Carlson and O'Regan, 1978) and "high level wellness" (Ardell, 1977). This perspective allows practitioners to work constructively to improve the health of those who do not feel well but have no obvious organic disease (by some estimates, 75 to 80 percent of those who come to primary-care physicians) and to help those who are functioning well to make still greater use of their faculties, as well as to treat those who have clinical illness.

5. *Holistic medicine emphasizes the promotion of health and the prevention of disease.* Only a few physicians—notably John Travis (1975)—restrict their attentions to the "well," but virtually all holistic practitioners would agree that health—not just the cure of illness—is the goal and that a preoccupation—whether personal or professional—with illness may itself be debilitating.

The histories that holistic practitioners take include extensive inquiries about their patients' goals and the obstacles in meeting them as well as about their past and present illnesses and "chief complaints." They want to know how the people who come to them live and feel, what they eat and smoke, how much they exercise, what kind of stress they have at work and at home, whether they are satisfied with their achievements and their relationships to other people. Some practitioners use standardized tests—health hazards appraisals, social readjustment rating scales, and wellness inventories (Holmes and Rahe, 1967; Travis, 1975) to help them and their patients determine whether or not they are likely to become ill. Much of their therapeutic work consists of helping people to see how their habits, attitudes, expectations, and the way they live, work, think, and feel affect their physical and emotional health and then assisting them to take steps not only to prevent disease but also to feel better.

6. *Holistic medicine emphasizes the responsibility of each individual for his or her health.* The practitioners of holistic medicine feel that we have the capacity to understand the psychobiological origins of our illness, to stimulate our innate healing processes, and to make changes in our lives that will promote health and prevent illness.

Many use psychotherapeutic techniques (such as Freudian free association, Jungian active imagination, Gestalt, role playing, hypnosis, and visualization) to help their patients become more aware of the ways they have translated psychological processes and interpersonal dynamics into physical symptoms. These explorations have confirmed what ordinary language has revealed: emotional burdens may "break people's backs," chronic stress may cause them "pains in the neck," and loss may indeed precipitate a broken heart (Holmes and Rahe, 1967; Parkes et al., 1969; Shealy, 1976; Bresler and Trubo, 1979).

Many of the therapeutic techniques that holistic practitioners use also rely primarily on the patient's rather than the physician's efforts. Inspired by the examples of the yogis and aided by contemporary psychological techniques and modern instrumentation, they have taught their patients to use biofeedback, autogenic training, meditation, and self-hypnosis to control blood pressure and flow, heart rate, and intestinal motility; to relieve migraine headaches and chronic pain; to reverse abnormal electroencephalographic patterns; and to stimulate an immune response (Green and Green, 1977; Gordon, Jaffe, and Bresler, in press).

7. *Holistic medicine uses therapeutic approaches that mobilize the individual's innate capacity for self-healing.* Practitioners view themselves as midwives to the body's own resources. Their job is to help restore what Hippocrates called the *vis medicatrix naturae,* the healing force of nature (the Chinese call it *chi* and the French philosopher Bergson labeled it *élan vital*), not primarily to relieve symptoms or combat disease. Instead of suppressing symptoms, holistic practitioners regard them as indicators of disharmony and arrows to the origins of distress. Instead of trying to eradicate an illness, they may attempt to strengthen the body so that it can rid itself of disease.

For example, holistic practitioners are unlikely to employ suppressive or palliative agents like steroids and aspirin to treat rheumatoid arthritis. They may instead use a variety of modalities to improve the physical and emotional well-being of the person with this condition. They may include guided-imagery techniques that, according to extrapolations from recent work (Stein, Schiavi, and Camerino, 1976), may activate the patient's immune system; biofeedback to teach the person to reduce the stress that precipitates acute attacks (Pelletier, 1977); nutritional counseling to alter the body's chemical balance; hydrotherapy, exercise, and massage to mobilize limbs and joints; and individual and family therapy to discover and dissolve intrapsychic and interpersonal patterns that encourage chronicity.

8. *Though none would deny the occasional necessity for swift and authoritative medical or surgical intervention, the emphasis in holistic medicine is on helping people to understand and to help themselves, on education and self-care rather than treatment and dependence.* Holistic practitioners tend to believe that each person is his or her own best source of care, that their job is to share rather than withhold or mystify their knowledge, to become resources rather than authorities. Some, following Sehnert's (1975) lead, have organized courses for "activated patients," while others provide instruction in self-care (Ferguson, 1979). Most offer their patients introductory talks about their approach to health care and the techniques they use. In addition, some, particularly those who have group practices or clinics, present a variety of courses on topics like stress reduction, interpersonal relations, and nutrition (Tubesing, 1979). Many of these classes, which change with the changing needs of people in the community, are run jointly by professionals and patients whom they have treated.

9. *Holistic medicine makes use of a variety of diagnostic methods and systems in addition to and sometimes in place of the standard laboratory examinations.* Practitioners are particularly concerned with reviving and extending the kind of clinical observation that has always been the hallmark of great diagnosticians (Reich, 1970; Dychtwald, 1977). They watch the way their patients stand, sit, and walk, attend to the fear or anger that a sunken chest or hunched shoulders may reveal. They listen carefully to the tone of voice their patients use to describe their symptoms and observe the color, feel the texture, and smell the odor of their skin.

Holistic practitioners are sensitive to the iatrogenic consequences of invasive diagnostic techniques and are, as a group, interested in exploring the utility of systems that purport to find holographic maps of internal functioning on the body's surface. According to preliminary investigations, several of these maps—which have been used by traditional Chinese physicians—including the radial pulse, the acupuncture meridians (Motoyama, 1978), and the external ear (Bresler et al., 1978), may be capable of yielding accurate information about disease states, sometimes even before they appear clinically. Other sites, including the iris, the foot, and the tongue, are used by practitioners who present anecdotal evidence for their utility.

10. *Physical contact between practitioner and patient is an important element of holistic medicine.* Touch, or the laying-on-of-hands, has been an overt or implied part of virtually all therapeutic systems (Krieger, in press) and is of vital impor-

tance in the early development of children (Klaus and Kennell, 1975). Though the technological armamentarium of Western medicine sometimes threatens to obscure it, patients, nurses, and physicians recognize the potency of touch. The physician's soft, parting touch, the careful dressing of wounds, the hand on the laboring woman's belly are all reassuring and intimate communications. Holistic medicine makes explicit use of the healing potential of touch. Robert Swearingen (1979), an orthopedist, finds a decreased need for analgesia when he reduces fractures or dislocations with a soft, almost meditative manipulative technique; and Dolores Krieger (in press) reports that nurses who have been taught a specific kind of "therapeutic touch" are able, in controlled studies, to raise their patients' hemoglobin levels significantly. Physical contact is, of course, the basis for a variety of "body therapies," including massage, chiropractic, Feldenkrais, rolfing, and others, that may be part of a holistic practice (see Feldenkrais, 1972; Rolf, 1977).

11. *Good health depends on good nutrition and regular exercise.* Over two thousand years ago Hippocrates declared that food should be our medicine and medicine our food. In the last decade holistic medicine has helped to resurrect nutrition from the obscurity to which biomedical education and practice had consigned it. Some holistic practitioners confine their dietary prescriptions within a framework erected by nutritional biochemists (Williams, 1977). Others have borrowed from the dietary regimes of other cultures, from U.S. naturopathy and clinical ecology (Dickey, 1976). Some use fasts or raw food to cleanse the body; others may eliminate foods like milk and wheat that seem to cause atypical allergic reactions, including emotional lability and depression in some people. All recognize the fundamental interdependence between food and health, and virtually all would urge their patients to follow the prescription of the U.S. Senate Select Committee on Nutrition and Human Needs (1977): cut down on processed, refined, and preserved foods; reduce sugar, artificial sweeteners, colorings, and flavorings; increase the amount of fiber, complex carbohydrates, and raw food in the diet; eat somewhat less red meat; and use stimulants like tea and coffee and depressants like alcohol in moderation.

Exercise is a natural complement to diet. The former burns off the calories that the latter provides and makes the body supple. Holistic practitioners use a variety of exercises from a number of different traditions to improve cardiopulmonary functions, muscle tone, and emotional stability (Ardell, in press). Many suggest jogging for depressed, overweight, or anxious patients (Kostrubala, 1977). Others prescribe oxygen-utilizing ("aerobic") exercises (Cooper, 1970) and still others find that psychological balance and emotional flexibility accompany the physical benefits of such meditative Eastern martial arts as tai chi and aikido. The most sophisticated practitioners tailor their prescriptions to the individual, perhaps jogging for the fearful asthmatic and tai chi for the awkward young woman or unbending old man.

12. *Holistic medicine includes an appreciation of and attention to sensuousness and sexuality.* At its best, medicine has always taught a respect for what Cannon

(1926) called "the wisdom of the body." Unfortunately this appreciation of the body's wisdom has rarely been accompanied by a delight in its sensual capacity. Holistic approaches to healing emphasize not only the marvels of the machine but the pleasures it may yield.

Freud's followers Reich (1960) and Groddeck (1977) were particularly conscious of the emotional penury and physical damage that resulted from dammed up sexuality, of the necessity for supplementing words and pharmacotherapy with physical approaches designed to remove these blocks. Modern holistic practitioners have been heavily influenced by Reich's work and its adumbration of the "human potential movement" of the 1960s and 1970s and have incorporated its insights and techniques into their clinical practice. They know, for example, that a clear chest with a negative X-ray is not necessarily a healthy one, that the emotional constriction that may be read in shallow breaths and hunched shoulders can cause as much chronic disability as more obvious organic pathology. Some have learned techniques like bioenergetic therapy (Lowen, 1975) and the Alexander method (Alexander, 1969) to help their patients discover the pleasure of deep oxygenating breaths, erect carriage, an open pelvis, and a graceful walk.

All tend to be more concerned with the quality of their patients' sexuality and their capacity for sensuousness. A couple's pleasure in touching and being touched as they make love is regarded as more important than the number of times they have intercourse. Providing information and counseling about sexuality is as much a part of a holistic physician's practice as treating diabetic impotence.

13. *Holistic medicine views illness as an opportunity for discovery as well as a misfortune.* Holistic practitioners help their patients understand the psychosocial stresses – loss, unemployment, or simply change – that may have precipitated an illness and the relationship between particular forms of organic pathology and particular emotional problems. They may help a patient to see the connection between feeling overburdened and having a bad back, between chronic genitourinary or gynecological problems and fear of or aggressive use of sex. They may use the overwhelming trauma of a heart attack as a lever to help the middle-aged man reevaluate the killing pace of his life and the destructiveness of some of his habits and attitudes. Some (Simonton, Matthews-Simonton, and Creighton, 1978) have even been able to help terminal cancer patients wrest an understanding of lifelong patterns of behavior and a sense of personal meaning from the illness that threatens to soon kill them.

14. *Holism includes an appreciation of the quality of life in each of its stages and an interest in improving it as well as knowledge of the illnesses that are common to it.* Holistic midwives or obstetricians are as prepared to help their patients deal with negative feelings – a mother's animosity or father's jealousy toward the developing fetus – as with first trimester bleeding or eclampsia. Instead of quickly referring a depressed middle-aged man to the psychiatrist or prescribing antidepressants for him, holistic practitioners will try to explore the man's preoccupation with waning physical or sexual powers or his concern about a career that once seemed hopeful and now seems a dead end. Holistic practitioners may set

up groups or individual sessions where older people can learn practices like deep breathing, relaxation, yoga, or tai chi to improve their physiological and psychological functioning. Instead of shunning death and "snowing" the dying with tranquilizing medication they will try to be present physically and psychologically to help their patients experience the last part of their lives.

15. *Holistic medicine emphasizes the potential therapeutic value of the setting in which health care takes place.* Even the most modern of hospitals tends to overwhelm and intimidate, to erect a barrier between those who come for help and those who provide it, to encourage patients to assume and maintain a sick role (Parsons, 1963). Though they recognize the hospital's utility in some acute life-threatening situations, holistic practitioners feel that the human experiences of birth and death, the treatment of chronic illness, check-ups, and counseling (which do not require high technology) should be removed from the relentlessly disease-oriented hospital, that those who come for help should have the opportunity to participate actively in their own care and, indeed, in the care of others.

The small centers that holistic practitioners have created for general health care are built on a more human scale and substitute respectful and responsive personal attention for a large, impersonal bureaucracy. Some are free standing, others occupy parts of such existing community institutions as churches or schools. All offer an opportunity for education and socializing as well as care in health and illness. Though holistic practitioners would of course use the personnel and technology of the hospital for a high-risk delivery or an acute life-threatening illness, they prefer to attend those who are giving birth or dying in the familiarity and intimacy of their own homes or in special birthing centers or hospices where family members are encouraged to participate in care.

16. *An understanding of and a commitment to change those social and economic conditions that perpetuate ill health are as much a part of holistic medicine as its emphasis on individual responsibility.* A holistic medical practitioner cannot consider individuals in isolation from their social, economic, and ecological context. Treatment of a lead-intoxicated child with chelating agents is doomed to failure unless the child's physical surroundings change; administration of vitamins is absurd in the face of a poverty that continues to make proper nutrition impossible and is inadequate in a society whose media daily encourage children to subsist on processed junk food.

In their commitment to change, some practitioners may confine their efforts to advocacy on behalf of, or in conjunction with, individual patients and to making the attitudes, principles, and techniques of holistic medicine more accessible to their colleagues. Others offer classes in self-help in their clinics, in local schools, or to community groups. Some testify against the health-denying nutritional and pharmacological practices that pervade many of our schools, hospitals, and retirement facilities. Some participate in groups like the Medical Committee for Human Rights or Physicians for Social Responsibility, which challenge economic, military, and industrial practices like war, nuclear development, poverty, and industrial pollution that threaten our health and, indeed, our lives.

17. *Holistic medicine transforms its practitioners as well as its patients.* In much of the ancient world and in many contemporary aboriginal societies the education of healers is at once technical and sacred (Mattson, 1978; Needleman, 1978). In these settings, a process designed to pare away psychological armor, anxiety, fears, and arrogance accompanies the accumulation of technical knowledge and enables young practitioners to handle their status as healers with modesty and wisdom. The long hours, low pay, persistent challenges, and intermittent abuse of internships and residency are a distant shadow of this kind of training. The personal analysis of a modern psychoanalyst is our closest contemporary analog.

Though there are no formal schools for holistic health care professionals, many individuals have begun to seek out this kind of psychological and spiritual refinement and nourishment – in continuing education programs sponsored by such newly formed groups as the American Holistic Medical Association, the Congress of Nurse Healers, and the Association for Holistic Health; in experiential seminars and retreats on humanistic medicine; and in an ever increasing variety of psychotherapeutic and meditative techniques. In these contexts some have grown more aware of the intrapsychic and interpersonal barriers that prevent them from providing effective and sensitive care. Many have learned to be less dogmatic with and more generous to their patients, to regard their consultations as an opportunity to learn about their own shortcomings as well as their patients' illnesses. Increasingly, they are taking seriously the Hippocratic tradition and its insistence that medicine is a sacred trust as well as a profession.

Conclusion

The holistic approach to medicine and health care that I have described synthesizes the ecological sensitivity of ancient healing traditions and the precision of modern science, techniques whose effectiveness has already been extensively documented and techniques we are just beginning to explore, our contemporary concern with personal responsibility and spiritual and emotional growth, and our urge to democratic cooperation and social and political activism. This holistic approach informs the contexts, animates the techniques, and is embodied in the programs described in the remainder of this volume. The future of our medicine and our health as a people will in part be determined by the ways this approach comes to shape the larger health care system, the training of the professionals who will work in that system, and the education of the citizens who must ultimately learn to take care of themselves.

References

Alexander, F. Mathias. *The Resurrection of the Body.* New York: Delta, 1969.
Ardell, Donald. *High Level Wellness.* Emmaus, Pa.: Rodale Press, 1977.

Ardell, Donald. Physical disciplines and health. In this volume and also in Arthur Hastings, James Fadiman, and James S. Gordon (Eds.), *Holistic Medicine*. Rockville, Md.: National Institute of Mental Health, in press.

Arms, Suzanne. *Immaculate Deception: A New Look at Women and Childbirth in America*. New York: Bantam, 1977.

Benson, Herbert. *The Relaxation Response*. New York: William Morrow, 1975.

Benson, Herbert. *The Mind/Body Effect*. New York: Simon and Schuster, 1979.

Benson, Herbert, and Epstein, Mark. The placebo effect: a neglected asset in the care of patients. *Journal of the American Medical Association*, June 23, 1975. **232**, 1225–1227.

Boston Women's Health Book Collective. *Our Bodies, Ourselves* (2nd ed.). New York: Simon and Schuster, 1976.

Boyd, Doug. *Rolling Thunder*. New York: Random House, 1974.

Brecher, Edward M., and the *Consumer Reports* editors. *Licit and Illicit Drugs: The Consumer's Union Report on Narcotics, Stimulants, Depressants, Inhalants, Hallucinogens, and Marijuana, Including Caffeine, Nicotine, and Alcohol*. Boston: Little, Brown, 1973.

Brenner, Harvey. *Estimating the Social Costs of National Economic Policy: Implications for Mental and Physical Health, and Criminal Aggression*. U.S. Congress Joint Economic Committee. Washington, D.C.: U.S. Government Printing Office, 1975.

Bresler, David E.; Oleson, Terrance D.; and Kroening, Richard J. *Ear Acupuncture Diagnosis in Musculoskeletal Pain*. San Francisco: Institute of Noetic Science, 1978.

Bresler, David E., and Trubo, Richard. *Freedom from Pain*. New York: Simon and Schuster, 1979.

Brody, Howard, and Sobel, David. A systems view of health and disease. In D. Sobel (Ed.), *Ways of Health: Holistic Approaches to Ancient and Contemporary Medicine*. New York: Harcourt, Brace, Jovanovich, 1979.

Brook, Robert H. et al. Effectiveness of non-emergency care via an emergency room. *Annals of Internal Medicine*, 1973. **78**, 333–339.

Bureau of the Census, U.S. Department of Commerce. *Statistical Abstract of the United States, 1977*. Washington, D.C.: U.S. Government Printing Office, 1977.

Cannon, Walter B. *The Wisdom of the Body*. New York: W. W. Norton, 1926.

Capra, Fritjof. *The Tao of Physics*. Berkeley, Calif.: Shambhala, 1975.

Carlson, Rick J. *The End of Medicine*. New York: Wiley-Interscience, 1975.

Carlson, Rick J., and O'Regan, Brendan. *The Superhealthy*. San Francisco: The Institute of Noetic Sciences, 1978.

Cooper, Kenneth H. *The New Aerobics*. New York: Bantam Books, 1970.

Dickey, Lawrence D. (Ed.). *Clinical Ecology*. Springfield, Ill.: Thomas, 1976.

Dubos, René. *Mirage of Health*. New York: Harper and Row, 1959.

Dubos, René. *So Human an Animal*. New York: Scribners, 1968.

Dychtwald, Kenneth. *Bodymind*. New York: Jove, 1977.

Ehrenreich, Barbara, and Ehrenreich, John. *The American Health Empire: Power, Profits, and Politics*. New York: Random House, 1970.

Eisenberg, Leon. Psychiatry and society: a sociobiologic synthesis. *New England Journal of Medicine*, 1977. **296 (16)**, 903–910.

Engel, George L. The need for a new medical model: a challenge for biomedicine. *Science*, April 8, 1977. **196**, 129–136.

Everson, T. C., and Cole, W. H. *Spontaneous Regression of Cancer*. Philadelphia: Saunders, 1966.

Feldenkrais, Moshe. *Awareness through Movement*. New York: Harper and Row, 1972.

Ferguson, Tom (Ed.). *Medical Self-Care: Access to Medical Tools.* New York: Summit Books, 1979.

Frank, Jerome. *Persuasion and Healing: A Comparative Study of Psychotherapy* (Revised ed.). Baltimore: The Johns Hopkins University Press, 1973.

Frank, Jerome. The medical power of faith. *Human Nature,* August 1978. 40–47.

Friedman, Meyer, and Rosenman, Ray. *Type A Behavior and Your Heart.* New York: Fawcett Crest, 1974.

Gajdusek, D. C., and Gibbs, C. J. Slow virus infections of the nervous system. In T. N. Chase (Ed.), *The Nervous System,* vol. 2, *The Clinical Neurosciences.* New York: Raven Press, 1975. 113–135.

Gordon, James S. Special study on alternative services. In President's Commission on Mental Health, *Report to the President.* Washington, D.C.: U.S. Government Printing Office, 1978.

Gordon, James S., and Haire, Doris. Alternatives in childbirth. In this volume and also in Arthur Hastings, James Fadiman, and James S. Gordon (Eds.), *Holistic Medicine.* Rockville, Md.: National Institute of Mental Heath, in press.

Gordon, James; Jaffe, Dennis; and Bresler, David (Eds.). *Mind, Body, and Health: Toward an Integral Medicine.* Rockville, Md.: National Institute of Mental Health, in press.

Grad, Bernard. Some biological effects of the "laying on of hands": a review of experiments with plants and animals. *Journal of the American Society for Psychical Research,* April 1965. **59** (2), 95–126.

Graettinger, John. The results of the NIRMP for 1977. *Journal of Medical Education,* 1978a. **53,** 83–91.

Graettinger, John. The results of the NIRMP for 1978. *Journal of Medical Education,* 1978b. **53,** 500–502.

Green, Elmer, and Green, Alyce. *Beyond Biofeedback.* New York: Delta, 1977.

Groddeck, Georg. *The Book of the It.* New York: International University Press, 1977.

Heisenberg, Werner. *Physics and Philosophy.* New York: Harper and Row, 1958.

Hoebel, F. C. Coronary artery disease and family interaction: a study of risk modification. In Paul Watzlawick and John Weakland (Eds.), *The Interactional View.* New York: W. W. Norton, 1977. 362–375.

Holmes, Thomas H., and Masuda, M. Life change and illness susceptibility, separation, and depression. *Science,* 1973. 161–186.

Holmes, Thomas, and Rahe, Richard. The social readjustment rating scale. *Journal of Psychosomatic Research,* 1967. **2,** 213–218.

Horn, Joshua S. *Away with All Pests: An English Surgeon in People's China, 1954–1969.* New York: Monthly Review Press, 1971.

Illich, Ivan. *Medical Nemesis.* New York: Pantheon, 1976.

Klaus, Marshall, and Kennell, John. *Maternal Infant Bonding.* St. Louis, Mo.: C. V. Mosby and Co., 1975.

Kleinman, Arthur; Eisenberg, Leon; and Good, Byron. Culture illness and care. *Annals of Internal Medicine,* 1978. **88,** 251–258.

Knowles, John (Ed.). *Doing Better and Feeling Worse: Health in the United States.* New York: W. W. Norton, 1977. Also in *Daedalus,* Winter 1977. **106** (1).

Kostrubala, Thaddeus. *The Joy of Running.* New York: Pocket Books, 1977.

Krieger, Dolores. Therapeutic touch: the imprimatur of nursing. *American Journal of Nursing,* May 1975. **75** (5), 784–787.

Krieger, Dolores. Therapeutic touch. *Mind, Body, and Health: Toward an Integral Medicine*

(J. Gordon, D. Jaffe, and D. Bresler, Eds.). Rockville, Md.: National Institute of Mental Health, in press.

LaLonde, Marc. *A New Perspective on the Health of Canadians.* Ottawa: Information Canada, 1975.

LeShan, Lawrence. *The Medium, The Mystic, and The Physicist.* New York: Viking Press, 1974.

LeShan, Lawrence, and Worthington, R. E. Some recurrent life history patterns observed in patients with malignant disease. *Journal of Nervous and Mental Diseases,* 1956. **124,** 460–465.

Lowen, Alexander. *Bioenergetics.* New York: Penguin, 1975.

Marti-Ibanez, Felix. Toward a history of medical thought. *International Record of Medicine,* 1952. **165,** 484–523.

Mather, H. G. et al. Acute myocardial infarction: home and hospital treatment. *British Medical Journal,* 1971. **3,** 334–338.

Mattson, Phyllis. *Holistic Health in Perspective.* San Francisco: Institute of Noetic Sciences, 1978.

McKeown, Thomas. *The Role of Medicine: Dream, Mirage, or Nemesis?* London: Rock Carling Fellowship, Nuffield Provincial Hospitals Trust, 1976.

Miller, Stuart et al. *Essays in Humanistic Medicine.* San Francisco: Institute for the Study of Humanistic Medicine, 1975.

Minuchin, Salvador; Rosman, Bernice; and Baker, Lester. *Psychosomatic Families.* Cambridge, Mass.: Harvard Press, 1978.

Motoyama, Hiroshi. *Science and the Evolution of Consciousness.* Brookline, Mass.: Autumn Press, 1978.

Needleman, Jacob. The two sciences of medicine. *Parabola,* 1978. **3 (3),** 34–55.

Parkes, C. N.; Benjamin, B.; and Fitzgerald, R. G. Broken heart: a statistical study of increased mortality among widowers. *British Medical Journal,* 1969. **1,** 740–743.

Parsons, Talcott. The sick role. *Social Structure and Personality.* Glencoe: Free Press, 1963.

Pelletier, Kenneth R. *Mind as Healer, Mind as Slayer: A Holistic Approach to Preventing Stress Disorders.* New York: Delta, 1977.

President's Commission on Mental Health. *Report to the President* (Vol. 1). Washington, D.C.: U.S. Government Printing Office, 1978.

Reich, Wilhelm. *Selected Writings: An Introduction to Orgonomy.* New York: Farrar, Straus, and Giroux, 1960.

Reich, Wilhelm. *The Mass Psychology of Fascism.* New York: Farrar, Straus, and Giroux, 1970.

Rolf, Ida P. *Rolfing.* Santa Monica, Calif.: Dennis Landman, 1977.

Schmale, A. H. Giving up as a final common pathway to changes in health. *Advances in Psychosomatic Medicine,* 1972. **8,** 20–40.

Schneiderman, Marvin A. Trends in cancer incidence and mortality in the United States. In U.S. Senate Committee on Human Resources, *Testimony before the Subcommittee on Health and Scientific Research.* Washington, D.C.: U.S. Government Printing Office, 1979.

Sehnert, Keith S. *How To Be Your Own Doctor (Sometimes).* New York: Grosset and Dunlap, 1975.

Selye, Hans. *The Stress of Life.* New York: McGraw-Hill, 1956.

Shapiro, Arthur K. Placebo effects in psychotherapy and psychoanalysis. *Journal of Clinical Pharmacology,* 1970. **10,** 73–78.

Shealy, C. Norman. *The Pain Game.* Millbrae, Calif.: Celestial Arts, 1976.

Sidel, Victor, and Sidel, Ruth. *Serve the People: Observations on Medicine in the People's Republic of China.* Boston: Beacon, 1974.

Simonton, O. Carl; Matthews-Simonton, Stephanie; and Creighton, James. *Getting Well Again.* Los Angeles: Tarcher, 1978.

Smith, M. J. Paranormal effects on enzyme activity through laying on of hands. *Human Dimensions,* Spring 1972. **1**, 15–19.

Smuts, Jan Christian. *Holism and Evolution.* New York: Macmillan, 1926.

Speck, Ross V., and Atteneave, Carolyn. *Family Networks.* New York: Vantage Books, 1973.

Stein, M.; Schiavi, R. C.; and Camerino, M. Influence of brain and behavior on the immune systems. *Science,* February 6, 1976. **191**, 435–440.

Swearingen, Robert. The ontogeny of healing. *Mind, Body, and Health: Toward an Integral Medicine* (J. Gordon, D. Jaffe, and D. Bresler, Eds.). Rockville, Md.: National Institute of Mental Health, 1979.

Thomas, Caroline B., and Duszynski, K. R. Closeness to parents and the family constellation in a prospective study of five disease states: suicide, mental illness, malignant tumor, hypertension, and coronary heart disease. *Johns Hopkins Medical Journal,* May 1974. **134 (5)**, 251–270.

Travis, John. *Wellness Inventory.* Mill Valley, Calif.: Wellness Center, 1975.

Tubesing, Donald A. *Wholistic Health: A Whole Person Approach to Primary Health Care.* New York: Human Sciences Press, 1979.

Turshen, Meredith. The political ecology of disease. *Review of Radical Political Economics,* Spring 1977. **9 (1)**, 45–60.

U.S. Department of Health, Education, and Welfare. Cited in *Business Week,* September 4, 1978.

U.S. House of Representatives, Committee on Interstate and Foreign Commerce. *Cost and Quality of Health Care: Unnecessary Surgery.* Washington, D.C.: U.S. Government Printing Office, 1976.

U.S. House of Representatives, Committee on Interstate and Foreign Commerce. *Surgical Performance: Necessity and Quality.* Washington, D.C.: U.S. Government Printing Office, 1978.

U.S. Senate Select Committee on Nutrition and Human Needs. *Dietary Goals for the United States.* Washington, D.C.: U.S. Government Printing Office, February 1977.

U.S. Surgeon General. *Report on Smoking and Health.* Washington, D.C.: U.S. Government Printing Office, 1964.

Williams, Roger. *The Wonderful World Within You: Your Inner Nutritional Environment.* New York: Bantam Books, 1977.

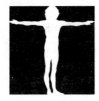 ANNOTATED BIBLIOGRAPHY

Berkeley Holistic Health Center. **The Holistic Health Handbook.** Berkeley: Berkeley Holistic Health Center, 1978.

This compendium of articles on holistic health was assembled by members of the Berkeley Holistic Health Center, a collectively run Northern California health program. It is divided into sections entitled Overview (the need for and paradigm of holistic health), Healing Systems (acupuncture, homoeopathy, etc.), Techniques and Practices (nutrition, chiropractic), Transitions (topics particularly related to life cycle and life style), and Legal and Social Issues. The articles range from reprints of previously published documents (such as Carl Simonton and Stephanie Matthews-Simonton's article on "Belief Systems and Management of the Emotional Aspects of Malignancy" and an excerpt from Elisabeth Kübler-Ross's *Death Does Not Exist*) through interviews and profiles (with John Travis, "Doctor of Wellness," and Patricia Sun, who heals through sound) to practical step-by-step brief instruction in such techniques as shiatsu and natural birth control.

Although the individual pieces are organized in a somewhat confusing way and suffer from a lack of documentation—which will disconcert the health care professional or scholar—this volume is a useful sampler of some of the systems, techniques, and perspectives that have been grouped under the rubric "holistic health." They give a feeling for the enthusiasm, the adventurousness, and the concern for self-care (as well as the evangelism) of some who are active in the movement for more holistic care.

Bloomfield, Harold H., and Kory, Robert B. **The Holistic Way to Health and Happiness.** New York: Simon and Schuster, 1978.

This book by Bloomfield (a psychiatrist and founder of the Center for Holistic Health in San Diego) and Kory (a health educator) shows how the principles of holistic medicine are applied in practice. Though they present some historical background and discuss a number of aspects of holistic health, the authors emphasize the importance of the "healing silence" (the practice of transcendental meditation) for reducing stress and promoting a feeling of well-being.

Boston Women's Health Book Collective. **Our Bodies, Ourselves** (2nd ed.). New York: Simon and Schuster, 1976.

This remarkable compilation of medical fact, personal experience, and political analysis provides a picture of the forces that shape the lives and health of women in the contemporary United States. Clearly written, well illustrated, and comprehensive, it discusses, among other topics, pregnancy, menopause, sexuality, nutrition, lesbian relationships, and aging. It has been instrumental in helping hundreds of thousands of women to understand and appreciate their physiology and their psychology, informing them about the limitations of the current health care system and helping them challenge it.

This book is particularly important for health professionals who wish to understand what their women patients "really want" and for women of all ages (including most especially adolescents) who want to understand themselves better.

Bricklin, Mark. **The Practical Encyclopedia of Natural Healing.** Emmaus, Pa.: Rodale Press, 1976.

Though this readable volume by the executive editor of *Prevention Magazine* is more practical than encyclopedic, it does offer excellent introductions to a variety of health-related topics. The alphabetized essays are about evenly distributed between discussions of disease states and natural therapies that may be used to remedy them. The chapter on herbs is particularly comprehensive.

Though parts of this book may make medical scientists wince, it is a useful introduction to a variety of illnesses and a number of unorthodox therapies.

Carlson, Rick J. **The End of Medicine.** New York: Wiley-Interscience, 1975.

In this book, Carlson (a lawyer, health care consultant, and political organizer) crisply presents the case against a system of medical care that he describes as costly, dangerous, misguided, and ineffective. He contends that this system will be replaced in time by one that emphasizes the promotion of health through careful attention to the relationships among human beings and between them and their environment.

With its wealth of careful documentation, *The End of Medicine* has proved enormously useful to health professionals and students who sense that there is something wrong with the quality of the care their professions offer and the ideology on which they are based. His sections on the future of health care are less strong but are still suggestive.

Carlson, Rick J., **The Frontiers of Science and Medicine.** Chicago: Henry Regnery, 1976.

This volume, a collection of the May 1975 lectures, is not very coherent. Topics range from "The Role of the Mind in Cancer Therapy" by Carl and Stephanie Simonton to an article on "Interpersonal Communication between Man and Plant" by Marcel Vogel. It provides, nevertheless, a fascinating overview of some of the research that is being conducted on the ability of the mind to control bodily functions and on the physical effects of "nonphysical" forces, such as thoughts, intentions, and faith.

Carlson, Rick J., and Cunningham, Robert (Eds.). **Future Directions in Health Care: A New Public Policy.** Cambridge, Mass.: Ballinger, 1978.

This collection of reports from a 1977 conference sponsored by the Blue Cross Association; the Health Policy Program of the University of California Medical School, San

Francisco; the Institute of Medicine; and the Rockefeller Foundation documents the medical establishment's efforts to enlarge its conceptualization of health care beyond contemporary biomedicine. It includes literate introductory essays ("Ill Health and Its Amelioration: Individual and Collective Choices" by Kerr White and "Behavioral and Environmental Determinants of Health and their Implications for Public Policy" by Thomas McKeown), a series of papers on the prevalence and prevention of hypertension, and a brilliant summary by Beverly Winikoff (then of the Rockefeller Institute) of some of the individual and collective nutritional problems that beset us.

Cousins, Norman. **Anatomy of an illness (as perceived by the patient).** *New England Journal of Medicine,* December 23, 1975. **295 (26),** 1458–1463.

In this fascinating and eminently readable essay, the former editor of *The Saturday Review* tells of his successful attempt to treat a complicated and potentially lethal collagen vascular disease that baffled his physicians. This article, which has already been widely circulated among the professional and lay community, demonstrates the importance of mental attitude in healing (Cousins prescribed Marx brothers movies for himself to improve his spirits), of the setting in which healing takes place (he left a rather depressing and exceedingly expensive hospital room for an attractive hotel room), and of cooperation between a respectful, highly trained physician and a patient determined to use such unorthodox healing techniques as large doses of laughter and vitamin C.

Dubos, René. **Mirage of Health.** New York: Harper and Row, 1959.

In this remarkable volume Dubos, a Rockefeller Institute microbiologist, demonstrates the interrelationship between the health and disease of individuals and the biological and social environment in which people live. Without slighting the achievements of the germ theory or modern biomedicine to which he has contributed substantially, Dubos manages to place them both in a larger context. He concludes that further improvements in the health of the peoples of developed nations will come not from new "magic bullets" designed to combat cancer and heart disease but from improvements in our capacity to change and to adapt to our environment.

This pioneering work has been instrumental in helping a generation of students develop some historical perspective on the achievements of modern biomedicine while catalyzing their own self-critical questioning. It continues to be an invaluable resource for health care professionals and lay people.

Eisenberg, Leon. **Psychiatry and society: a sociobiologic synthesis.** *New England Journal of Medicine,* 1977. **296 (16),** 903–910.

This learned, clearly written paper by the current chief of psychiatry at the Massachusetts General Hospital draws, among other subjects, on recent work on the epidemiology of kuru, a slow virus, to demonstrate the necessity for heeding the sociocultural context of conditions we may too easily label as physical or psychological. Many of the points that Eisenberg makes are similar to those made by George Engel.

Engel, George. **The need for a new medical model: a challenge for biomedicine.** *Science,* 1977. **196,** 129–136.

In this succinct, lucid, and influential critique, one of the most eminent figures in psychosomatic medicine draws on carefully chosen studies to detail some of the limitations of the biomedical model. He urges his physician colleagues not to diminish their intellectual and clinical stature and their patients' opportunities for health by ignoring the social and psychological dimensions of illness and health.

Frank, Jerome. **Persuasion and Healing: A Comparative Study of Psychotherapy.** (Revised ed.). Baltimore: Johns Hopkins University Press, 1973.

A now classic and still vivid account by a professor emeritus of psychiatry at Johns Hopkins Medical School of the mind's power to cure or to kill and of the therapeutic importance of the congruence between a healer's assumptions and his or her patient's beliefs. Frank's discussions of the power of faith healing and placebos and the analogies he draws between modern medicine and primitive shamanism have informed the work of a generation of investigators.

Gordon, James; Jaffe, Dennis; and Bresler, David (Eds.) **Mind, Body, and Health: Toward an Integral Medicine.** Rockville, Md.: National Institute of Mental Health, in press.

This is a collection of papers on the practice of "integral" (virtually synonymous with holistic) medicine, originally presented at a 1977 conference sponsored by the Center for Integral Medicine and the National Institute of Mental Health. Taken together these original articles provide an excellent introduction to the clinical applications of holistic approaches to medicine and health care. Contributors include C. Norman Shealy and David Bresler, who have pioneered in the development of holistic programs for treatment of chronic pain; Carl and Stephanie Simonton, who combine conventional cancer therapies with visualization techniques and individual, group, and family therapy; and Robert Swearingen, who uses relaxation techniques in orthopedic practice.

Groddeck, Georg. **The Book of the It.** New York: International University Press, 1977.

Groddeck, a student and colleague of Freud, was one of the first modern holistic practitioners. At his clinic in Germany he combined massage, diet, and hydrotherapy with a brilliant and penetrating psychoanalytic psychotherapy. Groddeck contended that the It (from which Freud borrowed his Id) was the expression of the total physical, psychological, and social being of the individual, that each disease process was a unique and particular form of self-expression.

This book was first published some fifty years ago and consists of letters from an alter ego (whom Groddeck called Patrik Troll) to an imaginary correspondent. If Groddeck sometimes seems to explain too much too easily, incessantly hammering home the truth of the Oedipus complex, his insights and his humor are still enormously valuable to anyone interested in the practice of holistic medicine.

Horn, Joshua S. **Away with All Pests: An English Surgeon in People's China, 1954–1969.** New York: Monthly Review Press, 1971.

Joshua Horn's elegiac account of his experiences in the People's Republic of China manages, without seeming dogmatic or even particularly romantic, to use stories and statistics to paint a picture of the responsive, humane, and effective health care system that has emerged in China since the 1949 revolution. Horn is particularly strong and affective in conveying the contrast between life before and after the revolution and in demonstrating how the Chinese have managed to improve and humanize health care, to train a remarkable corps of paraprofessionals (the barefoot doctors), and to achieve a synthesis between modern biomedicine and traditional Chinese health practices, including acupuncture and herbalism.

Illich, Ivan. **Medical Nemesis.** New York: Pantheon, 1976.

In this book Illich, who has elsewhere focused a finely critical eye on education, transportation, and social service, takes modern medicine to task. The heart of this densely written, meticulously documented polemic is that modern medicine has become a self-aggrandizing, imperialistic, and counterproductive enterprise that debilitates and demeans its patients as it gathers them into its domain.

When the book appeared Illich was excoriated both by the medical establishment – for his refusal to recognize the gains that modern biomedicine had made – and by the Left – for his insensitivity to the need for a collective response to the illnesses that our society visits disproportionately upon its poor. Neither these critiques nor Illich's own tendency to narrow the evidence to fit the lens of his argument diminish the fundamental importance of this book. Reading it is a humbling experience for physicians, frightening for lay people, and enlightening for all.

Kaslof, Leslie J. (Ed.). **Wholistic Dimensions in Healing.** New York: Doubleday, 1978.

This volume by Kaslof, an herbalist and director of the National Council on Wholistic Therapeutics, is a useful resource for those interested in exploring the dimensions of holistic medicine. The book is organized under eight headings and each is in turn subdivided. Thus, under "Nutrition and Herbs" there are several chapters, among them "Preventive Nutrition and Health Maintenance" and "Macrobiotic and Oriental Medicine." Each chapter consists of an introduction by an authority in that discipline and concludes with the names and addresses of practitioners, clinics, associations, and journals to which interested readers may refer further questions.

The essays are far too brief (approximately 1,500 words) to present a full picture of the disciplines they describe, far too sparsely documented, and at times too dogmatic to appeal to the skeptical, but they may often whet the appetites of the curious. The listings following the essays constitute the most comprehensive collection to date and are particularly useful. Two caveats to bear in mind when consulting them: (1) Kaslof has listed all those who claim to practice, teach, or educate in a particular discipline but has not selected those whom he regards as most competent, and (2) a number of the listings are already out of date.

Knowles, John (Ed.). **Doing Better and Feeling Worse: Health in the United States.** New York: W. W. Norton, 1977. Also in *Daedalus*, Winter 1977. **106 (1).**

This is a collection of essays by pillars of the American medical establishment on the current problems and future directions of our health care system. Although all of them are worth reading, the clearest and most sustained note is struck by the late John Knowles, formerly director of Massachusetts General Hospital and Rockefeller University. It is no longer enough, Knowles tells us, with ample documentation and much force, for American medicine to deal with sickness and disease. If we are to deal with the problems that beset us we must improve not our antibiotics or tranquilizers but our individual attitudes and our habits—how much we eat, drink, and smoke and how fast we drive. Although Knowles's focus seems overly individualistic and his tone relentlessly Calvinistic, his emphasis—in a society accustomed to excessive dependence on its physicians—is a welcome one.

Kuhn, Thomas S. **The Structure of Scientific Revolutions** (2nd ed.). Chicago: University of Chicago Press, 1970.

Kuhn, a philosopher and historian of science, begins this influential and elegant essay by distinguishing between "normal science," whose rules define the universe of professional inquiry; the unsettled time when "the profession can no longer evade anomalies that subvert the existing tradition of scientific practice"; and the "extraordinary investigations that lead the profession at last to a new set of commitments." He goes on to describe how this drama was played out in the scientific revolutions that we associate with Copernicus, Lavoisier, and Einstein, among others.

Though his work does not discuss new medical models, this essay on scientific paradigms and paradigm shifts has provided a yardstick against which many have measured the current shift from a biomedical to a holistic perspective on health and illness.

LaLonde, Marc. **A New Perspective on the Health of Canadians.** Ottawa: Information Canada, 1975.

This clear-thinking, elegantly written, brief (seventy-six pages) status report on the health of Canadians and what can be done to improve it has been an inspiration to health-policy planners since its publication. The "LaLonde Report" challenges the "generally accepted view" that "the art or science of medicine has been the fount from which all improvements in health have flowed." Without slighting the biomedicine it challenges, the report summarizes the illnesses with which Canadians are afflicted, notes that "self-imposed risks and the environment are the principal or important underlying factors in each of the five major causes of death between age 1 and 70," and concludes that "unless the environment is changed and the self-imposed risks reduced the death rate will not be significantly improved."

Mattson, Phyllis. **Holistic Health in Perspective.** San Francisco: Institute of Noetic Sciences, 1978.

Mattson, an anthropologist, tends to see holistic health as a splinter movement and a subculture rather than an enlarged approach to health and medical care, but she offers a good overview of the holistic health movement. She raises helpful questions in the last section of her paper about research, public policy, and the potential integration of holistic and allopathic medicine.

McKeown, Thomas. **The Role of Medicine: Dream, Mirage, or Nemesis?** London: Rock Carline Fellowship, Nuffield Provincial Hospitals Trust, 1976.

Although briefer statements of his position are available in other volumes, this book presents McKeown and his argument at their carefully documented, literary best. Drawing on information derived from mortality and morbidity statistics in England and Wales in the last three centuries, McKeown demonstrates the central importance of changes in the environment, in nutrition, and in behavior for improving health. He concludes that the "engineering" approach to health – managing and subduing illness when it arises – is both ineffective and, in the long run, destructive of our capacity to heal ourselves.

Pelletier, Kenneth R. **Mind as Healer, Mind as Slayer: A Holistic Approach to Preventing Stress Disorders.** New York: Delta, 1977.

This is a clear, straightforward presentation of much of the research that has been done on the effects of stress on the human body. It is also a good summary of nonpharmacological techniques that have been used to alleviate the effects of stress, including meditation, autogenic training, and biofeedback. Some of the explanations, particularly in the section on the psychophysiology of stress, may not be complete enough for the biomedical scientist, but this is an extremely useful overview for health care professionals or the lay person.

Popenoe, Cris. **Wellness,** Washington, D.C.: Yes! Inc., 1977.

This is an extremely useful and extensive listing of books related to holistic health; it is a catalog as well as a bibliography. Although important areas (such as biofeedback, autogenic training, psychosomatic medicine, and chiropractic) are omitted, there are impressive listings in such fields as nutrition, body work, cancer therapy, fasting, natural childbirth, and Reichian therapy. The annotations are useful and thoughtful. Yes! Inc., located at 1035 31st Street, N.W., Washington, D.C. 20007, plans to update this volume periodically.

Reich, Wilhelm. **Selected Writings: An Introduction to Orgonomy.** New York: Farrar, Straus, and Giroux, 1960.

Reich, Wilhelm. **The Mass Psychology of Fascism.** New York: Farrar, Straus, and Giroux, 1970.

Taken together these two books offer an excellent introduction to the work and thought of this psychoanalytic pioneer and maverick. His style is sometimes difficult to penetrate and many of his methods and conclusions will be disputed by all but the most dedicated of his disciples, but Reich is nonetheless enormously illuminating. He was the first to make explicit connections between political oppression, emotional illness, and disturbed biological functioning and was for years a leader in movements to alleviate all of them.

Samuels, Mike, and Bennett, Hal. **The Well-Body Book.** New York: Random House/Book Works, 1973.

This is the best of the medical self-care books that I have seen. Skillfully combining allopathic knowledge with meditative wisdom, Samuels and Bennett have produced a systematic, comprehensive, and truly holistic approach to maintaining health and treating illness. The book helps readers experience as well as understand their bodies and their emotions (and the connections between them) and offers medical and psychological tools to approach and in some cases to remedy a variety of common medical problems.

Samuels and Bennett offer thoughtful chapters on, among other topics, visualization exercises (the book is particularly strong in this area), preventive medicine, physical examinations, and your doctor as a resource. They include information on medical instruments, common diseases, and emergency medicine. This is a superb volume, one that will enlarge the practice and the perspective of physicians as much as it will help their patients.

Sobel, David S. **Ways of Health: Holistic Approaches to Ancient and Contemporary Medicine.** New York: Harcourt, Brace, Jovanovich, 1979.

In this collection a young physician offers his readers a historical and cross-cultural perspective from which they may view the achievements and limitations of contemporary biomedicine. Most of the essays are original contributions, designed to provide a broad overview and fresh interpretations of areas (systems theory, Chinese medicine, homoeopathy, etc.) that have been obscured by heavy-handed scholarship or overenthusiastic claims. Other contributions, like René Dubos's "Hippocrates in Modern Dress," and John Powles's "On the Limitations of Modern Medicine," have been published elsewhere, but until the appearance of Sobel's volume they were nearly impossible to locate.

   The range of topics sometimes threatens to make this more of a sampler than a unified volume, but Sobel's editorial hand and the genial spirit of René Dubos's essay manage to hold the book together. This is a useful introduction to holistic medicine for physicians, medical students, and other health care professionals.

Tinbergen, Nikolaas. **Ethology and stress diseases.** *Science,* 1974. **185,** 20–27.

Tinbergen's Nobel Prize acceptance speech emphasizes "the critical importance for medical science of open-minded observation – of 'watching and wondering,'" the centrality of stress in the etiology of many kinds of illness, and the virtues of a holistic approach to ourselves and our patients. His account of his work with autistic children reveals that a fundamental respect for each child's uniqueness may be the first step toward a long-denied mutuality. Tinbergen's descriptions of the increased physical and emotional well-being he and his family experienced after learning the "Alexander method" provide a nice insight into the transformative power of one simple but elegant kind of muscular re-education.

U.S. Senate Select Committee on Nutrition and Human Needs. **Dietary Goals for the United States.** Washington, D.C.: U.S. Government Printing Office, February 1977.

This document (generally known as the "McGovern Report" after the committee's chairman) presents findings about the American diet and its deleterious effect on the nation's health. It gives specific recommendations for dietary improvement: decreased use of saturated fats, sugar, salt, and cholesterol and an increased consumption of the complex carbohydrates (including fruits, vegetables, and grain products, once the staple of the American diet).

   Though this extremely even-handed report refrains from a thorough-going indictment of either American eating habits or the agribusiness that helps create them by pandering to the public, it does recommend some important changes in nutrition education, food labeling, and expanded federal research on human nutrition. In addition, it makes the extremely valuable point that hurried meals in frenzied restaurants or depressing institutional cafeterias may have as much effect on us as what we eat.

   The fact that Congress issued this report is as important as what it contains.

Part Two

THE CONTEXT
OF HEALTH

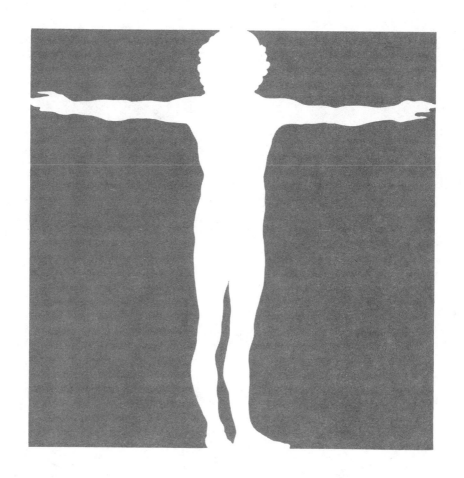

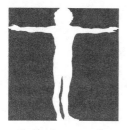

THE SOCIAL CONTEXT OF HEALTH

Leonard J. Duhl, M.D.

Common sense suggests and the data that have accumulated from years of long-term studies confirm the fact that a dynamic relationship between human beings and their social environments can be the cause of good or poor health (Churchman, 1972; Kitagawa and Hauser, 1973). These environments may be defined as the sum of those intangible interactions that exist between people. They are usually structured by prevailing political, economic, and cultural forces and are affected by and in turn affect the physical environment—the climate, the air people breathe, the houses they dwell in, whether they live in urban or rural places, the roads on which they commute (Proshansky et al., 1976).

Although the relationship between the socioenvironmental context and health status is sometimes immediately apparent, as for instance in the relationship between poor sanitation and the incidence of some infectious diseases, it is not always that simple. In some settings, the absence of good sanitation may be the result of an extremely complex group of factors, including scientific ignorance, local politics, lack of constructive skills, and lack of money. There may even be some political advantage to those in power in keeping people sick and anergic.

It is crucial then that health practitioners and policymakers who wish to be effective keep in mind the fact that health is embedded in a social context (because people are) (Duhl, 1963, 1968), that the causes of disease are not always strictly biological, and that healing cannot always depend on biomedical intervention, the future promises of biomedical intervention, or research (Somers, 1971).

Two Approaches to Social Context

There are two related but quite different approaches to the study of the impact of social environments on health. The first uses statistical and epidemiological techniques to correlate such factors as education, race, economic status, age, and occupation with the incidence of illness and injury (Kitagawa and Hauser, 1973). The second, a more broadly cultural approach to the relationship between social environment and health, considers the influence of "softer" factors on health and illness (Geiger, 1972). Among its concerns are the structure of social networks, the influence of the mass media on people's attitudes and beliefs, the presence or absence of freedom to grow and develop normally and naturally, the effects of community politics and participation, the ways in which social settings foster or frustrate self-esteem and confidence. Although the second approach makes use of some of the statistical information provided by the first approach, it tends to evade statistical analysis and must be defined in more intuitive, speculative ways. Both approaches, applied together, can help health planners and policymakers—and, indeed, individual practitioners—take action to affect the health of groups within their scope.

The analysis of social determinants of health rests on the simple observation that some groups of people are healthier than other groups. From studying these various groups and comparing them, a set of social, economic, and demographic characteristics can be derived that correlates strongly with either the absence of certain diseases or with higher mortality or morbidity.

Such studies have shown that income, age, and education are probably the three strongest influences on health and that all are interrelated. Higher *income* levels and better health, lower incomes and poorer health are consistently correlated. *Education* seems to affect health not only because it elevates economic status, but because it allows people better access to information about health and disease and about their bodies, because it helps them make more considered choices about matters that affect health.

Age also affects health in a variety of ways. Mortality statistics show that the first year of life is the most dangerous year of all below forty. But it is old age that most often emerges as an important social determinant of health. Our society now contains growing numbers of elderly persons who make great demands upon medical services, who are often poor and ill fed, and who are prone to accidents and the effects of loneliness and isolation. Thus to be old, poor, and uneducated almost always means to be ill.

Occupation, another major indicator of health, is related to income and education. But occupation is also directly related to health because of the accidents, poisonings, and exposures to contaminants and carcinogens that many jobs entail. The effects of occupation on housing, neighborhoods, commuting patterns, intercity moves, stress, and alcohol and tobacco use are less direct but universal. In addition there are special groups such as migrant workers, coal miners, and asbestos workers who suffer specific and often lethal occupational health hazards.

Ethnic and cultural background are also important determinants of health (Orleans and Ellis, 1971). Health problems among Blacks, Mexican Americans, Puerto Ricans, and Native Americans are of much concern to those groups and to public health workers generally. Some diseases like sickle cell anemia are biologically specific to racial groups. Many more are related to those general factors already mentioned—poverty, education, occupation, sanitation, housing, etc. There are also some ethnic and cultural groups that seem to experience good health, probably because of religious or cultural factors that affect their life-styles.

Other social determinants of health include geography, birth order, generation, sex, urban or rural residence, family structure, marital status, important "life events," and language barriers (Proshansky, 1976). Many such indicators can be observed simply and directly, but others take some fairly sophisticated epidemiological study to determine. For instance, the recent attention to factors that contribute to child abuse and neglect has revealed the importance of the mother's age at first pregnancy.

Although this kind of information is valuable and necessary, my personal attention as a psychiatrist and urban planner has been drawn to the softer issues that until recently have been neglected. The social context of health, in my view, may be defined as the entire set of relationships that exist among people and among the groups to which people belong. Health itself, rather than being simply the absence of disease or injury, I define more broadly as participation in a process of natural growth and development. These definitions may seem entirely too broad or vague to some, but I find they provide me with room in which to reconsider the relationship between society and health in a more holistic way (Duhl, 1976).

The Current Context

We are going through a period of rapid change and a heightening of contradictions in many aspects of public life. The economic situation is currently creating inflationary pressures on us, and the threat of a major recession seems always in the wings. Demographic changes are also underway. Several years ago we felt that the population of our country was getting increasingly younger; today with fewer children and more older people we find that the average age is creeping upward again. Americans are still on the move; major population shifts are bringing people into and out of the cities and into the Southwest and West. We change jobs, houses, neighborhoods, and regions more than any other people on the planet.

For many, work is the one thing that most orders and defines life. In many families both parents work in order to beat the high cost of living. Yet others—especially the young and most especially the young minorities—are denied the experience of work. For some minorities, unemployment is an experience that extends over the generations.

Education is also undergoing change. The system is producing some students who know more, think faster, and command events more ably than ever, while others who graduate cannot read or write, fill out a job application, make out a check, add up their budgets, or even communicate verbally. Teachers are beleaguered and bewildered; the educational bureaucracy is swollen and inefficient; schools are viciously vandalized.

Television has had a major impact on American lives. We know all too little about its effects and can only guess at what it means when millions spend anywhere from four to six or more hours a day watching television. While audiovisual communication gets more and more sophisticated, are we too becoming more sophisticated or more dull and apathetic?

The family seems threatened and under siege by many social factors—easy divorce, easy cohabitation, new sexual freedoms of many kinds, economic realities, the impact of feminism. All the stresses and strains of contemporary life affect the family and the health of its members one way or another, sometimes for good, sometimes for ill.

Urbanization, transportation, racial strife and inequality, crime, taxes, pollution, energy—the list of contemporary social problems is long, the items on the list inextricably interrelated, and their affects on health, particularly their contribution to the chronic diseases that beset so much of our population, profound. Within this context—this fast-moving, stressful and liberating, diverse and interlocked set of social, political, and personal changes—where do we begin to look for the signs of health or the mechanisms by which to enhance health?

Health and Disease

Often when I think about creating a social context that promotes individual health, I think about a unique experiment in health that took place in London more than forty years ago—the Pioneer Health Centre, founded by Drs. Scott Williamson and Innes Pearse in the working-class neighborhood of Peckham (Pioneer Health Centre, 1971; Williamson and Pearse, 1965). These physicians made an assumption much like Maslow's: no headway would be made into the understanding of health simply by researching the mechanisms of disease. They were aware that health itself has its own patterns of disease. To use their words, they expected the Peckham experiment (Pearse and Crocker, 1947) to show "that health is more powerful and infectious than disease."

Beginning with the assumption that there was indeed a state of "positive health," Drs. Williamson and Pearse built up a neighborhood center of sorts, a combination clubhouse, gymnasium, meeting room, theater, dance hall, library, and clinic. Peckham neighbors were eligible to join, with one stipulation—they would have to cooperate in an annual health "overhaul," which included an examination and subsequent discussion of its results with other family members and the doctors. An attempt was thus made to raise community sensitivity to health issues.

Out of the stipulated annual health overhauls came some interesting statistics. It was found that a little more than 10 percent of those examined really had nothing wrong with them at all; the other 90 percent had some diagnosable condition. However, more than 60 percent of those examined declared themselves to be "well"; that is, they had no complaints and felt no physical restrictions on their lives. The remaining 25 to 30 percent of those examined felt they were, by their own definition, "sick." (These figures, incidentally, were replicated later in other epidemiological studies.) I like to call the 10 percent or more of those who had no symptoms "the Alive"; the 60 percent or more who may have had this or that symptom but said they were "well," the "Survivors"; and the remaining 25 percent or more who said they were "sick," the "Ill or the Dying."

The Survivors are those who usually define health, who have the power to allocate health resources; they are the majority and have majority powers. The Ill or Dying are those who make most use of health resources, sometimes properly and beneficially, sometimes not. They also live their lives as if they were ill or dying and have particular attitudes toward health that are difficult to change. The Alive, on the other hand, are usually seen as deviants because they make demands for certain kinds of resources that the health system cannot provide. They demand change, growth opportunities, personal liberation, outlets for creativity and expression, significant encounters with the world and others, and so on. It seems that our society prefers to tolerate too many sick people, that it is made uncomfortable by the healthy ones and their disruptive demands.

Many recent writers (Alford, 1972, 1975; James, 1972; Satin, 1978) have stated that more has been accomplished in the fight against disease by social and political means than by strictly medical means. Changes in sanitation, housing, food, work places, population control, etc., have led to a reduction in disease and injury that could not have been accomplished as successfully any other way. At the same time, what the LaLonde Report (1974) calls the "dark side of economic progress"—the "ominous" and medically irremediable "counter forces" of pollution, urbanization, bad health habits (including abuse of tobacco, alcohol, and drugs), poor nutritional knowledge and practice—has done much to undermine health.

The medical care system is a net that catches the victims of social, political, and economic "illness," not a system that fosters and enhances health (Roemer and Friedman, 1971; Stevens, 1971). So the health and medical care system has been given credit for bettering health when other social institutions actually did more (Anderson, 1968), and it is blamed for not alleviating disorders that are actually the responsibility of other institutions.

At present, the health and medical care system of this country is overwhelmed by the responsibility for dealing with a host of social, political, and economic ills that do not belong to it (National Broadcasting Company, 1978). We are continually broadening instead of limiting our definition of illness and then telling the medical care institutions that they must deal with the growing number of symptoms displayed by Survivors and the life-defying and life-denying attitudes displayed by the Ill. Alcoholism, criminality, antisocial behaviors, drug abuse, mental retardation, anomie, fright, loneliness, stress, and all kinds of thwarted developmental issues are placed within the medical care system.

Along with relieving the medical care system of some responsibilities that have been wrongly given to it, we can begin to dispel some of the mystique of medicine and health care and some of the blind faith in medical practitioners and health professionals. A change in our dependency on the medical care system, a more realistic view of what it can and cannot, should or should not do will lead to an increased assumption of personal responsibility for growth and development.

One way to begin is by defining health in terms of the demands that are made by the Alive, by those whom Abraham Maslow (1970) called "self-actualizing." We ought to begin to define health in terms of growth and development, creativity, and the capacity to change and make change. Then we might begin to reorder the social system to provide for the demands of the Alive. One of the goals of social policy ought to be the maintenance of opportunities for growth and personal development, while the health care system by medical means ought to try to return those who are blocked from growth back to their normal growth cycles.

In other words, let the health care system continue as it is, but let us narrow its responsibilities. We have one of the best medical care systems in the world; it does superbly at applying scientific and technological interventions in disease and injury, at research, and at discovery. If we could find ways to lighten its load we might also find easier ways to finance what it can do best. But we cannot any longer let the Survivors and the Dying, with their necessarily limited point of view and their great needs, have total control over that system.

Some Alternatives

The task of creating a healthier social context and a more holistic attitude toward health care involves changes in the institutions where health and illness are dealt with, in the training of health professionals, and in the society as a whole. One important concept – and my special interest – that should be considered in this process of change is networking: the examination and activation of the social dynamics that exist in families, small groups, businesses, and even in entire societies and countries (Duhl, 1970, 1978).

There is a strong body of research and conceptual studies on networking that has been created by sociologists, social psychologists, anthropologists, political and social scientists, and urbanologists, among others. The interesting part of all this work is not so much that networks exist, exist so complexly, or exist in so many different forms, but that they seem to foster well-being among their members. This has been borne out quite specifically by some recent studies (Blum, 1974, 1976; Berkman and Syme, 1979) done in Alameda County, California, where it was shown that individuals with relevant social ties to other human beings were more healthy than individuals without such meaningful intercourse. Common-sense observations and statistics agree: a web of human relationships nurtures and protects an individual.

It follows that a breakdown of such nurturing relationships would have adverse effects on health. That this is so seems to be the point of the Thomas Holmes (Holmes and Masuda, 1973; Holmes and Rahe, n.d.; Rahe and Holmes, n.d.) "life event" scales, which show the relationship between significant life events and the incidence of illness. People who experience disruptive life events (like divorce, death of a partner or friend, loss of a job, a move from one city to another, and so forth) often become ill. Sometimes illness is also connected to important life events that are not necessarily negative — a wedding, a birth, a promotion. The key seems to be stress, induced by sudden major change, that is not buffered by supportive human relationships or that is caused by the loss of such human relationships.

A deep human need thus seems to exist for linkage to a dynamic network of other human beings as well as some sense of linkage to the network of all living beings. Perhaps well-being is related not only to our linkage to other human beings but also to the natural world — or even to some world of spiritual experience. I fear we know very little about the effect of these latter connections upon health.

The recent interest in and focus on preventive or "prospective" medicine often places too much emphasis on individual responsibility for health, leading to the syndrome of "blaming the victim." Individual change does not automatically lead to needed social change. The step from individual commitment to new definitions of health and new health practices is only the first step. The next step is to link these individual perceptions and changes into interpersonal networks in which the dialectical relationship between different perceptions and different stages of growth and development will lead to synergistic change effects. In other words, first, there must be a new understanding of what health means; next, networking must be created to build human groups to support and enhance the lives of their members.

We are a combination of the I and the U's. Sometimes we live as single I's, sometimes we enter into the U's, the social arena. One state is not better or worse than the other — both are needed if we are to be in balance, to be healthy. And both are needed if we are to be engaged in growth and development, if we are to be open to change and to make change.

So the social context of health begins with or builds on the personal context of health; the personal definition of and self-responsibility for health leads to linkage and networking, which are in themselves healthy and a sign of health. Through social linkage and participation in networks of change, we can together learn to effect change – in ourselves and in the world around us.

The hierarchy within a network, if it is a true network and not a rigid system, is fluid and organic. As networks grow and proliferate, new networks and new relationships are created, and the people in them will take on different roles and at times assume different relationships toward each other. At one moment and in one context a network member may be a leader, and in another context at another time he or she may be a follower. Usually, however, one will find in the network some people who take on the role of managers, who keep the others in touch with each other, who act to refer problems between network members and to spread the good news of the success of one network member to the others. There will also be others who function to link different networks, who have the ability to move in and out of different networks, to bring about alliances and to help networks work together for common goals.

Those who plan social change in the health and medical care field should become aware of and foster networking, should identify and support the network managers and network linkers who can initiate change. This may include helping self-help people (such as the ones that would have formed groups) to gain greater independence from the established medical system by learning new skills, linking groups together for such common purposes as improving housing or decreasing neighborhood crime, and facilitating their common interactions with and challenges to the policies and practices of boards of health, drug companies, hospitals, and other social institutions.

I like to call this the work of *making whole* (Duhl, in press). Social change, like individual change, most often comes about when one begins to achieve a balance between self- and group respect, an impact on the external world, and normal growth and development through time. Making whole – that is, creating a true holistic health policy and practice – is more than new or alternative techniques, beliefs, or approaches to treatment. It means working along all these lines together.

References

Alford, Robert R. The political economy of health care: dynamics without change. *Politics and Society,* Winter, 1972. 127–164.

Alford, Robert R. *Health Care Politics.* Chicago: University of Chicago Press, 1975.

Anderson, Odin W. *The Uneasy Equilibrium: Private and Public Financing of Health Services in the United States, 1875–1965.* New Haven, Conn.: College and University Press, 1968.

Berkman, Lisa F., and Syme, Leonard F. Social networks, host resistance, and mortality: a nine-year follow-up study of Alameda County residents. *American Journal of Epidemiology,* 1979. **109** (2), 186–204.

Blum, Henrik L. *Planning for Health: Development and Application of Social Change Theory.* New York: Human Science Press, 1974.

Blum, Henrik L. *Expanding Health Care Horizons.* Oakland, Calif.: Third Party Press, 1976.

Churchman, C. West. *Design of Inquiring Systems, Basic Concepts in Systems Analysis.* New York: Basic Books, 1972.

Duhl, Leonard J. *The Urban Condition: People and Policy in the Metropolis.* New York: Basic Books, 1963.

Duhl, Leonard J. *The poverty program: a national exercise in social change.* Mimeographed report, 1968. Available from author.

Duhl, Leonard J., assisted by Volkman, Janice. Participatory democracy: networks as a strategy for change. *Urban and Social Change Review,* Spring 1970. **3** (2), 11–14.

Duhl, Leonard J. The promotion and maintenance of health: myth and reality. Report of conference on Health Promotion through Designed Environment, October 5–7, 1976. Available from the Minister of Health and Welfare, Ottawa, Canada.

Duhl, Leonard J. The future of the mental health profession: plugging psychiatry into the healing network. *Psychiatry Annals,* May 1978. **8** (5), 102–109.

Duhl, Leonard J., with Den Boer, James. *Making Whole: Health for a New Epoch.* Elmsford, N.Y.: Pergamon Press, in press.

Geiger, H. Jack. A health center in Mississippi: a case study in social medicine. In Laurence Corey et al. (Eds.), *Medicine in a Changing Society.* St. Louis: C. V. Mosby, 1972.

Holmes, Thomas H., and Masuda, Minoru. Life change and illness susceptibility. In J. P. Scott and E. C. Senay (Eds.), *Separation and Depression.* Washington, D.C.: American Association for the Advancement of Science, 1973. 161–186.

Holmes, Thomas H., and Rahe, Richard H. Schedule of Recent Experience (SRE). Questionnaire published by the University of Washington, School of Medicine, Department of Psychiatry, Seattle, Washington, n.d.

James, Dorothy. *Poverty, Politics, and Change.* Englewood Cliffs, N.J.: Prentice Hall, 1972.

Kitagawa, Evelyn, and Hauser, Philip. *Differential Mortality in the United States: A Study in Socioeconomic Epidemiology.* Cambridge, Mass.: Harvard University Press, 1973.

LaLonde, Marc. *A New Perspective on the Health of Canadians.* Ottawa: Government of Canada 1974.

Maslow, Abraham H. *Motivation and Personality* (2nd ed). New York: Harper & Row, 1970.

National Broadcasting Company (Dan Conner, Executive Producer). Television special, Medicine in America: Life, Death, and Dollars. January 3, 1978.

Orleans, Peter, and Ellis, William R., Jr. Race research: "Up against the wall" in more ways than one. In Peter Orleans et al., *Race, Change, and Urban Society.* Beverly Hills, Calif.: Sage Publications, 1971.

Pearse, Innes H., and Crocker, Lucy H. *The Peckham Experiment: A Study of the Living Structure of Society.* London: George Allen and Unwin, Ltd., 1947.

Pioneer Health Centre. *Health of the Individual, of the Family, of Society.* Rotherfield, Sussex, England: Pioneer Health Centre, 1971.

Proshansky, Harold M. et al. *Environmental Psychology: People and Their Physical Settings.* New York: Holt, Rinehart and Winston, 1976.

Rahe, Richard H., and Holmes, Thomas H. *Life Crisis and Disease Onset: A Prospective Study of Life Crises and Health Changes.* Mimeographed report, Department of Psychiatry, University of Washington School of Medicine, Seattle, Washington, n.d.

Roemer, Milton J., and Friedman, Jay. *Doctors in Hospitals: Medical Staff Organizations and Hospital Performance.* Baltimore: Johns Hopkins Press, 1971.

Satin, Mark. *New Age Politics: Healing Self and Society,* West Vancouver, B.C.: Whitecap Books, 1978.

Somers, Anne R. *Health Care in Transition: Directions for the Future.* Chicago: Hospital Research and Educational Trust, 1971.

Stevens, Rosemary. *American Medicine and the Public Interest.* New Haven: Yale University Press, 1971.

Williamson, G. S., and Pearse, I. H. *Science, Synthesis, and Sanity.* London: Collins, 1965.

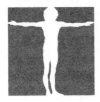 ANNOTATED BIBLIOGRAPHY

Berkman, Lisa F., and Syme, Leonard F. **Social Networks, host resistance, and mortality: a nine-year follow-up study of Alameda County residents.** *American Journal of Epidemiology,* 1979.

> Networks are critical issues in the phenomena of health and illness. People who are socially connected have less disease than those who are disconnected, suggesting some important social considerations for planning in the health area.

Blum, Henrik L. **Planning for Health: Development and Application of Social Change Theory.** New York: Human Science Press, 1974.

> The focus here is on the variety of processes in health, ranging from a definition of the problem to the techniques necessary to deal with the various issues. Blum describes the context within which health is accomplished.

Blum, Henrik L. **Expanding Health Care Horizons.** Oakland, Calif.: Third Party Press, 1976.

> The changing definition of health from medical care to the broader issues is the focus in this book. Dr. Blum looks at all aspects of the environment and the individual from a social, psychological, biological, and physical perspective.

Churchman, C. West. **Design of Inquiring Systems, Basic Concepts in Systems Analysis.** New York: Basic Books, 1972.

> This is a book on systems and how they operate, especially living systems, which are constantly in the process of change, much like the systems involved in the total environment as they impinge on the changing processes of health.

Conference on Future Directions in Health Care: The Dimensions of Medicine. Report of a conference sponsored by the Blue Cross Association, the Rockefeller Foundation, and the Health Policy Program, University of California School of Medicine, New York, December 10-11, 1975.

> This conference brought together many of the best thinkers of the establishment health care system and academia with the proponents of holistic and humanistic

medicine, including John H. Knowles, Philip R. Lee, Walter J. McNerney, Victor Fuchs, Thomas McKeown, Jerome Frank, Lewis Thomas, and Rick Carlson. These discussions about the future of health care in the United States provide some of the clearest expositions of the meaning of holistic health and holistic medical care. Throughout the discussions, there was an emphasis on the social context of these new directions for health.

Duhl, Leonard J. **The Urban Condition: People and Policy in the Metropolis.** New York: Basic Books, 1963.

A look at the urban scene from an ecological perspective, showing that health is related to environmental issues far beyond medical care.

Duhl, Leonard J., assisted by Volkman, Janice. **Participatory democracy: networks as a strategy for change.** *Urban and Social Change Review,* Spring 1970. 3 (2), 11–14.

A focus on networks and their potential role in social change.

Duhl, Leonard J. **The promotion and maintenance of health: myth and reality.** Report of conference on Health Promotion through Designed Environment, October 5–7, 1976. Available from the Minister of Health and Welfare, Ottawa, Canada.

This is part of a larger publication dealing with all aspects of the designed environment and how it impinges on health.

Duhl, Leonard J., with Den Boer, James. **Making Whole: Health for a New Epoch.** Elmsford, N.Y.: Pergamon Press, in press.

This book attempts to reconceptualize some of the issues of health within an environmental context, pointing to a new contextual understanding of health and medical care programs.

Geiger, H. Jack. **A health center in Mississippi: a case study in social medicine.** In Laurence Corey et al. (Eds.), *Medicine in a Changing Society.* St. Louis: C. V. Mosby, 1972.

Geiger's chapter in this book describes the creation of a health center with emphasis on housing, community organization, and social processes as part of the goal of achieving improved health.

Holmes, Thomas H., and Masuda, Minoru. **Life change and illness susceptibility.** In J. P. Scott and E. C. Senay (Eds.), *Separation and Depression,* Washington, D.C.: American Association for the Advancement of Science, 1973. 161–186.

This paper, plus other papers and questionnaires by Holmes and Rahe, shows how the accumulation of stresses that people have in their lives, both personally and environmentally, can lead to breakdown and illness.

Knowles, John (Ed.). **Doing Better and Feeling Worse: Health in the United States.** New York: W. W. Norton, 1977.

This collection of essays, which originally appeared as an issue of *Daedulus,* the journal of the American Academy of Arts and Sciences, provides a fairly current overview of the health status of the United States and renders in its title a catchy verdict. It includes essays by John Knowles, Renée Fox, Eli Ginsburg, and others who have been instrumental in forming health care policy in the past and will shape future policy as well. The collection is of use to both specialist and generalist.

Lalonde, Marc. **A New Perspective on the Health of Canadians.** Ottawa: Government of Canada, 1974.

The "LaLonde Report," authored by the Canadian government's minister of health, has had an impact on public health policy and planning that is almost without precedent in the last twenty-five years. The report argues that four major "fields" affect individual health: biological factors, health care services, environmental factors, and life-styles. A range of statistical data is given to show that biological factors and health services have little effect on health today, and that environmental and life-style factors cause the bulk of disease and injury. As a brief seminal statement, the LaLonde Report is necessary reading.

Michael, Donald N. **On Learning to Plan—and Planning to Learn.** San Francisco: Jossey-Bass Publishers, 1976.

All aspects of social change—including environmental change, Third World development, urbanization, and improved use of technology, transportation, energy, and health care—depend on an ability to learn methods for anticipating future change. Although this book does not focus on health or health planning, there is nevertheless much to learn here about long-range social planning. Michael examines the social-psychological aspects of individual and group resistance to change and the possibilities for breaking down these barriers, describing the planning process as a learning one. Instead of conceptualizing long-range social planning as the imposition of statistically oriented rationalizations on individual lives, he describes it as—at least potentially—a process of learning in its best sense, in which the end is not as important as the means.

Pearse, Innes H., and Crocker, Lucy H. **The Peckham Experiment: A Study of the Living Structure of Society.** London: George Allen and Unwin, 1947.

This book, as well as those published by the Pioneer Health Centre and by Williamson and Pearse (see the references for this chapter), focuses on the development of a neighborhood center concerned with health instead of illness. They describe the development of the project and the various findings that have emerged, including the community action of the participants.

Preventive Medicine U.S.A. Task force reports sponsored by the John E. Fogarty International Center for Advanced Study in the Health Sciences, National Institutes of Health, and the American College of Preventive Medicine. New York: Prodist, 1976.

This massive compilation of task force reports on preventive medicine includes sections on health promotion and consumer health education, personal health services, quality control and evaluation of preventive health services, health manpower education and training, environmental health, social determinants of human health, and the economic impact of preventive medicine as well as a short history of preventive medicine in the United States from 1900–1975. Neither a specialist's publication nor a popularization, this collection does provide an overview of the changing and nonreceptive attitude toward preventive health care that exists at the upper echelons of the establishment policymaking agencies.

Proshansky, Harold M. et al. **Environmental Psychology: People and Their Physical Settings.** New York: Holt, Rinehart and Winston, 1976.

A useful reader dealing with various aspects of environmental psychology.

Satin, Mark. **New Age Politics: Healing Self and Society.** West Vancouver, B.C.: Whitecap Books, 1978. (To be published by Dell Books, 1979.)

An attempt to bring together the activities in social change during the last fifteen years to devise a post-capitalist, post-Marxist view of social change in our current environment.

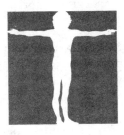

FAMILY THERAPY AND PHYSICAL ILLNESS

Richard Rabkin, M.D.

Family therapy is a method for treating the psychiatric problems of one or more members of a natural group by influencing the structure and processes within that group. Therapy sessions usually include all family or household members, but group composition has become more flexible in recent years. On occasion that group may be expanded to include family members living outside the household, such as grandparents. More rarely the entire network of family members, neighbors, friends, and significant others (physicians, clergymen, etc.) has been included in therapeutic sessions. Alternatively, group composition may be reduced to important threesomes or other variations. Although actual attendance at therapy sessions may vary, the therapist still continues to think in terms of influencing the entire family.

Family therapy began in the 1950s in several places, each of which lacked sufficient numbers of psychoanalytically trained therapists. Since each of the earliest family therapists came upon the idea of treating a natural group together ("conjointly") in his own way, there were many different approaches to family therapy. As the technique became more widely known and as communication among family therapists increased, two main schools of family therapy emerged. The Group for the Advancement of Psychiatry report, *The Field of Family Therapy* (1970), refers to them as the "Position A" and the "Position Z" family therapist. Most family therapists probably fall somewhere in between A and Z and are referred to as "Position M" family therapists.

Position A family therapists tend to come from academic backgrounds in which psychoanalysis is well received. They see family therapy as a *method* for dealing with the individual patient more effectively, a form of group therapy that may in academic settings be included in a "department of group and family therapy." Z family therapists tend to trace their roots to social psychology and U.S. pragmatism. They see family therapy as a new point of view toward psychological problems. For example, it is more likely for A family therapists to talk about indications and contraindications for the technique of family therapy, while Z family therapists consider all problems from a "family therapy" point of view.

Position A family therapists tend to think in terms of one patient's problems and how they affect the family, while Z family therapists consider the so-called "identified" or "index" patient simply as a symptom of family problems. Position A family therapists have as their goal the change of the individual patient's ideas; Z family therapists are more likely to try to modify sequences of events occurring in the family. Position A family therapists look at traumatic events in the individual's past and consider individual history to be very important. Z family therapists are totally ahistoric and consider only what is happening at the moment or view the history of the family over generations. The A family therapist makes an individual diagnosis, while the Z family therapist analyzes the family organization.

In short, Position A family therapy arises naturally from conventional psychiatric thinking, while Position Z family therapy is a total paradigmatic change, a change in the way problems are conceptualized and treated. The prospects for conceptualizing illness from a family perspective seem to lie at the moment with this Z family therapy, which is now often referred to as "systems-oriented" family therapy. Unfortunately, its usefulness has not been fully appreciated in establishment medical settings, which tend to include far larger numbers of Position A family therapists.

The best way to understand the relationship between Position Z family therapy and physical illness is to consider the influence of context on behavior. Raising an arm is considered a "voluntary" act. We generally say that it is under the control of the will. However, the concept of will upon which this distinction depends has been severely criticized. A more acceptable alternative, which I would like to suggest, is to consider arm raising and other such voluntary behavior "context independent" behavior. I can raise my arm when angry, when frightened, when running, when making love—in short I can raise my arm regardless of the social context and that is why I call it "voluntary." It is true that under hypnosis there have been demonstrations establishing that subjects cannot raise their arms. In most cases such subjects are asked to imagine that their arm is encased in a metal tube, etc.—that is, in a "context" that would make raising an arm impossible. In those cases in which there is no overt image from a hypnotist it has been discovered that the subjects adopt a similar image on their own. In general, physical restraints are not considered as "context."

When we shift our focus to another behavior such as sexual arousal (we might say "raising a penis" instead of "raising an arm") we find that that behavior is "not voluntary" or, to use the terminology being proposed here, sexual arousal is *context dependent.* In passing one might note that Saint Augustine, speculating on how sexual arousal might have been if man had not been banished from the Garden of Eden, postulated that one would raise a penis like one raised an arm, that God's punishment was to create for man context-dependent behavior. Sexual arousal since the Fall depends upon a very special atmosphere. It does not totally depend upon the display of anatomy since that same display in the operating room of a hospital fails to arouse. It is not dependent simply on specific stimuli but stimuli with a context or atmosphere. Quite frequently sexual problems arise because the participants are incompetent at the control of context. For example, one highly educated couple sought help for a sexual arousal problem. It was determined that they were attempting to have an erection as one might raise one's arm. While making love they would watch the bedside clock to time the erection, thus stripping themselves of the very context that might solve the problem. Once this was pointed out they had no problem with arousal.

Now let us consider another behavior such as an attack of asthma or ulcerative colitis. There are two schools of thought about this class of behavior. No one considers it a voluntary or context-independent behavior like raising one's arm. Raising an arm is a *desired* context-independent behavior. Asthma or colitis certainly is not an act that one can perform by desiring it. The question about these conditions is whether they are context dependent or part of another class of behaviors that is unrelated to will power or to context, one we might simply call "disease." So defined, disease is not voluntary, nor is it related to will power or to context. Z family therapy asks whether such a category of disease behavior exists or whether it is an illusion.

To return to asthma, a recent study showed that half of the pulmonary emergency admissions at Elmhurst Hospital in Queens, New York, were acute asthmatic attacks. When all of the asthmatic patients in the clinic were given a card with the telephone number of the pulmonary resident on call and were told that they could call and get immediate treatment—thus bypassing the emergency room with its strange doctors, long waits, etc.—the rate of acute asthmatic emergencies was decreased by 50 percent. The point is made in a different way by Molière, who noted we should never say that a patient died of a disease but rather (to paraphrase) of a disease, two doctors, three nurses, an emergency ward, several pharmacists (or pharmaceutical companies), a worried family, and a welfare system—in other words, a disease *and* a context.

Position Z family therapy takes the point of view that there are always *two factors* in sickness: pathological behavior of an organ or regulatory system and illness of the personal context—the family or natural group. Organ pathology is managed or cured; contextual problems are healed. The relationship between these two factors and their proper description constitute the crucial issues for Z family therapy, a vital source of information about the genesis, treatment, and perpetuation of pathology.

The Genesis of Illness

Patients begin their journey to a physician with the experience of a vague disease, a lack of comfort that is not localized to an organ system. In discussion with one's family (or significant others) the bodily changes that accompany almost every class of problem take on clearer definition. The prevailing contextual emphasis, what is considered important, determines whether one will go to a lawyer, clergyman, doctor, or the local drugstore. As options are narrowed down in the course of this negotiation, the "reality" of the problem is determined. If and when the patient meets with a physician, the "reality" is refined further.

Evidence supporting this point of view comes from both anecdotal and clinical studies. Balint's (1957) study of the construction of problems in the offices of family physicians in England was the first major contribution. A more recent report by Kleinman and colleagues (1978), while derivative, distinguishes between treating organic disease and the context that affects it. It describes in some detail this context, which they refer to as the "cultural construction of clinical reality."

The availability of other problem-solving methods besides the medical one makes it possible to divert those with problems from "medical-izing" their conditions. In New York City when a former mayor placed "little city halls" in health stations (general medical clinics), fully 60 percent of the people who were headed toward a process that would put a medical construction on their condition wound up diverted by a referral to the legal-political remedies available at the little city halls. No medical treatment was suggested or given. It is clear then that the capacity to reinterpret problems at this early stage of their development can radically change the flow of patients to medical institutions, and it is reasonable to believe that in many cases the family can control this "gate" into illness.

Treatment

Although there are studies to suggest that patients get better more quickly and have less complications from surgery if they like their surgeons, if their families are not anxious about the outcome, etc., most current medical treatments remain context independent. The general trend in medicine has been to ignore or deny context-dependent issues. Twenty years ago it was customary for an anesthesiologist to visit a patient the day before the surgery. Today it is the exception, not the rule.

The family that believes in context-independent disease usually produces passive patients who neither take note of their bodily condition nor attempt to do much about their health. They become habituated to medical visits. Most patients with psychosomatic illness can easily recall an early warning of impending difficulty; hours before they have an attack asthmatics often hear "squeaks" in their breathing. Many do absolutely nothing about it. Several interesting reports have suggested that, if the asthmatic takes certain action—for instance a relaxation exercise—he can learn to cut short the attack. Whether he does so or not seems to depend upon the prevailing atmosphere within his natural group.

The question that is now being raised insistently is whether all disease might not fit the model of context-dependent behaviors. Can cancer be conceptualized as a behavior of the immune system that is context dependent? Are there certain family ("context") characteristics that affect the immune system and hence protect or predispose to cancer?

This point of view is an extension of the one that considers disease susceptibility in relation not only to exposure but to *host factors.* Simply exposing people to cholera bacilli, even in high dosages, does not always produce cholera. Most exposed to the tuberculosis bacillus do not develop tuberculosis. Nor is disease uniformly distributed throughout the population. About 25 percent of the people have 50 percent of the disease episodes and another 25 percent have fewer than 10 percent of the disease episodes, a difference attributed to personal and environmental as well as *disease* variables.

Studies of disease patterns within families have suggested that some diseases seem to run a course, not only through a patient, but within a family. Woodyatt and Spetz (1942) described such a process for diabetes:

> This gives us the picture of diabetes appearing in a family (that has not exhibited it before so far as we knew) and running a definable clinical course but in the family as distinguished from the individual case. . . . The whole course can be run in two generations, but it is more commonly completed in three or four and rarely more. That is to say, we rarely find families with a history of diabetes in more than four generations.

In the course of studying such families, the phenomenon of "anticipation" has been described in which each successive generation has the disease at an earlier time and often as a more severe manifestation. Darwin described this phenomenon in 1894. Woodyatt and Spetz (1942) in their description of diabetes as a family disease continue as follows:

> In this picture, those patients that develop the disease in later life appear as cases of first or second generation. They are offshoots of a vine that has been affected for only a limited time—expressions of a young family of diabetes. On the other hand, juvenile diabetic patients appear as cases of following generations. In families that show rapid anticipation, they can be representatives of second generations but average rates are

more often of a third or fourth generation. They are shoots from a vine that has been diseased for a long time – expressions of an old family diabetes. Hence, the differences in the average course of diabetes in older and younger subjects.

Earlier and earlier expression of a disease will lead to the extinction of the family line.

The important point to emphasize is that the disease has changed "residence" in this conceptualization. It is seen as existing in the context rather than in the individual patient's body. It is in the entire vine or family tree, not only in the individual shoot or branch. Michael Kerr (1978) of the Georgetown Family Center, Washington, D.C., has been attempting to explore multigenerational family process in relationship to various diseases, including cancer. The question that is being posed is whether one can bring about some change in the organization of the family that might serve to treat the disease.

The Perpetuation of Pathology

Recovery from an illness episode is not a predetermined phenomenon but an idea: "I am now well." That decision is arrived at in much the same way that the decision "I am sick" is determined. Family and physicians participate. It is sometimes necessary for a physician to make a very unambiguous statement to the family and, perhaps, even a physical examination in their presence in order to make sure that, when a patient returns to his family, he is not placed in an invalid role. Heart attack victims, for example, can return to a family that takes special care not to aggravate the patient. For fear of causing another heart attack, they often fail to put limits on his behavior. Patients in such families find themselves without interpersonal "brakes" on their emotions, particularly on their rage. The result is that they are more likely to be enraged and to stress their hearts.

When current medical practitioners successfully convince the patient and his natural group that he is well, they often give the entire credit to the miraculous power of their medicine. It might be more helpful for the patient and his family if he left the hospital thinking "We beat that case of pneumonia" rather than "The doctors saved my life." The latter belief supports the medical establishment, while the former supports the natural group.

The Effect of Illness on the Family

Up to this point we have been talking about how family structure or beliefs can influence illness or treatment. The reverse is also true. Sometimes an illness might begin as the result of one factor but be *maintained* by another, in this case the way in which the family responds to the illness. During the 1700s there was a great wave of interest in tar water for the treatment of all diseases. Tar water, fresh water with a little bit of tar in it, was almost certainly effective because it led families to abandon the prior treatment method of bloodletting, not because it had any particular inherent beneficial properties. It was remarkably effective in a great many illnesses. We now believe that the host's capacity to cure its own disease was what caused the diseases to stop, but the tar water prevented the family from doing things that would have maintained the disease by weakening the host.

It has been noticed that families under stress are most likely to become extensively intertwined with each other. Each part of the family system becomes too reactive to each other part. If, when I am cold, I insist that my child put on his gloves, I am "fusing" with that child. We are enmeshed. This process makes every element of the natural group too vulnerable to every other member's projections and amplifies whatever deviance there might be in the individual patient. A family that is terrified of diabetes is more likely to adversely affect a diabetic child's health than a family that can maintain some perspective on the subject. This observation has led some family therapists (Minuchin, 1978) to work to disrupt the enmeshment that prolongs illness (and other stress) and has led others (Bowen, 1966) to study the effects of several generations of "fusion" on the mental and physical health of these families.

Summary

It is customary to give lip service to the idea that we treat people, not symptoms or diseases. When we place "that which we treat when we treat people" within the body in some undisclosed place, referring to it as if it were an organ (the mind) similar to the liver, we are making what has been considered a logical error. A "self" according to social psychology is the "envelope" of recurrent interactions with significant others. If we are to study or treat people then we must study and treat that set of transactions. Physically sick people are also what they do and who they are with significant others. If we are going to treat *people* with symptoms of physical disease then we must treat the natural group, most often the family, in which their significant interactions occur.

References

Balint, Michael. *The Doctor, His Patient, and Illness.* New York: International Universities Press, 1957.

Bowen, Murray. The use of family theory in clinical practice. *Comprehensive Psychiatry,* 1966. **7**, 354–474.

Group for the Advancement of Psychiatry. *The Field of Family Therapy.* March 1970, **7** (Report no. 78).

Kerr, Michael E. Emotional factors in physical illness, a multigenerational perspective. Unpublished paper, 1978.

Kleinman, Arthur; Eisenberg, Leon; and Good, Byron. Culture, illness, and care: clinical lessons from anthropologic and cross-cultural research. *Annals of Internal Medicine,* 1978. **88**, 251–258.

Minuchin, Salvador; Rosman, Bernice L.; and Baker, Lester. *Psychosomatic Families: Anorexia Nervosa in Context.* Cambridge, Mass.: Harvard University Press, 1978.

Woodyatt, R. T., and Spetz, M. Anticipation in the inheritance of diabetes. *Journal of the American Medical Association,* 1942. **120**, 602–605.

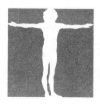 ANNOTATED BIBLIOGRAPHY

This list is based upon suggestions from the members of the editorial board of *Family Process* and four computer-assisted bibliographic searches. As far as I could determine, there is no review article that lists specific medical conditions and work done on family interactions in relation to those conditions.

Framo, James L. **Bibliography of Books and Journals Related to Marital and Family Therapy.** American Association of Marriage and Family Counselors, undated.

> This is an excellent selection of books relevant to family therapy up to about 1976. There are more than one hundred books and at least eleven journals listed specifically on family therapy. Available from C. Ray Fowler, Ph.D., 225 Yale Avenue, Claremont, California 91711.

Haley, Jay (Ed.). **Changing Families: A Family Therapy Reader.** New York: Grune and Stratton, 1971.

> This is a collection of the most important papers in family therapy. There are twenty-three contributions, including ones by Murray Bowen, Salvador Minuchin, Don Jackson, Milton Erickson, Lyman Wynne, Peter Laqueur, Virginia Satir, Carl Whitaker, and Ross Speck. Lynn Hoffman's "Deviation-Amplifying Processes in Natural Groups," which cannot be found elsewhere, is particularly relevant to the perpetuation of physical illness; it discusses vicious cycles and how they apply to the problems encountered by family therapists. The paper by Bowen is generally considered a definitive statement of his work on family history. Family therapy, conjoint family therapy, multiple family therapy, behavior therapy in the home, conflict-resolution family therapy, and social network intervention (with the extended family, friends, neighbors, etc.) are all included in this reader.

Haley, Jay. **Uncommon Therapy: The Psychiatric Techniques of Milton Erickson.** New York: Ballantine Books, 1973.

> Erickson (a psychiatrist who uses hypnosis, irony, and paradox) was an inspiration to early family therapists. Although they may be difficult to copy by the beginner, his

approaches and strategies are unique and unusual. In this remarkably useful discussion of his work, Jay Haley suggests that Erickson, working within the framework of a family's life history, finds that problems occur when the family's development is at a standstill. For example, problems may arise when parents find it difficult to give up their children, the so-called empty nest syndrome. Haley believes that Erickson's technique stimulates the healthy progress of family development, removing the symptoms or problems by removing the underlying source.

Haley, Jay. **Problem Solving Therapy: New Strategies for Effective Family Therapy.** San Francisco: Jossey-Bass, 1977.

This is a step-by-step guide for treating families by one of the founders of the family-therapy movement, who has discovered over the years that he is at his best when supervising family therapists from behind a one-way mirror. This book, the product of years of observation and instruction, is the very best introduction to the techniques of family therapy. It carefully goes over the first interview with a family, the process of giving directives to a family, the stages of family therapy, the problems in training therapists, and the ethical issues involved in this kind of family work. Haley, who is known for his wit, is rather restrained in this carefully and clearly worked-out guide.

Minuchin, Salvador; Rosman, Bernice L.; and Baker, Lester. **Psychosomatic Families: Anorexia Nervosa in Context.** Cambridge, Mass.: Harvard University Press, 1978.

Minuchin, recently described in *The New Yorker* as the "Horowitz" of family therapy, is its most acclaimed practitioner. This recent book, which reports on the results of ten years of work with psychosomatic children, has three purposes: to develop a new theory of psychosomatic disease based on the patient's context rather than on his or her intrapsychic forces, to confirm that theory with scientific data, and to show it unfolding in actual therapeutic situations with anorexia nervosa (self-starvation). Lengthy case histories demonstrate the effectiveness of a method that emphasizes the precipitation of crisis, which will first shake up the family system and subsequently allow it to reform in new and healthier patterns. Although anorexia is the focus of the book, its theories and techniques can be applied to many other conditions both psychosomatic and otherwise.

Rabkin, Richard. **Inner and Other Space: Introduction to a Theory of Social Psychiatry.** New York: W. W. Norton, 1970.

This book is a good introduction to the theory underlying the contextual point of view. While it does not deal directly with the techniques of family therapy, it introduces a way of thinking that is a prerequisite for treating families. It is organized along meta-psychological lines with chapters on structure, dynamics, topology, economics, genetics, diagnosis, and treatment. Each chapter briefly illustrates the intrapsychic point of view. For example, in the chapter on structure the concept of mind is discussed; the chapter then goes on to contrast the intrapsychic view with the family or systems point of view.

The book is not intended as a thorough elaboration of the field but merely as a literate and interesting introduction that offers a glimpse of how one might go about looking at people from a new point of view.

Rabkin, Richard. **Strategic Psychotherapy.** New York: Basic Books, 1977.

This book is intended as an introduction to family therapy from a systems-oriented point of view. The problem of treating a family is approached like chess. The treatment is divided into an opening, a midgame, and an endgame. Several chapters are devoted to each subject. The opening is considered the most important part of the treatment, as it is in chess. The goal of the opening is to get control of the family's expectations, boost their morale, and obtain some compliance to future suggestions. The midgame is the section of therapy in which specific suggestions are made. Some of these are discussed in the text with particular reference to depression and paranoia, both conditions that are often seen as intrapsychic. The endgame discusses termination of therapy and emphasizes that this, too, is a critical part of the treatment.

Watzlawick, Paul; Weakland, John; and Fisch, Richard. **Change, Principles of Problem Formation and Problem Resolution.** New York: W. W. Norton, 1974.

Instead of attempting to discover why a family problem occurred, these authors have found it effective to ask, What is maintaining the problem and how can these factors be changed? They see a family's problem as its need to change the strategy it is using for its problem. Most often it is this strategy that is backfiring and maintaining the problem. They discuss the theory behind their method and suggest various techniques, illustrating theory and method and making specific suggestions with case vignettes. Written in a highly readable style with intriguing references to philosophy and mathematics, this book is a milestone in family therapy.

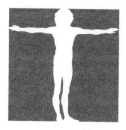

ECOLOGICAL FACTORS IN HEALTH

Stephen Lerner, Michael Lerner, Ph.D.,
and Jane Borchers, M.A.

Changes in Ecological Health Factors

The last thirty years have seen a vast increase in the existence and distribution of negative ecological factors affecting health. We are significantly more exposed to nuclear, petrochemical, and heavy metal pollutants. There has been a decline in the carrying capacities of the four biological systems that support life – croplands, oceans, forests, and grasslands – as increasing population and increasing consumption have diminished their capacity for sustained annual yields. There has also been a decrease in the nutrient value of the U.S. diet. In addition, an extraordinarily complex pattern of ecological changes in the U.S. life system has resulted from the introduction of television. These are just a few of the negative ecological developments of major significance that could be mentioned.

A disheartening proportion of young Americans raised during this period have shown marked evidence of biological and social disintegration. There has been a significant increase in this age group of chronic disease, accidents, suicides, violent crime, delinquency, family instability, male infertility, and educational decline. Some of these changes are perhaps reversible phenomena related to the transient demographic stresses of the "baby boom." Others are doubtless a function of the increase in major ecological stressors on the biological materials of the human family.

On the other hand, there has been a significant increase in positive ecological factors in health over the past thirty years—ecological sources of nurturance. Nutritious foods, adequate housing, adequate sanitation systems, and higher standards of living have enabled hitherto unthinkable proportions of the population in some countries to live in comfort.

In the United States—a major beneficiary of many of these positive as well as negative ecological changes—there has also been a substantial increase in voluntary efforts to improve the quality of individual ecosystems. Increased interest in health promotion—nutrition, stress reduction, fitness, and ecological sensitivity—is an example.

In evaluating ecological factors in health, we are faced with interlocking paradoxes. The environment as a whole is becoming more toxic and stressful with respect to major ecological systems. At the same time, there are many microenvironments serving substantial populations that have become more nurturant in important respects. Individuals living within these more stressful and more nurturant environments are increasingly choosing health promotion activities that increase resilience to the higher levels of ecological stress.

Ecological Treatment Modalities

Many therapeutic approaches explicitly utilize selective arrangement or manipulation of ecological factors in their treatment program. It is in principle possible to consider any therapeutic intervention an alteration of the ecological field. Pharmaceuticals are certainly an ecological factor in health, but so is psychotherapy. What is usually meant by "ecological intervention," however, is considerably narrower in scope. The emerging field of "health promotion" emphasizes the evaluation of sources of individual stress and nurturance over a range of areas including nutrition, fitness, psychological stress reduction, physiological stress reduction, occupational stress reduction, and awareness of ambient ecological stress factors. In each of these areas, the objective is not only to reduce inappropriate levels or kinds of stress but also to increase nurturance. The health promotion paradigm characteristically regards these ecological factors in health as profoundly interactive. Blood sugar, for example, feeds the brain and decisively affects mood. Nutrition can affect blood sugar but so can exercise and psychological, physiological, or occupational stress.

The objective of a high quality health promotion program is to educate the individual about the effects of all of these ecological factors in health and to help the individual develop an ecological stress profile. The health practitioner characteristically works with the client to identify specific areas in which excessive or inappropriate stress can be replaced with an increase in sources of nurturance.

Clinical ecology—the study and treatment of altered psychophysiological responses to foods, chemicals, and other environmental stressors—is another treatment modality in health that, along with health promotion programs, requires specific mention. Clinical ecologists broke away from the U.S. allergy and immunology establishment in the 1930s when allergies were redefined immunologically to focus on antigen-antibody interactions. The clinical ecologists resisted the new movement into the laboratories to study the biochemical mechanisms of allergic reactions. They retained a broad focus on *all* altered responses (literally "allergy") of the organism to a broad range of ecological stressors. Thus, while the mainstream allergists neglected individual susceptibilities to foods and chemicals, the clinical ecologists charted the clinical manifestations of food allergies and chemical hypersensitivities during a quarter of a century that witnessed dramatic changes in the nation's food supply and in the chemical environment.

Theron G. Randolph is considered the greatest theoretician of the clinical ecologists. He pioneered the "ecological unit," a hospital setting as devoid of antigenic substances as possible. His method is to isolate patients in an ecological unit and to fast them on spring water for approximately four days. He then reintroduces them to foods, chemicals, and other environmental stressors one at a time. Typically a patient who enters the ecological unit will experience an increase in symptomatology during the first days of the fast, followed by an abatement of symptoms toward the end of the fast. When the patient is reintroduced to a substance to which he is sensitive, he will experience an often dramatic symptomatic response.

Other methods for testing foods or chemicals utilized by clinical ecologists include a rotation diet, subcutaneous injection or sublingual administration of a food extract (chemicals should not be administered subcutaneously), or some modification of the Randolph fasting method outside the ecological unit. Much of the debate among clinical ecologists focuses on the technical issues arising from these different methods of testing reactions to foods and chemicals.

Dr. Ben Feingold's well-known work on the effects of food additives and salicylates on hyperactive children can be seen within the broader context of the clinical ecology tradition. While Feingold is not a clinical ecologist, his work fits within the theoretical and clinical parameters of clinical ecology.

The clinical ecologists also assert that weaker dilutions of antigenic substances administered sublingually or subcutaneously can provoke a more powerful symptomatic response in many cases than stronger dilutions of the extract. This finding is vigorously contested by traditional allergists. If the ecologists are correct, the finding suggests an intriguing link between clinical ecology and homoeopathy—which utilizes infinitesimally dilute substances for their purportedly profound biophysiological consequences—and casts grave doubt upon assumptions about safe thresholds for new toxic substances in our diet or the environment.

Ecological Concerns

The influence of ecological factors in health is so broad and so variously defined that no critical bibliography can isolate a few central references. Much of the standard literature on ecological factors in health focuses on relationships between specific environmental stressors and specific pathological conditions like the relationship between smoking and cancer; the specific health effects of lead, food additives, and noise; or the effects of a specific nutritional deficiency.

A second body of literature describes the health effects of broader environmental factors such as air ionization, climate, and nonionizing radiation. Another segment of the literature explores the health effects of specific configurations of psychosocial or life-style stressors, such as divorce, a death in the family, or a change in occupational status. And yet another segment of the literature evaluates the health effects of specific technologies or specific settings. The automobile, the television, the workplace, and hospitals are all ecological factors in health. An example from each category might be the health effects of sugar on a child, of a television transmitter on a pregnant woman, of the closing of a factory on the workers, and of eight years of intensive television viewing on a growing child.

We have developed seven useful dichotomies that focus attention on the different perspectives from which ecological factors in these four categories (and others) can be viewed. We can study:

- The effects of individual stressors or their synergistic effects
- Short-term effects or long-term effects
- Average effects on populations or subtle and widely varying effects on individuals
- Biological outcomes or psychobehavioral outcomes
- Specific medical pathologies or more subtle positive or negative adaptations

We can utilize:

- Methodologies that assume no important health effects in the absence of significant evidence to the contrary or methodologies that may sometimes start with a presumption of potential health hazard
- Widely varying theoretical perspectives, utilizing images of the human being that vary from the eternally adaptive to the relatively fragile

These seven dichotomies point to important sources of confusion in discourse on ecological factors in health. An investigator may see human beings as self-contained, resilient entities capable of absorbing quantities of toxins up to definable threshold limits unless defined clinical pathologies prove the contrary. Another investigator may regard human beings as subtle "dances of energy" interpenetrated by other energy fields, whose complex function should be presumed to be disturbed at levels beyond present identification by the untraceable interactions of technological-industrial stressors. The first investigator may regard people as healthy unless there is specific evidence of a pathology; the second may regard individuals as functioning on a continuously changing continuum of health and may regard clinical pathology as an inadequate index of true health status. These two investigators will not be able to communicate until they have clarified their positions on some of the questions raised by these dichotomies.

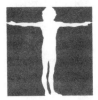 ANNOTATED BIBLIOGRAPHY

The annotated bibliography that follows reflects the diversity of important work on ecological factors in health. The largest group of works cited treat such specific stressors as food additives, pesticides, microwaves, and other environmental pollutants. There are also works on broader ecological factors such as air ionization, as well as a number of important references to the changing ecology of health in a changing technological-industrial system. The reader who fails to explore the diversity of ecological factors in health outlined in this introduction will not derive the greatest benefit from this very useful collection of materials.

Casarett, Louis J., and Doull, John (Eds.). **Toxicology: The Basic Science of Poisons.** New York: Macmillan, 1975.

This textbook was intended to accompany a graduate course in toxicology. It is primarily valuable as a source of history and development of the various branches of the science. The editors organize material into four units, using contributions from thirty-three associate editors. Unit 1 establishes a framework for studying the elements of toxicology and covers definitions, mechanisms, and basic principles. Unit 2 is unique among toxicology textbooks, analyzing the action of toxins on the various systems of the human body. Summaries and citations of the most current research material are included with particular attention to physiological and pharmacokinetic mechanisms of toxic action.

Unit 3 organizes toxic agents by chemical nature or by mode of occurrence (air pollutants, pesticides, metals, food additives, etc.). The format and degree of detail of the contributions in this unit vary greatly; one of the most interesting accounts is the chapter on the toxicology of plastics. Unit 4 discusses a few practical applications of toxicology in such disciplines as clinical, forensic, and veterinary medicine. A chapter on industrial toxicology covers such topics as laboratory administration, the role of the toxicologist in the corporate structure, and how to interpret legislation controlling toxic substances. An excellent chapter, "Toxicology and the Law," provides a valuable account of the enactment of legislation to control toxic substances and the development of regulatory agencies.

This is a useful work for those needing a perspective on the historical development and conventional approach to the study of toxicology. One would expect it to be cited by both the industrial toxicologist wishing to play down the hazard presented by his company's product and by the environmentalist wishing to avert a possible chemical catastrophe.

Some areas in which toxicology suffers from a paucity of theory and information are noted, though many others are not. The fact that we really know very little of the effects of various metabolites of many substances is pointed out, while the effects of chronic exposure to low levels of toxic substances is given short shrift or, at best, conventional dose-response treatment. The validity of the concept of "tolerable threshold concentration," a hotly debated issue today, had little currency in 1975 when this volume was edited. Another obvious omission was a discussion of risk analysis for assessment of the hazard presented by various toxic substances.

On balance, the book should be valuable to anyone in the field of toxicology for its useful bibliography and its historical perspective of the subject, if not for the selective view of various facets of the field.

Czerski, P., Shore, M. L. et al. (Eds.). **Biological Effects and Health Hazards of Microwave Radiation.** Warsaw: Polish Medical Publishers, 1974.

This volume is a compilation of papers given at an international symposium in Warsaw in October 1973. The symposium brought together for the first time scientists from nations known to have a research interest in the effects on health of exposure to microwave radiation in the 300 to 300,000 MHz range.

The book opens with a state-of-the-art commentary by J. C. Villforth, an expert on microwave radiation from the U.S. FDA Bureau of Radiological Health. In it Villforth identifies the current areas in this field that are under investigation: epidemiologic studies, pathologic studies, metabolic studies, neurophysiologic studies, genetic studies, and dosimetric studies.

Primarily presented for research-oriented professionals, the studies described in this volume would nevertheless be of interest to clinicians interested in being able to correctly diagnose microwave-induced pathologies and behavior disorders. Unfortunately, descriptions of health effects are often buried in highly technical articles that exhaustively detail experimental parameters and conditions.

In addition to the section on the general effects of microwave radiation, the session dealing with effects on the nervous system and behavior will be useful to health practitioners willing to extrapolate from animal studies the possible health implications for human populations. In a subsequent section devoted to occupational exposure and the public health aspects of microwave radiation, the health-effects data are somewhat more accessible. Of particular interest are U.S. ophthalmologist Milton Zaret's controversial findings on microwave-induced cataracts.

Two important debates about the effects of electromagnetic radiation can be detected by comparing the various papers presented at this conference. First, research that claims microwave pathologies are caused exclusively by the thermal effects of radiation are challenged by those who believe that there is a significant nonthermal health impact. Second, there is disagreement between U.S. (and western European) and Soviet (Eurasian) research about what constitutes safe microwave exposure levels, with the Americans concluding that the dangers of microwave technologies are less severe than the Russians claim. In this book, the debate surfaces in public for the first time.

In summary, this volume is a good introduction to the extremely complex and highly technical research in progress on the health effects of electromagnetic pollution.

Dickey, Lawrence D. (Ed.). **Clinical Ecology.** Springfield, Ill.: Thomas, 1976.

This is the standard and most readily accessible text on the field of clinical ecology. Clinical ecology is the clinical study of the effects of foods, chemicals, and other allergenic substances on the individual and of the widely varying psychophysiological function of human beings. It contains contributions from many of the foremost figures in the clinical ecology movement, including Theron Randolph, whose excellent contributions should be read sequentially since they constitute the theoretical and clinical heart of the work. There are also excellent contributions by Dickey, Lockey and Mandell. The theoretical structure of clinical ecology is discussed in the introduction to the bibliography.

Eckholm, Erik. **The Picture of Health: Environmental Sources of Disease.** New York: W. W. Norton, 1977.

This paperback book presents a picture of both traditional and modern environmental health threats on a worldwide scale. Discussed are the age-old problems of sanitation, undernutrition, and infant mortality, as well as the new health risks created by the life-styles and technologies of modern societies.

The dangers of the affluent diet, tobacco, and air pollution each receive a chapter. Cancer is looked at as the product of interactions between organisms and their environments. Occupational health hazards are examined and the industrial worker is said to have "unwittingly served as a toxic-substance early warning system." Eckholm gives numerous examples of environmental agents and their known or alleged health effects. He then discusses regulation and society's role in prevention.

The diseases of the poor complement the discussion of diseases of affluent nations. Schistosomiasis, a parasite disease that afflicts 200 million people in at least seventy-one countries, is used as an example of a widespread health problem that has not received adequate attention. Also touched upon are issues of population control, contraception, abortion, and family planning. Undernutrition is shown to be affecting perhaps one out of every six people in the world. Poor nutrition leads to a wide variety of illnesses and contributes substantially to infant mortality.

Eckholm concludes by charging every country with taking on environmental health priorities and keeping a close watch on the earth's life-support systems. He recommends surveillance of oceans, soils, air, plants, and animal and human populations for telltale changes so that human and environmental health can be preserved or achieved.

This book is a well-done general overview of environmental contributions to disease in both developing and affluent nations. It will be of interest to health practitioners and policymakers and is suitable for lay readers as well. Helpful for further study are a complete set of references, suggested readings, and a thorough index. The author presents a good deal of information in a readable, but not striking, form.

Ehrlich, Paul; Ehrlich, Anne; and Holdren, John. **Human Ecology.** San Francisco: W. H. Freeman, 1973.

This is a condensed introduction to the study of human relationships with the environment. Deriving its major tenets from its predecessor, *Population, Resources, En-*

vironment, this book has as its primary emphasis the biological and physical dimensions of the critical problems presently confronting the human race as a result of modern society's technologically abusive relationship to the earth. Among the interrelated aspects of the population-food-environment crisis the authors consider are: the exponential rate of present world population growth; urbanization; the carrying capacity of the earth's food, land, energy, and mineral resources; the synergistic effects of pollutants on society; and the upsetting of numerous natural ecosystems caused by current human consumption patterns.

At the heart of the book is the understanding that, given present use of technology and trends of human behavior, the earth is already overstressed in providing for its inhabitants. Population growth is examined as directly increasing the probability of worldwide plague and thermonuclear war. The intelligent application of technology to reduce pollution, facilitate communication, and control fertility is seen as providing valuable assistance, but the authors assert that dramatic and rapid changes in human attitudes toward population, economic growth, use of technology, and care of the environment are the determining factors in whether we resolve our ecological crisis or succumb to it.

Although their conclusions are pessimistic, the authors are committed to the view that the problems can be solved with everyone's help. They propose governmental responsibility in controlling population, designing a low-consumption economy in the United States, and channeling our energy and resources equitably to meet the needs of underdeveloped countries.

The book is a first-rate primer in basic ecological concerns. Views are presented lucidly and draw from a broad variety of sources. Although it concentrates on the United States' role in meeting the ecological crisis, it does so from a globally conscious perspective. It will prove a useful guide to anyone concerned with the present ecological crisis and with working toward its resolution.

Epstein, Samuel M., M.D. **The Politics of Cancer.** San Francisco: Sierra Club Books, 1978.

This is a comprehensive treatment of chemical environmental carcinogens, focusing on their regulation and nonregulation by government and industry. Epstein attacks various current myths about the prevalence of cancer in U.S. society and closely examines the scientific norms that govern inferences from animal and human experimental studies. Thirteen case studies of environmental carcinogens are presented, illustrating three separate areas of concern: (1) The Workplace, with studies on asbestos, vinyl chloride, bichloromethylether, and benzene; (2) Consumer Products, including tobacco, red dyes no. 2 and no. 40, saccharin, acrylonitrile, and female sex hormones; and (3) The General Environment, including the effects of pesticides, aldrin/dieldrin, chlordane/heptachlor, and nitrosamines. A final section discusses governmental policies and the agencies established to regulate particular aspects of the cancer problem, describes nongovernmental policies (what industry does), and concludes with a long section on what steps individuals can take to prevent cancer. In addition the book contains a lengthy set of useful appendixes that identify carcinogenic substances, list governmental reports and regulations, and provide the names of groups (governmental, private, and consumer oriented) involved in the cancer question.

The book is clearly oriented toward prevention, arguing that despite the billions of dollars spent in past decades on cancer treatment, little has been devoted to cancer prevention. Epstein argues forcefully that narrowly focused industrial economic concerns are central to our society's inability to develop successful cancer preventive strategies. The organization of industry into powerful special-interest groups severely limits the ability of government to effectively regulate the production and dissemination of carcinogens even in the face of existing legislation. The case studies abound with instances of industrial misuse of test data (to the point of falsification), destruction of personnel records to cripple epidemiological research, failure to transmit data on known hazards to workers, dissembling before governmental boards and commissions, and the routine production of vastly exaggerated projections concerning the economic consequences of regulation. The case studies also make clear that the most effective regulatory activity has come only at the instigation and insistence of consumer-oriented groups petitioning government agencies.

This is the most comprehensive examination to date of the various participants — governmental and industrial — who interact in the regulatory arenas overseeing cancer concerns. Epstein, a participant in many of these controversies, makes no apologies for his preventionist stance, permitting the weight of the evidence to justify that posture. The book meets high standards for the presentation and evaluation of evidence, and the combination of information presented is unavailable from any other single source.

Feingold, Ben. F., M.D. **Why Your Child is Hyperactive.** New York: Random House, 1975.

In this well-known book, Ben Feingold presents his theories on the causes of hyperkinesis — and its relationship to learning disabilities — and delineates a diet free of salicylates and artificial colors and flavors, which he feels is helpful in treating hyperactive children. Feingold believes that genetic and biochemical aberrations account for the behavior patterns of most hyperactive children, while a smaller percentage may have allergic reactions to food, food additives, or the increasing number of environmental pollutants.

Written for the parent and lay reader, the book combines case histories and practical advice with simplified explanations of the role of genetics, biochemistry, and allergies in behavior. Diet plans and recipes are given for persons wishing to try his elimination diet. Although representing one doctor's bias, this book gives parents and health care practitioners an alternative to drug management for some cases of hyperactivity.

Fritsch, Albert J. **The Household Pollutants Guide.** New York: Anchor, 1978.

This is an excellent paperback sponsored by the Center for Science in the Public Interest. The editor is an organic chemist and codirector of the center. This paperback is the best available guide on pollutants in the home for the health professional and layman. Topics covered include aerosol sprays, building materials, clothing and fabric-care products, emissions from heating and cooling devices, garbage, pesticides, disinfectants, laundry detergents, motor-vehicle products, oven cleaners, plastics, radiation pollution, utensil coatings, water contaminants, zoological wastes, and yuletide decorations. The book is particularly useful for any health practitioner seeking to become acquainted with chemicals to which hypersensitive patients may be responding psychologically or physiologically.

Fuchs, Victor R. **Who Shall Live? Health Economics and Social Choice.** New York: Basic Books, 1974.

For any health professional interested in ecological factors in health, this modern classic on health economics is essential reading. The author is professor of economics at Stanford University and of community medicine at Stanford Medical School. He is also research vice-president of the National Bureau of Economic Research, where he directs the Center for Economic Analysis of Human Behavior and Social Institutions. Fuchs demonstrates with brilliant control of economic data and health statistics that health in the United States has much less to do with how much is spent on medical care than with hereditary, environmental, and life-style factors. Nonetheless, it is the physician who makes the major choices among medical technologies and thus controls how much we pay for medical care. In one chapter Fuchs contrasts the health of the citizens of Nevada and Utah, two contiguous western states that are very much alike with respect to income, schooling, degree of urbanization, climate, and many other variables frequently thought to cause variations in mortality. Yet the inhabitants of Utah are among the healthiest of Americans, while those of Nevada are at the opposite end of the spectrum. For example, infant mortality is about 40 percent higher in Nevada than in Utah. "Lest the reader think that the higher rate in Nevada is attributable to the 'sinful' atmosphere of Reno and Las Vegas, we should note that infant mortality in the rest of the state is almost exactly the same as it is in these two cities. Rather, as was argued earlier in this chapter, infant death rates depend critically upon the physical and emotional condition of the mother."

Ginn, D. L., and Stevens, J.G.R. (Eds.). **Pesticides and Human Welfare.** Oxford, England: Oxford University Press, 1976.

This book was compiled by a group of pesticide experts and chemists at the request of ten European chemical companies in an attempt to combat misinformation arising in the current debate on pesticide dangers. The authors acknowledge that certain chemicals can cause serious damage to humans. For example, in cases of severe poisoning, methyl and ethyl mercury fungicides injure the nervous system; carbon tetrachloride and methyl bromide are harmful to the kidney and nervous system, respectively. However, the basic position taken is that cases of severe damage are the exception and generally pesticides toxic to mammals may produce acute reactions but tend to cause no permanent destruction of vital tissue. Common sense and careful handling are deemed appropriate measures for protection from most pesticides. The authors note that there is no epidemiological evidence supporting the position that exposure to pesticides causes cancer.

The volume discusses the current controversy over the relative merits of animal testing as a predictor of how toxic agents will affect humans. In general, it supports the position that test animals constitute good predictors of human responses. This conclusion is hedged, however, in the interpretation of data indicating possible liver cancers. Here the authors attest that the behavior of the lesions and the animals indicates these may not be "true" cancers—a position hotly contended by those outside the industries affected. The book concludes that governments and the companies themselves are doing much to reduce the hazards of pesticides.

The value of this book is limited by its obviously self-interested character. Much of the debate over the potential and actual health effects of pesticides focuses around the nature of the scientific testing that is or is not done to determine effects. The book makes an advocational contribution to one side of this debate rather than serving as a dispassionate scholarly treatment of the subject. It will be of use to those interested in the industry side of the pesticide argument.

Graham, Frank, Jr. **Since Silent Spring.** Boston: Houghton Mifflin, 1970.

This book is a chronological account of pesticide use from the 1962 publication of Rachel Carson's *Silent Spring* up to 1970. The first six chapters of Part 1 are devoted to a brief biography of the author, the publication of *Silent Spring,* and the ensuing public uproar. In Part 2 the health hazards to wildlife and humans are discussed. Graham presents evidence from British and U.S. scientific studies that suggests that bird populations declined with the increased use of insecticides.

More scientific knowledge has been gained about the health effects on wildlife and small animals than on humans, since direct human experiments are not possible. Nevertheless, some investigators posit that pesticides may increase the chance of mutations in man that may not show up for several generations. Others suggest that pesticides, particularly hydrocarbons, are carcinogenic. The most obvious human targets are those who handle pesticides directly: crop dusters, other pesticide appliers, pesticide manufacturing employees, and household users. There is a high rate for accidental poisonings of children.

Part 3 describes the pork-barrel politics of pesticide use and the aggressive sales efforts of the chemical industry. Although the 1965 report from the President's Science Advisory Committee recommended wider use of bio-environmental pesticide control methods in place of total reliance on chemical control, an absence of national awareness of the pesticide problems continues to prevail. Graham attributes this to an unwillingness on the part of the scientific community to speak out against pesticide use because of political pressures from above or ties to the chemical industry.

Part 4 gives an account of the first lawsuits opposing the use of DDT by Victor J. Yannacone, Jr., and a group of scientist-friends who eventually formed the Environmental Defense Fund. The appendix of the book suggests safer pesticides for commercial, home, and garden use and mentions persistent pesticides to avoid.

This book provides a comprehensive overview of the pesticide problem, the political forces shaping it, and the struggle between the chemical industry and environmentalists. The author takes a strongly argumentative position that chemical industry forces have inhibited progress toward safer pesticide regulation and usage. The book presents a lot of information, particularly on the effects of pesticides on bird life.

Hunter, Beatrice Trum. **Food Additives and Federal Policy: The Mirage of Safety.** New York: Scribner, 1976.

This is a superb and thoroughly researched study of the extremely complex political, scientific, and social issues involved in the use of food additives that are frequently carcinogenic, teratogenic, and mutagenic.

Joint FAO/WHO Expert Committee on Food Additives. **Toxicological Evaluation of Some Food Additives Including Anticaking Agents, Antimicrobials, Antioxidants, Emulsifiers and Thickening Agents** (Food Additive Series no. 5). Geneva: World Health Organization, 1974.

This volume is a compilation of monographs based on deliberations of the Joint

FAO/WHO Expert Committee on Food Additives, which met in Geneva from June 25 to July 4, 1973. The monographs provide in a condensed form the biochemical and toxicological data available at the time for more than one hundred particular food additives. Each entry includes the results of short- and long-term animal studies, observations in humans, an evaluation of the acceptable daily intake for man (when possible), and indicates further information and studies called for. The volume ends with a set of references. The index lists all the additives under their scientific and common names.

This is a useful reference for someone wishing access to information about the testing done on additives up to 1973. The manual is somewhat outdated, but it offers a sound, clearly presented summary of scientific evidence available at the time on the anticaking agents, antimicrobials, antioxidants, emulsifiers, and thickening agents. Not covered are food colorings, flavorings, and sweeteners. The WHO Food Additive Series is included as an important resource because it is one of the few publications that deals comprehensively with the health effects of specific food additives.

Lee, Douglas H. K. (Ed.). **Handbook of Physiology**, Section 9: **Reactions to Environmental Agents.** Bethesda, Md.: American Physiological Society, 1977.

This very scientific volume attempts to summarize much of what is known about the interactions of various toxic and potentially toxic environmental agents (natural and synthetic) and living organisms. The preface states: "The emphasis is on well-known environmental perturbations, particularly physical and chemical agents introduced by man, and the physiological responses evoked by these agents." Each chapter is an independent body of material, typically beginning with a basic description of the biophysics, pharmacokinetics, or physiology involved in analyzing the biological system in question. Most chapters include a referenced summary of pertinent research in the field, and some attempt to relate the whole to a toxicological model. Occasional cautionary recommendations for application are offered.

Physical agents covered are sound, heat, microwaves, and ionizing radiation. The chemical agents discussed include airborne pollutants, food additives and contaminants, chemical agents from occupational sources (e.g., arsenic, mercury, pesticides, plants, and plastics), medicines and drugs, and cigarette smoke. The remaining sections explore the physiology of the interactions of those agents with the organism at the various portals of entry (such as the lung and skin), transport and chemical transformation by the organism, and mechanisms of injury at a cellular level.

The book is research oriented; the articles are technically refined. It is a scholarly work intended mainly for the scientific community. Although there is some variation in detail and level of complexity from chapter to chapter, a solid foundation in the biological sciences is necessary to fully understand the material. The chapters are generally well written and richly documented; however, the lack of integration between chapters causes a sense of discontinuity. There are also some very obvious biases; for example, the chapter on food additives contains an interesting discussion of aflotoxins but it glosses over color additives without mentioning any specific associated toxicity. The authors of this chapter, who are all associated with the FDA, apparently find it sufficient to equate FDA approval of food colors with complete safety.

The chapters on sound, microwaves, food additives, and contaminants are of particular interest. There is much valuable, timely information here, and the resources for any basic search of the literature on the covered topics exist within its references.

Lee, Douglas H. K., and Kotin, Paul (Eds.). **Multiple Factors in the Causation of Environmentally Induced Disease.** New York: Academic Press, 1972.

Lee, Douglas H. K., and Minard, David (Eds.). **Physiology, Environment, and Man.** New York: Academic Press, 1970.

These two books are part of a series on environmental sciences published by the Academic Press and based on symposia conducted by various governmental agencies, including the National Academy of Sciences and the John E. Fogarty International Center at the National Institutes of Health.

Physiology, Environment, and Man contains the results of a conference sponsored by the National Academy of Sciences/National Research Council. In this volume are twenty-six essays on various aspects of the relationship between our environment and states of human health and disease. The book is at once a general discussion of environmental factors and human physiology and a compendium of articles focused on specific topics. Chapters cover such topics as the accumulation of environmental agents in the body, the interaction of environmental agents and drugs, and effects of environmental agents at the level of enzyme-forming systems. Also included are more distinctly conceptual pieces on human adaptation and cross-adaptation and the definition of an optimum environment.

Multiple Factors in the Causation of Environmentally Induced Disease is a shorter and more tightly organized work. The book contains a series of chapters focused on multiple causation in connection with a variety of diseases, such as cancer, cirrhosis of the liver, coronary artery disease, renal disease, and so on. Also included is a section dealing with some special environmental factors like DDT and lead, radioactivity, and mineral dusts. The book concludes with an essay by Lester Breslow addressing the "Implications of Multiple Factors for Prevention and Control."

Both of these books are important contributions to the literature on environmental causation of disease, but neither of them represents a conceptual breakthrough. Although they were published in the early 1970s, their saliency has probably not diminished. Each has numerous sources for more in-depth study.

Multiple Factors may be more valuable as a scientific work, as it is more directly targeted on a given subject (multiple causation) and because its organization makes the information easier to assimilate. *Physiology*, however, does contain some particularly useful essays on concepts of adaptation, which are of increasing importance since it appears that we cannot completely avoid or eliminate disease.

McKeown, Thomas. **The Role of Medicine: Dream, Mirage, or Nemesis?** London: Nuffield Provincial Hosptials Trust, 1976.

This recent book is already considered a classic in the discussion of the role of environmental factors in health and disease. The book includes cogent and revealing discussions of the roles of medical intervention, public health measures, and changes in the character of infectious diseases. It also considers such factors as improvements in nutrition and increases in food supplies and technology. The last chapter is an excellent discussion of *The Lives of a Cell* (Lewis Thomas), *Genes, Dreams and Reality* (Sir Macfarlane Burnet), *The Mirage of Health* (René Dubos), and *Medical Nemesis* (Ivan Illich). This slender volume should be high on the list of any health practitioner seriously interested in ecological factors in health.

National Research Council. **Drinking Water and Health.** Washington, D.C.: National Academy of Sciences, 1977.

This is a comprehensive review of the health effects of the contamination of drinking water by bacteria, viruses, and other microorganisms; solid particles, such as asbestos; trace metals and other inorganic solutes (arsenic, selenium, fluoride, sodium, nitrate, sulfate); organic solutes; and radioactivity. The book provides an overview of water testing and treatment practices for each pollutant and makes recommendations for further research. The chapter on "Safety and Risk Assessment" is an excellent presentation of the general problems surrounding extrapolation from laboratory animals to man. Each chapter has an extensive bibliography.

Randolph, Theron G., M.D. **Human Ecology and Susceptibility to the Chemical Environment.** Springfield, Ill.: Thomas, 1972.

This is the most accessible work of Dr. Randolph, one of the founders and certainly the greatest theorist of the clinical ecology school of allergy and hypersensitivity. While most scientists have focused on laboratory exploration of the effect of chemicals on human well-being, over the past twenty-five years Randolph has isolated more than 5,000 individuals suffering from a wide range of medical and psychological disorders in hospital environments specifically designed to be as free as possible of all chemical sources of pollution. Randolph's method is to have the patient fast on spring water for four days and then to systematically reintroduce the patient to foods and chemicals to which his ecological history suggests he may be allergic or hypersensitive. This text is primarily concerned with the description of the chemical environment and secondarily concerned with the clinical manifestations of the patient's response.

Randolph's major work on his remarkable theory of clinical responses to foods and chemicals is contained in the many chapters he contributed to Lawrence Dickey's textbook on clinical ecology, reviewed elsewhere in this bibliography. This volume contains the extensive questionnaire that Randolph utilizes to identify chemical additives and contaminants of air, food, water, drugs, and cosmetics. It contains a discussion of the interpretation of the questionnaire. Other chapters in the volume discuss the chemical environment in general, air pollution, chemical contamination of ingestants, drugs and cosmetics, treatment, case reports, and instructions for avoiding chemical pollutants.

Reiser, Stanley Joel. **Medicine and the Reign of Technology.** New York: Cambridge University Press, 1978.

One major ecological factor that has a very direct impact on health is medical technology. This is a superb historical study of the development of medical technology from the seventeenth to the twentieth century and its changing impact on health care and on the physician's conception of his role. The author has an excellent grasp of an important literature not heretofore gathered in one place.

Secretary's Commission on Pesticides and Their Relationship to Environmental Health. **Report of the Secretary's Commission.** Washington, D.C.: U.S. Department of Health, Education, and Welfare, December 1969.

This book assesses the benefits and risks of pesticides and recommends guidelines for continued use. The information in the report covers the uses and benefits of pesticides, their effects on nontarget organisms, and their carcinogenicity, mutagenicity, and teratogenicity. The report recommends that we should be: (a) promoting closer cooperation on pesticide problems between the departments of HEW, Agriculture, and the Interior; (b) eliminating the use of DDT and DDD in the United States; (c) restricting the use of certain persistent pesticides in the United States; (d) developing standards for pesticide content in food, water, and air; (e) developing a clearing house for pest information; (f) increasing federal research support on pesticides and their effects on human health and the ecosystem; (g) providing incentives for industry to develop more specific chemicals; and (h) promoting safe use of pesticides.

This detailed and informative volume on the effects of pesticides gives extensive coverage to research findings, particularly to studies on human subjects. The report concludes that insufficient research has been undertaken or completed on the relationship between pesticides and chronic diseases. For example, although a relationship between exposure to DDT and tissue concentration was found, there is still insufficient evidence to correlate tissue concentration with disease. Although the commission found no proof of the mutagenicity of pesticides, they concluded that each chemical used should be tested. If mutagenic, the pesticide should be removed from the market or severely restricted.

Although not organized for convenient lay study, the report is an excellent manual for those desiring more than an overview of the health effects of pesticides.

Select Committee on GRAS Substances of the Life Sciences Research Office, Federation of American Societies for Experimental Biology. **Evaluation of health aspects of GRAS food ingredients: lessons learned and questions unanswered.** *Federation Proceedings,* October 1977. **36**, 11.

This article details the procedures and problems that went into this committee's task of assessing the potential health hazard of some 400 food ingredients classified as "generally recognized as safe (GRAS)."

The report discusses the paucity of data regarding consumption of most food ingredients and additives. Information on fetal exposure was found to be deficient for more than four-fifths of the GRAS substances reviewed. The predictive value of current mutagenicity tests was discovered to be unreliable and inconsistent in many cases. The questions of carcinogenicity, allergenicity, hypertrophy of the liver, and enzyme induction are also reviewed briefly. It is suggested that serious consideration be given to the interaction of food ingredients with other food components and drugs.

The report concludes the sections describing the procedures used to arrive at judgments on health hazards, the process for translating scientific assessments into official regulation, and appendixes with lists of substances already reviewed and those in the process of being evaluated.

This report would be a useful introduction for a practitioner or layperson beginning a study of the human health effects of food additives. It presents a background for understanding how food ingredients are evaluated, using a conversational style that includes interesting examples. For specific evaluation reports a reader would have to consult other publications of the Life Sciences Research Office, Federation of American Societies for Experimental Biology.

Sidel, Victor W., and Sidel, Ruth. **A Healthy State: An International Perspective on the Crisis in United States Medical Care.** New York: Pantheon, 1977.

This is an excellent comparison of medical care in Sweden, Great Britain, the Soviet Union, China, and the United States. The form of health care systems is one of the critical ecological factors in human health. The Sidels take the strongly stated position that only a national health service based on centralized standards and local implementation can maximize health and provide the human care Americans need. One may disagree with their conclusions, but the contrast between the American health care system and that of other societies with far fewer resources is an important and thought-provoking one.

Soyka, Fred. **The Ion Effect.** New York: Bantam, 1977.

The literature on the health effects of different concentrations of negative and positive air ions is readily accessible in this recent paperback summarizing much of the research on air ions of Dr. Albert P. Krueger and others. Different concentrations of negative and positive air ions are caused by such natural phenomena as hot dry winds and by such technological-industrial phenomena as pollution, air treatment, the "dead" air spaces of sealed buildings, and the friction of synthetic clothes or synthetic fiber carpets that can generate excessive positive charges in a sealed-air environment.

Soyka's paperback is a readable and generally accurate introduction to the subject of air ionization. The specialist may wish to consult some of the following references:

Kimura, S.; Ashiba, M.; and Matsushima, L. Influences of the air lacking in light ions and the effect of its artificial ionization upon human beings in occupied rooms. *Japanese Journal of Medical Science,* 1939. **7**, 1–12. Cited in Krueger, 1969 (below).

Krueger, A. P. Preliminary consideration of the biological significance of air ions. *Scientia,* September–October 1969.

Krueger, A. P.; Andriese, P. C.; and Kotaka, S. Small air ions: their effect on blood levels of serotonin in terms of modern physical theory. *International Journal of Biometeorology,* 1968. **12 (3),** 225–239.

Krueger, A. P., and Kotaka, S. The effects of air ions on brain levels of serotonin in mice. *International Journal of Biometeorology,* 1969. **13 (1),** 25–38.

Krueger, A. P.; Kotaka, S.; and Reed, E. J. The course of experimental influenza in mice maintained in high concentrations of small negative air ions. *International Journal of Biometeorology,* 1971. **15 (1),** 5–10.

Krueger, A. P.; Kotaka, S.; Reed, E. J.; and Turner, S. The effect of air ions on bacterial and viral pneumonia in mice. *International Journal of Biometeorology,* 1970. **11,** 279–288.

Krueger, A. P., and Smith, R. F. The physiological significance of positive and negative ionization of the atmosphere. *Journal of the Royal Society of Health,* 1959. **79,** 642–648. Cited in Krueger, 1969 (above).

Stern, Arthur C. (Ed.). **Air Pollution** (Vol. 2, 3rd ed.). New York: Academic Press, 1977.

This volume is addressed to engineers, chemists, physicists, physicians, meteorologists, lawyers, economists, sociologists, agronomists, and toxicologists. As stated in its preface, the volume is concerned with "the cause, effect, transport, measurement and control of air pollution."

Three sections in Part B of this volume on the effects of biological systems will be of particular interest to professionals researching the health effects of air pollution. The first of these, "Biological Effects of Air Pollutants" by David L. Coffin and Herbert Stokinger, discusses the long- and short-term effects of photochemical oxidants, ozone, nitrogen dioxide, sulfur oxides, carbon monoxide, and particulate matter. Experiments with human subjects and animals are described, as are both pathological effects and physiological responses to those stressors. "Organic Particulate Pollutants – Chemical Analysis and Bioassays for Carcinogenicity" by Dietrich Hoffman and Ernst L. Wynder presents an exhaustive description of organic particulates in the air, followed by a discussion of how bioassays for organic environmental agents are carried out. They also describe studies of the tumorigenicity of urban air pollutants. "The Effects of Air Pollution on Human Health" by John R. Goldsmith and Lars T. Friberg provides an effective overview of some of the more esoteric earlier chapters, including those on routes of absorption, cause and effect relationships, and synergistic effects. Also discussed are particulate pollutants: asbestos, lead, cadmium, mercury, beryllium, arsenic, fluoride, chromium, and magnesium. The chapter ends with a description of air pollution as a causal factor in chronic disease and outlines its contribution to specific diseases such as bronchitis, emphysema, asthma, cardiovascular disease, nervous system disorders, hematological reactions, and chemical mutations.

Though not for the layman, this is a most useful reference book. It is highly technical, comprehensive, well documented, and extensively footnoted and indexed.

Tyler, Paul (Ed.). **Biological effects of nonionizing radiation.** *Annals of the New York Academy of Sciences,* 1975. **247,** 5–545.

This compilation of research studies concerning the biologic effects of microwaves is not unlike the Czerski et al. report from the 1973 Warsaw conference (reviewed earlier in this bibliography). However, by the time this symposium sponsored by the New York Academy of Sciences took place, a great deal more had been published in this field, reflecting the concurrent quantum leap in microwave technologies. By that time the debate about whether or not microwaves could produce nonthermal pathological and behavioral effects was also in full bloom.

Unfortunately, research in this area had come to have such important political and economic implications that some of the more controversial research was excluded from this conference or had had its funding revoked. Nevertheless, this volume contains useful information on ocular, nervous system, immunologic, genetic, and behavioral effects of microwaves. What emerges from a reading of these papers is a realization that while there has been a tremendous increase in the amount of research being done in this area, studies targeted directly on health impacts on humans are still scarce. Additionally, it becomes clear that the mechanism by which nonionizing radiation causes adverse health effects is still undefined; the research is still at a relatively early stage.

In contrast to the books produced from research conferences, Paul Brodeur, an investigative science reporter, has written a provocative book entitled *The Zapping of America* (New York: W. W. Norton, 1977). In it he charges that there has been a government cover-up of research demonstrating the danger to humans of nonionizing radiation. The usefulness of his book stems from Brodeur's presentation of case histories of industrial workers and military personnel who have presumably suffered ill effects from microwave-emitting technologies, thus giving clinicians an insight into the kind of people and situations where microwave-induced disease may manifest itself.

Another overview of the health implications of spreading microwave technologies has been published in *Working Papers* (March 1978), a newsletter on public health and the environment published by Commonweal, a nonprofit corporation in Bolinas, California. "Electromagnetic Smog: Bathing the Human Family in Microwaves" by Steve Lerner reviews much of the literature surrounding this topic and presents interviews with a number of the leading American researchers in the field. A useful overview of the regulation of and research on the health effects of microwaves, Lerner's article is aimed at translating a complex issue for the concerned layman.

Van Den Bosch, Robert. **The Pesticide Conspiracy.** New York: Doubleday, 1978.

This book, written by the late professor of entomology at the University of California, Berkeley, argues that a conspiracy exists within the agriculture and chemical industries to maintain chemical control of pests as the solitary form of pest management. Van Den Bosch saw a successful resolution of the pesticide question as paramount for the survival of the human species. He warned that the chemical system of control will ultimately pose a threat to human food sources. The danger to birds, bees, and wildlife is widespread. If humans do not learn to understand pests and to develop an ecologically sound pest control policy, insects may outlast them on the planet. In 1975 1,300 Californians received medical treatment for pesticide poisoning. This reported total may represent only 1 percent of the actual poisonings, according to the California Department of Public Health.

Van Den Bosch was very concerned about the use of chemical company salespeople as "advisors" to farmers on insect management, likening it to pharmaceutical companies prescribing drugs for patients. The author advocated Integrated Pest Management (IPM) as the best answer to pest control. This system includes dissemination of knowledge and information about the pests and crops, continuous monitoring of pest populations, establishing levels at which control methods are begun, and using methods and materials for pest management. The book describes several successful uses of IPM in California, Washington, and the Midwest in which there has been a notable reduction in pesticide use or pest-control cost.

Van Den Bosch contended that there is corruption within the chemical industry due to monetary greed and competition. He cited the repression of information and cover-ups as two techniques used to enforce a pro-industry status quo. Within the industry, marketing criteria often take precedence over chemical policies and concerns. Van Den Bosch saw the Environmental Protection Agency as having been "raped" by the Department of Agriculture and legislative interests. He advocated the establishment of a federal research institution on pest management and an effective watchdog commission as beginning steps toward reform. The book stresses the importance of creating changes in current philosophical stands.

The book is a personal account of Van Den Bosch's attempts to shape a sound pest-control policy. His anger and frustration may distract the reader, but further exploration reveals a knowledgeable rendering of pesticide facts. There is no index and no table of contents, which makes academic use of the book somewhat difficult.

Waldbott, George L. **The Health Effects of Environmental Pollutants.** St. Louis: C. V. Mosby Company, 1973.

Written for the practicing clinician, this volume is filled with useful data that can help doctors do the difficult detective work involved in tracking down the often delayed and disguised health effects of environmental pollutants—particularly airborne pollutants—in the population at large. Waldbott covers a wide spectrum of air pollutants including: pulmonary irritants (ozone and chlorine), fibrosis producing agents (silica, iron, cobalt, barium), asphyxiating pollutants (carbon monoxide and hydrogen sulphide), systemic poisons (lead, mercury, fluoride, and cadmium), allergic agents, radioactive contaminants, carcinogens, and mutagens, as well as smoke.

Typically, Waldbott introduces the reader to a pollutant by examining its sources: how much comes from natural sources and how much from man-made sources; of man-made pollution, what percentage is emitted into the atmosphere by moving as opposed to stationary sources; what are the agent's industrial and commercial applications; and where is it most likely to be found. Following a careful description of each environmental stressor, Waldbott examines the way in which each is ingested (uptake) and how the body's defenses mobilize to deal with the intrusion. Where applicable, a distinction is made between acute and chronic effects of a given pollutant, based on available animal tests and human exposures.

What is perhaps most refreshing about Waldbott's presentation is that he manages to tell when and where the ill effects of an air pollutant were first recognized without allowing anecdotal case histories to overwhelm the more formal and systematic studies that have been done on the effects of different toxic agents. Brief narrative accounts packed with relevant and accessible information punctuate an otherwise ponderous subject:

> In 1911 workers in Peruvian mines developed a disease characterized by irritation of the throat, eyes, and nose, and by a severe cough with pulmonary hemorrhages. In some the kidneys were involved with blood loss through urine and generalized anemia. Exposure to vanadium dust fumes was found to be responsible for the disease.

If any criticism can be leveled at this work, it is that when Waldbott gets away from air pollutants (his specialty), the treatment of vast subjects such as pesticides, radioactive contamination, and water pollution tends to be no more than introductory. Similarly, his concluding chapter, entitled "Prophylaxis and Treatment," is dealt with in a cursory fashion, when the subject could easily provide enough material for another book. In spite of these relatively minor criticisms, overall Waldbott's book is not only vastly informative but also stands out as eminently readable in a field known for its jargon-ridden and impenetrable prose.

Weiss, Bernard, and Laties, Victor G. **Behavioral Toxicology.** New York: Plenum Press, 1975.

This is a definitive collection of essays on behavioral toxicology, a young discipline in the United States that focuses on the effects of environmental pollutants and drugs on behavior and performance. Leading specialists on toxicology examine such topics as prenatal exposure to methylmercury, the effects of carbon monoxide, and the effects of pesticides and antibiotics.

Behavioral toxicologists recognize that the lesser effects of many environmental contaminants and chemicals may show up only as subtle functional disturbances not usually discovered by traditional medical evaluations. This collection grew out of a series of international conferences on chemical toxicity at the University of Rochester, sponsored "partly as a response to concern over the consequences to health of the rich chemical soup in which we live."

5

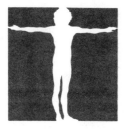

MEDICAL SELF-CARE:
SELF-RESPONSIBILITY FOR HEALTH

Tom Ferguson, M.D.

Most health care is – and has always been – self-care, as shown in Figure 5.1 (Levin, Katz, and Holst, 1976; Levin, 1977; Williamson and Danaher, 1978). Until recently, medical researchers had almost entirely ignored the potential resource represented by the large (and at present poorly trained) pool of unsung paramedical workers – health consumers themselves. Within the last five years, however, there has been an explosion of interest in this field. A cover story in *Medical World News* called self-care "medicine's fastest-rolling new bandwagon" (Yeager, 1977). More than six hundred self-care books have been published in the past few years (Rosenzweig, 1978). "One of the most exciting things that's going to happen in the next ten years," predicts Dr. B. Leslie Huffman, Jr., president of the American Academy of Family Physicians, "will be the increasing involvement of patients in their own health care" (Yeager, 1977).

Indeed, it has been suggested that the growing self-care movement will seek to replace the very word "patient" with "client" or "person" in the same way the civil rights movement worked to replace "Negro" with "Black" and the women's movement strove to replace "Mrs." and "Miss" with "Ms." (Travis, 1979; Sehnert, 1979a). Comparisons with these far-reaching social movements are much to the point, for self-care advocates feel that the self-care movement represents the extension of a broad contemporary change of consciousness (which includes the counterculture of the 1960s, the ecology movement, the consumer movement,

87

Figure 5.1
What People Do About Their Symptoms
(Source: Williamson and Danaher, 1978)

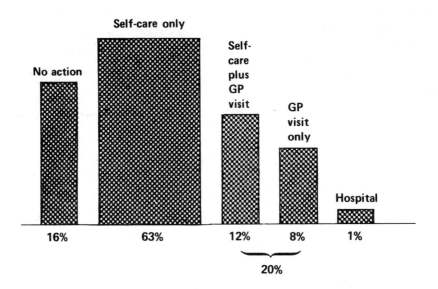

and the more recent taxpayers' revolt) into the realm of medicine (Levin, Katz, and Holst, 1976; Levin, 1977; Sehnert, 1979a).

What exactly is self-care? Levin (1977) offers the following working definition: "a process whereby a layperson can function effectively on his or her own behalf in health promotion and decision-making, in disease prevention, detection, and treatment *at the level of the primary health resource in the health-care system."*

Williamson and Danaher (1978) describe self-care as "a bimodal phenomenon, comprising *health maintenance,* which includes disease prevention, and *care of self in illness,* however loosely the latter is defined." There seems to be wide agreement that individuals can and should be better informed and take on increased responsibility in two distinct but overlapping areas that Travis has perceptively described as *illness* and *wellness* (Travis, 1977, 1979).

The self-care movement is suggesting that laypeople be encouraged to develop skills and knowledge for a wide variety of illness and wellness situations. The range of this expansion can be indicated by noting a few of the regular sections of the major journal of the self-care movement; *Medical Self-Care Magazine:* Being Your Own Paramedic, Clinical Sciences, Eating, Exercise,

Health Workers and Self-Care, Medical Consumerism, The Medical Literature/ Libraries, Stress/Unstress, and Therapy/Growth (Ferguson, 1976).

Self-Care and Holistic Health

One of the most common points of confusion is reflected in the question I am most commonly asked after making presentations on self-care: "Just what's the difference between self-care and holistic health?" If holistic health represents a change in the philosophical basis of health care, self-care represents a change in the basic patterns of responsibility and decision making.

For self-care advocates, the problem is that most laypeople know far too little about (1) evaluating and improving their health *without* waiting for serious symptoms to occur, and (2) coping with illness—both through self-care and by making *appropriate* use of health care facilities—when illness *does* occur. The self-care movement feels that we have depended too much on experts in health care, that with the proper training and self-study materials, individuals are capable of being their own paramedics, both in the prevention and in the treatment of common illnesses—in much the same way that China's barefoot doctors function as lay paramedics.

While self-care and holistic health are not identical, it is important to note that they are not antithetical. Holistic health proposes that our health care system needs a new map. Self-care suggests that the wrong person has been holding the map. This distinction can be expressed graphically as follows. First, we place instances of health care along a scale with traditional medical approaches at one end and alternative or holistic approaches at the other:

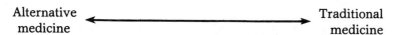

| Alternative medicine | ← | → | Traditional medicine |

We can also look at any instance of health care according to whether it is expert care or self-care:

Expert care ←————————————→ Self-care

Combining these two scales creates Figure 5.2. We can use this figure to plot any experience of health care. For example:

- If you go to a physician to have your sore throat examined or to have your gall bladder out, you would be making use of expert-administered traditional medical care, represented by the letter A.
- If you learned to use a blood pressure cuff and kept track of your own blood pressure, if you started keeping a copy of your own medical record, or if you used your stethoscope to listen to your child's lungs when she had

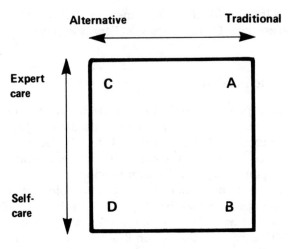

Figure 5.2

a bad cold, you would be practicing self-care using the tools of traditional medicine, letter B.

- If you consulted a spiritual leader, a practitioner of acupuncture, or a chiropractor, you would be making use of expert-delivered alternative health care, letter C.
- If you started an exercise program, practiced yoga, or began meditating, you would be practicing alternative self-care, letter D.

Teaching and Learning Self-Care

How are self-care skills and knowledge to be transferred? In four principal ways: (1) by an increased emphasis on self-care education in clinical settings; (2) by adult classes, study groups, and individual study; (3) by innovative school programs supporting a goal of universal health literacy; and (4) by making reliable self-care information more widely available—through publications, consumer health-resource centers, library collections, and other public sources. In addition, a number of institutions and businesses are becoming interested in sponsoring self-care education in the work place (Sehnert, 1978).

Self-Care in Clinical Settings

The clinician-client illness consultation is an excellent opportunity for the transfer of self-care information. Unfortunately, this opportunity is not always grasped. Responsibility for this failure must be shared by clinicians and clients alike. Clinician and client may have conflicting needs and expectations, as Williamson and Danaher (1978) have described so well:

Since patient and doctor are approaching diagnosis from different perspectives it may seem that the doctor is not listening, or that he is disregarding important facts, or that he is not even interested in the patient. The latter, being largely ignorant of modern medicine, is often confused by the doctor's questions or examination—"I only went with a face rash and he asked me to take my shoes and socks off!" The doctor, on the other hand, wants very specific information which will help him to make the diagnosis, and the time constraint will encourage him to be as quick as possible and to cut short any apparent diversion introduced by the patient, even though this might seem to be most significant to the latter. . . .

The doctor is effectively in charge of the conduct of the consultation. He controls all, or virtually all, of the means of treatment or help available to the sick person. He has the specialized knowledge to make sense of symptoms or complaints that the patient has found incomprehensible, and his decisions are frequently accepted as valid in themselves. The patient will only rarely argue; in any case the patient is fully aware of the fact that he may have to go back to the doctor at some future date, and so is likely to feign acquiescence on occasions. This diffidence may well be encouraged by the doctor.

On the other hand, as Williamson and Danaher point out, the client "has a good deal of power simply by the virtue of the fact that he or she is initiating the consultation." Clearly wide acceptance of self-care would require a very different clinician-client relationship than the kind described above. As Williamson and Danaher conclude, "Doctors will have to take on the role of educating their patients and guiding them through the mass of information which will be made available with or without medical approval so that rational decisions can be made by individuals. A major loss might be the placebo effect of the doctor's own personality, but perhaps in an informed and autonomous lay person such a phenomenon would be unnecessary."

As few examples of clinical facilities offering services in support of self-care have been described in the literature, a look at several different approaches may be of value.

Walt Stoll, M.D. Family practitioner Walt Stoll practices in Lexington, Kentucky. He has written the *Patient Brochure and Self-Help Manual* (1977), which he provides free of charge to his clients (and at cost to others). The book contains seven sections:

1. Prevention. Dr. Stoll encourages clients to strive for high-level wellness by undertaking one or more of the following: an exercise program, relaxation program, relaxation training, and a wise eating plan.
2. Clinic policies. This section spells out expectations and responsibilities of client and clinician alike. Two examples concern appointments and fees: "Our policy is to have no patient who has an appointment wait longer than 15 minutes. . . . You have a responsibility not to expect unrelated problems to be discussed during a visit contracted for a specific purpose. . . .

The fairest arrangement for charges is when you are charged what you think every service is worth. This includes charges for phone calls, sending medical records, helping you collect medical insurance, etc. . . . We do not charge more for office visits so that we can support clerical service. . . . Routine office visit—$11. Phone calls, when diagnosis, treatment, or advice is given over the phone—$5."

3. How the doctor's office should use the patient as a tool in his or her own health care. In this section Dr. Stoll states, "Counting its effect on compliance with instructions, patient education is the most powerful medication or treatment available in the doctor's office. Any health-care provider who doesn't use his or her most important tool cannot deliver quality care."

4. The doctor-patient relationship. Dr. Stoll says, "Doctors are not infallible. Unfortunately, there is often an assumption which both patients and doctors tend to accept—that the doctor not only has to know everything, but that he has to be right. . . . If the doctor is secure enough to know he is doing his best, and that his best is pretty good, defensiveness is no longer necessary. The 'God' image is not only a bar to effective communication, it is a straightjacket for effective decision-making."

5. How to choose and use a primary medical care provider.

6. How and when to use self-care and how and when to use the doctor's office for each of the thirteen complaints most commonly seen in Dr. Stoll's practice.

7. Additional services. This section contains brief descriptions of services available from several practitioners with whom Dr. Stoll works—a counselor and teachers of biofeedback, meditation, relaxation, and yoga.

Burnout Prevention for Doctors. Dr. John Travis, who directs a series of burnout prevention workshops at the Wellness Resource Center in Mill Valley, California, feels that the spreading enthusiasm for self-responsibility offers physicians a golden opportunity to re-examine their own frequently overextended schedules and to learn to take better care of *themselves.*

Most doctors are trained to try to rescue people—and most people go to the doctor to *be* rescued. . . . The doctor assumes total responsibility, and the client is a sort of uninvolved bystander. I like to call this the *pill fairy* model of health care. It's just as hard on the doctor as it is on the client. . . . That's why we feel it's so important for health workers to deal with issues of self-responsibility in their own lives before they can hope to help their clients with them (Travis, 1979).

Kaiser Health Plan's Health Education Library. Another notable example of self-care in a clinical setting is the Health Education Library for Patients, part of the comprehensive health care delivery system at the Oakland, California, facility of the Kaiser Permanente Medical Care Program, a large prepaid group practice in an urban ambulatory setting. According to the Kaiser model, incoming patients are routed "to sick care for discovered illness, to preventive maintenance care for early or asymptomatic disease, and to health care for health protection and maintenance information." The clinical facility is thus composed of the Sick Care Service, the Preventive Maintenance Service, and the Health Care Service. The library is a part of the Health Care Service.

The library collection is especially strong in audiovisual materials. There are twenty-four viewing booths, each equipped to show 16 millimeter and 8 millimeter films and sound filmstrips and containing cassettes, audio tapes, and slide carousels. There is a separate projection room for small groups and a facility for viewing videotapes. Many of the audiovisual programs are developed at Kaiser at the request of staff physicians, who then serve as consultants in their production. The subjects range from allergy to urology. The two most popular programs to date are family planning and prenatal care. There is also an extensive collection of printed material, including books, pamphlets, and clipping files on selected subjects.

About half the library users are referred by Kaiser clinicians. The other half are self-referred. The library also serves as a staff and community resource and as a resource for nearby community colleges. The library staff has helped to set up "mini-libraries" in other departments within the Kaiser complex and consults widely with groups seeking to set up similar health resource centers in other institutions (Collen and Soghikian, 1974).

Self-Care Classes

The first U.S. self-care class may have been the one Thomas Jefferson instituted at the University of Virginia, but the first of the modern breed of classes was taught in 1970 by family practitioner Keith Sehnert at the Reston-Herndon Medical Center in Herndon, Virginia. Sehnert developed a series of sixteen two-hour sessions in which he taught good health practices, how to handle common emergencies, illnesses, and injuries, the economics of medical care, prescription and over-the-counter drugs, childhood growth and development, and a variety of self-help and preventive skills to an audience of forty housewives, grandmothers, and a sprinkling of husbands and other interested men enrolled in the course. Sehnert went on to found the Center for Continuing Health Education at Georgetown University in 1972. The center taught self-care classes, developed support material, and trained health workers from around the country to teach similar courses in their home areas.

Sehnert and coworkers state the goals of their course as follows:

- To teach patients how to use health care resources more effectively
- To provide a better understanding of self-help and preventative medicine and emphasize the importance of *individual* responsibility
- To train patients to do certain easy procedures and to make better observations of clinical events in common illnesses and injuries

- To help patients save money when purchasing drugs, buying insurance, and obtaining medical care

Evaluations of the students in Sehnert's courses showed the following results (Sehnert, 1975b; Sehnert, 1977b):

- Increased confidence and ability of patients to handle illnesses, injuries, and emergencies, and a parallel lessening of the usual anxieties associated with them
- Some changes in the behavior of patients regarding improved eating habits, more regular exercise, and efforts to prevent illness
- Savings in drug costs and some types of medical expenses

The emotional impact of these classes is best described by Sehnert himself:

Until recently, the medical mystique was much like the religious mystique in the days of Martin Luther and the Protestant Reformation – the language of the laity was one world and the language of the clergy was another. They didn't even say their *prayers* in the same language. It was a priesthood. There were things that the layperson wasn't *supposed* to know about.

I think what we're seeing now – the demystification of medical language – is best understood seen in the context of the change that Luther made, in bringing Christianity into the language of the people.

That's the most important thing that happens in these self-care classes – first, you let people know that it's OK for them to step into this formerly forbidden area, and second, you guide them on their first few steps. So the main thing is not the class itself, but the fact that it can get people started (Sehnert, 1979a).

Self-care classes are currently being offered in forty states (Sehnert, 1979a). Sehnert and Eisenberg's (1975) book *How To Be Your Own Doctor (Sometimes)* was developed from lectures given in the early classes. It remains one of the best resources on – and one of the best textbooks for – self-care classes.

Sehnert and coworkers have also published a self-care class curriculum with special emphasis on the needs of elderly populations (Health Activation Network, 1977). Healthwise, Inc., of Boise, Idaho, has produced a textbook for self-care classes aimed at the parents of young children (Beard, Tinker, and Kemper, 1976). Karen Johnson has described a university-based course for a mixed population of adults (Johnson, 1979), and Ferguson has described a self-care–class curriculum for young adults as developed by the Self-Care Project at the Haight-Ashbury Free Medical Clinic (Ferguson, 1978). Current information on self-care classes and support materials can be found in two quarterly publications, *The Health Activation News* (Health Activation Network) and *Medical Self-Care Magazine*. The latter journal publishes a nationwide listing of self-care classes and contact people in each issue.

Health Education in the Schools

There is wide agreement that if self-care is to become a cornerstone of health policy, attention must be paid to very early learning about self-care. Recent work by Charles and Mary Ann Lewis at the UCLA School of Medicine in Los Angeles has shown that the general adult patterns of health care behavior are already evident in children by the early elementary grades (Lewis et al., 1977; Fink, 1979). Thus school health-education programs must attempt to reach children at the earliest possible age.

A number of innovative approaches have been made. Health Skills Associates of Dayton, Ohio, has established simultaneous programs for adults and children; while the parents attend a self-care class, their children spend time in a health learning center (Poley, 1979). Sehnert has described a self-care class for sixth graders (Sehnert, 1979b), and Ferguson talks about a class for first and second graders (Ferguson, 1978, 1979b). The American Health Foundation has developed a new school health-education project, "Know Your Body," for children aged ten to twelve, that focuses on eating, exercise, discouraging smoking, and controlling blood pressure (Kristein et al., 1977).

There is, in addition, a critical reappraisal of existing school health-education programs and the ways in which they may be actually *discouraging* self-responsibility in health. As Levin, Katz, and Holst (1976) write, "School health education, where available, has by and large perpetuated a view of health care which suppresses or severely limits the growth of values and beliefs that the individual is competent as the primary source of health maintenance. Health 'facts' are presented to children as secure and immutable, health professionals as possessing skills fixed and demarcated from those available to laypersons. 'Folk medicine' or home remedies and indigenous health customs are often denigrated as quaint, ineffective, and sometimes dangerous."

Another important approach to the self-care education of children is to make available high-quality health publications at a child's reading level—in the home, in the school, and in the public libraries. A fine example of this kind of book is Herman and Nina Schneider's *How Your Body Works* (Schneider and Schneider, 1949).

Self-Care Publications

The most thoughtful theoretical overviews of the issues and questions that an increased acceptance of self-care would force us to face are to be found in *Self-Care in Health* (Williamson and Danaher, 1978), *Self-Help in the Human Services* (Gartner and Riessman, 1977), and in the works of Lowell Levin. An excellent introduction to Levin's work can be found in his paper "Forces and Issues in the Revival of Interest in Self-Care" (Levin, 1977). This paper appeared in a special issue of *Health Education Monographs,* which also includes the following very useful papers: "Changes in Health Care Ideology in Relation to Self-Care by Families" (Pratt, 1977), "Self-Care in Urban Settings" (Milo, 1977), "Family and Self-Help Education in Isolated Rural Communities" (Grant, 1977), and "Research and Demonstration Issues in Self-Care: Measuring the Decline of Medicocentrism" (Green et al., 1977). The footnotes to these five papers comprise the most extensive listing of self-care publications in the professional literature. The most extensive annotated bibliographies of self-care publications are to be found in *Self-Care: Lay Initiatives in Health* (Levin, Katz, and Holst, 1976), *Self-Care in Health* (Williamson and Danaher, 1978), and in *Medical Self-Care: Access to Medical Tools* (Ferguson, 1979a). A listing of people involved in and articles on self-care are available from the Department of Health, Education, and Welfare's Bureau of Health Education (Ogden, 1977). The history of self-care is examined in *Medicine Without Doctors* (Risse et al., 1977).

Some of the best suggestions as to ways health workers can implement self-care are to be found in several papers by Sehnert (Sehnert, 1972, 1975a, 1975b, 1977a, 1979b). Sehnert has also done one of the few existing studies on the effectiveness of self-care classes (Sehnert, 1977b). An excellent short, popularly written book on self-care, *Help Yourself*, is available free (and in quantity) from the Blue Cross Association (Miller, 1978). Finally, the most wide-ranging single resource on self-care, containing interviews with and articles by many of the authors cited in this chapter, is *Medical Self-Care: Access to Medical Tools* (Ferguson, 1979a), an anthology and resource guide compiled by the editors of *Medical Self-Care Magazine*.

Why Self-Care Now?

In addition to the cultural/historical changes previously mentioned, the following historical changes have contributed to the present emergence of self-care:

- The rise in chronic morbidity from approximately 30 percent to the current 80 percent over the past four decades and the resulting shift from *cure* to *care*
- An increasing awareness of the effect of life-style on many of these chronic diseases
- The frequent inability of "high technology" medicine to deal with these chronic diseases
- The frequently dangerous side-effects of high-technology medicine
- Drastically rising health-care costs resulting from an excessive reliance on high-technology, late-stage medical intervention
- Increasing explorations of alternatives to the philosophical assumptions of traditional Western medicine
- The demystification of medicine as a result of the increasing numbers of nonphysicians now providing clinical services

- The growing reliance of large numbers of Americans on nonprofessional self-help groups

Issues

The following seem to be some of the principal issues raised by the burgeoning self-care movement:

- Will self-care result in increased quality of care?
- Will self-care result in economic savings?
- How will medical liability and defensive medicine be affected by an increased acceptance of self-care?
- What new problems will self-care create?
- Will self-care be used as an excuse not to provide high-quality professional care to presently underserved areas, notably to poor neighborhoods?
- What are the limits of self-care?
- What incentives would encourage professionals and individuals to practice and support self-care?
- To what extent will both professionals and individuals be able to change from a professional-centered to a person-centered model of health care and to embrace the self-care principles perhaps best stated by David Werner (1977)? Werner's principles are as follows:
  1. Health care is not only everybody's right but everybody's responsibility.
  2. Informed self-care should be the main goal of any health program or activity.
  3. Ordinary people provided with clear, simple information can prevent and treat most common health problems in their homes—earlier, cheaper, and often better than doctors.
  4. Medical knowledge should not be the guarded secret of a select few but should be freely shared by everyone.
  5. People with little formal education can be trusted as much as those with a lot. And they are just as smart.
  6. Basic health care should not be *delivered* but *encouraged*.

References

Beard, Toni Roberts; Tinker, Kathleen McIntosh; and Kemper, Donald W. *Healthwise Handbook*. Boise, Id.: Healthwise, Inc., 1976. (Healthwise, Inc. is located at 111 S. Sixth St., Boise, Idaho 83702.)

Collen, F. Bobbie, and Soghikian, Krikor. A health education library for patients. *Health Services Reports*, May–June 1974. **89 (3)**, 236–243.

Ferguson, Tom (Ed.). *Medical Self-Care Magazine*, 1976.

Ferguson, Tom. *Three Communications Projects in Medical Self-Care*. Unpublished M.D. Thesis, Yale University, 1978.

Ferguson, Tom. *Medical Self-Care: Access to Medical Tools*. New York: Summit Books, 1979a.

Ferguson, Tom. Teaching medicine to kids. In Tom Ferguson, *Medical Self-Care: Access to Medical Tools*. New York: Summit Books, 1979b.

Fink, Donald L. Self-Care and Children. In Tom Ferguson, *Medical Self-Care: Access to Medical Tools*. New York: Summit Books, 1979.

Gartner, Alan, and Riessman, Frank. *Self-Help in the Human Services*. San Francisco: Jossey-Bass, 1977.

Grant, Richard H. Family and self-help education in isolated rural communities. *Health Education Monographs*, Summer 1977. **5** (2), 145–160.

Green, Lawrence W. et al. Research and demonstration issues in self-care: measuring the decline of medicocentrism. *Health Education Monographs*, Summer 1977. **5** (2).

Health Activation Network. *Health Activation for Senior Citizens*, 1977.

Johnson, Karen. On teaching self-care. In Tom Ferguson, *Medical Self-Care: Access to Medical Tools*. New York: Summit Books, 1979.

Kristein, Marvin M. et al. Health economics and preventive care. *Science*, February 4, 1977. **195**, 457–462.

Levin, Lowell S. Forces and issues in the revival of interest in self-care. *Health Education Monographs*, Summer 1977. **5** (2), 115–120.

Levin, Lowell S.; Katz, Alfred H.; and Holst, Erik. *Self-Care: Lay Initiatives in Health*. New York: Prodist Press, 1976.

Lewis, Charles E. et al. Child-initiated care: the use of school nursing services by children in an "adult-free" system. *Pediatrics*, October 1977. **60 (4)**, 499–507.

Miller, Eddie (Ed.). *Help Yourself*. Chicago: Blue Cross Association, 1978. (Blue Cross Association is located at 840 N. Lake Shore Drive, Chicago, Illinois 60611.)

Milo, Nancy. Self-care in urban settings. *Health Education Monographs*, Summer 1977. **5** (2), 136–144.

Ogden, Horace G. *Self-Care Information Sheet*. Atlanta, Ga.: Bureau of Health Education, Public Health Service, Center for Disease Control, 1977.

Poley, Jane. Teaching kids health. In Tom Ferguson, *Medical Self-care: Access to Medical Tools*. New York: Summit Books, 1979.

Pratt, Lois. Changes in health care ideology in relation to self-care by families. *Health Education Monographs*, Summer 1977. **5** (2), 121–135.

Risse, Guenter B.; Numbers, Ronald A.; and Leavitt, Judith Walzer. *Medicine Without Doctors*. New York: Science History Publications, 1977.

Rosenzweig, Sandra. Learning to be your own M.D. *The New York Times Magazine*, April 2, 1978. 42–46.

Schneider, Herman, and Schneider, Nina. *How Your Body Works*. Reading, Mass.: William R. Scott Books/Addison-Wesley Publishing, 1949.

Sehnert, Keith W. The patient as a paramedical. *Virginia Medical Monthly*, April 1972. 409–413.

Sehnert, Keith W. A note to physicians. In Keith W. Sehnert and Howard Eisenberg, *How To Be Your Own Doctor (Sometimes)*. New York: Grosset and Dunlap, 1975a.

Sehnert, Keith W. Patient education: a new resource for family practice. *Delaware Medical Journal*, October 1975b. 487–494.

Sehnert, Keith W. Putting the pharmacist to work as a health educator. *American Druggist*, August 1977a. 53–58.

Sehnert, Keith W. A course for activated patients. *Social Policy*, November–December 1977b. **8 (3)**, 40–46.

Sehnert, Keith W. *How Business Can Promote Good Health for Employees and Their Families*. Washington, D.C.: The National Chamber Foundation, 1978.

Sehnert, Keith W. A Conversation with Keith Sehnert. In Tom Ferguson, *Medical Self-Care: Access to Medical Tools*. New York: Summit Books, 1979a.

Sehnert, Keith W. On teaching self-care to children. In Tom Ferguson, *Medical Self-Care: Access to Medical Tools*. New York: Summit Books, 1979b.

Sehnert, Keith W., and Eisenberg, Howard. *How To Be Your Own Doctor (Sometimes)*. New York: Grosset and Dunlap, 1975.

Stoll, Walt W., M.D. *Patient Brochure and Self-Help Manual*. Lexington, Ky.: author, 1977.

Travis, John W. *Wellness Workbook*. Mill Valley, Calif.: Wellness Resource Center, 1977.

Travis, John W. A conversation with John Travis. In Tom Ferguson, *Medical Self-Care: Access to Medical Tools*. New York: Summit Books, 1979.

Werner, David. *Where There Is No Doctor*. Palo Alto, Calif.: The Hesperian Foundation, 1977. (The Hesperian Foundation is located at P.O. Box 1692, Palo Alto, California 94302.)

Williamson, John D., and Danaher, Kate. *Self-Care in Health*. New York: Neale Watson Academic Publications, 1978.

Yeager, Robert C. The self-care surge. *Medical World News*, October 3, 1977. **18 (20)**, 43–54.

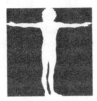 ANNOTATED BIBLIOGRAPHY

Boston Women's Health Book Collective. **Our Bodies, Ourselves** (2nd ed.). New York: Simon and Schuster, 1976.

A widely-known, readable, practical, and accurate popular guide to women's health. The first, and still one of the best, of the contemporary self-care books. An unmatched blending of the personal and the clinical. Recommended reading in the gynecology rotation at Yale School of Medicine.

Ferguson, Tom (Ed.). **Medical Self-Care Magazine.**

A quarterly journal for health workers and health consumers. Contains articles that teach self-care skills, interviews with self-care innovators, and reviews of popular and professional self-care publications. Each issue includes a national listing of current self-care classes and a "networking" column through which persons interested in self-care can contact others with similar interests. Available from *Medical Self-Care*, P.O. Box 717, Inverness, California 94937.

Ferguson, Tom. (Ed.). **Medical Self-Care: Access to Medical Tools.** New York: Summit Books, 1979.

The most wide-ranging single resource on self-care, containing interviews with and articles by many of the authors cited in this chapter. Ferguson includes information on teaching self-care skills, interviews with self-care innovators, and reviews of over three hundred self-care books. The chapters cover the following topics: The Self-Care Concept, Being Your Own Paramedic, Body Work, Birthing, Clinical Sciences, Couples, Drugs, Dying and Grieving, Eating, Elders, Health Workers and Self-Care, Human Sexuality, Kids, Exercise, Medical Consumerism, The Medical Literature, Men's Health, Midlife, Self-Care Classes, Sleep/Dreams, Stress/Unstress, Therapy/Growth, and Women's Health. Compiled by the editors of *Medical Self-Care Magazine*.

Gartner, Alan, and Riessman, Frank. **Self-Help in the Human Services.** San Francisco: Jossey-Bass, 1977.

A thoughtful examination of contemporary self-help groups in terms of the following assumptions: (1) that the proper basis of power in all human services lies with the client, not with the professional; (2) that most of the services in all human services are self-provided; (3) that both (1) and (2) listed above are inappropriately subordinated in the professional-dominated model of the human services; and (4) that a fundamental restructuring of human services is needed—and is fact taking place—through increasing reliance on self-help in a wide variety of human services. Includes a listing (with name, address, and focus) of 130 U.S. self-help groups and an extensive bibliography on self-help.

Grant, Richard H. **Family and self-help education in isolated rural communities.** *Health Education Monographs,* Summer 1977. **5 (2)**, 145–160.

Describes the objectives, implementation, and evaluation of a self-care education program in a medically underserved community in rural Oregon. Additional course materials are available from the author in care of Eastern Oregon Health Systems Agency, 1037 N. Sixth Street, Redmond, Oregon 97756.

Health Activation for Senior Citizens, 1977.

A detailed course syllabus for the self-care classes developed by Sehnert. Available from Health Activation Network, P.O. Box 923, Vienna, Virginia 22108.

Hoffman, Lloyd E. **Patient education: how we designed our own program.** *Group Practice,* September/October 1976. **25**, 21–24.

This paper describes the development of a learning resource center within a large multispeciality group practice. Twenty-three areas of instruction are summarized.

Lee, Philip R. **Self-care deserves strengthening—and physician support.** *Medical World News,* October 3, 1977. **18 (20)**, 77.

Lee is the former HEW assistant secretary for health and former dean of the School of Medicine, University of California at San Francisco. As the current director of the UCSF Health Policy Program, he urges physicians to "take the lead in promoting a greater understanding of self-care and in supporting development of public policies that make it more effective."

Levin, Arthur. **Talk Back to Your Doctor: How to Demand and Recognize High Quality Health Care.** New York: Doubleday, 1975.

A groundbreaking book on medical consumerism that does a remarkably fine job of describing the principles of good medical care.

Levin, Lowell S. **Forces and issues in the revival of interest in self-care.** *Health Education Monographs,* Summer 1977. **5 (2)**, 115–120.

Describes historical forces leading to the present emergence of self-care and lists research, ethical, legal, and practical questions that would be raised by a shift from a professional-centered to a client-centered health-care system.

Levin, Lowell S.; Katz, Alfred H.; Holst, Erik. **Self-Care Lay Initiatives in Health.** New York: Prodist Press, 1976.

> The report of a self-care conference held in Copenhagen in August 1976. Contains an extensive annotated bibliography of self-care publications through 1976.

Long, James W. **The Essential Guide to Prescription Drugs.** New York: Harper and Row, 1977.

> A detailed consumers' encyclopedia of the more than two hundred most commonly prescribed drugs. The author describes mode of action, side effects, contraindications, time required for benefit, recommended follow-up examinations, interactions with other drugs, use in pregnancy, and use in breastfeeding for the various drugs.

Milo, Nancy. **Self-care in urban settings.** *Health Education Monographs,* Summer 1977. **5** (2), 136–144.

> Describes the advantages and special problems involved in the development of self-care in the inner city.

Pender, Nola J. **Patient identification of health information received during hospitalization.** *Nursing Research,* May–June 1974. **23** (3), 262–276.

> One of the few studies that looks at health information received by clients during a clinical encounter with health workers. Eighty-five percent of the hospitalized persons studied received some health information. Approximately half of the conversations in which information transfer took place were initiated by health professionals. Fifty-eight percent of those receiving information felt that they needed more information on postdischarge self-care than they received.

Sehnert, Keith W., and Eisenberg, Howard. **How to Be Your Own Doctor (Sometimes).** New York: Grosset and Dunlap, 1975.

> The body of this book is adapted from class presentations in Sehnert's self-care course. It presents the author's concept of the Activated Patient, a layperson trained in basic paramedical skills and in preventive medicine, a Western version of China's barefoot doctors. It differs from most popular medical guides in that it assumes that the lay reader is capable of learning some basic clinical medicine. Appendixes include a 128-page self-help medical guide and "A Note to Physicians," describing how doctors can promote self-responsibility among their clients. An excerpt from this book appears in Ferguson, *Medical Self-Care: Access to Medical Tools* (above).

Sehnert, Keith W. **A "doctor" in every home.** In Eddie Miller (Ed.), *Help Yourself.* Chicago: Blue Cross Association, 1978.

> A good introduction to the idea of taking more responsibility for one's health by developing paramedical illness and wellness skills. Other articles in this free booklet encourage taking self-responsibility in such areas as eating, exercise, environmental health, and dealing with stress. The Blue Cross Association is located at 840 N. Lake Shore Drive, Chicago, Illinois 60611.

Stoll, Walt, W., M.D. **Patient Brochure and Self-Help Manual,** 1977.

A graphic portrait of one physician's efforts to integrate the principles of self-care into his clinical practice and a fine model for other physicians wishing to do likewise. Available from Walt Stoll, M.D., 1412 Broadway, Lexington, Kentucky 40505.

Williamson, John D., and Danaher, Kate. **Self-Care in Health.** New York: Neale Watson Academic Publications, 1978.

A practical-minded overview of ways to implement self-care in the existing health care system, along with a very close look at the characteristics of that system as it exists at present. A short excerpt from this book appears in *Medical Self-Care Magazine,* 5, and a longer excerpt appears in Ferguson, *Medical Self-Care: Access to Medical Tools* (above).

Yeager, Robert C. **The self-care surge.** *Medical World News,* October 3, 1977. **18 (20),** 43–54.

A good quick overview of U.S. self-care projects operating as of 1977.

Part Three

MODALITIES FOR HEALTH AND MENTAL HEALTH

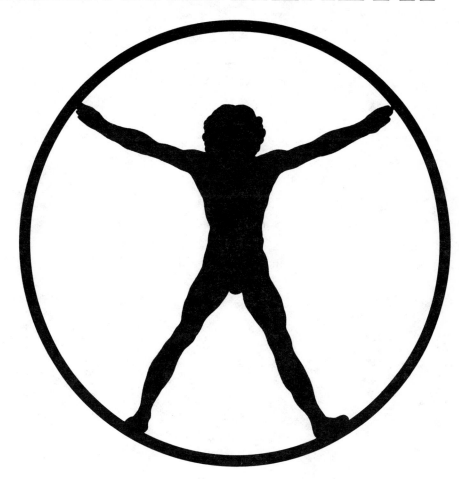

6

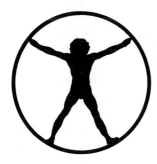

THE MIND IN HEALTH AND DISEASE

Kenneth R. Pelletier, Ph.D.

Since the Middle Ages, scientists and philosophers have tended to divide man into body, mind, and spirit. This split is apparent in the current structure of the healing professions. Physicians are dedicated to the treatment of the body; psychologists and psychiatrists are concerned with treating the mind; and the clergy are attendants to the soul and administer the practice of spiritual healing. While many other societies have created healing rituals that involve the whole person as well as the family and social matrix, Western healing practices have been characterized by specialization. If the prevention of pathology is the ultimate goal of the healing professions, then health practitioners and laymen need to address themselves to the entire person—mind and spirit as well as body—in relation to his or her total environment.

Holistic concepts in medicine extend back to the late Assyrian and Greek cultures. "Psychosomatic" itself is a Greek word: "psyche" means breath or spirit; "soma" means body. But a progressive division between mind and body has dominated recent Western medicine, and in the last century emphasis has been placed on the body, encouraged by the pathological findings of Virchow, the laboratory work of Pasteur, and the high success of asepsis, immunization, antibiotics, and chemical therapy in stemming disease.

Since the early 1960s, the enormous incidence of stress-related chronic conditions and an increasing awareness of the effects of emotional and psychological

107

states have helped reinstate the psychosomatic perspective on the causes and relief of disease. Within the healing professions today a more holistic approach is emerging. This approach considers the entire person rather than his or her fragmented parts and places emphasis on the psychosocial factors that contribute to disease or facilitate the healing process.

Stress disorders have long since replaced infectious diseases as the major health afflictions of postindustrial nations. Many of these afflictions of civilization, including cardiovascular disease, arthritis, respiratory disorders, cancer, and the ubiquitous depression, seem to be associated with particular kinds of personalities and particular kinds of stressful experiences. Pathogenic personality factors were hypothesized in the 1940s in the pioneering research of Flanders Dunbar and Franz Alexander. More recently cardiologists Meyer Friedman and Ray H. Rosenman (1974) have described the Type A personality who is predisposed toward cardiovascular disorders and Lawrence LeShan (1966) the carcinogenic personality who when subjected to extreme stress is likely to develop cancer. One of the most striking research studies in this area is a longitudinal sixteen-year prospective study of 1,337 medical students by Caroline Bedell Thomas and F. A. Murphy (1974). Their research focused upon the correlation between medical school personality profiles and later incidences of suicide, mental illness, hypertension, coronary heart disease, and malignant tumors. The most pathogenic and predictive personality pattern – a marked lack of closeness to parents – appeared in those medical students who later developed malignant tumors.

Increasingly, the research and clinical evidence suggests that all disease is psychosomatic and that just as it can be caused by emotional factors so it may be possible to help people to use their minds to restore themselves to health. In this context, symptoms can be seen as a warning, a sign that it is time for the individual to attempt to undergo a self-healing process, one that may be disrupted rather than enhanced by extreme interventions.

Throughout the history of medicine, practitioners have puzzled about the seemingly inexplicable recovery of mortally ill patients and the sudden morbidity of patients who should have fully recuperated. Among the subtle variables in this process are profound alterations in psychological outlook, life-style, and the interaction between mind and body. Beginning as early as the nineteenth century, the French neurologist Charcot explored the psychosomatic etiology of hysterical seizures. Freud, Sherrington, Pavlov, Cannon, Selye, and others have added to our understanding of the precise mechanisms and biochemical mediators by which psychological states, subjective imagery, and emotions effect the body.

Increasingly researchers have become concerned with the effects of mental and emotional states on health and illness with the possibility of treating the patient as an active and responsible participant in the healing process rather than as a passive victim of either the disorder or the treatment. This emphasis provides the context for using a variety of techniques – such as autogenic training, hypnosis, meditation, and clinical biofeedback—to help mobilize the individual's natural process of recovery. These techniques enable "ordinary" individuals to control heart rate, blood flow, pain perception, and the electrical activity of the brain itself. They have done much to dissolve arbitrary distinctions between the voluntary and involuntary nervous system, between what can be controlled by the mind and what can not.

The results of this work suggest that as yet unexplored capacities of the mind may exert more influence on an individual's creation of and response to illness than contemporary medicine has so far acknowledged. Psychological factors may thus be the basis of the spontaneous cancer remissions that have been documented by Everson and Cole (1966), of the "placebo effect," and of what Jerome Frank (1963) has termed "the faith that heals." Recent research (Snyder, 1977) suggests a particular biochemical procedure for this process—the newly discovered endogenous opiates or "endorphins." In studies of postoperative pain, placebo analgesia appeared to be induced by endorphin activity and reversed by naloxone, an opiate antagonist.

During the years ahead much of our attention should be directed toward trying to understand the far-ranging effects of our mental life on remissions from serious illness as well as on its creation and to explain why some individuals emerge from illness with increased rather than impaired functioning while others succumb easily to relatively minor illnesses. A truly holistic medicine cannot but emphasize the capacity of the mind to play a vital role in healing or slaying the individual.

References

Everson, Tilden C., and Cole, Warren H. *Spontaneous Regression of Cancer*. Philadelphia: Saunders, 1966.

Frank, Jerome. *Persuasion and Healing*. New York: Schocken, 1963.

Friedman, Meyer, and Rosenman, Ray H. *Type A Behavior and Your Heart*. New York: Alfred Knopf, 1974.

LeShan, Lawrence. An emotional life-history pattern associated with nephritic disease. *Annals of the New York Academy of Sciences*, 1966. **125** (3), 780–793.

Thomas, C. B., and Murphy, F. A. Closeness to parents and the family constellation in a prospective study of five disease states: suicide, mental illness, malignant tumor, hypertension, and coronary heart disease. *The Johns Hopkins Medical Journal*, May 1974. **134**, 251–270.

Snyder, Solomon H. The brain's own opiates. *Chemical and Engineering News*, November 28, 1977. 26–35.

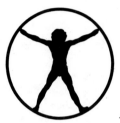

ANNOTATED BIBLIOGRAPHY

Achterberg, Jeanne, and Lawlis, G. Frank. **Imagery of Cancer.** Champaign, Ill.: Institute for Personality and Ability Testing, 1978.

This discussion of the use of visual imagery as a therapeutic tool in cancer management may be read as a companion book to O. Carl Simonton et al., *Getting Well Again* (below), or as a work in itself. It represents the first stage of an empirical evaluation of the role of imagery in cancer therapy. The authors have developed a replicable way (IMAGE-CA) of scoring a patient's imagery and of using these scores to predict outcomes. Examples of drawings of the images are included and the applicability of this scale to disorders other than cancer is discussed.

Bloomfield, Harold H., and Kory, Robert B. **The Holistic Way to Health and Happiness.** New York: Simon and Schuster, 1978.

This book demonstrates that individuals can prevent severe disorders particularly by using the power of the mind to guide their behavior and to reduce stress. Areas of health maintenance considered are meditation, stress management, diet, exercise, psychosomatic factors, and spiritual influences. Although the book is not referenced as fully as it could be, both practitioner and layman can benefit greatly by implementing the clear procedures that are outlined in it.

Cooper, Kenneth H. **The Aerobics Way.** New York: H. Evans and Company, 1977.

This book helps readers to develop a safe exercise program in clearly defined, gradual stages based upon periodic assessment of their aerobic – oxygen consuming – capacity. Cooper's excellent text makes the Royal Air Force program of exercise available to the general population and offers ways of applying its principles to a variety of physical activities. If Cooper shortchanges the emotional and spiritual side of exercise, he does pay attention to the interactions of exercise with age, sex, and diet.

Cousins, Norman. **Anatomy of an illness (as perceived by the patient).** *New England Journal of Medicine,* December 23, 1976. **295 (26),** 1458–1463.

This moving personal account of Cousins's recovery from a progressively degenerative condition contains extraordinary insight into such issues as placebo effects, vitamin C, diet, and the curative value of humor. It serves as a prototype for nonantagonistic cooperation between patient and doctor, biomedical system and individual, and – most importantly – between mind and body.

DeBakey, Michael, and Giotto, Antonio. **The Living Heart.** New York: Grosset and Dunlap, 1977.

This work provides clear and succinct information concerning all aspects of cardiovascular disorders, which are at present the major cause of death in the United States. It is a superb state-of-the-art overview by one of the world's most eminent heart surgeons and his research colleague. Most importantly, the book elucidates both the applications and limitations of purely biomedical approaches to cardiovascular disease. It enumerates both the primary (serum cholesterol, hypertension, smoking) and secondary (obesity, alcohol, stress, personality) risk factors and suggests that early intervention can be accomplished only through systematic reduction of the risk factors.

Engel, George L. **The need for a new medical model: a challenge for biomedicine.** *Science,* April 1977. **196 (4286),** 129–136.

This article clearly differentiates between purely biomedical approaches to health and those that consider these elements in a psychosocial context. It points out that consideration of psychosocial influences in health and disease has been excluded by convention and convenience, not by necessity. Engel proposes an extended model of medicine in which responsibility, decisions, and practices are shared by patients, social workers, psychologists, physicians, and researchers. This is an expansive and stimulating article that raises fundamental philosophical and pragmatic issues in a period of transition to a more inclusive model of health and disease.

Farquhar, John W. **The American Way of Life Need Not Be Hazardous to Your Health.** Stanford, Calif.: Stanford Alumni Association, 1978.

This overview of "life-style medicine" is replete with specific health maintenance directives for stress, exercise, nutrition, weight control, and smoking. Relying heavily on the development and use of positive mental imagery as a therapeutic principle, it is invaluable for both professionals and laymen.

Friedman, Meyer, and Rosenman, Ray H. **Type A Behavior and Your Heart.** New York: Alfred A. Knopf, 1974.

This classic study of the psychosocial precursors and concomitants of cardiovascular disease presents detailed analyses of the behavioral characteristics of those Type A people who are particularly vulnerable to hypertension and myocardial infarction. The book is useful in the psychological understanding and clinical management of patients with cardiac disorders and serves as a model for integrating biomedical and psychosocial investigations of disease states.

Gunderson, E. K. Eric, and Rahe, Richard H. (Eds.). **Life Stress and Illness.** Springfield, Ill.: Charles C. Thomas, 1974.

In 1972, NATO sponsored an international symposium on stress and its contribution to psychological disorders, myocardial infarction, depression, schizophrenia, and their underlying psychophysiological mechanisms. The product of that conference, this anthology lends empirical validity to the concept of a stress syndrome by providing research replicated in different laboratory and clinical contexts. There is an inevitable lack of cohesiveness among the essays, but they provide an impressive argument in favor of combining psychosocial and biochemical research as well as a ground plan for much of the work that needs to be done.

Knowles, John. **The responsibility of the individual.** In John Knowles (Ed.), *Doing Better and Feeling Worse: Health in the United States.* New York: W. W. Norton, 1977. Also in *Daedalus,* Winter 1977. **106 (1).**

To date, this is the best single attempt to differentiate individual, medical, and sociopolitical responsibility for health. Knowles presents striking evidence that biomedical technology, national health insurance, and more doctors are not the solution to improving health or reducing costs. He emphasizes the kinds of health maintenance activities that are documented in Marc LaLonde's *The Health of Canadians* and concludes that the "right" to health care should be replaced by "a moral obligation to preserve one's own health."

Pelletier, Kenneth R. **Mind as Healer, Mind as Slayer: A Holistic Approach to Preventing Stress Disorders.** New York: Delacorte and Delta, 1977.

Based upon extensive research data and clinical observation, this book proposes a model of the developmental etiology of stress disorders, including cardiovascular disease, arthritis, respiratory disorders, and cancer. Most importantly, it examines a stepwise sequence of multiple factors that result in specific disorders, from neurophysiological predispositions through life event assessments to psychological predispositions. This integration of medical and psychological research suggests specific interventions for stress disorders through stress alleviation, clinical biofeedback, autogenic training, nutrition, and exercise. Finally, the book provides a pragmatic basis for the implementation of a holistic approach to health care for individuals and institutions.

Samuels, Mike, and Samuels, Nancy. **Seeing with the Mind's Eye.** New York: Random House, 1975.

Applications of stress-management techniques and visualization have played an important role in the developing areas of psychosomatic medicine. The Samuels's abundantly illustrated volume is the best book for clinicians and laymen to use in acquainting themselves with visualization. In it the authors consider the historical, psychological, physiological, and metaphysical aspects of visualization and provide specific exercises and references for its therapeutic application. This is a useful book for anyone using visual imagery in clinical practice.

Saward, Ernest. **The current emphasis on preventive medicine.** *Science,* May 26, 1978. **200,** 889–894.

A leading proponent of health maintenance organizations, Saward emphasizes the need for a reallocation of financial and human resources from crisis intervention to prevention. His main point is that greater health at lower cost will result from reducing environmental hazards, improving nutrition, and adopting life-style practices conducive to health. Since the article convincingly addresses the cost benefits of such a program and has particular relevance to a time of budgetary restrictions, it is extremely important.

Simonton, O. Carl; Matthews-Simonton, Stephanie; and Creighton, James. **Getting Well Again.** Los Angeles: J. P. Tarcher, 1978.

This pioneering book concerns the application of visual imagery to the overall clinical management of cancer. The authors maintain that certain positive visual images—white blood cells destroying cancer—may help cancer patients to retard and halt the growth of their tumors as well as to feel better. Concepts covered include relaxation procedures, interpretation of visualizations, the issues of pain and fear of death, and the psychosomatic dimensions of cancer. Although the book has insufficient data on outcomes and presents no controlled studies, it is the single most important book for anyone who wishes to work with cancer patients in a holistic way.

Williams, Roger J. **Nutrition Against Disease.** New York: Bantam, 1973.

This book maintains a solid base in biochemistry as it elaborates basic data on every aspect of nutrition from the sociopolitical and environmental to the behavioral and the physiological. Among the areas covered are the role of diet in cardiovascular disease, obesity, dental disease, arthritis, longevity, alcoholism, and cancer. Although the book is somewhat dated, it is a solid approach by an eminent biochemist firmly committed to health maintenance.

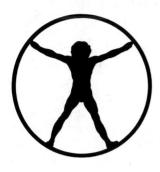

7

BIOFEEDBACK

Joe Kamiya, Ph.D.,
and Joanne Gardner Kamiya, M.A.

We can hardly question the general validity of one of the basic premises of "holistic health" and "alternative health care"—that behavioral and mental processes, along with their central nervous activities, are important in determining overall health. Such processes, after all, constitute a large part of the total range of health-relevant interactions of human organisms with their environment. However, when we consider the details of *how* the whole system is related to its parts, many unanswered questions arise. There is a need for much more specific knowledge at all levels of analysis of the complex social, behavioral, mental, biological and chemical systems constituting the domain of health.

In the last few decades, there has been much growth toward such detailed knowledge as well as a growing awareness of the nature of the various phenomena as parts of interlocked self-regulating systems. Contributing to this growth has been the field of psychophysiology, which addresses itself specifically to the interface between behavioral and physiological functions. From its beginnings it has studied how learning, perception, motivation, and emotion are reflected in physiological functions, especially those of the autonomic system. But it has also developed a new interest through the discovery that just as persons can learn to

The work leading to this publication was supported by grant number 5K02 MH-38897-10 awarded by the National Institute of Mental Health.

perceive the external world and to control their behavior with respect to it, they can to some degree learn to perceive the internal world of physiological activity and to control it voluntarily. The method developed to study these phenomena is called *biofeedback*.

This word was adopted in 1969 at a meeting of psychophysiological researchers to refer to a method of training individuals to enhance their discernment and voluntary control of one or more specific physiological functions (such as heart rate, muscle tension, or brain waves). Central to the method is providing the trainee with continuous information, via sensory signals, of the momentary fluctuations in physiological functions. Consider the case of heart rate. The small fluctuations in the time intervals between beats of the heart are continuously monitored and displayed visually or aurally to the trainee as a feedback signal. He is instructed to discover whatever internal activity is sufficient to control the fluctuations in the signal—to increase, decrease or regularize it. Several feedback sessions are often required for the development of maximum control, and the trainee must be sufficiently motivated to learn the task of control. Demonstration that the learned control can be exercised without the signal to a degree not seen before training confirms that a new skill has been acquired.

Biofeedback has been used with a variety of physiological measures. Heart rate, blood pressure, hand temperature, muscle tension, palmar skin conductance, and brain electrical activity are among the most widely known. The method is being used in studying physiological systems experimentally, in the study of brain-behavior relationships, in research on the nature of learning, and in attempts to quantify the relationships between conscious experience and physiological functions.

Biofeedback also shows promise when used as a therapeutic method in certain functional disorders and organically based dysfunctions. The disorders for which it has been tried cover a wide range. Common to many of the clinical applications are the following procedures:

- The patients are informed of the relationship between their symptom and its underlying physiological mechanisms.
- They are told that with the aid of an electronic biofeedback device they may be able to learn the internal activity necessary to achieve a sufficient degree of voluntary control of the physiology.
- They are told that repeated training sessions may be necessary for adequate learning to occur.
- They are shown the biofeedback equipment, the physiological transducers are put in place, and training begins.
- To help facilitate learning, they are given suggestions of general strategies of approach. Also, the sensitivity of the feedback signal is adjusted so that during the initial phases of training, easily produced small changes of the physiological activity in the desired direction cause signals indicating success. Readjustments are made to train for increasingly larger changes.

- As learning progresses, the patients are given gradually increased practice in controlling the physiological activity without the aid of the feedback signal. They are instructed to practice regularly at home, without feedback, between training sessions. In some instances, they are given portable feedback equipment to help them practice at home. Self-rating of success at the task and of symptom changes is generally used. This provides useful clinical data and also focuses the patient's attention on his task.
- Training is given from once a week to daily, each session lasting about thirty to sixty minutes, for periods ranging from one week to three months or more.

The clinical studies vary widely with regard to the extent to which the method is used by itself or adjunctively with other behaviorally based procedures. The variation in part is due to the orientation of the clinical investigators. Some focus on how much the patient can learn with biofeedback alone, as in the model of an operant-conditioning procedure for the training of a specific skill. At the opposite end of the spectrum, others see biofeedback merely as one tool in a more inclusive program of therapy, similar to the manner in which bathroom scales are used in monitoring a weight reducing program.

The actual clinical applications fall between these extremes. For stress-related disorders, there is a clear mix of both approaches. Biofeedback training is given for the control of that specific physiological measure related functionally to the presenting symptom, insofar as available instrumentation permits. In addition, the patient is given other training for general relaxation, with or without biofeedback. Exercises such as those developed for progressive relaxation and autogenic training are examples. The importance of regular and frequent relaxation practice in daily life outside the clinic is strongly emphasized. The non-stress-related disorders that have been treated with biofeedback involve more circumscribed responses than general relaxation of stress, and biofeedback training more closely approaches the operant-conditioning model.

To provide a brief overview of these applications, we list below the main disorders for which biofeedback has been most widely or most successfully used, together with the specific currently preferred biofeedback procedures. We also name several other applications that have been reported in the literature but are not yet as well known or widely used.

Stress-Related Disorders

The excessive stress of everyday life has a pervasive influence on many systems of the body. Operating through rather widely distributed control systems, such as the hypothalamus, the diffuse reticular activating systems, and the limbic structures that mediate emotion and motivation, stress may have such consequences as excessive chronic muscular contractions, constriction of blood flow, high blood pressure, insomnia, spastic colon, excessive stomach motility and hyperacidity, excessive sweating, and headaches.

A complete program of prevention and treatment of stress-related disorders optimally includes reducing the environmental stressors. Where this is not practical, the individual's internal response to the stressors can be modified to some degree reducing the adverse consequences. Health practitioners often recommend that their headache patients stay calm and relaxed, but all too often the patients are unable to achieve such calmness and relaxation. Biofeedback is frequently useful in such instances in that it provides a reasonably clear indicator of the actual degree of calmness and relaxation that the patient has achieved. The following are examples of how some stress-related disorders can be treated through biofeedback:

1. *Muscle contraction (tension) headache.* To teach relaxation of the head muscles, electrodes are usually attached to the forehead, and the electrical activity of the muscles in the frontal regions is amplified by an electromyographic (EMG) device. Usually both auditory and visual feedback signals are given (tones or clicks and meter displays) to reflect changes in the amplitude of the electrical activity. Headache relief following roughly ten to twenty half-hour sessions over a period of four to ten weeks has been well documented in a clinically significant proportion of chronic cases. The findings of studies comparing EMG biofeedback with instructed relaxation favors the feedback method. Among the stress-related disorders, tension headache has been the most successfully treated with biofeedback.

2. *Migraine.* This disorder is generally believed to result from excessive sympathetic discharge to the cranial vasculature, which leads to vasoconstriction and subsequent excessive reflex vasodilation. To prevent the onset of this sequence, training is focused on general reduction of stress and sympathetic activity. This is usually measured by an electronic thermometer placed on the hands or fingers to detect the warming effects of generalized vasomotor relaxation. Forehead EMG feedback is also often used, alone or in conjunction with hand temperature feedback. Earlier clinical results and the current widespread use of the method strongly suggest its utility, but how much this success depends specifically on the temperature feedback needs clarification.

3. *Essential hypertension.* For the treatment of high blood pressure, biofeedback has been given with blood pressure itself as the feedback variable. EMG and hand temperature feedback are sometimes also used. If direct blood pressure feedback is used, the momentary fluctuations in either systolic or diastolic pressure are monitored noninvasively. In the most commonly used method to date, the method uses a cuff that is partially inflated at a constant pressure near the prevailing median pressure. It monitors relative changes in blood pressure occurring at each heart beat during trial periods lasting for fifty or fewer successive beats. The median pressure of each trial is tracked over successive trials, thus providing an indication of progress over the total session. Other techniques

of monitoring the pressure that do not require a pressure cuff, such as pulse wave velocity, are under investigation.

The success of biofeedbck for the treatment of this disorder has been more limited than for the treatment of tension headaches. The various behavioral methods of relaxation training have been about equally effective. One reason for the limited success of behavioral treatment methods may be that the disorder can be symptomatic of a wide variety of dysfunctions, masked under one name. Also, high blood pressure does not produce immediate discomfort, and motivating sustained effort at keeping blood pressure low is often difficult. The results are promising enough, however, to merit further clinical investigation.

4. *Insomnia.* The two most common complaints of insomniacs are difficulty in falling asleep at the beginning of the night and difficulty in returning to sleep after spontaneous awakenings. Studies reveal that all-night electroencephalographic (EEG) sleep recordings are necessary to verify the complaints because of the highly unreliable nature of self-evaluation of sleep. Two biofeedback modalities have some promise in alleviating both kinds of insomnia. One modality is EMG biofeedback to induce general relaxation, and the other is biofeedback to increase the sensory motor rhythm (SMR), which is an EEG frequency of 12 to 15 Hz. SMR training is not given as part of a general relaxation training program. Although the "sleep spindle" at 13 to 14 Hz has been universally accepted as a sign of sleep, and its frequency is within the range of the SMR, the training is given to patients while they are fully awake. One of the effects of SMR training is an enhancement of the sleep spindle during sleep as well as improvement in sleep onset and disturbance. The number of insomnia cases treated with EMG and SMR biofeedback—especially SMR—is still small. The efficacy of these methods relative to instructed relaxation methods, which are also effective, has not yet been fully studied.

5. *Raynaud's disease.* The excessively cold hands characteristic of this disorder reflect restricted blood flow due to arterial and arteriolar contraction. In the primary idiopathic form of this disorder, the vasospastic attacks can be precipitated by emotional disturbances. Tolerance for cold temperatures is very low. Biofeedback training is given for voluntary warming of the hand as indicated by an electronic thermometer. Results have been quite encouraging. Following treatment elevated temperatures can, in many cases, be maintained despite cold ambient temperatures.

6. *Sinus tachycardia.* When the unusually rapid heart rate characteristic of this condition is not associated with other cardiac disease, the biofeedback approach is an effective means of aiding self-management for maintaining more normal heart rates. Feedback is given for the beat-by-beat fluctuations in heart rate. After learning how to maintain reduced heart rate in the clinic, patients are able to transfer their learning to daily life without the feedback.

7. *Other stress-related disorders.* In some conditions stress is not always considered the primary source of the disorder, but biofeedback training for general

stress reduction has been helpful in the treatment of bruxism (tooth grinding), bronchial asthma, functional colitis, stuttering, urinary retention, sexual dysfunctions, drug abuse, hyperactivity, anxiety, and phobias.

Disorders Not Caused by Stress

A characteristic of biofeedback training is that the changes it produces can be highly specific to the particular physiological function being trained. The rather generalized responses seen early in training tend to fade out, leaving only the specific response for which the feedback signal is given. For example, in finger temperature warming, the temperature of the specific finger on which the probe is placed will be more responsive than the other fingers as training continues. This feature helps in applying biofeedback to disorders that are caused not by diffuse stress responses but by malfunctions of more specifically localized physiological systems. We describe below some of the better-known examples of such highly specific feedback training.

1. *Neuromuscular dysfunctions.* Included in this group are disorders from peripheral nerve-muscle injury (Bell's palsy, neck muscle injury), spinal cord injury, spasmodic torticollis, hemiplegias following stroke, and cerebral palsy. The feedback given for rehabilitation of muscular functions is usually the electromyograph (EMG), which facilitates either increases or decreases in activity of specific muscle groups. Devices for detecting movement and posture are also used. A particularly dramatic example of biofeedback treatment in this area is for foot drop in victims of stroke. For these patients the problem is failure to lift the affected foot appropriately for normal walking. In one clinical series approximately three-fourths of the patients were able to discard their short leg brace entirely following three to twenty-five sessions of approximately thirty minutes of biofeedback training, and some of the patients were even able to discard their canes for the activities of daily living. Control of spasticity, initiating contractions, and gaining control of specific muscles is typically assisted by the therapist, who trains the patient to attend to the internal cues, encourages increases and decreases of the EMG signal, or positions the affected member for optimal learning of flexion or relaxation.

Application of these techniques in neuromuscular rehabilitation has become one of the most rapidly growing areas in the total field of biofeedback. As an adjunctive technique biofeedback has already earned a permanent place in many rehabilitation centers.

2. *Cardiac disease.* In a small number of patients, paroxysmal atrial tachycardia, atrial fibrillation, premature ventricular contractions, and Wolf-Parkinson-White disease have been treated with biofeedback, for speeding, regularizing, or eliminating abnormal heart beats. While the efficacy of biofeedback methods relative to other forms of treatment has not yet been determined, they deserve further serious attention.

3. *Epilepsy.* A variety of types of epilepsy manifest abnormal electrical brain activity patterns. Two of these are the relative absence of 12 to 15 Hz activity and the relative abundance of activity in the lowest frequencies (1 to 7 Hz). Biofeedback training to shift the EEG frequencies toward a normal pattern has been successful in reducing the frequency of seizures in a majority of heterogenous epileptic patient samples. Training is usually extended for at least a year with portable home-training units. It would now be possible to investigate the success of such techniques on a larger scale in clinical settings.

4. *Fecal incontinence.* This disorder is due to dysfunction in rectosphincteric responses, which is confirmed by pressure measurements with a rectal balloon. Training for external sphincter contraction synchronized with internal sphincter relaxation in response to rectal distension of the balloon is given repeatedly during single sessions, using the polygraph tracings of the two sphincteric responses as feedback. The benefits have been dramatic, and in consideration of the alternative treatments, biofeedback would be clearly the treatment of choice.

Evaluation of Biofeedback

The evaluation of the clinical uses of biofeedback shares many of the problems of evaluating all health programs in which self-help is a central feature. Efficacy, risks, time and effort required, costs, and posttreatment requirements are all relevant, and they must be compared with similar aspects for other available treatments.

There are three interrelated factors that determine evaluation and make it a more complex matter than is often recognized: the motivation of the patient to learn and sustain the necessary skills, the expectations of the patient, and the role of the therapist and the therapeutic setting.

1. *Motivation.* The effects of biofeedback cannot be evaluated as adequately as the effects of a pill. The electronic hardware of biofeedback does not do something to the patient; it is more like a physiological mirror or reflector that can, *if the patient wishes,* be used to his advantage. Since learning and sustaining a psychological state or a behavioral process with the aid of the mirror is critical to the method, biofeedback treatment necessarily includes the process of establishing motivation and cognitive orientations that are optimal for the treatment. Thus studies of biofeedback cannot provide a definitive answer on treatment efficacy unless the motivating conditions are optimal. If advances are made in physiological monitoring that allow us to improve motivation the efficacy of treatment should be improved. For example, better indications of the optimal sequences of physiological patterns leading to the control of a specific physiological process would promote faster learning.

2. *Expectations and the placebo effect.* It is easy to see that motivation should be optimal. However, we also need to recognize that the very procedures that optimize motivation create another difficulty for evaluation of biofeedback, since

they may produce some of the same effects sought by the biofeedback training. For example, giving encouragement and confidence that hand warming can be achieved may by itself result in reduced sympathetic activity and therefore in some warming of the hands, especially for those who may be anxious about their performance ability.

Two quite opposite stances have tempted clinical researchers faced with this apparent dilemma. One is that of designing experimental evaluations of biofeedback that attempt to eliminate all expectations by the trainee. The process consists of the feedback system, a simple instruction to try to change the feedback signal in a given direction, and little else. Great care is taken to minimize expectations of success and other cognitive processes supporting such expectations by avoiding suggestions of strategies, encouragement, evaluation of performance, opportunities for spontaneous reporting of impressions gained during training, or describing the relevance of the procedure to the trainee's concerns about health, insight, and so on. From our own experience and the results of many studies, this approach often results either in failure to learn control or in only slight degrees of control. One of the difficulties of this approach is that in the effort to eliminate expectations and supporting cognitive processes, the task of control is sometimes made more difficult or productive of performance anxiety. In the case of biofeedback for relaxation, such an effect can significantly impede success or even cause increased tension.

The other stance that has tempted clinical researchers is that of assuming since biofeedback seems to work best when all expectations and cognitive processes are given free reign that biofeedback should be regarded as a way of maximizing the placebo effect and that efforts to disentangle such effects from biofeedback are futile. Unfortunately this only begs the question of the degree to which biofeedback does in fact enhance the placebo effect.

A solution to the evaluative dilemma has not yet emerged in a form acceptable to all. More analysis of the complexities of this problem seems in order. For instance, there seem to be several kinds of expectations at issue, each operating at different points in the total biofeedback process. Expectations of successful performance in physiological control are distinguishable from expectations of the therapeutic utility of such performance, although the two expectations tend to support each other. Also, the therapeutic utility of sophisticated electronic devices operated by experts, quite apart from considerations of their mode of operations, are clearly distinguishable as another kind of expectation.

Some methods try to deal with the evaluative issues by including the use of control groups that are given the same treatment as experimental groups except that the signal used for feedback is actually unrelated to the trainee's physiological changes. In some studies this method is administered in a "double-blind" fashion, such that neither trainer nor trainee knows that the feedback may be false. The double-blind procedure has much to recommend it, but for measures such as muscle tension the subject can discover faulty signals by trying obviously large increases in muscle tension, thereby spoiling the study. In addition, double-blind procedures are difficult if not impossible to use in therapy settings where active coaching in strategies is part of the training sessions.

Another evaluative method is to use the trainee as his own control. At various stages of training the relationship of the feedback signal to the physiological activity is reversed. Again, in some studies the reversal is made without the knowledge of trainee or trainer. A difficulty of this method is that it can in some cases create confusion and frustration, thereby obscuring the effectiveness of the placebo control it might otherwise provide.

Still another approach is to use comparison groups that have been treated by alternative methods with similar objectives to those of biofeedback. Progressive relaxation and autogenic training are often compared to EMG and hand-temperature feedback for relaxation. These approaches do not control for the role of expectations that may be unique to biofeedback especially because of its impressive hardware.

3. *Characteristics of the therapist and the therapeutic setting.* In view of the importance of the total circumstances in which biofeedback training occurs, including the behavior of the therapist and the therapeutic setting, differences in results among studies from different clinics and laboratories are certain to occur. How much these factors contribute to differences in results is difficult to evaluate because in many if not most published reports the particular factors that may be important may not even have been recognized, let alone described.

Despite the evaluative difficulties of clinical biofeedback, there has been a growing consensus about the desirability of certain research design features. Extended pretraining assessment is important for both the time course of the symptoms to be treated as well as for the variability of the physiological measures on which training is to be given. Clinical evaluation is at best hazardous without some assessment of the symptoms that covers several weeks, months, or years prior to treatment. This is important because overly optimistic evaluations of treatment can occur as a result of the tendency of patients to seek treatment when the symptoms are most severe and to terminate treatment when the symptoms recede, regardless of whether the treatment itself was effective.

The pretreatment physiological variability also needs to be assessed so that it can be compared with the degree of control achieved by training. Of particular interest is the extent to which the patient can be induced to produce changes by various test conditions, including (but not limited to) specific instructions for voluntary control of the physiological measure of interest. Otherwise, there is no way of knowing if the result of biofeedback training is actually nothing more than a demonstration that the patient learned the relationship between the feedback signal and what he already knew how to do. If the relationship is relatively obscure, learning the rules defined by the signal contingency may take longer than learning how to improve the internal behavior itself and may be mistaken for the latter. An example of operant reinforcement of motor behavior may help clarify this point. If a person is given a slightly delayed token reward (which is, of course, a feedback signal) each time he blinks his eyes, and he is not informed of this contingency, it may well take hours before he learns voluntarily to blink his eyes as rapidly as possible. If instead he had merely been asked to do so, he could have obliged easily. The conclusion that it required hours for him to learn to blink his eyes rapidly would clearly be incorrect. Many past studies of biofeedback, especially in the area of stress reduction, have neglected this point.

Long-term follow-up of treatment success is another essential research design feature, in terms of symptoms as well as physiological measures. Follow-up of treatment failures may be useful in providing some information of the incidence and extent of spontaneous remission rates, although they will be confounded with possible delayed benefits traceable to components of training other than the feedback itself.

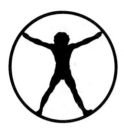 ANNOTATED BIBLIOGRAPHY

Barber, T. X.; DiCara, L.; Kamiya, J.; Miller, N.; Shapiro, D.; and Stoyva, J. (Eds.). **Bio-feedback and Self Control Annual** [Vols. 1970, 1971, 1972, 1973, 1974, 1975–76, 1976–77, and 1977–78]. Chicago: Aldine Atherton.

Each year the board of editors selects from the previous year's publications those jour-nal articles judged to be the most outstanding and representative of the current work in biofeedback and self-control. Space limitations do not permit the inclusion of ex-tremely lengthy articles, but these annuals otherwise reflect accurately the current state of the field and are a convenient way of referencing source material in a single volume. Each year a different member of the board serves as editor in chief and is listed as the first-named author.

Basmajian, J. V. (Ed.). **Biofeedback – Principles and Practice for Clinicians.** Baltimore: Williams and Wilkins, 1978.

At the time this review was written, Basmajian's volume was still in press. However, the depth and range of treatment, as well as the recognized standing of the con-tributors, are sufficient to recommend it as an outstanding up-to-date source on clini-cal principles and applications of biofeedback. Chapter topics and their respective authors are as follows: introduction (Basmajian), anatomical and physiological basis of biofeedback (Wolf), biofeedback strategies in the physical therapy clinic (Baker and Wolf), biofeedback strategies of the occupational therapist in total hand rehabilitation (Brown and Nahai), further applications of EMG muscle rehabilitation (Brown and Nahai), spasticity control (DeBacher), specific muscle retraining (Baker), training of general relaxation (Stoyva), biofeedback strategies in psychotherapy (Fair), headache treatment (Budzynski), thermal biofeedback (Green and Green), cardiovascular disorders (Engel), general psychiatry (Adler and Adler), psychosomatic disorders (Adler and Adler), disorders of voluntary movement (Cleeland), gastrointestinal motility (Schuster), biofeedback and biophysical monitoring during pregnancy and labor (Gregg), basic biofeedback electronics for the clinician (Cohen), equipment needs for the psychotherapist (Peffer), supplementary equipment needs in the rehabilitation setting (Fernando), and research and feedback in clinical practice (Schwartz).

Biofeedback and Self-Regulation, New York: Plenum Press.

A quarterly journal of the Biofeedback Society of America.

Biofeedback Society of America. The publications listed below are available from the BSA Central Office, University of Colorado Medical Center, C268, 4200 East Ninth Avenue, Denver, Colorado 80262. (Send for order forms.)

1. *Proceedings of the BSA Annual Meetings.* These are published in a softcover bound volume each year and contain long abstracts of all papers presented. These are a good source of information about recent developments in research and new applications.
2. *Membership Directory.* A listing of current national membership in the association.
3. *Task Force Reports.* Because of the wide professional and public interest in up-to-date accounts of biofeedback in its various areas of application, the Biofeedback Society of America appointed specialists in several areas to prepare state-of-the-art appraisals known as *Task Force Reports.* The first six listed below have been published in the society's journal, *Biofeedback and Self-Regulation,* 1978. **3 (4).** The other reports are currently available, though it was not possible to review them for this publication. The names given are those of the section chairpersons.

   - The use of biofeedback in the treatment of muscle-contraction (tension) headache. T. Budzynski.
   - The use of biofeedback in the treatment of vascular headache. S. Diamond.
   - The use of biofeedback in the treatment of vasoconstrictive syndromes. E. Taub and C. Stroebel.
   - The use of biofeedback in the treatment of psychogenic disorders. S. Fotopoulos.
   - The use of biofeedback in the treatment of gastrointestinal disorders. W. Whitehead.
   - Physical medicine and rehabilitation. C. K. Fernando and J. Basmajian.
   - Pediatrics. W. Finley.
   - Geriatrics. K. Gaarder.
   - Athletic applications of biofeedback. J. Sandweiss.
   - Stress management. J. Abbondanza.
   - Biofeedback and self-regulation and respiratory disorders. R. Kinsman.
   - Applications of a systems approach to self-regulation training in alcoholism treatment. J. Troiani.
   - Pain. C. N. Shealy.
   - Biofeedback as a research tool. J. Carlson.
   - Biofeedback as an adjunct to sex therapy. J. Perry.
   - Biofeedback and dysmenorrhea. D. Culver.
   - Biofeedback and clinical outcome. C. Wright.

4. *Biofeedback Equipment Manufacturers List.* This list is the most complete and up-to-date list of its kind available. At the time of this writing it was current through December 1978.
5. *Relaxation: A Bibliography.* D. Waterman, B. Tandy, and E. Peper. This bibliogra-

phy contains much of the literature in the area of relaxation from 1966 through 1976.

Blanchard, E., and Epstein, L. **A Biofeedback Primer.** Reading, Mass.: Addison Wesley, 1978.

An introductory overview in paperback, including a twelve-page bibliography.

Butler, Francine. **Biofeedback: A Survey of the Literature.** New York: Plenum Press, 1978.

This volume contains the most complete current bibliography of the total field of biofeedback in both its experimental research and clinical applications. Replacing a 1973 bibliography by Butler and Stoyva (850 references), the present volume reflects the growth of the field, listing 2,300 references as of January 1978. The convenient topical index, based on more than three hundred words drawn from the reference titles, provides an invaluable aid for scanning the research and clinical literature in specific areas. This bibliography also includes the titles of papers given at the 1978 annual meeting of the Biofeedback Society of America.

Gaarder, Kenneth, and Montgomery, Penelope. **Clinical Feedback: A Procedural Manual.** Baltimore: Williams and Wilkins, 1977.

This volume is a carefully prepared text and manual for the practitioner. It also is an excellent beginning point for those who want to evaluate biofeedback as a total social, personal, and physiological process, since it gives an integrated picture of how variables at each of these levels determine therapeutic outcomes. It begins with analysis of the scientific foundations of biofeedback therapy, giving a detailed description of the major components characterizing human homeostatic adaptive control systems. It relates the role of biofeedback to the information flow and state changes in the system. In a very different approach from most analysts, who confine their view to the biological level, the authors then focus on the nature of the therapeutic relationship and explicitly recognize how the "contract" between patient and therapist is very much a part of biofeedback and plays a central role in determining its success. The choice of patients and the structuring of a treatment program with consideration of the assessment and modification of treatment are topics that complete the first half of the volume. Next they discuss ways of developing a biofeedack therapy program, how to learn the practice of biofeedback, how to administer general relaxation and biofeedback procedures, and how to aid treatment by use of tape recordings for relaxation and mental imagery exercises. The volume ends with a description of instrumentation techniques and criteria for selection of biofeedback equipment. Author and subject indexes make the volume easy to use as a manual.

Hassett, J. **A Primer of Psychophysiology.** San Francisco: W. H. Freeman, 1975.

This is an excellent introduction to psychophysiology, the general discipline of which biofeedback is an applied part. The most commonly recorded human physiological functions, along with their basic physiology, are described in six separate chapters: the activity of the sweat gland as seen in electrodermal measures, the cardiovascular system, the respiratory and digestive systems, the eyes, the muscles, and the brain. Technical notes on recording these activities are given in separate appendixes.

Kamiya, J.; Barber, T. X.; DiCara, L.; Miller, N.; Shapiro, D.; and Stoyva, J. (Eds.). **Biofeedback and Self-Control.** Chicago: Aldine Atherton, 1971.

Included in this reader are many of the seminal papers in the field of biofeedback published before 1970. The major chapter topics covered are: heart rate; blood pressure and vasomotor responses; electrodermal activity; salivation; urine formation; gastric motility; electroencephalographic activity; electromyographic activity; methodology and conditioning; classical conditioning; yoga, zen, and autogenic training; voluntary control and hypnosis; voluntary control, consciousness, and physiology.

Psychophysiology. Madison, Wisc.: Society for Psychophysiological Research.

A bimonthly journal of the Society for Psychophysiological Research.

Schwartz, Gary E., and Beatty, J. (Eds.). **Biofeedback, Theory and Research.** New York: Academic Press, 1977.

A collection of eighteen original chapters on current issues in biofeedback, this volume primarily addresses itself to theoretical and research questions. It includes chapters on biofeedback as a scientific tool (Mulholland), sensory and perceptual determinants of voluntary visceral control (Brener), cognitive analysis of biofeedback control (Lazarus), operant learning theory (Black, Cott, and Pavloski), issues in therapeutic applications of biofeedback (Miller and Dworkin), biofeedback and performance (Lawrence and Johnson), biofeedback and patterning of autonomic and central processes (Schwartz), visceral learning in the curarized rat (Dworkin and Miller), long-term cardiovascular studies in primates (Harris and Brady), learned regulation of EEG alpha and theta activity in humans (Beatty), the meaning of operantly conditioned changes in evoked responses (Rosenfeld), and learned control of single motor units (Basmajian).

Of more direct clinical relevance are Taub's comprehensive treatment of human skin temperature regulation; Rosen's chapter on human sexual responses; Shapiro, Mainardi, and Surwit's discussion of biofeedback and essential hypertension; Sterman's chapter on EEG biofeedback and epilepsy; and Budzynski's chapter on clinical implications of electromyographic training.

Schwartz, G., and Shapiro, D. (Eds.). **Consciousness and Self-Regulation.** New York: Plenum Press, 1976.

Contributing original chapters for this work are some of the foremost researchers in the areas of consciousness and self-regulation. The intent is to present current research along with relevant theoretical issues, integrating psychological and physiological approaches. The major topics include: a model of consciousness (John); self-consciousness and intentionality (Pribram); self-regulation of stimulus intensity (Buchsbaum); neodissociation theory of multiple cognitive control systems (Hilgard); hypnotic susceptibility, EEG-alpha, and self-regulation (Engstrom); toward a cognitive theory of self-control (Meichenbaum); physiological and cognitive processes in the regulation of anxiety (Borkovec); dreaming: experimental investigation of representational and adaptive properties (Cohen); and biofeedback and the twilight states of consciousness (Budzynski).

Sterman, M. B.; Finley, W. W.; Kuhlman, W. H.; Allison, T.; Wyler, A. R.; and Lubar, J. F. **Symposium on operant conditioning and epilepsy.** *Pavlovian Journal of Biological Sciences* 1977. **12** (**2, 3**), 63–185.

The authors contributed five papers on epilepsy and EEG feedback at the November 1975 meeting of the Pavlovian Society of Los Angeles, California. They were prepared as articles in the referenced journal. This is the best single reference source on this topic to date.

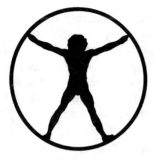

8

AUTOGENIC THERAPY

Erik Peper, Ph.D., and Elizabeth Ann Williams

Autogenic training (AT) is a highly systematized technique designed to generate a state of psychophysiologic relaxation–a state diametrically opposed to that elicited by stress. Through the generation of this state, termed the autogenic (self-generated) state, the recuperative and self-healing processes of the trainee are facilitated, presumably through effects on the autonomic nervous system. This technique forms the foundation for the more inclusive system known as autogenic therapy.

AT grew out of work in the late nineteenth century by O. Vogt and K. Brodmann of the Berlin Neuro-Biological Institute. In the course of their studies with sleep and hypnosis, they observed that patients were able to put themselves into a state similar to hypnosis–autohypnosis–and that this state had positive, recuperative effects. J. H. Schultz, psychiatrist and neurologist in Berlin, was stimulated by their work to investigate the therapeutic potential of hypnosis. He observed that there were certain experiences common to his hypnotized patients (e.g., heaviness and warmth in the extremities) and that those patients who were most successful in relaxing were those that assumed a casual (i.e., passive, non-striving) attitude. Based on these observations and on his desire to decrease the client's dependency on the therapist, Schultz developed autogenic training. In subsequent work, Schultz, along with W. Luthe and others, developed the adjunctive autogenic methods that, along with autogenic training, make up the techniques of AT.

Standard Exercises

Six standard exercises or orientations form the foundation of autogenic training. These exercises are taught in a structured fashion. Following the completion of a detailed medical/psychological history, the trainee is instructed in a specific training posture (intended to reduce to a minimum any distracting stimuli), the proper mode of terminating the exercises, and the phrases themselves (discussed below). The trainee then practices these techniques for several minutes at least three times a day and keeps a log of his or her experiences. The trainer/therapist monitors the trainee's progress and determines from observations of the trainee and his or her reports from the training sessions and from home practice (log entries) whether the trainee is ready to move on to the next exercise. When appropriate, the trainer offers suggestions to enhance the learning of passive attention and the autogenic shift (entry into the autogenic state) or suggests the use of an adjunctive technique. Hence, despite the structured approach, through the trainee-trainer interaction, AT allows for adaptation to the individual needs of the trainee.

Each exercise involves the use of a specified phrase intended to generate a particular physiological state. While practicing, the trainee is instructed to passively attend to a particular body part while mentally repeating one of the phrases. For example, the first exercise is concerned with the generation of heaviness in the extremities. The trainee begins by passively attending to his dominant arm and mentally repeating a number of times "my right (left) arm is heavy." Following the focus on the dominant arm, the trainee is encouraged to generalize the heaviness to all limbs (i.e., "my left (right) arm is heavy," "both arms are heavy," "my arms and legs are heavy") before moving on to the second exercise. Table 8.1 summarizes the six standard exercises.

Adjunctive Techniques

The four adjunctive techniques of AT are autogenic modification, autogenic neutralization, autogenic meditation, and interdisciplinary techniques.

1. *Autogenic modification* uses the autogenic state as a vehicle for effecting changes of a specific nature. This approach involves a phrase, used in addition to or in combination with the standard exercises, that focuses either on physiologic change (an organ-specific formula) or on attitudinal or behavioral change (an intentional formula). Using an organ-specific formula, a trainee with chronic constipation added the phrase "my lower abdomen is warm" to the standard exercises in order to stimulate peristalsis in the colon (Luthe, 1977). The use of "breath carries the words" by a stutterer (Rosa, 1976) and "I am satiated" by an obese individual (Luthe and Schultz, 1969, vol. 2) are examples of intentional formulas.

In the process of practicing AT, the trainee may experience again some of the

Table 8.1
Six Standard AT Exercises

Standard Exercise	Physiological State	Phrase
1	heaviness in the extremities	"my arms and legs are heavy"
2	warmth in the extremities	"my arms and legs are warm"
3	calm and regular function of the heart	"my heart is calm and regular"
4	calm and regular respiration	"my breath is calm and regular" or "it breathes me"
5	solar plexus warm	"my solar plexus is warm"
6	forehead cool	"my forehead is cool"

sensations associated with a past event (i.e., experience discharge of material that has nothing to do with the content of the standard exercises). For example, during the practice of the second AT exercise a twenty-eight-year-old male trainee experienced the image of his partially paralyzed, drooling grandmother as he let go of his habitually clenched jaw. He was confronted with his early decision to always hold his jaw tight, lest he be like his grandmother (Peper, 1976).

2. *Autogenic neutralization* allows the structured release of material in order to neutralize or reduce its disturbing effects. The trainee is encouraged to verbalize either material related to a theme (autogenic verbalization) or whatever comes to mind (autogenic abreaction). Of crucial importance in the practice of these techniques is the maintenance of an attitude of passive acceptance by both trainee and trainer – an attitude of neither suppressing nor enhancing the sensations, allowing the sensations to be while continuing AT. For example, when aggressive dynamics were found to underlie an obese individual's drive to overeat, autogenic verbalization around the theme of hostility was found to be useful (Luthe and Schultz, 1969, vol. 2).

3. *Autogenic meditation* consists of a series of seven exercises begun only after the trainee has developed the ability to maintain passive concentration for at least thirty minutes (usually after at least six months of AT practice). The focus of the exercises progresses from color, concrete objects and images, feelings, and persons to a state where the trainee directly poses questions to the unconscious.

4. *Interdisciplinary techniques* have been developed that integrate AT with other therapeutic techniques. These techniques include autogenic biofeedback,

autogenic behavior therapy, and graduated active hypnosis. For example, temperature biofeedback training has been used with modified autogenic phrases for the successful treatment of migraines (Sargent, Green, and Walters, 1973).

Precautions

Clinical experience suggests certain areas where caution should be exercised in the application of AT (Luthe, 1977). The International Committee on Autogenic Therapy states that "autogenic therapy is a psychophysiological form of medical treatment. The application of this therapy requires a medical evaluation of the prospective trainee, critical adaptation of the method, clinical guidance, and regular control of the patient's technique and progress by a qualified physician" (International Committee on Autogenic Therapy, 1961). It is important that any individual teaching AT be aware of cautionary areas; in fact, these precautions may apply equally well to other relaxation techniques, meditation practices, and biofeedback. Briefly, situations where the training is not recommended include those where (1) the trainee cannot or will not follow instructions (e.g., acute schizophrenics, children less than five years of age, and unmotivated individuals); (2) where differential diagnosis must be established in order to differentiate a discharge from a clinical symptom (e.g., a heart patient may have angina or a pain in the chest that is not angina as an autogenic discharge); (3) where pathology is present and its course cannot be monitored to indicate whether there is a worsening of the symptoms of the disease process (e.g., hypertension, diabetes, or glaucoma).

Conditions where the trainee should either omit or postpone a phrase include those where (1) the trainee reports the experience of an undesirable reaction (e.g., while repeating the phrase "my heart is calm and regular," the trainee experiences tachycardia or major vasodilation causing flushing of the face); (2) the formula focuses on an area of pathology or concern (e.g., with peptic ulcer, the trainee should skip "my solar plexus is warm" or with cardiac neurosis, the trainee should skip "my heart is calm and regular"); (3) a unique situation exists (e.g., omission of "my solar plexus is warm" by pregnant women).

Research and Theory

Although there has been little controlled research, the clinical evidence is suggestive that AT is efficacious, both as a primary and as a supportive technique, in promoting healing in a broad range of illnesses such as gastritis, hypertension, asthma, diabetes mellitus, arthritis, premature ejaculation, sinus tachycardia, anxiety reaction, and alcoholism. Autogenic therapy is not an instant cure; it requires practice over a long period (from two to six months) in most cases for the reversal of pathology. In addition to this remedial use, AT has application both in preventive and self-growth areas. Specifically, AT has been used in the areas of education, industry, and sports where such variables as performance, ability to concentrate, endurance, and anxiety level have been explored (Luthe and Schultz, 1969, vols. 2 and 3).

Although on the surface AT appears to be mainly verbal formula and techniques, in fact it is an encompassing system with a broad philosophical foundation. Many of its beliefs, assumptions, and goals are common to other relaxation and meditative techniques. They include:

- The body has an innate capacity for self-healing and it is this capacity that is allowed to become operative in the autogenic state. Neither the trainer nor trainee has the wisdom necessary to direct the course of the self-balancing process; hence, the capacity is allowed to occur and not be directed.
- Homeostatic self-regulation is encouraged.
- Much of the learning is done by the trainee at home; hence, responsibility for the training lies primarily with the trainee.
- The trainer must be self-experienced in the practice.
- The attitude necessary for successful practice is one of passive attention; active striving and concern with results impedes the learning process. An attitude of acceptance is cultivated, letting be whatever comes up. This quality of attention is known as "mindfulness" in meditative traditions.

A major and unique contribution of AT has been the systematic investigation and follow-up of trainees. Out of this practice have come over 2,600 scientific publications discussing the procedures, efficacy, applications, and precautions of AT, most reported in Luthe and Schultz (1969). Both this vast literature and the highly systematic approach make AT a rich tool for the interested professional.

References

International Committee on Autogenic Therapy, ICAT Regulations. *Proceedings of the Third World Congress of Psychiatry* (Vol. 3). Montreal: University of Toronto and McGill University Press, 1961.

Luthe, W. *Introduction to the Methods of Autogenic Therapy.* Manual for a workshop sponsored by the Biofeedback Society of America in Orlando, Florida, March 8–10, 1977. Denver, Colo.: Biofeedback Society of America, 1977.

Luthe, W., and Schultz, J. H. *Autogenic Therapy* (Vols 1–6). New York: Grune and Stratton, 1969.

Peper, E. Unpublished case study, 1976.

Rosa, K. R. *You and AT.* New York: Saturday Review Press/E. P. Dutton, 1976.

Sargent, J. D.; Green, E. E.; and Walters, E. D. Preliminary report on the use of autogenic feedback training in the treatment of migraine and tension headaches. *Psychosomatic Medicine,* 1973. **35**, 129–135.

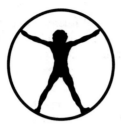 ANNOTATED BIBLIOGRAPHY

Lindemann, Hannes. **Relieve Tension the Autogenic Way.** New York: Peter H. Wydon, 1974.

> This is a guide and review of autogenic therapy for the lay reader with a number of suggestions for clinical applicability.

Luthe, Wolfgang. **A Training Workshop for Professionals: Introduction to the Methods of Autogenic Therapy.** Denver, Colo.: Biofeedback Society of America, 1977.

> This provides a concise description and summary of autogenic therapy. It includes a detailed guide to errors in posture and provides samples of medical history forms and a summary of precautions. This workbook is an expanded version of "Autogenic Therapy," by W. Luthe and S. R. Blumberger in E. D. Wittkower and H. Warnes (Eds.), *Psychosomatic Medicine: Its Clinical Applications.* New York: Harper and Row, 1977.

Luthe, Wolfgang, and Schultz, J. H. **Autogenic Therapy** (Vols. 1–6). New York: Grune and Stratton, 1969.

> These volumes are the basic and essential literature on autogenic therapy. Poorly written and often difficult to read, they nevertheless provide the most extensive compilation of methods, applications, effects, and precautions of the autogenic techniques.
> Volume 1: *Autogenic Methods.* This summarizes the actual methods of autogenic therapy with emphasis on the standard exercises. It includes detailed case reports of trainees' subjective experiences.
> Volume 2: *Medical Applications.* This volume covers the applications of autogenic therapy to medical disorders, organized in terms of functional systems. Evaluations of effectiveness are included.
> Volume 3: *Applications to Psychotherapy.* The uses of autogenic therapy in psychotherapy are described, organized by illness category. The volume includes discussions of efficacy.
> Volume 4: *Research and Theory.* This volume contains studies of psychophysiological changes concomitant with the practice of autogenic training.

Volume 5: *Dynamics of Autogenic Neutralization.* This is an exhaustive discussion of the process and dynamics of autogenic neutralizations, with extensive subjective reports of patients.

Volume 6: *Treatment with Autogenic Neutralization.* The use of autogenic neutralization in treatment is discussed with special focus on the resistance process.

Rosa, K. R. **You and AT.** New York: Saturday Review Press/E. P. Dutton, 1976.

A practical guide for the lay reader to the system of autogenic therapy, this book emphasizes the autonomy of the trainee.

Shealy, Norman. **Ninety Days to Self-Health.** New York: Dial, 1977.

A self-help guide that is based upon a greatly modified autogenic therapy structure. It includes many self-help exercises.

Information about Autogenic Therapy may be obtained from:

International Center for Autogenic Therapy
Medical Center
5300 Cotes des Neiges, Room 550
Montreal H3T 1YE
Canada

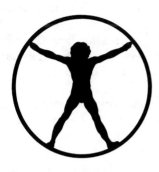

9

HYPNOSIS

David B. Cheek, M.D.

Hypnosis has been used for medical and therapeutic purposes during most of its history. In ancient Egypt and Greece, trance states were evoked by the priest-doctors of healing temples. States resembling hypnosis were used by Native Americans for reducing the effects of pain (Estabrooks, 1957). In the late eighteenth century, around the time of the American Revolution, hypnosis played a part in the "magnetic" treatments of Viennese doctor Franz Mesmer. Hypnosis was refined and practiced throughout the nineteenth century, and Scottish physician James Esdaile (1957) used hypnosis successfully in 3,000 surgical operations. At the turn of the century, French physicians Liebeault, Bernheim, and others used hypnosis for treating physical and nervous disorders (Bernheim, 1895).

With improved physical medicine, interest in hypnosis has fluctuated, but there has always been a continuity of clinical and therapeutic use, and this chapter will focus on the current applications of hypnosis in medicine and therapy.

Concepts of Hypnosis

Definitions and theories of hypnosis are almost as numerous as the physicians, dentists, psychologists, and lay people who have been interested in it. Most authorities seem now to be agreed that hypnosis brings about some sort of altered awareness and behavior as compared with the presumably normal awake state. Various definitions say that attention is more focused or more mobile in this state, there is a diminishing of the general reality orientation, and there is a greater response to suggestions of the hypnotist. However, most definitions have been limited by the conditions of laboratory research and are based on states induced by one human being in another human being.

The idea that hypnosis only occurs when one person brings it about through repetitive mesmeric passes or verbal suggestions appears to me a very restricted view. If we understand the appearance, the behavior, and the thinking processes associated with hypnosis we will find them occurring spontaneously under a variety of circumstances. A hypnotic state may occur spontaneously when people are frightened, disoriented in space, unconscious, very ill, or starving. Bernheim (1895) observed the phenomenon with typhoid patients. Estabrooks (1957) remarked on this matter, and Milechnin (1962) has given a beautiful description of its appearance with starving Russian prisoners in German camps. We should be able to recognize spontaneous hypnosis when we see it, and to use its potentials for good, and to help our patients avoid its great dangers.

A hypnotic state also occurs spontaneously when a person is driving long distances along a straight road that does not require alert behavior. It occurs when wisps of fog, rain drops, or evenly spaced white lines on the road draw the driver's eyes repetitively downward. It occurs with repetitive flashes of light and shadow, as helicopter pilots know. Poplar trees at regular intervals along a road may be a menace for drivers in the early morning or late afternoon on sunny days. The danger of hypnosis on the highway is that our movements become slower; we may not move the wheel fast enough at a turn in the road. We may develop tunnel vision and fail to see a car coming in from the side until it is too late.

Theories of Hypnosis

Hypnosis has been explained in terms of trance states, role playing, conditioning, and ego regression, but no theory is currently widely accepted. I find that much hypnotic behavior can be understood in terms of biological survival mechanisms. The slowing down and the immobilization of physical and sensory processes is a natural defense mechanism when flight or fight is not possible and further assists in recovery after trauma. The reticular activating system receives information from the complex nerve network extending among all tissues and sense organs. This system controls messages to the cortex and is able to influence how much conscious and unconscious attention is paid to stimuli from both the external and internal environment (Magoun, 1950, Hernandez-Peon et al., 1956). It is likely that this system is being utilized whenever we work with attention, memory, and subconscious experiences under hypnosis.

The Appearance and General Responses of Hypnosis

There are great variations in the phenomena we can see in both induced and spontaneously occurring hypnosis. The variations depend on the genetic background of the individual as well as on his personal experiences with stress during prenatal life, at birth, and in the two or three years that precede the origin of conscious memory. Possibly the most common changes occurring with hypnosis are as follows:

- There is a loss of animation in facial expression.
- Muscular action is made more slowly and may cease.
- Speaking becomes increasingly difficult as the hypnotic state deepens.
- There is great economy in the use of words. Adjectives and adverbs are left out.
- Understandings of words change. There is a regressed type of understanding that is typical of childhood. The more emotionally charged of two interpretations will be taken with such statements as "You can leave the hospital in five days *if all goes well."*
- There is an increasing tendency to hold a position, even an uncomfortable one, as the hypnotic state deepens. We call this catalepsy.
- Similarly, there is a tendency to continue an action that has been promoted by the hypnotist, such as the twiddling of one's thumbs or revolving of one hand around the other.
- At the beginning of a hypnotic state there may be evidence of increased autonomic activity. The respiration may accelerate, and perspiration may appear on the subject's forehead or the palms of the hands. (In my experience this usually relates to a consciously unrecognized flashback to a stress event and can be a major factor preventing a subject from going on with the hypnotic state [Cheek, 1960]. It can be removed either by having the subject go in and come out of hypnosis a number of times to learn that it can be comfortable, or the therapist can help the subject to discover the original stressful event and can help him or her to find it unnecessary to relive that trouble.)
- As hypnosis deepens there is a slowing of physiological processes. The skin cools. Respiration and heart rate become slower. There is an increasing inhibition in response to a normally painful stimulus. Disturbed motility of the gut (such as vomiting and diarrhea) eventually stops. Reactions of hypersensitivity as manifested by asthma and hay fever tend to diminish and disappear. Bleeding from wounds or from mucous membranes of the nose, rectosigmoid, bladder, and uterus diminishes and may cease.

Those using hypnosis clinically in the healing arts often suggest to the patient that one or more of these possibilities will occur. This is all right and it probably improves the prestige of the hypnotist who tells the patient what would happen anyhow without suggestion.

Who Can Be Hypnotized?

Much thought has gone into the consideration of who is susceptible to hypnotic suggestion (Hilgard, 1965), and scales have been developed to measure this susceptibility. However, these are derived from behavior of students in university centers under relatively nonthreatening circumstances. Tests of susceptibility are not necessary in a clinical setting where the patient recognizes at some level of awareness that hypnosis may be of value. From the standpoint of the holistic healing arts, therefore, I suggest that we give up consideration of whether or not a person can be hypnotized and focus rather on the remarkable things that all people are capable of doing when they receive adequate instruction and are subconsciously willing to let us help. Willingness for change is necessary, and we must know how to evaluate and possibly remove unconscious resistance to change. I believe that all people will use the potential help of hypnotic behavior when their survival depends on it.

The Induction of a Hypnotic State

The production of a hypnotic state by mesmeric passes in the old style took up to an hour, and production of very profound states today may require several hours. Spontaneous states may occur very rapidly in response to a physical or mental shock.

Most of the textbook types of inductions take from ten to twenty minutes. Generally they begin with some of the tests of hypnotic suggestibility (Hilgard, 1965), such as arm levitation, immobilizing clasped hands, or eye closure. If these are done successfully, the state is already present in the person. The hypnotist then follows with repetitive instructions and suggestions to the subject to relax and become drowsy but nevertheless to continue listening to the instruction of the hypnotist. The hypnotist may count from one to ten to symbolize the depth of the state and to assist the person to go deeper. For samples of induction procedure see Crasilneck and Hall (1975).

In contrast, these procedures are cumbersome and unsubtle compared to the use of an already potential hypnotic state in a person who is, say, critically ill or traumatized or compared to the unobtrusive interactions used by Erickson, which develop hypnosis in the process of an apparently normal communication (Erickson, 1958; Haley, 1967). There are also very rapid inductions used by stage hypnotists with selected subjects, but the methods are not really good for the relationship between a psychologist, physician, or dentist and a client or patient.

An approach that I use extensively is LeCron's method of questioning with a Chevreul pendulum, which obtains an ideomotor response from the patient. This will produce a hypnotic state almost immediately after the patient has selected symbol movements for the pendulum's answers. The use of this technique will be described in a later section.

Suggested Explorations and Uses of Hypnosis

When we are using hypnosis we are taking advantage of the mind's ability to store an enormous wealth of information that passes unrecognized by those who conduct their investigative and therapeutic activity on the limited horizon of "objective observation," as "scientists" relying on conscious-level reporting. Much of the literature extolling or denying the virtues of hypnosis reflects only the ability or failure of the author to mitigate the influences of faulty understandings, fear, and hopelessness in the individual being treated. We can use the individual's behavior with hypnosis as a control for behavior without it, but we cannot really come to meaningful decision with large groups of people to satisfy the appetite of a computer or statistician. With hypnosis we can:

- Explore early life attitudes of the individual toward parents, self, and the external world
- Help the individual improve self-confidence and learning abilities early in life before difficulties become entrenched
- Discover and eradicate the origins of imprinted triggering mechanisms responsible for the continuation or recurrence of disease
- Impart confidence in being able to use helpful physiological responses in place of disturbed ones, using hypnosis for "instant biofeedback"
- Explore the advantages and dangers of ideation in deeper levels of sleep

General Approaches

There are three general approaches. First, we can use suggestion with hypnotized subjects to directly relieve symptoms and to help override any unconscious resistance that might stand in the way of success. For example, we can use hypnosis for reducing pain. There are some serious problems that can arise from this type of use, however, particularly if the symptom is serving to prevent the individual from doing violence to himself or to someone else or if it is a reflection of a systemic or larger malfunction.

Second, we can use hypnosis as a medium for substituting good physical responses in place of disturbed ones. For example, we may use familiar experiences, such as the memory of hunger during a peaceful time in life, to help a patient overcome severe vomiting in pregnancy. Much of the time we obtain an automatically beneficial response simply by inducing a hypnotic state and using the standard calming suggestions.

Third, we can use the selective memory available in hypnosis to reveal cause and effect relationships for physical and emotional problems. Ideomotor questioning can be combined with hypnosis in such a way as to discover the origins of inappropriate behaviors, fears, factors of guilt, self-punishment, and passive acceptance. Often patients are able to change their reactions as soon as the causes are discovered; in other cases they are able to use their own reasoning processes to reassess the original situation and to learn to eliminate its harmful effects.

Pain

The experience of pain can be removed or substantially reduced through direct hypnotic suggestion and often simply through the induction of the hypnotic state with its concomitant physiological characteristics. Pain and inflammation of wounds are not necessary for the survival of patients suffering from angina or coronary artery occlusion. The same is true for the pain of a broken bone or the postoperative discomfort of a sterile surgical procedure. Hypnosis can be used effectively in such cases with beneficial effects beyond the relief of pain (Cheek and LeCron, 1968).

James Esdaile (1957), a Scottish physician, observed in 1845 that the three cardinal signs of inflammation disappeared when pain was relieved by his method of inducing hypnosis with long continued mesmeric passes. Redness, swelling, and local heat disappeared. Even more important was the drop in surgical mortality from 50 percent (standard at that time) to 5 percent, when he used hypnosis for surgical operations. Something positive happened to the immune responses of his patients who were relaxed under hypnosis and whose traumatic reactions to his surgical intervention were apparently turned off. The general surgical mortality rate did not drop to Esdaile's level until half a century later when sterilization procedures were accepted.

"Pain relieving" drugs are not necessarily as effective as hypnosis in managing the effects of pain. They influence conscious awareness but do not block subconscious circuits that continue to stimulate the release of inflammatory enzymes at the injury. I have used the term "subconscious pain" for this element (Cheek, 1962b). It is a sense of discomfort that is not accessible to the verbal level but may be retrieved at an ideomotor or physical response level. For example, a liver abscess may be consciously painless yet involve the usual tissue changes of inflammation that would occur with a very painful boil on the surface of the skin. Further, in tests at the Stanford hypnosis laboratory, Hilgard (1977) found that a part of the hypnotized person's mind was very much aware of a painful stimulus, even though consciously he did not report a painful sensation.

Hypnotic Awareness Under Anesthesia

One of the important discoveries made through the use of hypnosis and ideomotor question techniques is that patients in surgical planes of general anesthesia can hear and react to meaningful messages that relate to their condition, and if this message is interpreted as pessimistic this may be incorporated as if it were a hypnotic suggestion to be carried out (Cheek 1959, 1961b, 1962a; Levinson, 1965). Awareness was first suggested by George Crile (1947) in 1908, who accidentally learned that nitrous oxide anesthesia does not eliminate the ability to hear, and more recently was noted by Milton Erickson (1954) and Leslie LeCron (1954a). David Elman (1962) told me of his discovery in 1948 that the continued distress of a woman after surgery was caused by a disturbing remark of her surgeon.

We recommend that surgeons, anesthesiologists, and all the staff who work with patients who are in anesthesia be careful about what they say and how it might be understood by their patients. If in doubt about the effect of some remark, they should explain their comments to and reassure their seemingly insensate patients.

Another finding relating to hypnosis and surgical anesthesia comes from my study of the subjective impressions of 3,000 patients as they lost consciousness and as they went through the rest of the surgical experience. There are three moments in which traumatic fear reactions may occur. The first is usually at the beginning of the loss of consciousness when patients may have a spontaneous flashback to a frightening earlier experience with a badly given anesthetic for a childhood surgery. The second is a feeling of panic at being unable to use respiratory muscles during the moments after a muscle relaxant is given intravenously to make possible the introduction of a tracheal airway. This reponse is not universal, but when it occurs it has always related to respiratory difficulty at birth, a near-drowning incident, or an infantile experience of choking on food. It can be avoided by preparing the patient with explanations about what to expect and the value of this procedure for maximum efficiency of the anesthetic. The third frequent fearful event occurs when an anesthetized patient is jolted without forewarning. This may occur when positioning the patient on the table for surgery, or when the recovering patient is jolted during transfer to a carriage or into bed. The jolt can produce a hypnotic state so deep that the surgical team may mistake it for cardiac arrest. However, the patient will recover quickly if congratulated about relaxing so well and told to take a deep breath and resume his normal bodily processes.

Communication with the Unconscious or Critically Ill Patient

A person who has suffered a traumatic injury or who is critically ill can be considered to be in a spontaneous hypnotic state. Frightened people need no formal induction to hypnosis; they are already in the hypnotic state when we see them. This makes them wonderfully responsive to helpful suggestion, even though they may appear apathetic or even unconscious.

These principles may be helpful in using this state for the benefit of the patient (Cheek, 1969):

- Learn to recognize and enhance the signs of hypnotic behavior in the critically ill.
- Use all your power to communicate hope and optimism; do it sincerely because phony reassurance is easily recognized by the critically ill.
- Collect your thoughts and marshal a plan of action; don't be rushed. Give some instructions to bystanders before touching or speaking to the patient. This allows time to regain your poise.
- Tell the patient what has happened and that he will be all right. Outline what you are doing and what your reason for doing it is. Tell what your plan is for him tomorrow and in the future. With unconscious people, even if they show no pupilar reflex to light, give instruction and promises of a future. Congratulate the person for being so relaxed. Tell him specifically how long you expect him to remain relaxed before awakening with feelings of hunger or thoughts of food. Give instructions for the body to relax and for it to deal as necessary with physical needs and recovery.
- Give medication for pain if possible. Tell the patient what you are giving and why. This communicates constructive action.
- Get a conscious patient to talk about work, hobbies, family, and experiences if he is able to talk. This directs the mind to concern itself with times and places where pain and fear did not exist.

Obstetrical Uses of Hypnosis

Probably every professional person concerned with the welfare of obstetrical patients uses variants of suggestion much of the time. It would be wonderful if this were always done in a constructive way, but often it is done in the reverse. The doctor may tell a bleeding patient, "Don't worry about this. If the embryo is abnormal you will abort, but you will carry on *if it is O.K.*" To the patient this means, "My doctor thinks my baby may be abnormal. If it is I don't want to carry on."

Hypnosis is very satisfying for both mother and her obstetrician when it works successfully as the sole means of comfort during labor. The chances for this are rather slim in our modern obstetrical hospitals where "team approach," oxytocin challenge tests for adequacy of placental circulation, artificial induction of labor, and fetal monitoring are ways of scientifically keeping up-to-date. If hypnosis or its cousins, "natural childbirth" and Lamaze techniques, were adequately recognized we would be seeing a drop in Caesarean section incidence.

Instead, Caesarean rates have nearly doubled in many parts of the United States since the wide acceptance of fetal monitoring in labor. Obstetricians are now saving babies from the complications that we may often have initiated by our atmosphere of pessimistic expectation. As Grantly Dick-Read and Frederick Leboyer have observed, obstetricians and obstetrical nursing staffs have been treating labor as a disease instead of as a natural process.

In the modern hospital the laboring woman's attention is so centered on what her uterus and its contents are doing that it is difficult for her to relax and dissociate her awareness for the benefit of an easy labor and birth of an infant that recognizes it has caused no trouble. Even in this setting, however, it is possible to use hypnosis constructively when an emergency arises. Should contractions accelerate to the point of great distress, should there be a sudden rise in blood pressure, or should there be unexpected vaginal bleeding, the patient enters a ready-made hypnotic state brought on by her apprehensiveness; she becomes hypersuggestible. A good approach to this situation was invented by Milton Erickson*, a great pioneer in the therapeutic uses of hypnosis. We can walk into the room and ask, "Have you been anywhere recently for a drive in an automobile?" A surprised affirmative answer can be followed up rapidly by requests for information regarding the time of day she got into the car, what she was wearing, how she got to her destination, what she did there. Further components in this approach work toward successfully reversing unfavorable physiological reactions, mitigating fear, and eventually, eliminating pain.

The steps take place very rapidly. First, the patient is taken off guard by the seeming inappropriateness of the questioning. She wonders why this is taking place. Next, she realizes the doctor must have some purpose that will eventually be helpful. Perhaps it has something to do with the trouble she has just been having. She becomes a bit confused while trying to keep up with the interrogation. This brings on a light hypnotic state that deepens while she tries to remember sequential events. Her orientation is displaced to a time and place where she was comfortable, where there was no labor, no bleeding. Her limbic and reticular activating system are now tuned into what was happening back then instead of what was going on before the questions began.

Ordinary Training for Delivery

Far better value can be obtained for hypnosis if we have a chance to use it early in pregnancy to evaluate the woman's readiness for pregnancy, her unconscious identifications, and her fears. A valuable way of uncovering fear is to use a Chevreul pendulum or ideomotor responses of fingers to the question, "Does the inner part of your mind know the sex of your baby?" Women who fear for themselves or their baby will not commit themselves on subconsciously "knowing" the sex of their baby (Cheek, 1961a).

*Editors' note: Dr. Erickson died March 25, 1980, as this book went to press.

We can train the patient during the second trimester to use autohypnosis and to be aware of finger movements in answer to questions. This permits use of hypnosis over the telephone in case she awakens at two or three o'clock in the morning with profuse vaginal bleeding or rhythmic abdominal pains that might presage premature labor. The time to act is right then. It may be too late by the time she gets to the hospital. We can say, "Let's see, now, which is your 'yes' finger?" This indicates to the patient that we are in some sort of control. Her thought is directed to answering the question and away from the bleeding or the pain. We can then ask her to review the thoughts and dreams that have preceded onset of the symptoms. She will discover that there have been repeated troubled thought sequences. In the light of conscious reason these thoughts usually appear foolish. She can then be asked to give a designated signal when she knows she has turned off the bleeding or the pain and can sleep constructively for the sake of her baby (Cheek, 1965).

During the third trimester a patient can be rehearsed with the conduct of labor from the early contractions through the admission to the hospital, the enema, and the easy, relaxed labor of two or three hours. She is told that she has been able to reduce the feeling of her contractions to 50 percent, that labor means just work, that soon she will see her healthy baby. After saying hello to her baby she will look over to one side and see the nurse writing up the date, the sex of her baby, and its weight as well as the total length of labor. It is reassuring to the obstetrician when he gets a solid commitment on these vital statistics. Unwillingness to see the blackboard or the writing means that there are some unresolved and consciously unrecognized fears that need discovery and correction. The patient can be asked to orient her thoughts to the moment she got the idea that she could not select a date for her delivery. The reason is usually simple and easily corrected. Husbands should be included in the training and told how to keep their wives occupied with memories of places they went and meals they had during their honeymoon. They can be of enormous help with their contributions during labor. People do not panic when they know each step in a series of events and what to do with each one.

Gynecological Uses of Hypnosis

Probably most of the endrocrine and functional disturbances of the female urogenital system are psychological in origin. The interested reader may wish to search the wealth of literature on this subject documented by Flanders Dunbar (1954). The major sources of trouble start with birth and are augmented during adolescence. We need to know whether or not the baby felt welcome as a girl at birth, whether or not the birth of a subsequent sibling affected whatever self-image the child held. We need to know whether the adolescent girl had become a tomboy in order to please a seemingly rejecting father, whether or not she was taller than the boys in her class at school, and what her reactions were to menstruation. We need to know what parental inhibitions and rigidities about sexual matters were passed on to the child.

In a search of factors contributing to a healthy multiorgasmic adult life, Cheek (1976) found that all such patients had felt welcome as girls at birth, they were all nursed by their mothers, their hands were not slapped when they explored their genital feelings as babies, and they escaped the outraged discovery by adults of their innocent mutual explorations of neighborhood children in the backyard. The most important feature of their development was the association of pleasurable sexual feelings with an atmosphere of loving acceptance and trust. The concept that there are special areas to stimulate, special physical buttons to press seems not to justify the attention paid them by the followers of Masters and Johnson, for it was clear from these studies that mature orgasmic responsiveness is almost purely a cerebral experience. The female children feeling accepted as such and growing older in a continuum of acceptance experienced dreams of identification with leading ladies in movies and television shows. They experienced orgasms in these dreams simply with demonstrations of love by the leading man in the play. No genital stimulus was necessary. These learning processes occurred around the ages of six to ten years.

Conversely, adult nonorgasmic patients from inhibited parentage could remember no such orgasmic dreams during age-regression studies. It appears that the same factors helping us inhibit the urge to urinate while asleep will terminate potentially helpful sexual fantasies during sleep. The inhibited teenager will see her angry mother looking through the window as she is on the point of orgasm just as the youngster with a full bladder will find the dreamed-of toilet blocked or no longer there when on the point of voiding. A major part of hypnotic therapy to correct troubled beginnings involves encouraging the patient to recognize that sexual feelings are normal and healthy. The next step is to give the patient permission to dream freely and without guilt.

Studies made by the author with the help of ideomotor questioning methods have strongly suggested a correlation between troubled sexual attitudes and dysmenorrhea, endometriosis, uterine myomas, genital viral infections, and vulvovaginal inflammation due to *Trichomonas*, yeast, and the influenza bacillus. The stresses of unhappy work relationships and the anxieties of feeling "used" by male companions seem largely responsible for the sequences of cervical dysplasia, which can revert to a normal cytologic appearance when the stresses are recognized, but may lead on to surgical intervention in an atmosphere of professional apprehension about the potential development of cancer.

Habitual abortion and the inability to become pregnant are usually medically handled from the standpoint of endocrine disturbance without any consideration of the possibility that the hypothalamic releasing substances for appropriate hormones may be inhibited because of unconscious fears, identifications, and hostilities. Large teaching centers are concerned about female immune reactions against the sperm of their sexual partner, but they overlook the possible existence of consciously unrecognized emotional factors that might be making the woman react immunologically against her partner's sperm. These are areas that need to be researched using methods now available for exploring the levels of physiological response to subconscious perceptions. The conscious impressions of women about their problems may be helpful, but they are often misleading because memory does not extend to the very significant impressions gained before the origins of conscious memory.

Ideomotor Questioning Methods

Ideomotor questioning is a simple method of uncovering information that otherwise is very hard to reach, including inner feelings and motivations, forgotten traumatic experiences, and material heard while in unconscious states. The methods have been outlined by Leslie M. LeCron (1954b, 1961, 1964) and by Cheek and LeCron (1968).

In one method the patient holds a pendulum—a weight on a string—and under the direction of the hypnotist or himself instructs the pendulum to swing in response to questions. The individual selects a particular direction of movement to represent "yes," "no," and other answers. The pendulum then responds to subconscious motor impulses and provides answers to inquiries (e.g., "Is there a significant event in your life that contributes to the fears that you are having now?"). In another method, one of the patient's fingers is designated as a "yes" finger and another as a "no" finger. The fingers then are instructed to move automatically in response to the questions.

The value of ideomotor questioning is that through it we may obtain information that is not conscious or accessible to verbal report. Speech, the most highly developed and the most recently evolved means of communication, is of no value when we search for information that has been pushed into the subconscious, experiences that antedate the beginning of talking ability around age eighteen months, or when we want to know about things that have happened while a person has been unconscious. When we request a verbal report on such items the hypnotized subject may become confused, shrug his shoulders, or try to please the hypnotist by making up a story that might satisfy an uncritical investigator.

Using ideomotor questioning we can identify the existence of an amnesic period and request the subject to re-experience it at a subconscious or "inner" level, requesting an ideomotor signal to indicate the beginning and the ending of the reliving. One or more repetitions of the event in this manner may help the patient elevate it to a talking level of awareness. The secret lies in refraining from the temptation to ask for a verbalized report until we recognize that the patient is able to do so.

People with deep-resting information stored in primitive parts of the brain's memory reservoir often become troubled when prematurely asked to elevate the information to a speech level. They respond better when we go only part of the way toward this memory by asking for physiological action given unconsciously from muscles that are not usually part of verbal communication. By watching carefully, we will see that a troublesome experience is first revealed at a physiological level. Neck pulsations accelerate, as do respiratory movements. Tiny droplets of perspiration may appear on the finger that will eventually lift unconsciously. This all happens before skeletal muscles become active and speech can be evoked, and it may take a varying number of sweeps of the subconscious information. In one of my cases, it took thirteen repetitions of an entire appendectomy experience before we completely uncovered and eliminated the harmful effects of disturbing comments made during the operation (Cheek, 1959).

Ideomotor techniques are useful because they can operate gradually to bring information to consciousness and because they can be used easily without formal hypnotic inductions. They require skill and experience, and the role of the therapist is to keep the subject from centering on anxiety, fear of failure, and hopelessness. The therapist is there to set constructive goals after eliminating the destructive physical and emotional factors in disease.

The Status of Hypnosis Today

Many medical schools in the United States now have courses for students and postgraduates on hypnotic theory and techniques, and hypnosis is recognized by the American Medical Association as an accepted therapeutic technique. There are two societies in the United States concerned with clinical and experimental hypnosis. Both the International Society of Clinical and Experimental Hypnosis and the American Society of Clinical Hypnosis have journals, and their combined membership is about 2,800. Both are recognized by the American Medical Association and the courses of instruction given by members of their Educational and Research Divisions are recognized for Category I credit. Psychologists and dentists also can take these courses. There are hypnosis societies in England, Sweden, Japan, and Australia as well. Similar societies under the name of "sophrology" exist in Italy, Spain, and Brazil. A search of the medical literature between 1974 and 1978 has revealed more than eight hundred published scientific papers dealing with hypnosis.

References

Bernheim, H. *Suggestive Therapeutics.* (2nd ed., C. Herter, trans.). New York: G. P. Putnam's Sons, 1895. (Originally published in 1888.)

Cheek, David B. Unconscious perception of meaningful sounds during surgical anesthesia as revealed under hypnosis. *American Journal of Clinical Hypnosis,* 1959. **1**, 101–113.

Cheek, David B. Removal of subconscious resistance to hypnosis during ideomotor questioning. *American Journal of Clinical Hypnosis,* 1960. **3**, 103–107.

Cheek, David B. LeCron technique of prenatal sex determination for uncovering subconscious fear in obstetrical patients. *International Journal of Clinical and Experimental Hypnosis*, 1961a. **9**, 249–258.

Cheek, David B. Unconscious reactions and surgical risk. (Editorial by invitation). *Western Journal of Surgery, Obstetrics and Gynecology*, 1961b. **69**. 325–328.

Cheek, David B. Areas of research into psychosomatic aspects of surgical tragedies now open through use of hypnosis and ideomotor questioning. *Western Journal of Surgery, Obstetrics and Gynecology*, 1962a. **70**, 137–142.

Cheek, David B. Ideomotor questioning for investigation of subconscious "pain" and target organ vulnerability. *American Journal of Clinical Hypnosis*, 1962b. **5**, 30–41.

Cheek, David B. Some newer understandings of dreams in relation to threatened abortion and premature labor. *Pacific Medicine and Surgery*, 1965. **73**, 379–384.

Cheek, David B. Communication with the critically ill. *American Journal of Clinical Hypnosis*, 1969. **12**, 75–85.

Cheek, David. B. Short term hypnotherapy for frigidity using exploration of early life attitudes. *American Journal of Clinical Hypnosis*, 1976. **19**, 20–27.

Cheek, David B., and LeCron, Leslie M. *Clinical Hypnotherapy*. New York: Grune and Stratton, 1968.

Crasilneck, Harold B., and Hall, James A. *Clinical Hypnosis: Principles and Applications*. New York: Grune and Stratton, 1975.

Crile, George. *George Crile, An Autobiography*. Philadelphia: Lippincott, 1947.

Dunbar, Flanders. *Emotions and Bodily Changes* (4th ed.). New York: Columbia University Press, 1954.

Elman, David. Personal communication. 1962.

Erickson, Milton H. Personal communication, 1954.

Erickson, Milton H. Naturalistic techniques of hypnosis. *American Journal of Clinical Hypnosis*, 1958. **1**, 25–29.

Esdaile, James. *Hypnosis in Medicine and Surgery*. New York: Julian Press, 1957. (Originally published as *Mesmerism in India*, 1850.)

Estabrooks, G. H. *Hypnotism*. New York: E. P. Dutton, 1957.

Haley, Jay (ed.). *Advanced Techniques of Hypnosis and Therapy: Selected Papers of Milton H. Erickson*. New York: Grune and Stratton, 1967.

Hernandez-Peon, R.; Scherrer, H.; Jouvet, M. Modification of electric activity in cochlear nucleus during "attention" in unanesthetized cats. *Science*, 1956. **123**, 331–332.

Hilgard, Ernest R. *Hypnotic Susceptibility*. New York: Harcourt Brace, 1965.

Hilgard, Ernest R. *Divided Consciousness*. New York: Wiley, 1977.

LeCron, Leslie M. Personal communication, 1954a.

LeCron, Leslie M. A hypnotic technique for uncovering unconscious material. *Journal of Clinical and Experimental Hypnosis*, 1954b. **2**, 76–79.

LeCron, Leslie M. *Techniques of Hypnotherapy*. New York: Julian Press, 1961.

LeCron, Leslie M. *Self Hypnotism*. Englewood Cliffs, N.J.: Prentice-Hall, 1964.

Levinson, Bernard. States of awareness under general anesthesia: primary communication. *British Journal of Anesthesiology*, 1965. **37**, 544–546.

Magoun, H. W. Caudal and cephalic influences of the brain stem reticular formation. *Physiological Review*, 1950. **30**, 459–473.

Milechnin, Anatol. The Pavlovian syndrome: a trance state developing in starvation victims. *American Journal of Clinical Hypnosis*, 1962. **4**, 162–168. [Reprinted as a chapter in Anatol Milechnin, *Hypnosis* (Galina Solovey, trans.). Bristol: John Wright and Sons, 1967.]

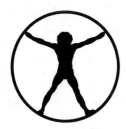

ANNOTATED BIBLIOGRAPHY

August, Ralph. **Hypnosis in Obstetrics**. New York: McGraw-Hill, 1968.

The author reports on the successful use of hypnosis in 1,000 consecutive deliveries. August takes an authoritative approach that is effective in the group setting. He trained his patients in small groups with support from his staff associates. His results speak for themselves: a Caesarean-section rate of 2.2 percent. Emotional factors possibly causing abortion, premature labor, and stillbirth are not discussed in this otherwise excellent book, but neither are they considered in the standard obstetrical texts used by medical students and the modern hospitals where Caesarean rates are now approaching 20 percent. A 33⅓ rpm recording of the author's voice is included with the book and illustrates his approach.

Chapman, L. F.; Goodell, Helen; and Wolff, H. G. **Changes in tissue vulnerability induced during hypnotic suggestion.** *Journal of Psychosomatic Research*, 1959. **4**, 99–105.

Thirteen subjects were hypnotized in forty experiments. In twelve experiments the subjects were told that one arm would have normal sensitivity but that the other arm would be very sensitive and vulnerable to the thermal stimulus to be applied. Nine of the twelve had greater tissue damage on the "vulnerable" arm. One showed more tissue damage on the "normal" arm. Two showed equal responses on both arms. (I have found this frequently with subjects who did not know they had once been left-handed.)

In twenty-seven experiments it was suggested that one arm would be very sensitive to injury and the other arm would be anesthetic. In one of these experiments there was great damage on the "anesthetic" side. In six the reactions were equal for both arms. However, in twenty of this series the inflammatory reaction was greater on the side of suggested heightened vulnerability. The reader interested in pain and inflammation is referred to other work by this group that demonstrates that local tissue reaction can be modified by higher nervous system control.

The authors were not aware that primal handedness often is converted before the origin of conscious memory and that confusion can occur with spontaneous regression to earlier handedness orientation as the subject enters a hypnotic state. This could account for some variability in their observations.

Cheek, David, and LeCron, Leslie M. **Clinical Hypnotherapy**. New York: Grune and Stratton, 1968.

This book was designed by the authors as a handbook for students of hypnosis symposiums offered by LeCron from 1956–1970. This and *Techniques of Hypnotherapy*, (now out of print), edited by LeCron, are the only books in the English language that include discussions and directions for using ideomotor (subverbal) responses to reveal cause and effect relationships in disease, whether emotional or physical. Bibliographical references are limited to those pertinent to material offered in the symposiums. Emphasis is placed on utilization rather than on the formalizing of hypnotic induction.

Chapters include recognition and alteration of factors in pain states, exploration of ideation in deep levels of sleep, recognition of the factors behind "high risk" pregnancy, emergency uses of hypnosis in shock and hemorrhage, recognition and strategies for overcoming resistances to therapy, a discussion of preparing patients for surgery, and evidence that anesthetized people are able to hear meaningful conversations in the operating room.

Like Volgyesi and Milechnin the authors look on human hypnosis as a species-selected biological survival mechanism rather than as a tool for laboratory investigation. At times of food privation the animal has to shut down metabolism. At times of great danger an animal needs instant replay of information having to do with previous escape. Similarly, in hypnosis deeply recessed information can be retrieved and the evidence tested for validity with ideomotor questioning methods.

Crasilneck, Harold B., and Hall, James A. **Clinical Hypnosis: Principles and Applications**. New York: Grune and Stratton, 1975.

Crasilneck, a psychoanalytically oriented psychologist, and Hall, a Jungian psychiatrist, have put together an excellent survey of significant literature relating to history, theory, inductions, and applications of hypnosis. Specific induction techniques are carefully described in the beginning of the book, but the term "hypnosis" is used in a way that suggests only a helpful state during which good things happen. The authors evidently expected interested readers to search out the source material with the help of the bibliography in order to critically evaluate hypnotic applications in the many special areas outlined in the book. A good report is given of the dramatic results with burn patients that were first published by Crasilneck, Stirman, and Wilson in the *Journal of the American Medical Association*, 1955. **158**, 103–106. Crasilneck was able to relieve pain and help the patients eat and sleep. The subject of ideomotor questioning methods and the power of short-term learning comparable to "imprinting" are not found in the text or in the index.

Erickson, Milton H. **Development of apparent unconsciousness during hypnotic reliving of a traumatic experience**. *Archives of Neurology and Psychiatry*, 1937. **38**, 1282–1288.

Erickson's contributions are so many and so varied that it is hard to select one or two. This one is not included in Haley's collection of Erickson's papers (see below). The author discusses the need for repetitive subconscious review before a hypnotized subject can reveal information about a period of unconsciousness (in one case, caused by drugs and a beating with the intent to kill). Sequential events preceding the amnesiac period had to be recalled in their chronological order. It was not enough to try to isolate the main experience. This principle of exploration with the help of ideomotor review has permitted rapid and consistently fruitful explorations of experiences that occurred during surgical anesthesia and birth.

Erickson, Milton H., and Erickson, Elizabeth M. **Concerning the nature and character of post-hypnotic behavior.** *Journal of General Psychology,* 1941. **2**, 95–133.

This classic paper has been reprinted in Haley's collection of Erickson's papers (see below). Classic posthypnotic suggestion involves a hypnotic state of sufficient depth to assure amnesia after the trance has been ended. Suggestions accepted by the hypnotized subject go into action in accordance with a signal included during the suggestion period. At this point the subject has a compulsion to carry out the suggestion, which may be totally irrelevant to circumstances of that moment. In order to get the assigned job done, the subject must rationalize a means for doing so. Herbert Spiegel has called this "the compulsive triad" and likens it to the characteristics of a neurosis. The Ericksons have pointed out that the subject goes back into a hypnotized state at the moment of carrying out a posthypnotic suggestion. Milton Erickson made use of this observation to further develop his subject's ability to use hypnosis and to achieve deeper levels of hypnosis.

Esdaile, James. **Hypnosis in Medicine and Surgery**. New York: Julian Press, 1957.

The original title of this book was *Mesmerism in India.* The U.S. edition (printed by the Psychic Research Company, Chicago, 1902), is rarely available. As a British surgeon in a prison hospital, Esdaile discovered the protective powers of the deep hypnotic state that occurs with prolonged mesmeric passes. He was the first to show that swelling, redness, and local heat disappeared when pain was removed. It took twenty years before Joseph Lister was able to approach Esdaile's 5 percent surgical mortality rate through the use of antisepsis techniques. It was more than a century before the Cornell research group, under direction of Harold Wolff, was able to demonstrate the basic reason for Esdaile's observations—the diminution of "neurokinin" release at the site of injury when painful stimuli to the brain were blocked through use of hypnotically suggested analgesia. The first experiments are reported in detail. His surgical results in those days of universally infected wounds before the advent of general anesthesia were not equalled anywhere in the world.

Haley, Jay (ed.). **Advanced Techniques of Hypnosis and Therapy: Selected Papers of Milton H. Erickson**. New York: Grune and Stratton, 1967.

As Haley explains in his introduction, this is a book that evolved over a ten-year period. It started with the desire of a young psychiatrist, Bernard E. Gorton, to collect all of Erickson's papers and supplement them with tape recordings. Gorton included André M. Weitzenhoffer, Jay Haley, and Milton Erickson himself in the effort. Gorton died tragically in 1959. Weitzenhoffer carried on with the project part of the way, but its completion took the devoted efforts of Jay Haley. This is a book for the experienced hypnotherapist, but it is also a valuable resource book for psychologists and psychiatrists who are ready to learn what one of the world's greatest observers has offered us with regard to human behavior. Erickson strives always to enhance the self-respect of his patients. He takes their behavior as offered and then works his magic.

The original goal of publishing all of Erickson's papers was dropped and only those that the editor felt to be most instructive were included.

Haley, Jay. **Uncommon Therapy: The Psychiatric Techniques of Milton H. Erickson**. New York: W. W. Norton, 1973.

The complex and sometimes bewildering art of Milton Erickson has been carefully and lucidly analyzed by Haley. The arrangement of chapters is structured around the evolution of the family with all of its many impingements on external forces. Haley's explanations are augmented by Erickson's own verbatim discussions of strategies used to help troubled people grow and function well in a complex world. This is not a "how-to-do-it" book. Only a clone of Erickson could do it his way. It will stimulate the reader, however, into thinking about human behavior in global terms rather than in the usually restricted clinical way.

Hilgard, Earnest, and Hilgard, Josephine. **Hypnosis in the Relief of Pain.** Los Altos: William Kaufmann, 1975.

The Hilgards are to be congratulated for gaining recognition for the fact that hypnosis can be used successfully in the treatment of pain states. Acupuncture has long been included in books and university-sponsored seminars on pain, but any mention of hypnosis has been hard to find. It is to be hoped that this book will remedy past oversights.

The authors report extensive laboratory experiments showing significant alleviation and control of pain through hypnotic suggestion. They have drawn attention to the "hidden observer," a part of the subject's awareness that is covertly aware of a pain stimulus, even though there is no overt sensation of discomfort. This "subconscious pain" may affect reactions to injury and conditioned hypersensitivity of tissues.

An exclusion that should be corrected in the next edition of this book is the omission of any reference to the monumental work by Harold Wolff's staff at Cornell, which showed that local inflammatory reaction is modulated by the highest nervous system centers through neurohumoral release of "neurokinin," an enzyme that is believed different from "bradykinin", the inflammatory enzyme released by local mild heat application to the skin (see Chapman, Goodell, and Wolff above). "Plasmin" or "fibrinolysin", as it is called in the United States, is another pain-producing enzyme not found in the text or index. It is the enzyme responsible for shock—and sometimes death—in fallopian pregnancies. It also causes the occasional severe pain of "mittleschmerz," when blood leaks into the abdominal cavity from a ruptured corpus luteum or follicle cyst of the ovary. On its constructive side fibrinolysin dissolves blood clots in vessels and lungs, but it seems to be the major factor in the disabling arthritis resulting from hemophilia. Fibrinolysin release seems also to be modulated by the action of higher nervous centers when subjects are under hypnosis.

Kroger, William S. **Clinical and Experimental Hypnosis**. Philadelphia: J. B. Lippincott, 1977.

Kroger, who started practice as an obstetrician in Chicago, is one of the pioneers in teaching and writing about the values of hypnosis. This updated edition of his 1963 book should be in the library of all those using hypnosis in the healing arts. He, like

Milechnin (see below), pays respect to the elaborate computer mechanisms of the limbic and reticular activating systems. Theoretical and clinical aspects of hypnosis are carefully considered, and the list of appropriate references is exhaustive. In addition, the author contributes from his own personal experience ways of stopping vomiting in pregnancy, terminating hemorrhage in obstetrical patients, and using hypnosis as the sole anesthetic for thyroidectomy and hysterectomy, among other possibilities.

Levinson, Bernard. **States of awareness under general anesthesia: primary communication.** *British Journal of Anesthesiology*, 1965. 37, 544–546.

As of 1978 this study made by an anesthesiologist-turned-psychiatrist is the only one that has used truly meaningful remarks as a test of ability to hear and remember while under the influence of a general anesthetic. Studies by other researchers all involved tape recordings of voices that were not pertinent to the tested patient, whose reticular activating system is trained on the voices of the anesthetist and the surgeons. "Stop the operation! I don't like the color of this patient. His lips are blue," were meaningful statements made by the anesthetist. Levinson was criticized by those who continued to believe anesthetized people cannot hear. However, four of Levinson's ten test patients recalled almost verbatim the remarks of the anesthetist. One recalled the expressed alarm of the surgeon over excessive bleeding during the operation. The remaining five patients could not be assessed because they either repressed the information or came out of hypnosis and refused to go over the experience. This was a retrospective study three weeks after surgery.

Milechnin, Anatol. **Hypnosis.** (Galena Solovey, trans). Bristol: Wright and Sons, 1967.

Hypnosis is treated in this book as a biological survival mechanism controlled through the limbic and reticular activating systems. The author draws parallels between human and animal hypnoticlike behavior at times of great emotional and physical stress and at times of food deprivation. This concept is shared by Volgyesi but is notably absent from the writings and considerations of most psychologists searching for meaning in nonmeaningful tests with volunteers "hypnotized" in nonthreatening circumstances. The 1967 edition contains a reprint of the author's classic report on the "Pavlovian syndrome"–hypnoticlike behavior observed under circumstances of privation in a German prison camp during World War II. Prisoners who were just beyond those who received a little food either became wild and irrational or collapsed in a faint. The references given in this book are excellent.

Volgyesi, Ferenc András. **Hypnosis of Man and Animals** (2nd ed., revised with Gerhard Klumbies). Baltimore: Williams and Wilkins, 1966.

Volgyesi was a physician in combat areas in both world wars. He was a student of Pavlov and a pioneer in extensive research with animals, ranging from lizards, crocodiles, swans, and owls, to primates of various sorts. The reader of this very special book will derive a broad view of hypnotic behavior not found in psychology classes or standard textbooks of hypnosis. The author looked on hypnosis as a multifaceted phenomenon involving shifting activation and inhibition of cerebral activity mediated through the primitive parts of the brain. The book is replete with photographic illustrations of methods and results with animals and humans.

Werbel, Ernest W. **One Surgeon's Experience with Hypnosis**. New York: Pageant Press, 1965.

The author, now a surgeon in San Luis Obispo, gives first-hand descriptions of his extensive experience with hypnosis since attending a course given by Leslie LeCron, Milton H. Erickson, and Aaron Moss early in 1954. The book contains helpful verbalizations used in preparing his patients for surgery and his uses of hypnosis in emergency situations. Werbel was among the first to demonstrate that postoperative hypnosis can permit painless recovery from hemorrhoidectomy. The author's background of training in malignant disease and general practice followed by specialty training in surgery in addition to active duty in the Pacific Theater in World War II (where he attained the rank of lieutenant colonel) lends authority to his observations.

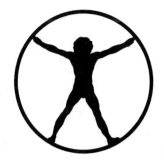

10

MEDITATION AND HOLISTIC MEDICINE

Deane H. Shapiro, Jr., Ph.D.

Reports of altered states of consciousness and extraordinary feats of bodily control by Zen and yoga masters have been filtering into the West for the past several decades. However, it is only within the last fifteen years that Western scientists and health care professionals have begun to look seriously at Eastern techniques, such as meditation, to determine their possible efficacy in mental and physical health-related matters. This interest in Eastern techniques has been spurred on by two different factors: (1) increased sophistication in scientific instrumentation that has made it possible to replicate and verify heretofore unsubstantiated reports, and (2) increased awareness of the need to find ways to help patients and clients develop more responsibility for their own lives and their own health care and to find nonpharmacological approaches to stress and tension management.

Out of this context, there has been an exponential increase in the number of studies looking at the potential psychotherapeutic, educational, and health-related benefits that may be obtained from the practice of meditation. In this chapter we will look briefly at what meditation is (and isn't), some of the specific research findings that have been reported when meditation is used as a self-regulation strategy, some of the research findings that have been reported when meditation is viewed as an altered state of consciousness, and finally, the areas of future research that seem important to explore (e.g., what are the negative effects of meditation, and who does meditation work best or least for?).

What is Meditation?

Meditation refers to a family of techniques that have in common a conscious attempt to focus attention. Sometimes attention is focused exclusively on one particular object (e.g., a candle or a mantra—a word, a picture of a teacher, the tip of the nose), and all other objects are excluded from awareness. This is called concentrative meditation. Sometimes attention is focused on no particular object, and the meditator tries to remain open to all stimuli in the internal and external environment. This is often referred to as "opening up" or "mindfulness" meditation. Both of these types of meditation have in common the fact that attention is focused in a nonanalytical, nonlogical way. An attempt is made to reduce discursive, ruminating thought.

These two types of meditation can be nicely contrasted by the results of two experiments, one that took place in India and one that took place in Japan. The study in India took place in the early 1960s with Raj yoga and illustrates the effects of concentrative meditation. Raj yogis, who meditate with their eyes closed, focus attention on the tip of their nose or the back of their skull. They were hooked up to equipment that monitored their brain-wave patterns. Soon after beginning meditation, alpha waves appeared in all four brain regions. Alpha waves are thought to be a sign that the individual is in a relaxed state. The experimenters then put the yogis' hands in cold water; there was no alpha blockage. In other words, the yogis did not feel the water because their attention was focused so completely on their object of concentration. The experimenters then administered the following types of external stimuli to the yogis: photic (strong light), auditory (loud banging noise), thermal (touching with a hot glass tube), and vibration (tuning fork). The experimenters note, "None of these stimuli produced any blockage of alpha activity when the yogis were in meditation" (Anand, Chhina, and Singh, 1961).

The study in Japan was done with Zen monks who practiced opening-up meditation (Kasamatsu and Hirai, 1966). As with the Raj yogis, soon after the onset of meditation (within fifty seconds), alpha waves were recorded in all brain regions. However, when a click sound was made, there was alpha blockage (i.e., the monks heard the click). Within two or three seconds, alpha resumed. The experimenters made the click sound twenty different times. Each time there was alpha blockage followed by a resumption of alpha. In other words, the Zen monks did not habituate to the stimuli and were able, in the words of Zen, to see the flower the five hundreth time as they saw it the first time. This, of course, presents a marked contrast to the results of the experiment with the Raj yogis, whose alpha waves showed no blockage even though very strong stimuli were presented.

Sometimes there are techniques of meditation that integrate elements of both concentrative and opening-up meditation. For example, a person may focus on his breathing (Zen meditation) or a mantra (transcendental meditation) but be willing to allow other thoughts to come up, watch those thoughts, and then return to the breathing (or mantra). In other words, he remains open to other stimuli but has an "anchor" that holds and focuses his attention.

Levels of Meditation

Meditation as a Self-Regulation Strategy

Western research has primarily focused upon meditation as a clinical self-regulation strategy. This research was initially interested in the physiological changes that occur during meditation. During the act of meditation itself, certain physiological changes have been rather consistently reported: reduced heart rate, decreased oxygen consumption, decreased blood pressure, increased skin resistance, and increased regularity and amplitude of alpha activity (Woolfolk, 1975; Davidson, 1976). Because the above parameters represent a state of quietness in the autonomic nervous system, it was suggested that meditation would be a useful self-regulation technique for relaxation training (Wallace, Benson, and Wilson, 1971). The clinical research has borne this out. In a recent review of the psychotherapeutic and health-related effects of meditation, it has been shown to be a promising clinical intervention strategy in (a) reducing stress and tension, (b) decreasing addictive behaviors, and (c) lowering blood pressure (Shapiro and Giber, 1978).

In the stress-related studies, meditators showed both subjective reports of decreased feelings of stress and anxiety as well as physiological indications based on the galvanic skin response (GSR) – that is, faster recovery time after a stressful stimulus (Goleman and Schwartz, 1976), faster habituation of GSR to tones, fewer multiple responses during habituation, and fewer spontaneous GSRs (Orme-Johnson, 1973). In studies of addictions, which have been conducted with both retrospective and longitudinal types of design, meditators consistently report a larger decrease of usage than nonmeditators for drugs ranging from alcohol and marijuana to LSD and heroin (Benson and Wallace, 1971; Shafii, Lavely, and Jaffe, 1975). Finally, with regard to the hypertension research, studies consistently indicate a reduction in blood pressure in the treatment group, a reduction in the use of hypertensive medication, and a reduction in reports of somatic symptoms (Patel, 1975; Stone and DeLeo, 1976). In addition, meditation seems to have potential psychotherapeutic value for the therapist – it helps the therapist become more open and receptive to the client's concerns (Lesh, 1970; Leung, 1973) – for patients in a psychiatric hospital (Glueck and Stroebel, 1975) and for patients with "psychoneurotic disorders" who seem resistant to other types of treatment (Vahia, Doongaji, and Jeste, 1973).

Meditation as an Altered State of Consciousness

Most research in the West has been carried out in laboratories and field settings with relatively short-term meditators. Further, Western research has looked almost exclusively at dependent variables related to meditation as a self-regulation strategy. It is important to note, however, that meditation was initially and originally conceived as a technique within a philosophical-religious context of the Eastern spiritual disciplines. It was a technique utilized primarily as a means for inducing altered states of consciousness, for changing an individual's ordinary perception of the world, and for developing a more intimate, unified, and accepting view of oneself, of nature, and of other people. The research literature on meditation as an altered state of consciousness suggests that there are, in fact, subjective phenomenological changes that occur during meditation, and they can range from relatively strong alterations in perception in short-term meditators (Deikman, 1969; Maupin, 1965) to more pronounced feelings of "self-transcendence," "felt meaning in the world," and "a heightened sense of con-nectedness with the world and with others, a sense of purpose and mean-ingfulness, deep positive emotion" (Osis, Bokert, and Carlson, 1973; Kohr, 1977). These very powerful subjective experiences have obvious implications for men-tal health because they influence the way individuals relate not only to themselves but also to other people and to the world around them.

There are many different types of meditation, and the research is not yet clear as to which type of meditation may be more appropriate for which in-dividual. Currently, we are doing research in our laboratory to determine whether individuals with certain strong representational systems (e.g., visual, auditory, tactile, etc.) would be better off with an object of meditation that either is or is not in that same representational system. Further, there is some question about whether individuals would be better off learning concentrative meditation versus mindfulness meditation or both, and if both, in which sequence. For those persons interested in learning meditation, the best advice is to pick the technique that feels most comfortable. This may involve a bit of experimentation, and it should be understood that there is no "right" technique. In the bibliography there are two books that provide instruction for different types of meditation (Benson, 1975; Shapiro, 1977) as well as two sets of taped instructions that individuals might find useful (Goleman, 1976; Shapiro, 1977). In addition to written or taped instructions, individuals may wish to choose a specific organization to teach them a particular system of meditation. This is not at all a bad idea. I often recommend that individuals contact organizations such as a transcendental meditation group (Student International Meditation Society). This group has the advantage of social support and instructors who can check to ensure that the meditation is going properly. For beginning instruction, this is certainly useful, although one must be cautious if any organization attempts to promote its par-ticular type of meditation as the one right path.

Summary and Future Research

As can be seen from the above discussion, meditation may be conceptualized as a self-regulation strategy for clinical and health-related problems. In addition, meditation may be conceptualized as an altered state of consciousness for inducing powerful subjective changes in one's view of one's self, of nature, and of other people (Shapiro, 1977). When meditation is conceptualized as a self-regulated strategy, it needs to be compared with other self-regulation strategies for its clinical effectiveness. Research suggests that there are several different relaxation techniques (e.g., hypnosis and deep muscle relaxation) that can produce the same physiological changes (Walrath and Hamilton, 1975; Curtis and Wessberg, 1975–1976; Morse et al., 1977; Benson, 1975) and the same clinical changes as meditation, whether it be in the area of anxiety reduction (Beiman et al., 1979; Smith, 1976) or alcohol consumption (Marlatt et al., in press).

Some researchers have argued that the kind of physiological measures that are being used in the studies cited above are not sufficiently sophisticated to ferret out the unique aspects of meditation as compared to other self-regulation strategies (Jevening and O'Halloran, 1979). From a clinical standpoint, some researchers are also saying that we need to discriminate more precisely between dependent variables, such as anxiety. For example, Davidson and Schwartz suggest that meditation might be useful for certain types of anxiety (cognitive anxiety), but not as useful for other types (somatic anxiety). The one study they have done in this area shows promising results (Schwartz, Davidson, and Goleman, 1978).

Other researchers are suggesting that not all aspects of the technique of meditation are equally important in its effectiveness and that a component analysis is necessary in order to determine the relative efficacy of different aspects. For example, how much of the effect of meditation is due to the expectation effects of the subjects (Smith, 1976) or to the demand characteristics of the teacher or training organization (Malec and Sipprelle, 1977)? How much of the effect of meditation is due to the various aspects of the behavior of meditation itself: for example, the attentional focus (Davidson, Goleman, and Schwartz, 1976), the posture (Ikegami, 1974), the mantra (Smith, 1976), or long-term adherence? Or how much of the effect of meditation is due to what happens after a person is finished meditating (e.g., saying to oneself, "I am a meditator, therefore I am more relaxed"), the feelings of increased self-responsibility and self-control, or the people that one meets and becomes involved with who are also meditators? Future research needs to be more precise about these different components and more precise about which type of self-regulation strategy is more effective with which type of clinical problem and with which type of individual (Beiman, et al., 1979; Otis, 1979; Smith, 1976). This evaluation should be made for those cases where meditation does not work as well as for those where it is effective.

Finally, in addition to being more precise, future research needs to be more visionary. It needs to look at the altered states of consciousness and profound subjective changes and experiences of long-term meditators. It should look at the life-style changes and the new vision of human potential toward which meditation and its philosophical and spiritual context can direct us.

References

Anand, B. K.; Chhina, E. S.; and Singh, B. Some aspects of electroencephalographic studies in yogis. *EEG and Clinical Neurophysiology*, 1961. **13**, 452–456.

Beiman, I.; Majestic, H.; Johnson, S. A.; Puente, A.; and Graham, L. E. Transcendental meditation versus behavior therapy: a controlled investigation. In D. Shapiro and R. Walsh (Eds.), *Meditation: Self-regulation Strategy and Altered State of Consciousness*. New York: Aldine, in press.

Benson, H. *The Relaxation Response*. New York: William Morrow, 1975.

Benson, H., and Wallace, R. K. Decreased drug abuse with transcendental meditation: a study of 1,862 subjects (U.S. House of Representatives, *Congressional Record*, Hearings before the Select Committee on Crime, Serial Number 92-1). Washington, D.C.: U.S. Government Printing Office, 1971.

Curtis, W. D., and Wessberg, H. W. A comparison of heart rate, respiration, and galvanic skin response among meditators, relaxers, and controls. *Journal of Altered States of Consciousness*, 1975–1976. **2 (4)**, 319–324.

Davidson, J. The physiology of meditation and mystical states of consciousness. *Perspectives in Biology and Medicine*, 1976. **19 (3)**, 345–379.

Davidson, R.; Goleman, D.; and Schwartz, G. Attentional and affective concomitants of meditation. *Journal of Abnormal Psychology*, 1976. **85**, 235–238.

Deikman, A. Experimental meditation. In C. Tart (Ed.), *Altered States of Consciousness*. New York: Wiley, 1969.

Glueck, D. C., and Stroebel, C. F. Biofeedback in meditation in the treatment of psychiatric illness. *Comprehensive Psychiatry*, 1975. **16 (4)**, 303–321.

Goleman, D. Meditation instructions. New York: *Psychology Today*, Cassette Department, 1976.

Goleman, D., and Schwartz, G. Meditation as an intervention in stress reactivity. *Journal of Clinical and Consulting Psychology*, 1976. **44 (3)**, 456–466.

Ikegami, R. Psychological study of Zen posture. *Bulletin of the Faculty of Literature, Kyushu University*, 1974. **5**, 105–135.

Jevening, R., and O'Halloran, D. Metabolic effects of transcendental meditation. In D. Shapiro and R. Walsh (Eds.), *Meditation: Self-regulation Strategy and Altered States of Consciousness*. New York: Aldine, in press.

Kasamatsu, A., and Hirai, T. An electroencephalographic study of Zen meditation. *Folia Psychiatria et Neurologica Japonica*, 1966. **20**, 315–336.

Kohr, R. Dimensionality in the meditative experience: a replication. *Journal of Transpersonal Psychology*, 1977. **9 (2)**, 193–203.

Lesh, T. Zen meditation and the development of empathy in counselors. *Journal of Humanistic Psychology*, 1970. **10**, 39–74.

Leung, P. Comparative effects of training in external and internal concentration on two counseling behaviors. *Journal of Counseling Psychology*, 1973. **20**, 227–234.

Malec, J., and Sipprelle, C. Physiological and subjective effects of Zen meditation and demand characteristics. *Journal of Consulting and Clinical Psychology*, 1977. **45 (2)**, 339–340.

Marlatt, Alan et al. Effects of meditation and relaxation training on alcohol abuse among male social drinkers. In Deane Shapiro and Roger Walsh (Eds.), *Meditation: Self-regulation Strategy and Altered State of Consciousness*. New York: Aldine, in press.

Maupin, E. Individual differences in response to a Zen meditation exercise. *Journal of*

Consulting Psychology, 1965. **29**, 139–145.

Morse, R.; Martin, J. S.; Furst, M. L.; and Dubin, L. L. A physiological and subjective evaluation of meditation, hypnosis, and relaxation. *Psychosomatic Medicine,* 1977. **39** (5), 304–324.

Orme-Johnson, D. Autonomic stability in transcendental meditation. *Psychosomatic Medicine,* 1973. **35** (4), 341–349.

Osis, K.; Bokert, E.; and Carlson, M. L. Dimensions of the meditative experience. *Journal of Transpersonal Psychology,* 1973. **5**, 109–135.

Otis, L. Adverse effects of transcendental meditation. In D. Shapiro and R. Walsh (Eds.), *Meditation: Self-regulation Strategy and Altered States of Consciousness.* New York: Aldine, in press.

Patel, C. H. Randomized control trial of yoga and biofeedback in management of hypertension. *Lancet,* 1975. **2**, 93–95.

Schwartz, G.; Davidson, R.; and Goleman, D. Patterning of cognitive and somatic processes in the self-regulation of anxiety: effects of meditation vs. exercise. *Psychosomatic Medicine,* 1978. **40** (4), 321–328.

Shafii, M.; Lavely, R.; and Jaffe, R. Meditation and the prevention of alcohol abuse. *American Journal of Psychiatry,* 1975. **132** (9), 942–945.

Shapiro, D. *Precision Nirvana.* Englewood Cliffs, N.J.: Prentice-Hall, 1977.

Shapiro, D., and Giber, D. Meditation and psychotherapeutic effects. *Archives of General Psychiatry,* 1978. **35**, 294–302.

Smith, J. Psychotherapeutic effects of transcendental meditation with controls for expectation of relief and daily sitting. *Journal of Consulting and Clinical Psychology,* 1976. **44** (4), 630–637.

Stone, R. A., and DeLeo, J. Psychotherapeutic control of hypertension. *The New England Journal of Medicine,* 1976. **294**, 80–84.

Vahia, N. S.; Doongaji, D. R.; and Jeste, D. V. Further explorations with a therapy based upon concepts of Patanjali in the treatment of psychiatric disorders. *Indian Journal of Psychiatry,* 1973. **15**, 32–37.

Wallace, R. K.; Benson, H.; and Wilson, A. F. A wakeful hypometabolic physiological state. *American Journal of Physiology,* 1971. **221** (3), 795–799.

Walrath, L., and Hamilton, D. Autonomic correlates of meditation and hypnosis. *The American Journal of Clinical Hypnosis,* 1975. **17** (3), 190–197.

Woolfolk, R. Physiological correlates of meditation. *Archives of General Psychiatry,* 1975. **32**, 1326–1333.

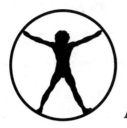 ANNOTATED BIBLIOGRAPHY

General Readings

Shapiro, D., and Walsh, R. **Meditation: Self-regulation Strategy and Altered State of Consciousness.** New York: Aldine, in press.

> This book brings together in one volume the major articles dealing with meditation as a self-regulation strategy (including stress management, addictions, hypertension, psychotherapeutic effects for the client, and effects for the therapist) as well as studies dealing with meditation as an altered state of consciousness. The collection includes physiological studies showing the changes occurring during meditation and a comparison of meditation with other self-regulation strategies. This is the most comprehensive, complete book on the subject to date.

Meditation

Benson, H. **The Relaxation Response.** New York: William Morrow, 1975.

> A useful book summarizing a meditationlike technique and describing the physiological changes that can occur with the practice of this technique.

Goleman, D. **The Varieties of the Meditative Experience.** New York: E. P. Dutton, 1977.

> A clear, well-written, nonbiased review of most of the major types of meditative practice. Goleman provides a clear introduction to different forms of meditation.

Naranjo, C., and Ornstein, R. **The Psychology of Meditation.** New York: Viking/Esalen, 1971.

> One of the first books to provide a Western psychological framework for understanding both the goals and the effects of meditation.

Shapiro, D. **Precision Nirvana.** Englewood Cliffs, N.J.: Prentice-Hall, 1978.

> This book describes both practical instructions for the practice of meditation as well

as the goals of meditation in terms of increased harmony with oneself, with others, and with nature. Certain chapters relate these Eastern goals to, and try to integrate them with, the goals of Western psychological health. Articles cited in the text are useful in providing further information about meditation – they are all reprinted in Shapiro and Walsh, *Meditation* (above).

General Reviews

Psychotherapeutic

Shapiro, D., and Giber, D. **Meditation and psychotherapeutic effects.** *Archives of General Psychiatry,* 1978. **35**, 294–302.

The most complete review of the therapeutic effects of meditation to date. The studies considered cover the effects of meditation on stress and tension; on addictions, hypertension, fears, and phobias; and on inducing altered states of consciousness. They also examine the concurrent validity for subjective changes and subjective reports of changes in attitudes and perceptions after meditation.

Smith, J. **Meditation as psychotherapy: a review of the literature.** *Psychological Bulletin,* 1975. **82**, 558–564.

A critical review that looks at some of the components of meditation, such as expectation effects and just sitting as possible explanations for the effects of meditation.

Physiological

Davidson, J. **The physiology of meditation and mystical states of consciousness.** *Perspectives in Biology and Medicine,* 1976. **19** (3), 345–379.

A very useful and informative review that not only looks at the physiological changes during meditation but also tries to come up with a theoretical explanation for the altered/mystical states of consciousness that meditation can sometimes induce.

Woolfolk, R. **Physiological correlates of meditation.** *Archives of General Psychiatry,* 1975. **32**, 1326–1333.

A review of the physiological effects of meditation in order to determine whether there are different types of physiological changes that occur with different types of meditation.

Comparison with Other Strategies

Davidson, R., and Goleman, D. **Meditation and hypnosis, a psycho-biological approach to the transformation of consciousness.** *International Journal of Clinical and Experimental Hypnosis,* 1977. **25** (4), 291–308.

An interesting article that compares the pre-state, and within-state, and after-state effects of meditation and hypnosis. It discusses the changes of consciousness that occur in meditation and in hypnosis and compares the two modalities.

Davidson, R., and Schwartz, G. **The psycho-biology of relaxation and related states: multi-process theory.** In D. I. Mostofsky (Ed.), *Behavioral Control and the Modification of Physiological Processes*. Englewood Cliffs, N.J.: Prentice-Hall, 1976.

> A very informative and useful review of the relaxation literature. It makes a primary distinction between cognitive anxiety and somatic anxiety and suggests a theoretical model to determine which types of self-regulation techniques may be most useful for which types of anxiety behavior.

Shapiro, D., and Zifferblatt, S. **Zen meditation and behavioral self-control: similarities, differences, and clinical applications.** *American Psychologist*, 1976. **31**, 519–532.

> A comparison of meditation and behavioral self-control strategies, both in terms of the actual procedures used (including the goals of the techniques) and the methods for possibly integrating the techniques in a treatment package.

How to Practice Meditation

Two books that give instructions on how to practice meditation are listed in the general readings: Herbert Benson's *The Relaxation Response* and Deane Shapiro's *Precision Nirvana*. In addition there are two tapes that give practical instruction for meditation that individuals may find helpful: Daniel Goleman (1976), "Meditation instructions," *Psychology Today*, Cassette Department, One Park Avenue, New York, New York; and Deane Shapiro (1977), "Instructions for the practice of meditation and behavioral self-control," in Cyril Frank's (Ed.), Behavior Therapy Tape Series, BMA Publications, available from IAHB-Media, P.O. Box 2288, Stanford, California 94305.

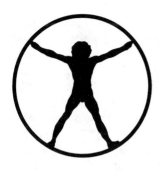

PSYCHIC HEALING

Stanley Krippner, Ph.D.

"Psychic healing" is used to describe incidents of physical healing that cannot be explained in purely medical, physical, or psychological terms, such as a surprisingly rapid rate of healing or a complete reversal of symptoms that is beyond medical expectations. Assignment to this category is generally restricted to cases in which a "healing" was performed by another individual (minister, shaman, medicine man, psychic, etc.), a nonphysical entity (deity, spirit), a group (prayer group, healing group, church group), or by the patient's presence at a place noted for miraculous cures (such as Lourdes). A wide variety of techniques is associated with psychic healing, including prayer, laying-on-of-hands, religious rituals, meditation, and psychic surgery.

While anecdotal accounts of psychic healing and miraculous cures date back to biblical times, attempts to rigorously document them have generally been inconclusive. See, for example, West (1957). Often the medical data before and after the healing are insufficient to eliminate alternative explanations, or the cured diseases are ones that are easily misdiagnosed or are known to have psychosomatic components. Still, there are many first-hand accounts by credible observers that, while not conclusive by current scientific standards, are impressive enough to suggest the need for further studies. These accounts include such cases as the spontaneous remission of cancer following a visit to a healer (Hintze and Pratt, 1975) and an unexplained growth of bone following a "healing service" (Fitzherbert, 1971). For further cases, see LeShan (1974) and Krippner and Villoldo (1976).

The strongest evidence of psychic healing comes from a small body of laboratory research, where the effects of suggestion are eliminated or at least minimized, baselines are established, before-and-after conditions are measured, control groups are used, and results are quantified. Measurable healing effects in controlled research designs with single- and double-blind conditions have been noted on plants (Grad, 1965), fungi (Barry, 1968), enzymes (Smith, 1972), and mice (Grad, 1965; Watkins and Watkins, 1971; Watkins, Watkins, and Wells, 1972; Wells and Klein, 1972). Working with humans, Krieger (1975) reports significant changes in hemoglobin values for a "healed" group (laying-on-of-hands) over a series of experiments. This list essentially exhausts the published laboratory research confirming psychic healing effects. These results must therefore be considered tentative, although they speak clearly of the need for major research efforts in this area.

While we await more definitive laboratory research, one thing at least is certain. Psychic healers, particularly in non-Western countries, provide a major holistic health-care resource for society, treating a wide variety of complaints with a combination of medicinal, psychological, and spiritual cures. These healers play a social role in situations where healing is expected. Furthermore, they are often part of a cultural group that contributes social support for their type of healing, providing an accessibility frequently lacking in orthodox medicine.

Some of the evidence suggests that careful study of psychic healers may lead us to a better understanding of healing processes in humans or may suggest ways in which to improve Western health care (Frank, 1973; LeShan, 1974). For example, touching the patient is common in psychic healing but rare in Western medicine, and there is evidence (Grad, 1965; Krieger, 1975; Smith, 1972) of beneficial effects of touch in healing. Two of the authors cited here, Krieger and LeShan, have experimented with training others to perform psychic healing (laying-on-of-hands and meditation) based upon their own studies of gifted healers. Here, too, we can only conclude that more research is needed to confirm their reported success. Frank also points out that even when the patient does not experience relief from physical disease, he or she often feels a sense of spiritual renewal after the healing.

We might infer that it would help any healing treatment to incorporate more physical touch in diagnosis and therapy, to find ways of communicating concern and healing intentions, and to promote the patient's belief and the clinician's belief in the efficacy of the healing process. Psychic healing effects in the laboratory appear not to be due to those factors alone, but they may be especially compatible with humanistic rather than technological contexts, and the increased use of these human psychological and support elements may promote healing beyond medical expectations.

References

Barry, Jean. General and comparative study of the psychokinetic effect on a fungus culture. *Journal of Parapsychology,* December 1968. **32 (4)**, 237–243.

Fitzherbert, Joan. The nature of hypnosis and paranormal healing. *Journal of the Society for Psychical Research,* 1971. **46**, 1–14.

Frank, Jerome D. *Persuasion and Healing: A Comparative Study of Psychotherapy* (Revised ed.). Baltimore: Johns Hopkins University Press, 1973. See Chapter 3, Nonmedical healings: religious and secular, 46–77.

Grad, Bernard. Some biological effects of the "Laying on of Hands": a review of experiments with animals and plants. *Journal of the American Society for Psychical Research,* April 1965. **59 (2)**, 95–126.

Hintze, Naomi, and Pratt, J. G. *The Psychic Realm: What Can We Believe?* New York: Random House, 1975.

Krieger, Dolores. Therapeutic touch: the imprimatur of nursing. *American Journal of Nursing,* May 1975. **75 (5)**, 784–787.

Krippner, Stanley, and Villoldo, Alberto. *The Realms of Healing.* Millbrae, Calif.: Celestial Arts, 1976.

LeShan, Lawrence. *The Medium, the Mystic and the Physicist.* New York: Viking Press, 1974.

Smith, M. J. Paranormal effects on enzyme activity through laying on of hands. *Human Dimensions,* Spring 1972. **1**, 15–19.

Watkins, Graham K., and Watkins, Anita M. Possible PK influence on the resuscitation of anesthetized mice. *Journal of Parapsychology,* December 1971. **35 (4)**, 257–272.

Watkins, Graham K.; Watkins, Anita M.; and Wells, Roger A. Further studies on the resuscitation of anesthetized mice. In W. G. Roll, R. L. Morris, and J. D. Morris (Eds.), *Research in Parapsychology, 1972.* Metuchen, N. J.: The Scarecrow Press, 1973. 157–159.

Wells, Roger, and Klein, Judith. A replication of a "psychic healing" paradigm. *Journal of Parapsychology,* June 1972. **36 (2)**, 1944–1949.

West, D. J. *Eleven Lourdes Miracles.* London: Duckworth, 1957.

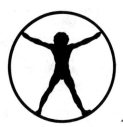 ANNOTATED BIBLIOGRAPHY

In the following bibliography, the articles included constitute the majority of the published experimental evidence for psychic healing. Additional conceptual support can be found in numerous studies of psychokinesis (or telekinesis) on living organisms in the *Journal of Parapsychology*, College Station, Durham, North Carolina 27708, and the *Journal of the American Society for Psychical Research*, 5 West 73rd St., New York, New York 10023. The mice experiments are the most interesting for establishing an effect on a complex organism (Grad; Watkins and Watkins; Watkins, Watkins, and Wells; Wells and Klein), the last three cited are particularly interesting since the healings were done at a distance and some interesting "lag effects" were noted after systematically varying the conditions. The Krieger article is notable for the reproducibility across experiments and for the implication that healing ability may be widespread in humans.

For a more general look at the scientific problems and possibilities posed by psychic healing, the Fosshage and Olsen volume is excellent. Krippner and Villoldo give a valuable critical examination of a variety of psychic healers around the world as well as a detailed discussion of building a theory (partially reproduced in Fosshage and Olsen). LeShan and Frank have both identified some common features of psychic healing that may be valuable to Western psychotherapists and medical personnel.

Barry, Jean. **General and comparative study of the psychokinetic effect on a fungus culture.** *Journal of Parapsychology*, December 1968. **32 (4)**, 237–243.

In this French experiment to "discover the effect of thought on the growth of a fungus," subjects tried to inhibit fungus growth in experimental petri dishes containing *Rhizoetonia solani* from a distance of 1.5 meters, while attempting to ignore the control dishes. Since this polyphagous parasite causes disease, the experiment is relevant to healing. The results, assessed by weighing paper tracings of each of the colonies by a naive assistant, showed the experimental dishes to have less growth than the controls thirty-three out of a total of thirty-nine trials, suggesting a definite influence by the subjects.

Fitzherbert, Joan. **The nature of hypnosis and paranormal healing.** *Journal of the Society for Psychical Research,* 1971. **46**, 1–14.

The author, a psychoanalyst, investigated the results of a "healing service" in Great Britain and found two cases of apparent paranormal healing: an instantaneous disappearance of a inoperable goiter, and the instantaneous growth of a piece of bone.

Fosshage, James L., and Olsen, Paul (Eds.). **Healing: Implications for Psychotherapy.** New York: Human Sciences Press, 1978.

This is currently the best available, up-to-date summary of psychological components of healing. The first section of this book, "Psychic Healing: Research, Theory and Practice," is a well-balanced account of psychic healing practices from three different perspectives. Jerome Frank provides the opening essay, drawing on his work with psychotherapy and placebo effects (see the review of his *Persuasion and Healing* below) and giving an excellent account of the problems of using traditional scientific methodology to study psychic healing. He encourages continued research on the work of healers and healings to achieve better understanding of the healing processes, but he is pessimistic of ever absolutely establishing the existence of the "healing power" in which he himself personally believes.

The second contribution presents the parapsychological point of view. Stanley Krippner reviews a wide variety of topics, from the role of models in science through healings associated with hypnosis and biofeedback, as well as electrically stimulated limb regeneration in amphibians and possible applications of psychic healing in the Western setting. He illustrates three models of the person—physical, psychological, and psychic—and describes how each one "explains" healing. This is a good overview of the frontiers within a frontier science and, although quite speculative at times, it gives the reader much to think about. Like Frank, Krippner is aware of the problems of sleight-of-hand (which some well-meaning healers use to reinforce their patients' belief systems) and the paucity of solid research to date, but he portrays a more optimistic view for research in the future.

The section ends with an article by Joyce Goodrich, a healer/researcher, who outlines the development and theoretical framework of Lawrence LeShan's training program for healers. This article, in contrast to the first two, is rich in anecdotal accounts, drawn from the author's personal experiences as a healee, healer, and researcher of paranormal healing. No attempt is made to establish the existence of psychic healing; indeed she, like Frank, questions whether this is possible. Nevertheless many research questions are raised here, some of them pointed toward testing the model on which LeShan's training is based. The main ideas, based upon subjective experiences with LeShan healing, are: (1) healing ability is natural in humans, probably varying only in degree; (2) it can be developed through training and practice; and (3) much research needs to be done to gain an understanding of this type of healing so that its potential may be realized and so that it may become a useful adjunct to Western medicine.

Frank, Jerome D. **Nonmedical healings: religious and secular.** Chapter 3 in Jerome D. Frank, *Persuasion and Healing: A Comparative Study of Psychotherapy* (Revised ed.). Baltimore: The Johns Hopkins University Press, 1973.

Frank presents an overview of a variety of healing practices that lie outside of the scientifically based medicine of Western society, including shamanistic healing in so-called primitive societies, religious healing in Western society, and some secular approaches like homoeopathy, osteopathy, and faith healing. The focus is on the shared features of these practices, particularly those that illuminate aspects of human functioning that are relevant to psychotherapy. Descriptions of shamanistic healing ceremonies and the Lourdes miracle healings are presented as illustrations of the mobilization of healing forces through the arousal of hope, emotional stirring, and strengthening ties with a supportive group – a process which may itself be at the core of the physical healing that takes place. On the topic of psychic healing, Frank finds compelling the evidence "that some healers serve as a kind of a conduit for a healing force in the universe, often called a life force, that, for want of a better term, must be called supernatural."

Grad, Bernard. **Some biological effects of the "laying on of hands": a review of experiments with animals and plants.** *Journal of the American Society for Psychical Research,* April 1965. **59 (2)**, 95–126.

Wounds were inflicted on 300 female mice by cutting an oval of skin, approximately 0.4×0.8 inches, from their backs. The mice were assigned to groups of three according to the size of their wounds, and the groups were then randomly assigned to one of three treatment procedures: (1) treatment E, in which a gifted healer (Mr. E) held the caged mice between his hands for fifteen minutes twice daily, five hours apart; (2) treatment M, in which different individuals (medical students) held the caged mice between their hands each day as in the E treatment; or (3) treatment O in which the caged mice were allowed to rest undisturbed on a table during treatment periods. "Healers" were allowed to hold half their charges in an open bag directly between their hands; the rest of the mice were held in a closed bag. The animals were housed in ten rooms (randomized blocks) in racks segregated by treatment group, with caretakers blind to the groups. Wounds were traced and measured by planimetry on a fixed schedule. Analysis of variance showed significant treatment effects (no interactions) on days fifteen and sixteen for the open-bag condition. The wounds of the E treatment group were significantly smaller than those of the M or O treatment groups and the contrast between M and O was insignificant. Heterogeneity of variances made it impossible to compare the closed-bag condition with the open-bag condition.

Following this, a series of plant experiments was conducted in which twenty-four peat pots containing twenty barley seeds each were watered with a saline solution, dried for forty-eight hours, and then set out in a room where they were watered every other day for thirteen days. Half of the pots, randomly assigned and blind to the caretakers, were initially watered with saline solution that had been "treated" by the laying-on-of-hands (fifteen minutes) by a gifted healer, Mr. E, while the other half received untreated saline solution. There were significant differences between the groups in the predicted direction with regard to the number of plants, average height of plants, and total yield (height). Five more experiments followed, all of which showed significant effects in the predicted direction. Spectrophotometer analysis showed differences in the transmission spectra (between 3,000 and 2,800 millicrons) of the control versus the treated saline solutions in the last three experiments. The authors attribute these significant treatment effects to some influence of Mr. E, which resulted in an increased healing rate in the animals and improved growth rate in the plants treated by him.

Hintze, Naomi, and Pratt, J. G. **The Psychic Realm: What Can We Believe?** New York: Random House, 1975.

This collaboration between Pratt, a leading parapsychologist, and Hintze, a popular author, includes a discussion of psychic healing that presents some cases of apparently paranormal healing and suggests that psi (parapsychological factors) may play some role in them.

Krieger, Dolores. **Therapeutic touch: the imprimatur of nursing.** *American Journal of Nursing,* May 1975. **75,** 784–787.

After a brief history of the laying-on-of-hands and a summary of recent scientific work, the author, a professor of nursing at New York University, describes a series of experiments she conducted in which she repeatedly found significant increases in blood hemoglobin values in human patients after a laying-on-of-hands treatment by healers. Control groups have shown no such changes. A pilot, a confirmatory study, and a third study that controlled for possible intervening variables (exercise, smoking, etc.) all showed significant effects from a gifted laying-on-of-hands healer. In a fourth study, selected nurses were trained to act as healers using therapeutic touch through laying-on-of-hands, and again there were significant increases in the hemoglobin values of the experimental group as compared to the control group. The author believes the requisite healing ability for effecting these changes is natural and widespread among humans. In some of these experiments, the hands were not physically touching the patient but were simply held near the person.

Krippner, Stanley, and Villoldo, Alberto. **The Realms of Healing.** Millbrae, Calif.: Celestial Arts, 1976.

The authors present the results of their extensive studies of "paranormal" healers in North America, Brazil, Peru, Czechoslovakia, and the Philippines. Detailed, frank accounts of their observations of healings performed on themselves and others are provided in an objective manner. The background, development, and belief system of each of the healers is explored, making this a rich overview of these phenomena. There is a brief review of laboratory research supporting psychic healing, and the last chapter provides a lengthy discussion (partially reproduced in the Fosshage and Olsen volume) of how these phenomena might be investigated and incorporated within a scientific framework. This is a commentary on the frontiers of our knowledge of the healing processes—physical, psychological, and psychic—and how they may eventually be united. To this end, the authors discuss E. H. Walker's quantum mechanical theory of consciousness and its implications for understanding psychic healing.

LeShan, Lawrence. **The Medium, the Mystic and the Physicist.** New York: Viking Press, 1974.

LeShan, a medical psychologist, outlines the rudiments of a general theory of the paranormal based on what he calls the "clairvoyant reality," a state in which time and space are no longer limits on knowing. In Chapter 7, he describes how he tested this model by training himself to heal by going into the clairvoyant reality. He distinguishes between "type-one" healing, in which the healer places himself or herself into a condition of "oneness" with the universe together with the healee, and "type-two" healing, in which there is a "laying-on-of-hands" or "healing energy" directed or channeled to the healee. He includes qualitative accounts of a number of case histories that compelled him to believe that healing was aided in some of the cases. This is a clear, detailed, critical exposition of his experiences and observations with psychic healing, valuable for the distinctions he draws between "type-one" and "type-two" healings. It will be of interest to psychotherapists and physicians who wish to explore these techniques for their own practices.

Smith, M. J. **Paranormal effects on enzyme activity through laying on of hands.** *Human Dimensions,* Spring 1972. **1**, 15–19.

A report of a double-blind study in which four aliquots of the enzyme trypsin were divided into the following treatments: (1) "wounding" by high ultraviolet rays followed by seventy-five minutes per day of laying-on-of-hands by a gifted healer, Mr. E.; (2) laying-on-of-hands by Mr. E; (3) exposure to a high magnetic field (which is known to increase enzyme activity level); and (4) no treatment. Conditions 2 and 3 showed similar patterns of increased enzyme activity levels, while Condition 1 showed smaller increases in the daily activity level. Working with the enzymes nicotinamide-adenine dinucleotide (NA) and amylase-amylose, Smith noted significant decreases in the first enzyme and no change in the second after laying-on-of-hands; both results were predicted as being beneficial to their functions in the human body.

Watkins, Graham K., and Watkins, Anita M. **Possible PK influence on the resuscitation of anesthetized mice.** *Journal of Parapsychology,* December 1971. **35** (4), 257–272.

A series of three experiments was run in which pairs of mice (one pair per trial, fifteen trials per experiment) were simultaneously rendered unconscious in identical etherizers, after which a human subject (nine "talented" psychics and three "non-talented" persons) attempted to mentally influence one of them to awaken more quickly, while the other mouse served as control. In Experiment 1, the experimental mouse and healer were in one room, the control mouse in another. In Experiment 2, experimental and control mice were brought into the same room and placed on a table divided by a screen so that the healer could see only the experimental mouse. Both experiments produced significantly shorter resuscitation times for the experimental versus the control mice. In Experiment 3, the healer was placed outside the room and viewed the mice through a one-way glass. Significantly shorter resuscitation times were found in six of these fifteen trials (no difference on the others) for the experimental group. The effects were also correlated with one particular person who timed the revival of the mice and with the left side of the table. While a timing bias could have inflated the striking results of the first two experiments, Experiment 3 (particularly the last four runs) points toward a psychokinetic influence by either experimenter or healer on the resuscitation of the mice.

Watkins, Graham K.; Watkins, Anita M.; and Wells, Roger A. **Further studies on the resuscitation of anesthetized mice.** In W. G. Roll, R. L. Morris, and J. D. Morris (Eds.), *Research in Parapsychology, 1972.* Metuchen, N.J.: The Scarecrow Press, 1973.

A summary of the results of seven series of experiments involving the basic procedure of simultaneously etherizing two mice per trial and placing them on a table, one on each side, while a "healer" concentrates on one of the mice (predesignated, unknown to the experimenters) from behind a one-way mirror in an attempt to accelerate resuscitation. The results are impressive—the first two series show significantly faster resuscitation for the experimental mice. In the third series, which used "nontalented" healers, chance results were obtained, but significant relationships were noted between the resuscitation time differential and two factors from an attitude questionnaire. The next two studies again yielded significantly accelerated resuscitation times for target mice, as well as significant physiological arousal states in the healers (especially in successful ones) during the sessions. The final two series showed evidence of a "lag" or "position" effect where an apparent healing influence on one trial continued to have an effect in the next trial for the same side of the table.

Wells, Roger, and Klein, Judith. **A replication of a "psychic healing" paradigm.** *Journal of Parapsychology,* June 1972. **36 (2)**, 1944–1949.

This is a direct replication of the Watkins and Watkins study involving two different experimenters (one of them not experienced in parasychological research) at the same laboratory. Anita Watkins selected the pairs of mice to be used for each trial, remaining throughout the experiments in the mouse colony room. Her presence raises the possibility of a parapsychological (psychokinetic or precognitive) experimenter effect. Eight 24-trial experiments were run with various groups (or solos) of four previously tested "talented" healers. Seven of the eight experiments showed faster resuscitation time differences for the target mice, two of the times being statistically significant. The total 192 trials had a mean difference of 5.52 seconds revival time between target and control mice, which while significant is less so than Experiment 3 of the Watkins and Watkins study on which this study was modeled.

West, D. J. **Eleven Lourdes Miracles.** London: Duckworth, 1957.

West presents a detailed examination of some purportedly miraculous cures taken from the records of the Lourdes Bureau. Taking the approach of a scientist looking closely at the facts to see what they suggest, West finds the evidence paltry at best, with most of the cures being explainable in terms of suggestion, placebo effects, misdiagnosis, and inadequate reporting. This little volume contains a great deal of interesting information about the history of Lourdes and previous attempts to validate the reports of cures, as well as some insight into the problems of studying healing from clinical case histories.

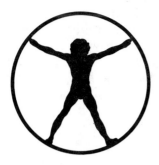

12

THE PLACEBO EFFECT:
A NEGLECTED ASSET
IN THE CARE OF PATIENTS

Herbert Benson, M.D., and Mark D. Epstein

The placebo effect is a neglected and berated asset of patient care. As new health care delivery systems evolve, it is imperative that we recognize the value of the placebo effect so that provisions can be made for its incorporation and proper use. Any health care system that minimizes or fragments the relationship between the physician and the patient will lessen the effects of this asset to health care.

Disdain for the placebo effect is the prevalent attitude in medicine today. However, throughout the history of medicine—at least until the nineteenth century—the placebo effect was the most a physician was able to offer his patients (Lesse, 1962; Shapiro, 1964), and it was relied on to maintain the physician's reputation. Despite patients' submission to "purging, puking, poisoning, puncturing, cutting, cupping, blistering, bleeding, leeching, heating, freezing, sweating, and shocking," the doctor or healer managed to retain his respected position throughout the ages (Shapiro, 1964). Although medicine has since developed therapies based on valid scientific data, there is little reason to assume that the placebo effect is no longer operative.

The disdain for the placebo effect became prominent in medicine with the

Reprinted with permission from the *Journal of the American Medical Association*, June 23, 1975. **232**, 1225–1227. Copyright 1975, American Medical Association.

introduction of controlled drug investigations in the 1950s. These investigations recognized the potency of the placebo and established controls for it. However, most investigations failed to assess the placebo effect itself as a therapeutic intervention, for they did not incorporate nontreatment controls. In the effort to quantify the effects of active drugs, most investigators have eliminated the placebo effect itself, ignoring its often remarkable benefits. Drugs yielding beneficial results similar to those of a placebo are rejected as being ineffective. The placebo effect is considered merely as a variable to be controlled and hence is ignored.

Definition

The significance of the placebo has been minimized by such narrow definitions as "an active substance or preparation given to satisfy the patient's symbolic need for drug therapy and used in controlled studies to determine the efficacy of medicinal substances. Also, a procedure with no intrinsic therapeutic value, performed for such purposes" (*Dorland's Illustrated Medical Dictionary*, 1974). Recognizing the potential benefits of nonspecific factors in any treatment, Shapiro (1964) has adopted a broader view of the placebo and its effects. He defines the placebo as

> any therapeutic procedure (or that component of any therapeutic procedure) which is given deliberately to have an effect, or unknowingly has an effect on a patient, symptom, syndrome, or disease, but which is objectively without *specific* activity for the condition being treated. The therapeutic procedure may be given with or without conscious knowledge that the procedure is a placebo, may be an active (non-inert) or nonactive (inert) procedure, and includes, therefore, all medical procedures no matter how specific – oral and parenteral medication, topical preparations, inhalants, and mechanical, surgical and psychotherapeutic procedures. The placebo must be differentiated from the placebo effect which may or may not occur and which may be favorable or unfavorable. The placebo effect is defined as the changes produced by placebos. The placebo is also used to describe an adequate control in research.

The Placebo Effect in Various Diseases

The existence of the placebo effect in the treatment of a variety of diseases is well-substantiated, although it is unknown how much of the effect attributed to the placebo is in fact due to spontaneous changes in the disease process. Chronic diseases have far more frequently been the subject of investigations employing placebos than have acute diseases for which specific treatments are available. This has led some (Bourne, 1971) to hypothesize that placebos are optimally effective in the treatment of chronic diseases, a conclusion for which there is little experimental evidence.

Reactions to placebos may involve practically any organ system in the body. For example, placebos have provided relief in cases of angina pectoris (Amsterdam, Wolfson, and Gorlin, 1969; Evans and Hoyle, 1933) rheumatoid and degenerative arthritis (Traut and Passarelli, 1957), pain (Beecher, 1955), hayfever (Baldwin, 1954), headache (Beecher, 1955), cough (Gravenstein, Devloo, and Beecher, 1954), peptic ulcer (Bäckman, Kalliola, and Östling, 1960), and essential hypertension (Grenfell, Briggs, and Holland, 1963). In a review of fifteen studies (including seven of his own), Beecher (1955) found that an average of 35.2 percent $\pm$ 2.2 percent of 1,082 patients investigated benefited from placebo treatment. Positive reports of placebo effects in the treatment of anxiety and depression have been prevalent. With placebo treatment, psychiatric patients' anxiety and tension decrease (Bourne, 1971; Uhlenhuth, Canter, Neustadt et al., 1959), their depression is alleviated (Malitz and Kanzler, 1971), and even patients with schizophrenia respond positively (Hankoff, Engelhardt, and Freedman, 1960). A comparison of supportive psychotherapy and placebo therapy for a group of patients mainly diagnosed as psychoneurotics showed a similar lessening of symptoms (Gliedman, Nash, Imber et al., 1958). In fact, supportive psychotherapy has been depicted as being quite similar to the placebo effect (Rosenthal and Frank, 1956).

The Doctor-Patient Relationship

The placebo effect seems to be derived from a combination of factors involving the patient, the physician, and the relationship between the two. A meaningful doctor-patient interaction is of utmost importance, allowing the transfer of the patient's concerns to an acknowledged scientist and healer, the physician (Shapiro, 1964). The placebo effect is not merely the result of taking an inert medication; it may commence before the actual administration of a pill (Nash, Frank, Imber et al., 1964), which illustrates the significance of the entire doctor-patient interaction. If the patient reacts adversely to a therapeutic encounter, symptoms can be exacerbated and side effects manifested by anxiety can be observed (Shapiro, 1964; Wolf, 1950).

The psychological state of the patient affects his response to both active and nonactive drugs (von Felsinger, Lasagna, and Beecher, 1955). The higher the level of patient concern and the greater the discomfort, the more likely it is that relief from a placebo will occur (Nash, Frank, Imber et al., 1964; Beecher, 1956; Beecher, 1960). Moreover, patients' expectations and convictions of the efficacy of treatment exert strong influences on the amount of relief afforded by a placebo (Liberman, 1962; Rosenthal and Frank, 1956; Wolf, 1950). "The largest number of possible placebo reactions are obtained in those patients who manifest an unreserved desire for and expectancy that relief from particular signs and symptoms will occur as the result of a specific drug or procedure" (Lesse, 1962).

The milieu in which drugs are given may also affect the patient's response to therapeutic treatment (Chessick, McFarland, Clark et al., 1966). The act of going to a physician to receive treatment or removing the patient from the surroundings in which he has been ill can beneficially affect the illness (Gliedman, Gantt, and Teitelbaum, 1954). "The doctor's reasonable hope for cure rests on making such environmental changes as will alter the emotional status of his patient. The environmental factor of most moment is likely to be the physician himself" (Houston, 1938). The type of therapeutic situation influences receptivity to treatment (Klerman, 1963). Also, a nontherapeutic, investigative situation may have positive effects. Improvement in up to 80 percent of schizophrenic patients has been found in response to the increased attention provided by a special research unit (Rashkis and Smarr, 1957). This phenomenon is similar to what has become known in the industry as the "Hawthorne effect" (Roethlisberger and Dickson, 1961), whereby the efficiency of factory workers was found to improve as a direct result of the increased attention received during investigation.

In addition to the attitudes, expectancies, hopes, and fears that a patient brings with him into any therapeutic encounter, the physician also exerts a profound influence on the course of treatment as a result of his own biases, attitudes, expectancies, and methods of communication. Physicians who have faith in the efficacy of their treatments allow that enthusiasm to be communicated, have strong expectations of specific effects, are self-confident and attentive, and are the most successful in producing positive placebo effects (Lesse, 1962; Wheatley, 1967). The length of time spent with the patient (Bogdanoff, Nichols, Klein et al., 1965) and the demeanor of the physician (Kast and Loesch, 1959; Shapiro, 1970) are pertinent factors.

Both the physician and the patient contribute to the placebo effect, but their actual interaction is probably most responsible for the effect (Houston, 1938; Bogdanoff, Nichols, Klein et al., 1965). "There can be no doubt that the placebo derives its power from the vast potential of the emotion relationship between the omnipotent physician and the needs of the patient" (Fischer and Dlin, 1956). In order for the nonspecific effects to be maximized, there must be congruence between the doctor's approach to therapy and the patient's attitudes toward illness and expectations from treatment (Freedman, Engelhardt, Hankoff et al., 1958). When that congruence is lacking, no favorable placebo effects are observed (Hankoff, Engelhardt, and Freedman, 1960). When the patient is able to freely express his emotions, especially during the taking of the history, it allows the doctor to understand the important developmental and situational highlights of the patient's life, thus establishing a satisfying and helpful doctor-patient relationship (Bogdanoff, Nichols, Klein et al., 1965).

Comment

As I have noted, in recent years the placebo effect has been viewed with disdain because of the way it is used in controlled drug trials to test the efficacy of new drugs. Yet, if a placebo and the tested new medication produce equally positive effects, does it make sense to report the nonspecificity of the medication and disregard both the medication and the placebo? Since the beneficial effect is the desired result, should not the placebo effect be further investigated so that we might better explain its worthwhile consequences? For example, the physiology of the placebo effect remains a relatively unexplored area (Wolf, 1950). There are substantiated, specific physiologic changes associated with the placebo effect that await further definition.

Patient and physician attitudes that create a sound doctor-patient relationship contribute to the production of the placebo effect. The placebo effect in most instances enhances the well-being of the patient and thus is an essential aspect of medicine. The growing trend toward decreasing doctor-patient contact (for example, through the use of computer facilities for obtaining histories) should be viewed critically. More emphasis on the potency of the placebo and its positive effects is needed. Research and instruction of efficient methods of establishing the appropriate doctor-patient relationship conducive to the placebo effect should be initiated (Werner and Schneider, 1974). The placebo effect demands greater study and must be allowed to survive if medicine is to provide optimal care for patients.

References

Amsterdam, E. A.; Wolfson, S.; and Gorlin, R. New aspects of the placebo response in angina pectoris. *American Journal of Cardiology*, 1969. **24**, 305–306.

Bäckman, H.; Kalliola, H.; and Östling, G. Placebo effect in peptic ulcer and other gastroduodenal disorders. *Gastroenterologia*, 1960. **94**, 11–20.

Baldwin, H.S. How to evaluate a new drug. *American Journal of Medicine*, 1954. **17**, 722–727.

Beecher, Henry K. The powerful placebo. *Journal of the American Medical Association*, 1955. **159**, 1602–1606.

Beecher, Henry K. Evidence for increased effectiveness of placebos with increased stress. *American Journal of Physiology*, 1956. **187**, 163–169.

Beecher, Henry K. Increased stress and effectiveness of placebos and "active" drugs. *Science*, 1960. **132**, 91–92.

Bogdanoff, M. D.; Nichols, C. R.; Klein, R. F. et al. The doctor-patient relationship. *Journal of the American Medical Association*, 1965. **192**, 45–48.

Bourne, H. R. The placebo – a poorly understood and neglected therapeutic agent. *Rational Drug Therapy*, 1971. **5**, 1–6.

Chessick, R. D.; McFarland, R. L.; Clark, R. K. et al. The effect of morphine, chlorpromazine, pentobarbital, and placebo in anxiety. *Journal of Nervous Mental Disorders*, 1966. **141**, 540–548.

Dorland's Illustrated Medical Dictionary. Philadelphia: W. B. Saunders, 1974.

Evans, W., and Hoyle, C. The comparative value of drugs used in the continuous treatment of angina pectoris. *Quarterly Journal of Medicine*, 1933. **2**, 311–338.

Fischer, H. K., and Dlin, B. M. The dynamics of placebo therapy: a clinical study. *American Journal of Medical Science*, 1956. **232**, 504–512.

Freedman, N.; Engelhardt, D. M.; Hankoff, L. D. et al. Drop-out from outpatient psychiatric treatment. *Archives of Neurological Psychiatry*, 1958. **80**, 657–666.

Gliedman, L. H.; Gantt, W. H.; and Teitelbaum, H. A. Some implications of conditional reflex studies for placebo research. *American Journal of Psychiatry*, 1954. **113**, 1103–1107.

Gliedman, L. H.; Nash, E. H.; Imber, S. D. et al. Reduction of symptoms by pharmacologically inert substances and by short-term psychotherapy. *Archives of Neurological Psychiatry*, 1958. **79**, 345–351.

Gravenstein, J. S.; Devloo, R. A.; and Beecher, H. K. Effect of antitussive agents on experimental and pathological cough in man. *Journal of Applied Psychology*, 1954. **7**, 119–139.

Grenfell, R. F.; Briggs, A. H.; and Holland, W. C. Antihypertensive drugs evaluated in a controlled double-blind study. *Southern Medical Journal*, 1963. **56**, 1410–1416.

Hankoff, L. D.; Engelhardt, D. M.; and Freedman, N. Placebo response in schizophrenic outpatients. *Archives of General Psychiatry*, 1960. **2**, 43–52.

Houston, W. R. The doctor himself as a therapeutic agent. *Annals of Internal Medicine*, 1938. **11**, 1416–1425.

Kast, E. C., and Loesch, J. A contribution to the methodology of clinical appraisal of drug action. *Psychosomatic Medicine*, 1959. **21**, 228–234.

Klerman, G. L. Assessing the influence of the hospital milieu upon the effectiveness of psychiatric drug therapy: problems of conceptualization and of research methodology. *Journal of Nervous and Mental Diseases*, 1963. **137**, 143–154.

Lesse, S. Placebo reactions in psychotherapy. *Diseases of the Nervous System*, 1962. **23**, 313–319.

Liberman, R. An analysis of the placebo phenomenon. *Journal of Chronic Diseases*, 1962. **15**, 761–783.

Malitz, S., and Kanzler, M. Are antidepressants better than placebo? *American Journal of Psychiatry*, 1971. **127**, 1605–1611.

Nash, E. H.; Frank, J. D.; Imber, S. D. et al. Selected effects of inert medication on psychiatric outpatients. *American Journal of Psychotherapy*, 1964. Supplement **1**, 33–48.

Rashkis, H. A., and Smarr, E. R. Psychopharamacotherapeutic research: a triadistic approach. *Archives of Neurological Psychiatry*, 1957. **77**, 202–209.

Roethlisberger, F. J., and Dickson, W. J. *Management and the Worker.* Cambridge, Mass.: Harvard University Press, 1961.

Rosenthal, D., and Frank, J. D. Psychotherapy and the placebo effect. *Psychological Bulletin*, 1956. **53**, 294–301.

Shapiro, A. K. Factors contributing to the placebo effect: their implications for psychotherapy. *American Journal of Psychotherapy*, 1964. **18**, 73–88.

Shapiro, A. K. Placebo effects in psychotherapy and psychoanalysis. *Journal of Clinical Pharmacology*, 1970. **10**, 73–78.

Traut, E. F., and Passarelli, E. W. Placebos in the treatment of rheumatoid arthritis and other rheumatic conditions. *Annals of Rheumatic Diseases*, 1957. **16**, 18–21.

Uhlenhuth, E. H.; Canter, A.; Neustadt, J. O. et al. The symptomatic relief of anxiety with meprobamate, phenobarbital and placebos. *American Journal of Psychiatry*, 1959. **115**, 905–910.

von Felsinger, J. M.; Lasagna, L.; and Beecher, H. K. Drug-induced mood changes in man:

2. Personality and reactions to drugs. *Journal of American Medical Association,* 1955. **157**, 1113–1119.

Werner, A., and Schneider, J. M. Teaching medical students interactional skills: a research-based course in the doctor-patient relationship. *New England Journal of Medicine,* 1974. **290**, 1232–1237.

Wheatley, D. Influence of doctors' and patients' attitudes in treatment of neurotic illness. *Lancet,* 1967. **2**, 1133–1135.

Wolf, S. Effects of suggestion and conditioning on the action of chemical agents in human subjects: the pharmacology of placebos. *Journal of Clinical Investigation,* 1950. **29**, 100–109.

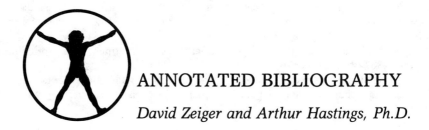

ANNOTATED BIBLIOGRAPHY

David Zeiger and Arthur Hastings, Ph.D.

Beecher, Henry K. **The powerful placebo.** *Journal of the American Medical Association,* 1955. **159**, 1602–1606.

The author reviews fifteen studies of placebo effects, involving 1,082 patients, and reports that placebos produced a therapeutic effect in 35 percent of the cases, including severe pain, headache, seasickness, anxiety, cough, and the common cold. Placebos produce objective physiological changes as well as subjective ones and have been known to result in toxic side effects such as drowsiness, nausea, and dermatitis. Beecher makes the important observation that the effects of a presumably active drug (e.g., morphine) may likely include its placebo effects. The total drug effect equals its "active" effect plus its "placebo" effect. The article is an excellent summary of evidence on effects of placebos and their therapeutic uses.

Beecher, Henry K. **Evidence for increased effectiveness of placebos with increased stress.** *American Journal of Physiology,* 1956. **187**, 163–169.

This research report presents evidence that placebos are effective in reducing pain, particularly when stress is great. Patients stressed by severe postoperative wound pain were divided into two groups that received alternating 10mg/70kg body weight dosages of morphine and placebo: group A in morphine, placebo order, and group B in placebo, morphine order. The dosages were given four times about seven hours apart. Patients described their degree of relief at intervals of forty-five and ninety minutes after each dosage, with relief defined as at least 50 percent reduction of pain.

The results indicated that the first dose of morphine relieved 52 percent of the patients, whereas the first dose of placebo relieved 40 percent. That is, when the pain was severest, the placebo's effectiveness was 77 percent that of morphine. At the fourth dosage, with less pain present, the placebo relief was 29 percent that of morphine. The study indicated that the differences between morphine and placebo appeared not to be due to learning or increased discrimination of the agents used. Beecher notes that a placebo can cause the adrenals to fire in anxious individuals and can mimic the effects of ACTH with normal patients. The more severe the disease state, the greater the placebo effect is on the adrenals.

Beecher, Henry K. **Increased stress and effectiveness of placebos and "active" drugs.** *Science*, 1960. **132**, 91–92.

This later study by Beecher continues his work with interactions of stress and placebo effects. The author compares two pain states: pathological pain (e.g., from injuries or wounds) and experimentally contrived pain (e.g., electric shock). The former produces a stronger psychopathological state (anxiety) than does the latter. Relief from the placebo is stronger in the higher anxiety state, suggesting that certain drugs (including presumably active ones) are effective in relieving visceral sensations only if an essential psychological state is present.

Dinnerstein, Albert J., and Halm, Jerome. **Modification of placebo effects by means of drugs: effects of aspirin and placebos on self-rated moods.** *Journal of Abnormal Psychology*, 1970. **75**, 308–314.

The authors report on an experiment to explore the interaction of "active" drugs and placebo effects – giving aspirin with various placebo instructions and testing the effects on the subjects' moods. In one set of conditions, the subjects received aspirin plus a placebo described as either a "tranquilizer" or an "energizer." The "tranquilizer" instructions resulted in friendly intoxication, while the "energizer" instructions resulted in a more sober, clear-headed depression.

The aspirin did not simply amplify the placebo effect. The aspirin plus the placebo treatment produced a qualitatively different mood state from either placebo treatment or aspirin itself. The authors conclude that a person's expectancies and the drug interact to produce the psychoactive effects, and the "real" effects of the drug depend on the patient's purpose and expectancies, the contextual setting, and the actual physiological effects. Thus drugs can modify the placebo effect and vice versa.

Hankoff, L. D.; Engelhardt, D. M.; and Freedman, N. **Placebo response in schizophrenic outpatients.** *Archives of General Psychiatry*, 1960. **2**, 43–52.

This article reports a study of 103 schizophrenic outpatients who were treated with a placebo in a psychopharmacological clinic. Forty-two patients demonstrated a positive or favorable response, defined in terms of improvement in their presenting symptomatology. In forty-one patients, no response was seen, and in twenty-one a negative response or worsening condition occurred. Negative responses and no responses correlated with treatment failures – i.e. drop-outs or rehospitalizations. Among the sixty-one patients in these two categories, fifty-three (86.8 percent) were treatment failures as compared to twenty-three (54.7 percent) treatment failures that occurred among the forty-two patients showing a positive placebo response.

A favorable placebo response was predictive of success in treatment and was also correlated with a high degree of denial of mental illness. This held for patients coming to the clinic after a recent hospitalization but not for outpatient referrals. Therefore, a positive placebo response was found to be correlated with the patient's defense mechanism (denial), the intake situation (recent hospitalization), and a favorable outcome for clinic treatment.

The placebo response appears to come from a matrix of factors, some existing before and some resulting from treatment. This matrix can be conceptualized as a nonverbal communication between doctor/therapist and patient in a specified treatment setting, the affective response to therapy being displaced to the ever-available pill. The placebo response helps define the treatment relationship and to predict its course. The authors also note the practical implications of their observations for the treatment of lower-class patients and chronic schizophrenics, where the therapeutic setting is often radically different from the conventional one.

Houston, W. R. **The doctor himself as a therapeutic agent.** *Annals of Internal Medicine,* 1938. **11**, 1416–1425.

In a 1938 address that remains relevant to a holistic medical approach, Dr. Houston spoke to the American College of Physicians on the subject of the doctor-patient relationship – its origins, its influence in healing, and its function as a mechanism of operation. Dr. Houston saw that relationship as declining but he was positive for the future of medicine if that decline was corrected.

The doctor-patient relationship is explored as one of love, faith, and understanding of the individual patient as a whole person. The dynamic of healing occurs when the doctor is able to help the patient modify his external view of his health environment. The placebo is a symbol of this interaction between the doctor and patient, a means through which the doctor can guide and counsel the patient toward a more positive picture of personal health. Houston also discusses possible avenues toward the study of the stress and emotional factors that influence the physiological well-being of patients.

Shapiro, A. K. **Factors contributing to the placebo effect: their implications for psychotherapy.** *American Journal of Psychotherapy,* 1964. **18**, 73–88.

The paper reviews the literature and draws inferential and implied deductions on the nature of the elements contributing to the placebo effect. These elements include the doctor-patient relationship, the doctor, the patient, and the treatment situation. The doctor-patient relationship is characterized by the act of transference by the patient to the physician. The patient may relate positively to the doctor as a good parent, a benevolent god, or a kindly magician, or he may relate negatively to the doctor as a devil, a sorcerer, or a bad parent. The doctor's countertransference with the patient is also important. Both affect the magnitude of the placebo reaction and the direction of the reaction (positive, negative, or absent), and both influence the outcome of the treatment.

Looking more carefully at the individual elements of doctor and patient, it is easy to see how the doctor can exert either a negative or positive influence on the patient's placebo response. A positive response is usually elicited by a doctor who imparts confidence, sincere interest in improvement, and enthusiasm for a particular treatment. Negative results occur if the patient perceives the doctor to be anxious, guilty, or in conflict about the patient or his treatment. Some additional factors that effect the patient are the degree of anxiety, sex, age, and faith. The symbolism (catharsis) of treatment and medication may help to expiate various degrees of guilt (e.g., enemas and purges).

Finally, there are situational factors that involve staff attitudes. Staff with high positive expectations were reported as a more significant factor than tranquilizing drugs in the number of patients discharged from mental hospitals. The size, color, texture, and shape of tablets, the form of medication, and particularly impressive machines or procedures will also have profound effects on the placebo response of a patient.

13

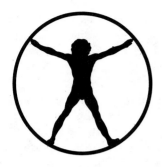

THE PHYSICAL DISCIPLINES AND HEALTH

Donald B. Ardell, Ph.D.

During the last ten years, there has been an explosive growth of interest and participation in a variety of physical disciplines (Institute of Medicine, 1978; Gellman, Lachaine, and Law, 1977; New York Academy of Sciences, 1976). The motivation for this activity is a belief among the participants that the discipline of their choice helps them to stay healthy, look young, feel good, and have fun (Leaf, 1973). In addition, this surge of involvement in participatory forms of exercise is related to a growing belief that what people do for their own health and well-being is vastly more consequential than what health professionals can do in this regard—and a lot less painful and expensive (Geannette, 1979).

The purpose of this chapter is to introduce health professionals to the range of ways in which physical disciplines can be used as partial pathways to wholeness—for the healthy as well as for the ill, for health care professionals themselves as well as for their clients and patients. In describing some of the connections between physical disciplines and health, we will look at relationships between various physical activities and well-being, comment on cultural norms affecting prevalent attitudes toward exercise, highlight the scientific evidence that supports the link between varied disciplines and improved health status, and outline strategies for transforming our individual and societal well-being through the promotion of physical disciplines by health professionals.

191

The Fitness Boom

During the past several years, large numbers of people of all ages and sizes have taken to the streets, tracks, and trails to run or jog – some for distances that others would reserve for jet travel. At present 24 percent of the United States' 224 million people are estimated by the Gallup pollsters to be exercising regularly in this fashion (Cantwell, 1978). For every jogger/runner, there are two others who engage regularly in some other physical discipline like aquatics (swimming, water polo); aerobics (including dance); cycling; handball; fencing; racket sports such as tennis, squash, and racquetball; team games (basketball, football); tai chi chuan and other non-Western martial arts (such as aikido and karate); yoga; and so on. Although there is a certain amount of faddism and sizable profit to be made – 9 million pairs of running shoes worth $147 million and $236 million worth of warm-up suits were sold in 1977 (Kirkpatrick, 1978) – neither fad nor fashion is the prime motivator. Most of us who pursue these various disciplines do so for a combination of two reasons: enjoyment, and illness prevention/health promotion (Kuntzleman, 1978).

How did things get to the point where nearly half the population participates in some form of physical discipline? Among the factors that have contributed substantially to our current interest and concern with fitness are the following:

- Studies and popular reports on the relationship between bodily dissolution and chronic diseases. See the annotated bibliography at the conclusion of this chapter for the sources of these studies and claims.
- President Kennedy's support for fitness. The late president's leadership and his image of vitality through staying fit made exercise "fashionable" for many Americans.
- The aerobics movement, led by Kenneth Cooper's books and lectures (1968, 1970). Millions have become acquainted with the concepts of "target heart rate," "training effect," "long slow distance," and similar phrases connected with Cooper's popularization of the fundamental elements of effective cardiovascular conditioning.
- The sedentary nature of most jobs and the reaction against the debilitating hazards of sedentary living. In the past, people used to get the exercise they needed just making a living and otherwise coping with a non-automated environment in a labor-intensive, low technology economy where citizens walked, cut logs, rode horses, and so on.
- The victory of Frank Shorter at Munich in the 1972 Olympic marathon. As we watched an American match strides with the world's greatest distance runners for more than twenty-six miles – and circle the Olympic stadium alone – many of us were inspired to explore anew our own potentials.

- The "new games" spearheaded by Stuart Brand (creator of the *Whole Earth Catalog*). The "have fun, play hard, be fair, everybody participates, nobody loses, everybody wins, nobody gets hurt" ethic felt good.
- The emergence of the martial arts as yet another available alternative to the competitive Western sports emphasis. Popular movies, such as those by Bruce Lee, and popularization in magazines and newspapers led to classes, clubs, and other centers where the form and defensive aspects of these arts were taught.
- The continued success of the YMCA, health clubs and other forms of association oriented to the pursuit of health and satisfaction (Myers, Golding, and Sinning, 1973).

In short, for highly varied reasons, a great many Americans have concluded that sedentary living is bad and fitness is good—and they are acting accordingly.

There is already evidence that this change in attitude and behavior has the potential of reducing the incidence of coronary heart disease, high blood pressure, obesity, boredom, depression, and most of what does or could ail you (Hammer and Fulton, n.d.; Brown, n.d.). It is not perfect, but it beats the relaxation that comes from the "happy hour" in bars, hours in front of the TV, and all other manifestations of what I call "low level worseness."

Unfortunately, this life-style "revolution" has not affected (i.e., involved) those members of the society for whom, by definition, it could do the most good—the hard-core unfit. In the future, the greatest challenge to professionals will be to find ways to motivate these people—who figure prominently among their clients and patients—to consider this form of self-therapy and renewal.

The Variety of Physical Disciplines

While some exercise physiologists rank cross-country skiing as the optimal physical exercise because of the number of muscle groups involved and the oxygen demands required (particularly at high altitudes), the President's Council on Physical Fitness and Sports has shown that jogging, cycling, swimming, and skating are the prime modes for regular aerobic conditioning. In a study of fourteen popular physical disciplines ranked by seven experts, each exercise was reviewed from the standpoint of heart and lung endurance, muscular endurance, muscular strength, flexibility, balance, and general well-being (weight control, muscle definition, digestion, sleep). Each of the seven panelists graded the fourteen types of exercise on a point scale from zero to three. An exercise that was of maximum benefit for muscle endurance would have a total score of twenty-one (three points from each of the seven experts). The overall ratings (total scores of each exercise for each element of physical fitness and general well-being) were then compiled. Here are the ratings (Conrad, 1976):

Exercise	Total Rating
Jogging	148
Bicyling	142
Swimming	140
Skating	140
Handball/squash	140
Skiing (Nordic)	139
Basketball	134
Skiing (Alpine)	134
Tennis	128
Calisthenics	126
Walking	102
Golf (cart)	66
Softball	64
Bowling	51

The list of actual forms of fitness expressions is mind-boggling. Consider, for example, the list of individual and team activities from which college students can select elective courses at Oral Roberts University (1977), where the emphasis is upon developing "a life-style in which an education takes place":

Advanced lifesaving	European team sports	Recreational aquatics
Aerobics I	Exercise and weight control	Self defense
Aerobics II	Fencing	SCUBA Diving
Archery	Field hockey	Skin Diving
Backpacking	Flag football	Soccer (T)
Badminton	Golf	Softball
Baseball	Gymnastics	Tennis
Basketball	Intermediate swimming	Track and field
Beginning swimming	Judo	Trampoline and tumbling
Body conditioning	Karate	Varsity sports
Bowling	Korfball	Volleyball
Cheerleading	Racquetball/handball	Water Safety
Cycling	Recreational activities	Wrestling

There are still other physical disciplines that are attracting a growing number of participants: hang gliding, wind surfing, skydiving, rock climbing, soaring, and skateboarding. The availability of new materials and technologies has revived hang gliding and skateboarding, both of which have been around for at least a decade. Equipment advances (new wing designs and fabrics for hang gliding, urethane wheels and "trucks" for mounting wheels on skateboards) have sparked and enlarged interest in these activities. Skateboarding alone is a $500 million-a-year business with at least 20 million riders worldwide (as estimated by the International Skateboard Association). The list could go on. One fitness director showed me charts on the aerobic benefits of sexual intercourse, and she suggested that such activity "is not only good for you but is also fun and does not re-quire expensive shoes!"

Another form of physical activity that has grown in popularity is tai chi chuan and a host of related but quite distinct non-Western disciplines, including judo, karate, kung fu, aikido, and jow ga kung fu, among others. Tai chi, as it is best known, is considered one of the most healthful and versatile of the martial arts. The purpose is to obtain exercise and harmony between mind and body. It is credited with developing faster reflexes and better awareness, is said to make the practitioner more sensitive to impending conflicts and more adept at their avoidance. Many of us have seen tai chi adherents, especially in the early morning, gracefully moving their hands, arms, and legs in slow circular rhythms with no evident starting or ending positions. Mark Tager, a physician and practitioner of this art and related disciplines, maintains that tai chi is a valuable health maintenance program for older people in that it teaches balance and unconscious weight transfer skills, and this reduces the chances of falls (Tager and Jennings, 1978).

Factors contributing to the growth of tai chi and the varied weaponless fighting arts of Asia are as difficult to identify as the key variables leading to greater participation in Western disciplines. However, a few events and persons have left their mark, including the inclusion of judo in the 1964 Olympic Games, renewed curiosity about Asian philosophies, books by certain Western writers (e.g., George Leonard on aikido), a rising crime rate and attendant interest in self-defense, well-promoted tournaments in varied martial arts, and television shows and popular movies (like Bruce Lee's "Fist of Fury" and Tom Loughlin's "Billy Jack"), which show evildoers vanquished by virtuous practitioners of the martial arts. There are thousands of schools throughout the United States where one may obtain instruction in these disciplines.

Another discipline associated with and valued for its health benefits is yoga, long practiced as a means of exercise and fitness through flexibility and relaxation. In practicing yoga, the individual seeks to establish a balance of body and mind in which health will naturally occur. Yoga is designed to encourage the individual to develop a passive attitude for stress management, to become more sensitive to areas of constriction in the body, to become more aware of weaknesses and strengths, and to enlarge the person's potentials for expansion and ease of movement. These physical experiences, in turn, make those who practice yoga more aware of habits and choices regarding food, exercise, stress, and life purposes. Since (Western) scientists began to measure its effects, yoga has been shown to be associated with many desirable and measurable physical indices of well-being, among them: reduced blood pressure, lower pulse rates, diminished fat levels in the blood, better regulation of menstrual flow, diminished stress, less joint pain and dysfunction, and an added sense of well-being. Yoga is a system of movements well suited for any age or physical condition (Christensen and Raskin, 1977).

Prevailing Attitudes and Norms

Until quite recently, the medical establishment had failed to actively promote participation in physical disciplines. A former president of the American Medical Association remarked several years ago that "thus far, physicians have shown little objective interest in promoting health and preventive care" (Todd, 1978). Dr. Kenneth Cooper (1968, 1970) has noted that he was warned by the medical establishment in 1968 that aerobic exercises would cause people (especially those over age forty) to die by the thousands. In fact, few died participating in the varied physical disciplines compared to the number who probably died from *not* participating.

While the medical establishment has been neutral or nonsupportive, U.S. industry has been highly supportive of all kinds of physical disciplines for employees (Cundiff, 1977; Life Style, 1977). Approximately five hundred companies have full-time fitness directors on their staffs, and recent articles suggest that firms are investing millions in physical disciplines as a strategy for reducing health care costs. Among the companies known to have made extensive commitments for employee fitness are Arco, Chase Manhattan, Motorola, Kimberly-Clark, Sentry Insurance, Western Electric, the Ford Motor Company, Exxon, General Foods, Firestone, Goodyear, Phillips Petroleum, Metropolitan Life, Boeing, Xerox, Rockwell International, Merrill Lynch, and the Continental Bank (Kattus, 1972). In addition, several insurance companies are offering dramatic rate reductions to persons who meet basic fitness standards.

While the reaction to and support for physical disciplines from the health professions was weak only a few years ago, it is rapidly increasing today. Theodore G. Klumpp, M.D., chairman of the board of the National Association for Human Development, has recently shown that routine exercise can offset numerous ailments and dramatically reduce health care costs (*Journal of American Insurance*, 1977–1978), and the 15 percent decrease in deaths from heart attacks since 1968 has been attributed in part to improvement in the exercise habits of Americans. Meanwhile, the new medical field of sports medicine has provided a forum within the medical community for research and comment on the appropriate use of physical disciplines for health enhancement and therapy. Increasingly health care professionals are considering and investigating the benefits of the physical disciplines for people who come to them with a variety of physical and mental health disturbances (Belloc and Breslow, 1972; Nolewajka, Kostuk, Rechnitzer et al., 1978; Wilhelmsen, Sanne, Elmfeldt et al., 1975; Cunningham, Ingram, Rechnitzer et al., 1977; Corrigan and Fitch, 1972; Vuori, Mäkäräinen, and Jääskeläinen, 1978).

Physical Disciplines and Better Health

During the past ten years, there has been an impressive series of studies linking various physical disciplines to higher levels of well-being, particularly to beneficial metabolic and cardiovascular changes (Castelli, Doyle, Gordon et al., 1977; Paffenbarger, Hale, Brand, and Hyde, 1977; Abu-Zeid, 1977; Fentem and Gould, 1978). In addition, the anecdotal literature and testimonials from the true believers and their spokespeople could fill a small library. The results have been followed with interest by the federal government. The Department of Health, Education, and Welfare's (1976) Public Health Service *Forward Plan for Health— 1977–1981*, for example, includes the following statement:

> Habitual inactivity is thought to contribute to hypertension, chronic fatigue, and resulting physical inefficiency, premature aging, poor musculature and lack of flexibility, which are the major causes of lower back pain and injury, mental tension, coronary heart disease, and obesity. By contrast, studies have reported that regular exercise can lower triglycerides, reduce the clinical manifestations of heart disease, improve the efficiency of the heart and circulation, and reduce blood pressure levels in individuals with hypertension.

The federal government has, in fact, instituted programs for its own employees based on the belief that the available evidence demonstrates that fitness will lead to reduced employee mortality and morbidity rates. A number of studies have suggested that regular participation in selected physical disciplines (jogging, cross-country skiing, swimming, bicycling, and nonstatic isokinetic training) may yield impressive physical benefits. Among the results of a ten-week study of middle-aged men and women who exercised were gains in overall body strength, flexibility, cardiovascular endurance, and decreased blood sugar, cholesterol, and triglyceride levels (Cantwell, 1978; Monkerud, 1978). A second longer-term study (National Jogging Association, 1971) showed that regular physical exercise improved heart muscle function, reduced blood pressure and tension levels, lowered body fat, and increased breathing capacity in older males, and a third (Fletcher and Cantwell, 1974) graphically demonstrated that high fitness is significantly correlated with more healthy physiological measurements (see Table 13.1).

Of the fifteen variables that affect the chances of someone having a heart attack—blood pressure, activity level, weight, mood and coping style, fasting blood sugar, triglycerides, fibrinolysins, cigarette smoking, diet, EKG readings, uric acid, pulmonary function, glucose tolerance, heredity, and cholesterol, all but one (heredity) can be positively affected by exercising vigorously at 80 percent of the heart's capacity for twenty-five minutes a day.

Conversely, some investigators have noted a dramatic drop-off in health indices when fit people discontinue their physical activities. The National Jogging Association (1978) reported a study by Dr. Ancel Keyes, who required healthy young men to spend several weeks in bed. He found that they developed a generalized weakness and atrophy of their muscles, lost blood volume and calcium, and their muscle protein was depleted of potassium, various vitamins, phosphorus, total sulphur, nitrogen, and sodium. A second study by Dr. John

Table 13.1
Physical Fitness of 835 People

| | Fitness Class[a] | | Significance |
	Very Low	High	
Weight, kg	85.9	75.1	P < .001
Percent body fat	19.6	14.9	P < .001
Triglyceride, mg/dl	184.6	100.4	P < .001
High density lipoprotein, mg/dl	46.0	58.5	P < .002
Blood pressure, mm Hg			
Systolic	136.8	129.1	P < .001
Distolic	89.3	81.5	
Lung function, liters			
Vital capacity	3.99	4.41	P < .001
FEV[b]	3.27	3.75	

[a]Based on oxygen uptake.
[b]FEV indicates forced expiratory volume in one second.

Dietrick of Cornell University Medical College yielded similar results.

There is little dispute today that exercise strengthens and improves the efficiency of the heart, blood vessels, and lungs; produces healthier body tissues, and better appestat mechanism, and a lower resting heart rate; facilitates increased lung capacity; reduces stored (versus essential) fat; and enables better digestion of food and more efficient elimination of waste. In short, exercise is a good thing and ought to be promoted on a larger scale (Paffenbarger and Hale, 1976; Paffenbarger, Wing, and Hyde, 1977; Fletcher and Cantwell, 1974).

Other studies (Wirth et al., 1978) also suggest that certain physical disciplines can relieve many of the common complaints of pregnancy. For example, running has been shown to reduce constipation, hemorrhoidal swelling, the complications of varicose veins, and insomnia. Babies born to fit mothers are benefited as well. One Scandanavian study showed that such children have lower blood acidity, less chance of asphyxiation at birth, and superior oxygen/carbon dioxide exchange. Finally, fit mothers who exercized were less likely to feel sick and were better able to perceive their pregnancy as a healthy life process.

Most of the other evidence for psychological improvement is anecdotal, but there is a lot of it—and a few research reports with "harder" data as well (Cantwell and Watt, 1974). The anecdotal evidence includes claims in books and in the popular press by varied authorities that fitness routines enable people to do more work, to feel and look better, to feel more spontaneity and joy in life, and to minimize their high risk behaviors. Psychiatrists and other mental health professionals committed to various physical disciplines also claim that regular participation lessens depression, improves self-image, diminishes hypochondriacal behaviors, and mitigates muscle tensions and anxieties. Dr. Ron Lawrence, president of the American Medical Joggers Association, states in *The Runner's Handbook* (Glover and Sheperd, 1978) that this discipline

> enhances the quality of life. It changes your whole lifestyle. You quit smoking. Your consumption of alcohol drops. Eating habits change because good nutrition is an integral part of aerobic exercise. Your total well-being improves. Your sex life is enhanced. You sleep better but require less sleep. Anxieties decrease and you're better prepared to cope with stress. Work productivity improves. You get away from TV and begin seeing a new world around you.

Dr. Kenneth Cooper claims that observations at his Aerobics Center in Dallas and elsewhere support his view that physically-fit people are also psychologically fit. Although he steers clear of a cause and effect explanation, Dr. Robert Brown at the University of Virginia states that neither he nor his colleagues have ever treated a physically-fit depressed person. And recent studies describe the prescription of distance training for insomnia (Kelling, 1978).

Thaddeus Kostrubala (1977), a psychiatrist and the author of *The Joy of Running*, goes farther than most. He claims that running can—in some cases—cure mental illness. In an article by the same title that appeared in *Runners' World* (January 1978) Kostrubala is quoted as suggesting a running regimen for patients with depression, anxiety, insomnia, or inability to cope, as well as for those diagnosed as schizophrenic. The article cites two studies. The first study at the University of Missouri involved 100 teachers who participated in swimming, weight lifting, cycling, and jogging. It indicated that all those who evidenced emotional depression in testing before the six-week program showed an improved state of mind at the end of the experimental period. The second study, conducted with prisoners and police officers in training under the direction of Dr. William P. Morgan of the University of Wisconsin yielded similar results.

Practitioners of fitness disciplines have also reported states of extreme calm or centeredness, oneness with the universe, and transcendence. This is often the case with marathon or distance runners, but it also occurs with tai chi, swimming, and other disciplines (Murphy and White, 1978). Until these studies are replicated with appropriate controls, we can only speculate about their implications. Perhaps the physical disciplines provide an opportunity for out-of-balance people to escape the stress and daily pressures of life and to burn up energy that would otherwise be available for anxiety. Perhaps physical disciplines work as muscle relaxants—simply offering decreased biological levels of tension—without the unpleasant, counterproductive side effects of tranquilizers. In any event, those mental health professionals who also pursue fitness regimens and attempt to integrate the physical disciplines in their work with patients and clients do not hesitate to mention that Freud was a great walker and that Jung practiced yoga exercises to counterbalance a preoccupation with the intellectual side of life.

Strategies for the Transformation

At a minimum, the growing mass participation in varied physical disciplines should be of personal and professional interest even to the most skeptical health care provider. There is enough information already available to suggest that it would be useful to explore the applications of exercise to a variety of physical and emotional dysfunctions. How else can one assess the claims of joggers and other physical enthusiasts? How else are we to determine how much of the alleged benefit is placebo derived and how much is directly associated with the individual disciplines?

For those who have experienced the satisfactions of physical excellence as a way of life and who believe that some of the physical disciplines can be of measurable aid to the well-being of those they serve, a number of strategies come to mind. All share a common goal—the promotion of a wider understanding and appreciation of the relationship of physical fitness to physical, emotional, and mental health—and all assume that for exercise to become enjoyable and self-reinforcing it must be chosen according to the unique preference of the individual. Among the strategies are the following:

1. Doctors, psychologists, counselors, and others in the helping professions should dwell less on client problems and more on the positive, life-enriching things the individual can do for him- or herself. Sometimes getting the person off his adipose gluteus maximus can be the best "medicine" or advice for feeling better and coping more effectively. Of course, this will not work if the motivation to assume responsibility is not present or cannot be instilled by the health professional. But it does seem a sound beginning, one that will be feasible in particular cases. An important part of such an effort would be to make as attractive as possible the option of exercising, providing a support system for initiating the patient into one or more physical disciplines. Exercise routines as therapy could change the structure, format, and process of treatment and delivery programs—and perhaps the impact on clients.

2. Mental health centers and certain other treatment facilities should be reorganized to promote positive health and to minimize the attention devoted to symptoms and negative life situations. Instead of just dispensing drugs and analyzing present and past failures, the multidisciplinary staff would deal with headaches, conflicts, anxieties, and depression through such active means as yoga, relaxation, massage, biofeedback, nutrition, and fitness regimens. Self-help would be emphasized as an alternative to continuing crises and dependencies on professional and societal helpers. The logical outcome might be mental-health–based wellness support centers.

3. The nature of traditional screening programs could be changed to emphasize those tests and indices that measure the client's understanding of

the value of varied physical disciplines and overall health. Among those instruments included would be some form of health assessment that emphasizes the importance of life-style (e.g., the health hazards appraisal instruments), pulmonary function measures, nutritional profiles, treadmill stress tests for fitness levels, hydrostatic or immersion tank measurements for determining percent of body fat, stress scales, and variations on purpose-in-life and well-being tests. The technologies are available now for administering all of these positive health measures.

4. New directions in research should be established. The current data on the effects of physical disciplines is highly fragmented and often open to challenge, as is the entire body of literature on positive health. The dominant focus on illness and the societal disinterest in healthy people is partly responsible but so too are the added complexities of defining and quantifying levels of positive functioning. An interest in fitness, exercise, and the entire range of physical disciplines as pathways to well-being carries with it the need to devote greater attention to measuring the potentials that Maslow, Horney, Rogers, and others began to describe. Some tests and measures for assessing positive health already exist — it is just a matter of developing variations and generating an appreciation for their use in specific health settings.

5. Finally, an effort can be made to use the physical fitness dimension as a stepping stone to an integrated life-style of total well-being. One approach, described as high level wellness (Ardell, 1979), often begins with the physical disciplines and grows into a conscious commitment to one's own best potentials for physical, emotional, and mental well-being. It is a positive approach tailored to the needs and capacities of each individual, pursued because it is more rewarding than the alternatives (such as muddling through or low level worseness). The five key areas are self-responsibility, fitness, stress awareness and management, nutritional awareness, and environmental sensitivity.

This kind of integrated approach to wellness is now being promoted by a third of the nation's health-planning agencies, by numerous corporations, by several hospitals, and by many university health programs. It is the focus of attention at mental health centers in at least six states — and it is growing. Wellness may thus be the logical outcome of the growing influence the physical disciplines are having on the health system and its practitioners.

References

Abu-Zeid, A.H.H. Hemoglobin level and ischemic heart disease: relationship to known risk factors. *Preventive Medicine*, 1977. **6**, 120–129.

Ardell, Donald B. *High Level Wellness: An Alternative to Doctors, Drugs, and Disease.* New York: Bantam Books, 1979.

Belloc, N. B., and Breslow, L. Relationship of physical health status and health practice. *Preventive Medicine,* 1972. **1**, 409–421.

Brown, B. S. *Effects of non-static isokinetic training.* Fayetteville, Ark.: University of Arkansas, n.d.

Cantwell, J. D. Running. *Journal of the American Medical Association,* September 22, 1978. **239**, 1409–1410.

Cantwell, J. D., and Watt, E. W. Extreme cardiovascular fitness in old age. *Chest,* 1974. **65**, 357–359.

Castelli, W. P.; Doyle, J. T.; Gordon, T. et al. High density lipoprotein cholesterol and other lipids in coronary heart disease. *Circulation,* 1977. **55**, 767–772.

Christensen, A., and Raskin, D. *Easy Does It Yoga for People Over Sixty.* Cleveland, Ohio: Light on Yoga Society, 1977.

Conrad, C. C. How different sports rate in promoting physical fitness. *Resident Staff Physician,* 1976. **22**, 43–50.

Cooper, Kenneth H. *Aerobics.* New York: Bantam Books, 1968.

Cooper, Kenneth H. *The New Aerobics.* New York: Bantam Books, 1970.

Corrigan, A. B., and Fitch, K. D. Complications of jogging. *Medical Journal of Australia,* 1972. **2**, 363–368.

Cundiff, David. Industrialization and lifestyle. *Innovations and Research,* February 23, 1977. 17–18.

Cunningham, D. A.; Ingram, K. G.; Rechnitzer, P. A. et al. Effect of a two-year program of exercise training on cardiovascular fitness and recurrence rates in postmyocardial infarct patients: an interim report. *Science Abstracts,* 1977. **62**, 136.

Fentem, P., and Gould, D. Does exercise train muscles or heart? *New Scientist,* October 1978. **26**, 256–261.

Fletcher, G. F., and Cantwell, J. D. *Exercise and Coronary Heart Disease.* Springfield, Ill.: Charles C. Thomas, 1974.

Geannette, Gloria. Inside the corporate gymnasium. *American Way,* January 1979. 20–23.

Gellman, D. D.; Lachaine, R.; and Law, M. M. The Canadian approach to health policies and programs. *Preventive Medicine,* 1977. **6**, 265–275.

Glover, Bob, and Sheperd, Jack. *The Runner's Handbook.* New York: Viking, 1978.

Hammer, D. C., and Fulton, C. D. *The effect of a circuit isokinetic and bicycle ergometer exercise on cardiovascular conditioning.* De Kalb, Ill.: Northern Illinois University, n.d.

Institute of Medicine. *Perspectives on Health Promotion and Disease Prevention in the United States.* Washington, D.C.: National Academy of Sciences, January 1978.

Journal of American Insurance. Find your own fitness quotient. Winter 1977–1978. 5–6.

Kattus, A. A. *Exercise Testing and Training of Apparently Healthy Individuals.* New York: American Heart Association, 1972.

Kelling, George, M.D. Long, sleepy distance running solution. *Runners' World,* October 1978. 30–34.

Kirkpatrick. T. The fitness boom. *Eugene* (Oreg.) *Register,* November 5, 1978.

Kostrubala, Thaddeus. *The Joy of Running.* New York: Pocket Books, 1977.

Kuntzleman, C. *The Exerciser's Handbook.* New York: David McKay, 1978.

Leaf, A. Getting old. *Scientific American,* 1973. **229**, 44–52.

Life Style. Oklahoma Journal for Employer/Employee Programs of Leisure, Recreation, Fitness, and Education. Summer, 1977.

Monkerud, D. Running into consciousness: caution–running may be good for your health. *New Realities,* August 1978. **11 (3),** 48–53.

Murphy, Michael, and White, Rhea. *The Psychic Side of Sports.* Reading, Mass.: Addison Wesley, 1978.

Myers, C. R.; Golding, K.; and Sinning, W. *The Y's Way to Physical Fitness.* Emmaus, Pa.: Rodale Press and National YMCA Board of Directors, 1973.

National Jogging Association. *The Jogger.* October 1971, 20.

National Jogging Association. *The Jogger.* October 1978, 2.

New York Academy of Sciences. *The Marathon.* New York: Academy of Sciences, 1976.

Nolewajka, G.; Kostuk, W. J.; Rechnitzer, P. et al. Assessment of collateral circulation and left ventricular function in the postmyocardial infarct patient before and after physical training. *American Journal of Cardiology.* 1978. **41,** 412.

Oral Roberts University. *The Aerobics Program at Oral Roberts University.* Tulsa, Okla.: Author, 1977.

Paffenbarger, R. S., Jr., and Hale, W. E. Work activity and coronary heart disease. *New England Journal of Medicine,* 1976. **292,** 545–550.

Paffenbarger, R. S., Jr.; Hale, W. E.; Brand, R. J.; and Hyde, R. T. Work energy level, personal characteristics, and fatal heart attack. *American Journal of Epidemiology,* 1977. **105,** 200–213.

Paffenbarger, R. S., Jr.; Wing, A. L.; and Hyde, R. T. Contemporary physical activity and incidence of heart attack in college men. *Circulation,* 1977. **56,** 3–15. (Abstract)

Runners' World. The joy of running. January 1978, 36–43.

Tager, Mark, and Jennings, Charles. *Whole Person Health.* Portland, Oreg.: Victoria House, 1978.

Todd, Malcolm C., M.D. The need for a new health program. *The Holistic Health Handbook.* Berkeley, Calif.: Holistic Health Press, 1978.

U.S. Department of Health, Education, and Welfare, *Forward Plan for Health–1977–1981.* Washington, D.C.: U.S. Government Printing Office, 1976.

Vuori, I.; Mäkäräinen, M.; and Jääskeläimen, A. Sudden death and physical activity. *Cardiology,* 1978. **63,** 287–304.

Wilhelmsen, L.; Sanne, H.; Elmfeldt, D. et al. A controlled trial of physical training after myocardial infarction: effects on risk factors, nonfatal reinfarction and death. *Preventive Medicine,* 1975. **4,** 491–508.

Wirth, Victoria; Emmons, Patty; and Larson, Daniel. Running through pregnancy. *Runners' World,* November 1978. 54–59.

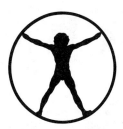

ANNOTATED BIBLIOGRAPHY

Anderson, Bob. **Stretching.** Fullerton, Calif.: Anderson Kramer, 1975.

The author presents an encyclopedic treatise, replete with clear and helpful illustrations (by Jean Anderson) for people concerned with movement, relaxation, injury prevention, and muscle toning. The tension-reducing benefits of a good stretch are convincingly demonstrated, and instructions are given for specific stretches of gradually increasing strenuousness for the back before and after running, cycling, skiing, racket ball, or varied team sports. This book is useful for sports physicians, coaches, and athletes of all varieties.

Brattnäs, Berit, and Gullers, K. W. **Fit for Fun: A Swedish Message.** Chicago: Blue Cross Association, 1973.

The "made for America" version of the Swedish approach to the physical disciplines. The authors describe why the Swedish government devotes the largest share of the national budget to health and fitness education, how it helps Swedes to live longer and healthier lives than Americans, and what we have to learn from them. Sections on running, nutrition, stretching, walking, cross-country skiing, and more are concluded with pages of entertaining and useful tips ("Go walk the dog. Even if you don't have a dog."). Good reading; recommended by the President's Council on Physical Fitness.

Cooper, Kenneth H. **The New Aerobics.** New York: Bantam Books, 1970.

Cooper describes the nature and success of the aerobics system he created, which emphasizes maximizing the amount and role of oxygen the body uses. The results of an aerobic training program—which may include swimming, running, dance, etc.—include strengthened respiration, less air-flow resistance, improved cardiac efficiency, greater oxygen transfer, generalized improvement of muscle tone, decreased blood pressure, and increased blood circulation.

Dilfer, Carol. **Your Baby, Your Body.** New York: Crown Publishers, 1977.

If you are pregnant, have friends who are pregnant, or are involved in the health care of pregnant women, this book is required reading. Carol Dilfer distinguishes "fat" from pregnant, describes and illustrates exercises that can and should be done regularly during pregnancy, provides plentiful tips on posture, and offers special exercises for the kinds of aches, pains, and muscle strains that often accompany pregnancy.

Donaldson, Rory. **Guidelines for Successful Jogging.** Washington, D.C.: National Jogging Association, 1977.

> An excellent primer for the novice jogger, *Guidelines* is a comprehensive manual containing hints, tips, recommendations, and adages for being a successful exerciser. Special sections are included on "whole life" considerations (stretching, diet, rest, and perspective), athletics for women, and routines geared for different ages.

Fixx, James F. **The Complete Book of Running.** New York: London House, 1977.

> Since this is the most overrated and oversold book you can buy on the running phase of the physical disciplines, it warrants a commentary in this overview. *The Complete Book of Running* is, of course, not complete. It does, however, contain lots of useful information, including material linking the physical disciplines to health, mental health, and longevity. It also has useful sections dealing with female runners, age-group considerations, gear, nutrition, and the broken heart club. Unfortunately, the book also contains excessive hucksterism for running. The benefits may or may not turn out to be as dramatic as Fixx suggests. There are too many photos and sketches of Fixx for my taste. The hype aside, it is a good–if overpriced–book. Borrow a copy.

Fluegelman, Andrew (Ed.). **The New Games Book.** Garden City, N.Y.: Doubleday, 1976.

> "Play hard, play fair, and nobody hurt" is the theme for two hundred new physical disciplines described and illustrated in this book. The emphasis is upon participation in games that allow all to play, none to lose, and everybody to be on the first string. In addition to interesting descriptions of the new games, the book contains chapters on the history and philosophy of the new-game concept, instructions for referees wishing to manage these games, and essays on the implications of "new-games thinking" for the physical disciplines.

Frankel, Laurence J., and Richard, Betty Byed. **Be Alive As Long As You Live: Mobility Exercises for the Older Person.** Charleston, W. Va.: Preventicare Publications, 1977.

> Exercise is one certain method of improving the quality of life for senior citizens. It helps to slow many of the chronic diseases of aging and thus prevents premature dependency. The authors introduce their concept of "preventicare," illustrate and discuss a variety of exercises for older people, and describe workout routines for the chairbound and bedridden. Special attention is given to nutrition, the hazards of obesity, proper breathing, and the values of music and laughter. In sum, this is an extremely useful book for older people.

Glasser, William. **Positive Addiction.** New York: Harper and Row, 1976.

> Having described how to "get hooked," Glasser takes a long look at the "positive" addictions that people have to a variety of physical disciplines. In contrast to their negative counterparts–drugs, alcohol, tobacco–these positive addictions reinforce desired

behavior and promote self-esteem, self-awareness, and increased confidence. The methods for pursuing an addiction are unconventional but the rationale is solid. If you want to get hooked on some activity you suspect is good for you, Glasser will show you how to proceed.

Herrigel, Eugen. **Zen and the Art of Archery.** New York: Random House, 1971.

The author of this classic piece on the relationship of mind and performance has inspired contemporary writers on a variety of sports. It was Herrigel who first helped sportsmen to understand that the harmonious interrelationship between themselves, their instruments, and the games they played was far more satisfying than the struggle to do better or to win. If you would achieve success, he seems to be saying, be content with failure.

Herrigel's experience can be applied to any sport. If you are, for example, a handball player, notice what happens when you execute a perfect "kill" shot. Note the ease, rightness, and truth of the act – the feeling of harmony with the universe that fills that moment. If you open yourself to this experience, the flight of the ball becomes part of your reality, and its perfection will fill you.

Jackson, Ian. **Yoga and the Athlete.** Mountain View, Calif.: World Publications, 1975.

A highly personalized account of the author's journey from competitive jock to *afficionado* of the calming and centering possibilities of the physical disciplines. Jackson describes his physical and emotional rehabilitation through yoga after an automobile accident. Illustrated with lots of photos of the author, the story is not easy reading, but it is interesting, nevertheless.

Kostrubala, Thaddeus. **The Joy of Running.** New York: Pocket Books, 1977.

As much as any book in this bibliography, this one makes a convincing case for physical disciplines as a vital element in physical and mental health. Kostrubala is a psychiatrist and a self-described former fat, anxious, and discontented being. The book chronicles his own transformation through running – and that of many of his patients, whose fitness regimes are described and evaluated. It is good for the historical account it gives of the connection between physical disciplines and excellence in life, between body and mind, soul and physique. It is also of value for the medical advice provided, the discussion of psychological effects of running, the bibliography, and Kostrubala's interesting theories on running and mental health.

Kuntzleman, C. T., and *Consumer Guide* Editors. **Rating the Exercises.** New York: Penguin, 1980.

Charles Kuntzleman is a former national director of YMCA athletic programs, including the popular and effective Fitness Finders Program. He is the author of several other fitness books and has experience in designing specific physical regimes for varied groups throughout the United States. I worked with him one summer and enjoyed his approaches and techniques in person as much as I enjoyed his books.

In this book, possibly his best, Dr. Kuntzleman rates every major exercise program from aerobics to yoga. He identifies fuzzy thinking, transparent claims, ripoff approaches, poor research, and old wives' tales. His most important criterion for effectiveness is whether an exercise provides adequate cardiovascular effects. Steamrooms, saunas, hot tubs, and other passive devices are enjoyable but unproductive for strengthening the heart, lungs, and major muscle groups; for decreasing body weight; or for increasing the ratio of lean muscle to fat content. The book, which devotes an entire chapter to discussing the utility of health spas and other health and fitness enterprises, is especially valuable as a reference document.

Leonard, George. **The Ultimate Athlete.** New York: Viking Press, 1974.

This book deals with the potentials of the physical disciplines to help individuals move beyond the limited perspectives of competition and conflict (inherent in contemporary sports) into larger games, new dimensions, and a way of basing their physical activities on enjoyments and celebrations. To help us on our quest, Leonard provides detached insights on a wide variety of disciplines, anecdotes about his own transformation, and exercises designed to enhance the flow of energy in the body.

Morehouse, Laurence E., and Gross, Leonard. **Maximum Performance.** New York: Simon and Schuster, 1977.

The authors make the same errors in this book that marred their earlier success (*Total Fitness in 30 Minutes a Week*), namely exaggerated promises and condescension to their readers. Nevertheless, *Maximum Performance* still comes out a winner. Morehouse and Gross help those who would "do better" to stop trying so hard (to use techniques of muscle relaxation, to worry less about perfection, to utilize anxiety for positive results, and to quiet the mind). In many ways, this book has the quality of *The Inner Game of Tennis* or *Zen and the Art of Archery*.

More standardized but equally helpful suggestions are provided in chapters on conditioning for maximum performance, pulse rate, monitoring, fitness exercise movements, diet, injury avoidance, and a reinterpretation of the concept of winning (e.g., "If you want to win, forget about winning"). It is a good book to help you make the most of your inner capabilities.

Orlick, Terry. **Challenge Without Competition.** New York: Pantheon, 1978.

A highly readable book with attractive, plentiful illustrations, *Challenge Without Competition* is designed to persuade us that games can be structured so that everybody wins and nobody gets hurt, physically or emotionally. Orlick shows us that challenge does not require that players be irrevocably locked in conflict and that playing the game is more satisfying than winning it.

At least one hundred games are outlined that challenge participants while promoting interpersonal acceptance and sharing. Imagination and a joyful attitude are prerequisites, but equipment needs are minimal for Orlick's invigorating exercise patterns.

Sheehan, George. **Running and Being: The Total Experience.** New York: Simon and Schuster, 1978.

A collection of *Runners' World* columns by the New Jersey sports physician on the joy of physical disciplines in general and on the art of running in particular. The emphasis is on the relationship between mind and body, fitness and true "youthfulness," and intellectual insights, spiritual ease, and physical excellence.

When Sheehan is good he is very, very good – as when he recounts how an emotional letdown that resulted from a weekend of playing hero and guru ended only when he realized that "life is not a problem to be solved." When Sheehan is bad, on the other hand, he is embarrassingly awful, as when he unburdens himself on such lines as "While a world composed solely of runners would be unworkable, a world without them would be unlivable." If you can put up with disconcerting lines like this and a lot of nonsense about predetermination of personality based on body-type, you might enjoy the book quite a lot.

Smith, David. **The East/West Exercise Book.** New York: McGraw-Hill, 1976.

David Smith wrote this book for people who have started but chosen not to continue other exercise programs. His approach is different. You are asked to visualize an exercise before embarking on it, to move slowly and mindfully from simple easy exercises to more difficult and intricate programs. The set of activities is designed to relax key tension points, develop balance, flexibility, coordination, strength, and endurance. Correct breathing is emphasized and described, as are techniques to increase awareness and a feeling of "centeredness." Smith borrows from hatha yoga, tai chi, Arica, bioenergetics, endurance training, isometrics, and isotonics. The book contains many photos, enjoyable "games to freedom," exercises for school and office, and a reference guide for special problem areas. It is easy to read and thoroughly useful for the layman or for health care professionals who may want to suggest interesting and relaxing exercises to their patients.

Ullyot, Joan. **Women Running.** Mountain View, Calif.: World Publications, 1976.

A physician and exercise physiologist, Dr. Ullyot has written the first major treatment of running for women. She clearly describes the principles (adaptation to overload and consistency) of fitness training in a manner tailored to the concerns of beginners and injury-prone people. Ullyot's chatty and personalized account of training plans, her advice on basic considerations (shoes, diet, safety), and her lessons on fundamentals (e.g., fat as body fuel) are highlights of the book. Also of interest to all runners are answers to often-asked questions (for example, what to do about "stitches"), conversion tables (miles to meters), and a recommended reading list. The book is somewhat dated (the records have been broken several times and the race descriptions seem like ancient history), but overall it is well worth reading.

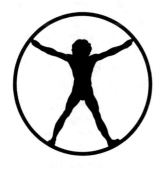

14

TOUCH: WORKING WITH THE BODY

Robert Frager, Ph.D.

Touching is one of the most natural human activities. We touch to comfort, to arouse, and to communicate. Systematic therapeutic uses of touch range from the extremely simple to the extraordinarily complex, from rubbing a bruise to releasing a lifetime accumulation of chronic tension.

The importance of touch is usually underrated. In his book, *Touching*, Ashley Montagu (1971) cites considerable evidence for the therapeutic effectiveness of touch. For example, numerous studies of both animal and human infants have found that lack of touch leads to serious impairment of physical, sexual, and social functioning. Montagu reminds us that the skin is one of the more complex and critical human organ systems, an organ capable of extraordinary sensitivity and responsiveness to external stimulation.

Most of the touch-oriented systems of body work are based on a holistic approach to human functioning. If we assume that all mental and physical processes are parts of a single, interrelated system, it becomes obvious that any system of body work that significantly improves one aspect of physical functioning is also likely to have important benefits for general health improvement. Although the prevalence of a psychosomatic component in "physical" disease is now generally acknowledged, there is as yet relatively little recognition of the obvious corollary—that there is a "somatopsychic" component to psychological functioning. That is, mental or emotional tension is virtually always correlated with physical tension, and relieving tension in any one area will tend to alleviate tension and promote more effective functioning in other areas.

We can divide the systems covered in this chapter into four major categories:

1. *Practices designed to promote greater relaxation.* This refers primarily to various forms of massage. However, many if not most systems of body work include relaxation and tension reduction as important components of their work.
2. *Disciplines aimed at improving body alignment and functioning.* By alignment I mean the spatial relationship of the major body parts – head, neck, spine, pelvis, etc. In rolfing, for example, great emphasis is placed on attaining a posture deemed optimal for functioning in our gravitational field.
3. *Techniques for enhancing sensory awareness.* This field was pioneered in the United States by Charlotte Selver. Her approach has been to focus on the process of sensing our own bodies and our environment. This is generally accomplished by exquisitely simple exercises designed to focus and clarify our awareness.
4. *Psychotherapeutic body work.* This area was first developed by Wilhelm Reich, who discovered the intimate connection between chronic physical tension, or armoring, and chronic psychological defenses. His work has influenced many other therapists, most notably Alexander Lowen and the field of bioenergetics.

There is considerable overlap among these four areas. For instance, shiatsu (Japanese finger-pressure massage) is primarily oriented toward muscle relaxation, but certain shiatsu treatments are designed to improve body alignment, enhance sexual functioning, and treat various specific illnesses.

Relaxation

Massage

Massage refers to ways of kneading or rubbing various parts of the body, usually with the hands, in order to stimulate circulation, relieve muscle tension, and enhance joint flexibility. Massage styles range from sensual stroking to moderately painful digging into sore or tense muscles. Swedish massage primarily involves fairly heavy pressure designed to relax and tone up the muscles. Esalen-style massage (Downing, 1972) is a soft and gentle approach focused on enhancing relaxation through smooth and rhythmical stroking of the skin. One major advantage of the Esalen approach is that it can be learned quickly and easily, and even for beginners this style of massage is effective in reducing tension.

Shiatsu

Shiatsu (Namikoshi, 1972) is a highly specialized form of massage. It is designed to relieve muscle tension and fatigue through direct pressure. Shiatsu treatments consists of pressure on a specific sequence of points, designed to affect certain muscle systems. The theoretical basis for shiatsu is derived in part from Chinese medicine, which holds that the roots of physical disease can be found in energy imbalances in different major organ systems of the body. One cause of energy blockage is muscular tension, and alleviating that tension brings the affected organ system back to more normal functioning. From centuries of Japanese clinical practice, shiatsu treatments have been successfully devised to relieve a wide variety of physical illnesses.

Body Alignment and Use

Rolfing

One of the best known systems for improving body alignment is structural integration or rolfing. This system was developed more than forty years ago by the late Ida Rolf (1977). Rolf received a Ph.D. in biochemistry and physiology in 1920 and worked in biochemistry at the Rockefeller Institute for twelve years. Rolfing is based on the concept of an ideally aligned body, one that enables the individual to function more effectively and with less muscular effort because the body structure is balanced and aligned in its gravitational field. According to Rolf, the basic pattern or orderliness inherent in the human body is inevitably disturbed in the course of growing up. Physical and emotional traumas, chronic tension, and the like all have permanent effects on physical posture. Rolf says that these influences tend to create "random bodies" and that structural integration treatments serve to organize the body into a more ordered, balanced, and efficient pattern. A series of ten sessions systematically focuses on different areas of the body (Schutz and Turner, 1977). Change is brought about through deep tissue massage, mainly through stretching the fascial tissue to reestablish balance, muscle movement, and flexibility. Most of the rolfing work involves lengthening and stretching tissues that have grown together or become unnaturally thickened as a result of past trauma and poor postural and movement habits.

Several methods have been employed to measure the effectiveness of structural integration. Before and after photographs provide considerable qualitative evidence in Ida Rolf's (1977) classic discussion of her work. Experimental studies, using electromyrographic recordings, have also provided statistically significant quantitative measures of changes produced by structural integration. Hunt and Massey (1977) found improved organization and greater balance in the neuromuscular system following rolfing intervention. Silverman et al. (1973) found increased amplitudes of evoked response waveforms and reduction in responsiveness on the augmenting reducing slope following structural integration, which they interpret as improved receptivity and responsiveness to environmental stimuli.

Alexander Technique

Another system designed to improve alignment and use of the body is the Alexander technique (Alexander, 1969; Barlow, 1973). Its main purpose is to improve awareness of one's habits of body movement and to attend to the process of body usage rather than to a goal or end result of a movement, such as sitting down or arriving at the top of the stairs. Alexander's ideas have far-reaching implications for education, health, and related fields; many prominent scientists and scholars became his pupils and were impressed with his ideas, including Aldous Huxley, George Bernard Shaw, John Dewey, and Nikolaas Tinbergen. Half of Tinbergen's Nobel prize acceptance speech was devoted to Alexander's work (Tinbergen, 1974).

F. Mathias Alexander was an Australian Shakespearian actor and monologist who originated this system in the late nineteenth century. He suffered from recurring loss of voice for which there seemed to be no organic cause. Alexander spent nine years of painstaking self-observation and self-study using a three-way mirror. He discovered that his loss of voice was related to a habit of holding his head up in a way that resulted in backward and downward pressure on the neck. By learning to inhibit this tendency, Alexander no longer lost his voice. In addition, reducing pressure on his neck had positive effects throughout his body. From this, Alexander developed a broad philosophy about learning and human functioning based on the concept of inhibiting habitual, inefficient movements and allowing new and more natural and effective ways of physical functioning to occur.

The Alexander work involves a natural upward lengthening of the spine. Special attention is devoted to neck and head alignment. Students move toward a sense of freeing the neck, feeling the head float forward and up, and sensing the back lengthen and widen. After years of training, an Alexander teacher can sense through his hands on a student's neck or back subtle tensions and movement inhibitions. Through both verbal and physical feedback, students are gradually reeducated to freer, more effective movement. The actual techniques of Alexander work have not been described in detail in the literature because of the system's stress on the importance of a finely trained sensitivity on the part of a teacher as opposed to the mechanical mastering of specific techniques.

Jones (1976) reports a variety of empirical studies of the effectiveness of the Alexander work. His research includes studies employing multiple image photographs analyzing body movement under the guidance of an Alexander teacher as compared to habitual movement patterns. He also used X-ray, photography, electromyography, and subjective judgments of effort. The movement patterns obtained through multiple image photography were analyzed graphically and statistically and demonstrated a significant improvement in coordination and functioning under Alexander guidance.

Feldenkrais

In harmony with Alexander's ideals, Moshe Feldenkrais is also concerned with developing greater awareness and, through this awareness, a more efficient use of the body (Feldenkrais, 1970, 1972, 1977). Exercises developed by Feldenkrais break down habitual movements into smaller, more subtle component parts. With an attitude of playful experimentation, the student learns new possibilities for movement, often involving more of the body. The new movements are performed with greater integration, sensitivity, and awareness.

Feldenkrais exercises are designed to re-establish connections between the motor cortex and the muscular and nervous systems, connections that have been short-circuited or rerouted by bad habits, chronic tension, and physical trauma. As the motor cortex becomes quieter and more balanced through attention to small, natural movements, the individual becomes more sensitive and more aware of the subtle differences in stimulation.

Feldenkrais developed his system in the 1940s. His work owes some debt to Alexander but even more to his own unique background. Feldenkrais is a mathematician and scientist with a doctorate in physics from the Sorbonne. He also opened the first Judo school in Europe and taught Judo for more than thirty years. Feldenkrais began by working on himself in order to alleviate a serious knee injury.

There are two distinct aspects to Feldenkrais's work: (1) awareness through movement and (2) functional integration. Awareness through movement is a system of exercises that can be done with large groups led through verbal instructions. Functional integration is more directly therapeutic in nature and requires one-to-one work. The individual work involves direct sensory experiences; increased awareness and a natural readjustment of posture, muscle tension, and body image are facilitated through the touch of the therapist. Both the exercises and the clinical work are described in greater detail in the annotated bibliography that follows this chapter.

Sensory Awareness

Sensory awareness work (Brooks, 1974) centers on relaxation and focusing attention on immediate experience. In many ways, the ideal is to become again as a child—deeply absorbed in experiencing the world in a free and playful way.

Work in sensory awareness brings many of the benefits found in the practice of formal meditation – in particular, stress and tension reduction. In addition, learning to experience both one's own body and the external world more clearly and deeply can be astonishingly rich and gratifying.

Sensory awareness has been taught in the United States primarily by Charlotte Selver, who was trained in Europe by Elsa Gindler and Heinrich Jacoby. Many of the exercises deal with the basic human activities of lying, sitting, standing, and walking. These activities provide an opportunity for developing greater conscious awareness of the body and senses. Exercises in interaction with others include learning to touch another and to receive touch.

Selver's work has strongly influenced the human potential movement (Schutz, 1967) through Bernard Gunther's (1968) best-selling book *Sense Relaxation*. Gunther's book includes a variety of exercises designed to help people become more sensitive to their bodies and senses, to accept touch and touching, caring and being cared for. Gunther's work is not as slow, subtle, and demanding as Selver's; however, it has attracted more attention, partly because the exercises can be led by virtually anyone who has read his book. These exercises have been adopted by many psychotherapists and human potential group leaders throughout the country. They are powerful tools for bringing people to a deeper awareness of themselves and of the world around them.

Psychotherapeutic Body Work

Reichian Therapy

The founder of psychotherapeutic body work was Wilhelm Reich, the first Freudian analyst to recognize that the ego, id, and superego inhabit a body (Reich, 1961, 1973, 1975; Baker, 1974; Boadella, 1974). Reich began as a highly respected Freudian psychoanalyst. His strong interest in psychotherapeutic techniques (he was in charge of training young analysts for several years) led him to stress the importance of analyzing the patient's character structure as an interrelated whole rather than focusing only on a neurosis or problem. Later in his career, Reich discovered that patterns of chronic muscular tension were closely related to character structure. By character structure, Reich meant an individual's habitual attitudes and consistent pattern of responses to various situations. In particular, Reich was interested in the ways in which an individual's ego defenses combine to form a mutually supportive, interrelated pattern. He found each pattern of defenses to be associated with a particular pattern of chronic muscular tension. By directly relieving the muscular tensions, Reich was able to speed up the psychotherapeutic work.

Reich also pioneered in sex education and counseling. In fact, it was his interest in sexuality that first led him to Freud. When Reich insisted that all neurotic patients were unable to enjoy full, unblocked sexual orgasm, his work was rejected by his fellow analysts. Although this is not considered as shocking today as it was when Reich first proposed it, his stress on attaining "full orgastic potency" is still controversial.

Reich gradually came to view therapy as a process of freeing the flow of energy throughout the body by systematically dissolving blocks of muscular tension or armoring. He developed the theory of orgone energy, which includes not only libidinal-muscular energy but also biological and cosmic energy found in all living things and in all matter. Reich's later work involved orgone physics, orgone energy accumulators, and a host of similar ideas.

There is a considerable body of clinical and experimental findings supportive of Reich's ideas that is reported in Reich's books and in Reichian journals. Because of the controversial nature of Reich's theories—his later work in particular—his research and that of his students has been professionally ignored rather than critically evaluated or refuted. However, his earlier theories of character armoring and body work in therapy have been major influences on other theories and therapeutic systems.

Bioenergetics

The system most directly influenced by Reich is bioenergetics. It was founded by Alexander Lowen (1969, 1971, 1975, 1977), originally a practicing Reichian psychiatrist. Bioenergetics includes many of Reich's physical and emotional release techniques, such as having patients cry, scream, and strike out. A central feature of bioenergetics is the use of various physical postures designed to energize different parts of the body. Some postures open up the chest and diaphragm and facilitate deeper breathing. Others are designed to increase tension in different parts of the body until the chronically tense body parts eventually let go and relax. Many therapists who are not fully trained bioenergetic practitioners have fruitfully adopted some aspects of Lowen's work in their own therapy.

Summary

The systems of body work discussed here share certain basic assumptions about the nature of human functioning. They all stress that health and efficient functioning are the normal and natural condition of the body. This state is disturbed or distorted in various ways by internal or environmental influences. Each system emphasizes certain means of eliminating such negative influences in order to restore a normal state of health and effectiveness. These systems are all based on holistic principles of the interconnectedness of all of physical functioning. Improving one or more aspects of physical functioning promotes significant improvement in other areas. For example, working to relax or align the body has been found to affect self-confidence, concentration, sexual behavior, and efficiency of movement.

Each system tends to work directly on different areas. Shiatsu seeks to tonify and relax specific muscle patterns, rolfing to readjust the fascia, Alexander work to re-educate the individual to new movement patterns through direct touch, Feldenkrais to promote re-education through attention to extremely subtle details of movement, and sensory awareness to allow changes to blossom naturally from new and deeper ways of experiencing oneself and the world. Because of the differences in emphasis, these systems are more complementary than contradictory. They also supplement effectively much of traditional medical and psychological therapy.

Research in these areas has been sparse. The originators and major practitioners of these systems are less interested in empirical than in clinical confirmation of their work. Empirical work has generally been done by experimenters who are untrained in the techniques they have studied, and so far the research has had little recognition either scientifically or within the discipline studies. It is hoped that this state of affairs will be remedied in the future as the potentials of these techniques receive wider recognition.

References

Alexander, F. Mathias. *The Resurrection of the Body.* New York: Delta, 1969.

Baker, Elsworth, M.D. *Man in the Trap: The Causes of Blocked Sexual Energy.* New York: Avon, 1974.

Barlow, Wilfred. *The Alexander Technique.* New York: Knopf, 1973.

Boadella, David. *Wilhelm Reich: The Evolution of His Work.* London: Vision, 1974.

Brooks, Charles. *Sensory Awareness.* New York: Viking, 1974.

Downing, George. *The Massage Book.* New York: Random House, 1972.

Feldenkrais, Moshe. *Body and Mature Behavior: A Study of Anxiety, Sex, Gravitation and Learning.* New York: International Universities Press, 1970.

Feldenkrais, Moshe. *Awareness Through Movement.* New York: Harper and Row, 1972.

Feldenkrais, Moshe. *The Case of Nora: Body-Awareness as Healing Therapy.* New York: Harper and Row, 1977.

Gunther, Bernard. *Sense Relaxation.* New York: Collier, 1968.

Hunt, Valerie, and Massey, Wayne. Electromyographic evaluation of structural integration techniques. *Psychoenergetic Systems,* 1977. **2**, 199–210.

Jones, Franklin. *Body Awareness in Action.* New York: Schocken, 1976.

Lowen, Alexander. *The Betrayal of the Body.* New York: Macmillan, 1969.

Lowen, Alexander. *The Language of the Body.* New York: Macmillan, 1971.

Lowen, Alexander. *Bioenergetics.* New York: Penguin, 1975.

Lowen, Alexander, and Lowen, Leslie. *The Way to Vibrant Health: A Manual of Bioenergetic Exercises.* New York: Harper and Row, 1977.

Montagu, Ashley. *Touching*. New York: Harper and Row, 1971.

Namikoshi, Tokujiro. *Shiatsu: Japanese Finger-Pressure Therapy*. San Francisco: Japan Publications, 1972.

Reich, Wilhelm. *Character Analysis*. New York: Farrar, Straus and Giroux, 1961.

Reich, Wilhelm. *Selected Writings*. New York: Noonday, 1973.

Reich, Wilhelm. *The Function of the Orgasm*. New York: Pocket Books, 1975.

Rolf, Ida. *Rolfing: The Integration of Human Structures*. Santa Monica, Calif.: Dennis-Landman, 1977.

Schutz, Will. *Joy*. New York: Grove, 1967.

Schutz, Will, and Turner, Evelyn. *Body Fantasy*. New York: Harper and Row, 1977.

Silverman, J.; Rappaport, M.; Hopkins, H. K.; Ellman, G.; Hubbard, R.; Belleza, T.; Baldwin, T.; Griffin, R.; and Kling, R. Stress intensity control and the structural integration techniques. *Confinia Psychiatrics*, 1973. **16**, 209–219.

Tinbergen, Nikolaas. Ethology and stress diseases. *Science*, 1974. **185**, 20–27.

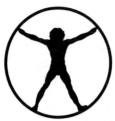 ANNOTATED BIBLIOGRAPHY

Alexander, F. Mathias. **The Resurrection of the Body.** New York: Delta, 1969.

This is an edited selection of Alexander's works, also including three pieces on the Alexander work by John Dewey, one of Alexander's best known students. There is a long introduction dealing with the history of Alexander's work and his teaching. Chapters by Alexander himself include case histories, discussions of breathing, exercise, concentration, and emotions. Alexander's writing style is difficult but his ideas make the effort worthwhile.

Alexander's work consists of re-educating the individual in how he uses his body. Through light touch and verbal guidance, an Alexander teacher helps make the student aware of habitual patterns of movement and usage and guides the student into new patterns and a new sense of self. Alexander describes how he himself came to develop the technique and outlines in many different ways his central notion of letting go of specific goal orientation. The desire for a certain end result makes it impossible for the individual to sense and understand the means – the very process – he is using to attain his ends. In many different contexts, Alexander points out the prevalence of the attitude of "end-gaining" and the ways that this attitude creates hit-and-miss, unconscious, mechanical behavior.

The first chapter was most fascinating to me. It consists of short aphorisms taken down by Alexander's students from his actual teaching sessions and gives a clear sense of the thrust of his ideas. The following is a short selection:

I see at last that if I don't breathe, I breathe.
If I breathe as I understand breathing, I am doing something wrong.
Change involves carrying out an activity against the habit of life.
When you are asked not to do something, instead of making the decision not to do it, you try to prevent yourself from doing it. But this only means that you decide to do it, and then use muscle tension to prevent yourself from doing it.
All the damned fools in the world believe they are actually doing what they think they are doing.
If your neck feels stiff, that is not to say your neck "is" stiff.

The book is an excellent introduction to Alexander's basic philosophy. It does not give any of the details of the Alexander technique of body work, however – there is no book that teaches the specific techniques of Alexander work. Alexander practitioners believe strongly that the work must be learned through personal instruction. Without the sensitivity developed through training, the Alexander work can only be superficially imitated.

Baker, Elsworth, M.D. **Man in the Trap: The Causes of Blocked Sexual Energy.** New York: Avon, 1974.

An excellent introduction to the practice of Reichian therapy. Dr. Baker is a practicing psychiatrist and one of the leading students of Wilhelm Reich. The book has four parts: Part 1 is concerned with character formation and the factors in body and character armoring; Part 2 deals with the various character types and the effects of armoring; Part 3 focuses on therapeutic techniques for the removal of armoring; and Part 4 deals with ways of preventing armoring in prenatal and infant care.

In terms of psychodynamics, the theoretical approach is basically Freudian. To the psychoanalytic conception of character types and dynamics, Baker adds a detailed and sophisticated discussion of the role of the body in development and maintenance of character structure. He also discusses several new character types. To me, the most interesting is his discussion of the ocular stage as the first stage of psychosexual development, linking this with the formation of ocular character types, in particular various schizoid characters. He also devotes a chapter to Reich's theories of socio-political character types, which is interesting, although it has little relevance to Reichian body work.

Baker is at his best in his discussions of the actual processes of therapy. The book is rich in case histories, and there are also detailed discussions of the processes of removing armoring in each of the major blocks in the body postulated by Reich – eyes, mouth, throat, chest, diaphragm, abdomen, and pelvis. In addition, Baker discusses his own psychotherapeutic procedures – including the initial examination, therapeutic goals, and the end phase of therapy.

His three basic principles in therapy are: "(1) increasing the inner push in the organism by building up its energy by breathing; (2) directly attacking the spastic muscles to free the contraction; and (3) maintaining the cooperation of the patient by bringing into the open and overcoming his resistance to therapy and the therapist" (p. 73).

Man in the Trap can provide practical ideas and approaches for those already involved in the practice of mind-body therapy. It will not make you into a Reichian therapist; that requires substantial training as well as hours in Reichian therapy.

Brooks, Charles. **Sensory Awareness.** New York: Viking, 1974.

This book reflects the subtle feeling of sensory awareness work in its powerful and simple style and in the many rich photographs that supplement the text. Introductory chapters discuss the underlying philosophy of the work. Accompanying photography of infants engaged in play and exploration provide beautiful examples of sensing and experiencing the world in a free and playful yet deeply absorbed way.

The second part of the book is devoted to what Brooks calls "the four dignities of man" – walking, standing, sitting, and lying. Each chapter describes an exercise or, more precisely, a set of suggestions that provides a framework and orientation for a particular kind of sensory exploration. More important are descriptions of the experiences that Brooks and his students have had with each of these basic human activities.

The third section of the book is entitled "Toward a More Sensitive Relating." Chapters include yawning, stretching, relating with others through touch and play, tasting, and working with objects. Rather than attempting to teach specific techniques of how to sense, Brooks generally describes in each chapter a particularly vivid example of the sensory awareness work. He is able to give the flavor of the core of sensory awareness—slowing down, coming more fully into the present moment, and then suddenly perceiving in a deeper and often qualitatively different way.

Downing, George. **The Massage Book.** New York: Random House, 1972.

This is a well-written, clearly illustrated introduction to soft, Esalen-style massage. The book is easy to work with and to learn from—a rarity among books that attempt to teach physical skills. It has introductory chapters with practical information about massage, including information on oils, powders, and massage tables; how to prepare a physical setting conducive to massage; how to apply oil; and so on. Then comes the main body of the book—sections describing different strokes for each part of the body, including head and neck, arms, legs, hands, feet, back, buttocks, chest, and stomach. Downing also includes sections discussing tension, ticklishness, self-massage, massage for animals, massage for lovers, anatomy, and other aspects of massage.

The theoretical material is light. The book is designed to teach practical skills of massaging, and it does that extremely well. The profuse illustrations and superb layout enhance its effectiveness in communicating the feelings and attitudes integral to this kind of massage work as well as the concrete, practical details of massage technique.

Feldenkrais, Moshe. **Awareness Through Movement.** New York: Harper and Row, 1972.

This book provides an introduction to Feldenkrais's system of learning through a progressive series of muscle and body movements. Feldenkrais begins with a theoretical section; the second, larger part of the book (more than 100 pages) is devoted to twelve lessons in awareness through movement. The theoretical chapters include discussions of self-image and its psychological and physical effects, the developmental sequences of human functioning, structures and function, and progress through the development of awareness. The lessons were selected from literally hundreds given by Feldenkrais. They were chosen primarily to illustrate various aspects of the author's systems and techniques. They include lessons on posture, breathing, coordination of flexors and extensors, differentiation of pelvic movements, self-image, carriage of the head, eye movements, gaining awareness of various parts of the body, and thinking and breathing. These techniques can be practiced individually and are also taught or learned in a group through verbal instructions.

It takes some effort to gain real benefit from this book. The lessons must be experienced to be appreciated; I have found that the more exposure I have had to these lessons through practice and teaching, the greater has been my understanding and learning. In the theoretical section, Feldenkrais presents a tremendous wealth of sophisticated ideas in a terse, elliptical style. It is easy to skim through these chapters, nodding in general agreement, without really getting the implications of Feldenkrais's ideas. I consider Feldenkrais by far the most innovative, brilliant, and provocative theorist working with the body today. This book is worth reading and savoring *slowly*, spending at least as much time reflecting on his ideas as reading them.

Feldenkrais, Moshe. **The Case of Nora: Body-Awareness as Healing Therapy.** New York: Harper and Row, 1977.

Feldenkrais has written up a single case study that reads like a detective story. He is first introduced to Nora after treatment at one of the world's finest neurological clinics has failed. Her speech and movement are impaired and her ability to read and write have been totally lost. Feldenkrais takes the reader through each stage of his examination, diagnosis, and treatment. At the end, we find Nora recovered enough to lead a normal, productive life. He shares his mistakes as well as his triumphs and frequently uses the case as a springboard for enormously valuable theoretical discussions.

> When I am presented with a trouble in function, I make a special effort not to think in words. I try not to think logically and in correctly formed sentences. It has become a habit with me to imagine the relevant nervous structures by seeing them with my mind's eye. I imagine a part which produces a flow of fluid. Part of the travel of the fluid is electrical, then becomes chemical, and again electrical. . . .
>
> I have found this way of imagining so fruitful that I cannot do without it. It often shows me where my knowledge is insufficient so that I know exactly what I am after. . . . I start each case as if it were my first, and ask myself more questions than any of my assistants or critics ever do (p. 27).

Feldenkrais describes how he painstakingly investigated the smallest details of Nora's behavior, eventually coming to the realization that her basic spatial orientation was disturbed, and this led to her other impairments. He describes her re-education process, beginning with the developing of greater awareness of her own body and gradually regaining a sense of right and left in her own body. Then Feldenkrais slowly taught her to transfer this body awareness to differentiating external objects. Next, Feldenkrais describes the process of re-educating her eyes, enabling them to focus properly and to recognize printed words and letters. Finally, he recreates in Nora the entire process of learning to write. The details of the techniques Feldenkrais describes are fascinating, but even more useful is the insight this book provides into his basic principles and underlying method of working.

Gunther, Bernard. **Sense Relaxation.** New York: Collier, 1968.

Gunther's book has been a major influence on many psychotherapists, counselors, and group facilitators. He offers a wide variety of individual and group exercises designed to create a greater sense of personal awareness and aliveness. *Sense Relaxation* is also a lovely picture book filled with stunning photos taken by noted photographer Paul Fusco. Fusco has captured the mood and feeling of each exercise. Many photographs are full page, and often there are three or four photographs illustrating a single exercise.

Simple and clearly written instructions for each exercise enable the reader to try out or to teach the exercise with a minimum of worry or confusion. At the beginning of each section of the book, Gunther provides a poetic, philosophical, and theoretical orientation in more or less blank verse. The section on self-awarness includes exercises for touching, tapping, lifting, stretching, and slapping different parts of your own body, along with suggestions for making sounds, breathing, or focusing on inner awareness where appropriate. The next section deals with two-person exercises duplicating much of the solo work. A chapter on sensory awareness emphasizes intense, present-centered awareness of commonplace activities, such as washing, drinking, stretching, touching, and eating.

One chapter is devoted to partnership touching exercises, including touching back to back, feet to feet, and touching with hands a partner's head, face, and entire body. The book closes with a chapter on group exercises – milling and touching, hand-to-hand and back-to-back exercises, group lifting and group passing of an individual member, a blind walk, crawling, chanting, tasting, and touching together. The joy, relaxation, and freedom evident on participants' faces make it clear how powerful these simple exercises can be, and how well they complement more traditional psychotherapeutic or medical forms of treatment.

Jones, Franklin. **Body Awareness in Action.** New York: Schocken, 1976.

The aim of this book is to introduce readers to the Alexander technique of body re-education. Jones weaves a discussion of Alexander's basic ideas into his history of the growth and development of Alexander's teachings. In the historical chapters, Jones mentions many of the great men of letters and science who supported Alexander's work and who often derived great personal benefit from working with him, including George Bernard Shaw, Aldous Huxley, Sir Charles Sherrington, and John Dewey. Of particular interest are the chapters outlining Jones's years of experimental research on the technique.

Jones's experimental work involved some innovative and fascinating methodology. He employed multiple-image, stroboscopic photography to measure and compare habitual movement patterns with the patterns of body movement resulting from Alexander lessons. In other studies, Jones employed electromyography, subjective questionnaires administered to subjects undergoing Alexander lessons, sound spectrographs, X-ray photographs, and a strain-gauge force platform (to measure the amount of force exerted in various movements). The extensive bibliography includes references to all the major research done on the Alexander technique as well as the theoretical writings of Alexander and others.

Lowen, Alexander. **Bioenergetics.** New York: Penguin, 1975.

This book is more personal and also more revealing of the techniques and therapeutic process of bioenergetics than any of Lowen's earlier works. In the first chapter, Lowen discusses his years of therapy with Reich, his own work as a Reichian therapist, and the development of bioenergetics. Other chapters include discussions of the energy concept, body language, character types, sexuality, and consciousness. Lowen also includes a variety of bioenergetic exercises and demonstrations for the reader to try out in order to experience his concepts. The book is rich in case studies, and Lowen's discussions always emphasize the theme of viewing physical and psychological processes in an integrated way.

In Lowen's discussion of character types (Chapter 5) he uses a schematic representation of the body as a six-sided star. The six points represent the head, two hands, two feet, and genitals. Each character type is described psychologically, physically (characteristic tension, rigidity; typical posture, body type, etc.), bioenergetically (energy blocks and their effects), and graphically (in terms of the star diagram). This integration is typical of Lowen's approach throughout the book.

Bioenergetics provides an excellent introduction to the techniques and basic principles of bioenergetics as well as an excellent example of one way of perceiving the functional unity of the emotional, physical, and energetic aspects of the individual.

Lowen, Alexander, and Lowen, Leslie. **The Way to Vibrant Health: A Manual of Bioenergetic Exercises.** New York: Harper, 1977.

This is basically a how-to manual. More than one hundred basic bioenergetic exercises are well presented, with excellent, clear illustrations for virtually every exercise. The Lowens devote two short chapters to introductory theory, covering basic definitions of bioenergetics, bodily vibration, and grounding. Following chapters cover breathing, sexuality, self-possession and self-expression, and being in touch. They combine both theory and exercises for practice.

Virtually all the rest of the book is devoted to the exercises. There are warm-up stretching and loosening exercises, exercises for the feet and legs, hips and pelvis, arms and shoulders, head and neck. There are standing up, sitting, and lying down exercises as well as exercises with the bioenergetic stool, massage, and exercises devoted to emotional expression and to enhanced sexuality.

The book is extremely clear and easy to follow. Anyone can begin bioenergetic work on themselves or begin to integrate bioenergetic exercises into a clinical practice with this book, although it will probably be most useful to those who have already had some bioenergetic work and can use it to continue on their own.

Namikoshi, Tokujiro. **Shiatsu: Japanese Finger-Pressure Therapy.** San Francisco: Japan Publications, 1972.

There are a number of good books written on shiatsu, representing different schools, theories, and styles of practice. Namikoshi is the man who almost singly-handedly popularized shiatsu in Japan. He claims to have successfully treated more than 100,000 patients, and his school has trained more than 20,000 practitioners. The book is primarily devoted to practice rather than theory. Basically, Namikoshi claims that shiatsu pressure on fatigued muscles causes reconversion of lactic acid into glycogen, eliminating fatigue and improper muscular contraction.

The first section of the book deals with basic theory, correct use of fingers and hands, and basic pressure points. The second section is devoted to techniques for general health improvement, including relief from fatigue, stiff arms and shoulders, insomnia, and high blood pressure. The third section is devoted to shiatsu treatments designed to improve sexual performance and sex-related functions. The fourth and final section outlines treatment for a wide variety of specific illnesses, including diarrhea, colds, headache, rheumatism, whiplash injuries, and asthma.

The instructions are simple and readable, accompanied by both photographs and extremely clear and specific drawings giving proper hand and pressure-point positions. This is an excellent book for learning the practice of shiatsu.

Reich, Wilhelm. **Selected Writings.** New York: Noonday, 1973.

This anthology is an excellent introduction to the full range of Reich's writings and theories. It includes excerpts from the classic *Character Analysis,* written while Reich was still a highly respected Freudian analyst. The book also contains Reich's discussion of his pioneering work in body-oriented psychotherapy as well as his more controversial writings—reports of his laboratory research with orgone energy, discussions of cosmic orgone energy, and social and philosophical writings.

The volume includes a section of Reich's orgasm theory, describing how it logically evolved out of traditional psychoanalytic theory. There are also chapters on character analysis and psychotherapy. More than half of the book is devoted to Reich's later orgone research—the discovery of orgone, experiments in orgone physics, and discussion of orgone in nature and the cosmos. Other chapters include Reich's applications of his theories to more philosophical issues—mysticism and mechanism, reason, truth, and consciousness.

It is advisable to read Reich's work, rather than simply to dismiss him on the basis of highly biased critiques written by orthodox psychoanalysts and conservative psychologists. The chapters on therapy are thought provoking and solidly grounded in Reich's years of successful clinical work. His theories of energy flow within the organism still seem ahead of their time today. Although most persons will not easily accept Reich's later work with orgone energy, when viewed along with his earlier work these writings fall into a meaningful context and enable the reader to see Reich as a serious scientist, however much one might disagree with his findings.

Rolf, Ida F. **Rolfing: The Integration of Human Structures.** Santa Monica. Calif: Dennis-Landman, 1977.

This is *the* definitive theoretical book on rolfing. The late Dr. Rolf has succeeded in the very difficult task of writing a book that is clear enough to be understandable to lay people, yet detailed enough (especially in the captions for illustrations and photographs) to satisfy medical readers or physiologically trained psychologists. The heart of the book consists of chapters concentrating on various parts of the body—feet, spine, pelvis, head, neck, etc.—along with detailed discussions of the effects of malalignment.

The book is rich in illustrations, presenting a more functional and dynamic view of the body than is customarily found in anatomy texts. There are also a great many photographs; reading *Rolfing* is an excellent education in viewing bodies, learning to see the effects of a tilted pelvis, constricted hamstrings, everted (toed out) feet, etc. Virtually every photograph has an accompanying caption calling the viewers' attention to various subtle details of posture and its effects. Also, the frequent pairing of before-and-after photographs is enough to make a good case for the value and efficacy of rolfing.

I have some caveats, but they are minor. Rolf's use of the term "random bodies" for all bodies that have not undergone rolfing seems to me to be imprecise, overgeneralized, and almost smacks of a sales pitch for rolfing. Secondly, Rolf hints at both the beginning and end of the book that rolfing is intimately involved with energy flow and subtle energies in the body. Unfortunately, she leaves the concept of energy undefined or only hinted at.

Rolf is suggestive of the results to be achieved in discussing the effects of postural changes on emotional and psychologial processes, but her theory seems oversimplistic in suggesting that developing a more upright posture will automatically enhance self-image, for example. One drawback often mentioned about rolfing is the issue of the permanence of change. Many persons have felt that they have lost much of the benefits of rolfing within a year or two, as they returned to habitual postures and ways of moving. However, in others I have seen major changes that have lasted for five to six years. Unfortunately, Rolf did not even address this issue. Nonetheless, *Rolfing* is a basic reference work and a reading must for any professional seriously interested in posture, movement, or the psychology of the body.

Schutz, Will, and Turner, Evelyn. **Body Fantasy.** New York: Harper and Row, 1977.

This is the case study of a single patient undergoing structural integration (rolfing) combined with guided fantasy. Included are descriptions of the physical work done in each session plus the physical changes observed by the therapist and reported by Evy, the patient. Schutz employed guided fantasy in working with psychological material. The patient (and co-author of the book) describes the fantasy experience and subsequent reactions in selections from the journal she kept throughout the course of treatment. For example, during the session devoted to releasing chronic tensions in the face, the patient was able to release her perpetual fixed smile. Schutz comments: "A perpetual smile usually covers up other feelings, typically fear, sadness, and anger. Considerable physical effort is required to hold this unnatural position, and the facial muscles become chronically contracted" (p. 84). During the session, Evy recalls painful childhood memories and becomes more fully aware of her need to please and her fear of disapproval from others.

The book provides relatively little theory about structural integration or psychotherapy. It is an excellent, detailed case study of mind-body interaction indicating how various repressed memories and suppressed emotions become conscious during each stage of the rolfing process. Schutz's comments on the relationship between the physical work and psychological process are clear, sophisticated, and helpful to anyone who wants to work in this area.

15

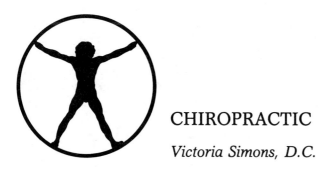

CHIROPRACTIC
Victoria Simons, D.C.

Introduction

Manipulation of the spine and joints has been an integral part of healing since the beginnings of recorded history and the practice persists in numerous systems throughout the world. In the late nineteenth century, at a time when the biomedical model of disease was capturing the imagination and allegiance of orthodox physicians, two Americans revived the therapeutic use of manipulation and elaborated its techniques in the schools of chiropractic and osteopathy. Chiropractic emphasized the centrality and integrity of the nervous system as the crucial element in proper bodily functioning and osteopathy focused on the importance of unimpeded circulation. The originators of both practices were concerned with creating systems that would help restore the integrity of the person rather than remedy a particular pathological process.

Since 1874, when the physician Andrew Still created osteopathy, manipulative therapy has undergone many changes. Some aspects have become incorporated into the practice of orthopedics, particularly in the area of rehabilitative medicine (Maigne, 1972), and manipulation of the temporomandibular joint has been incorporated into dentistry. Although some osteopaths have continued to refine the manipulative aspects of their profession, many more have come to regard the techniques and practice of manipulation as secondary to the use of pharmacological agents and surgery. In fact, in some states the licensing procedures for D.O.'s (osteopaths) and M.D.'s are identical.

Chiropractic, however, has tended to maintain its separate identity as a manipulative practice. Although most practitioners work on the spine as a whole, others have explored techniques that deal primarily with the sacrum and the occiput or with the upper cervical area. Some chiropractors have adopted a comprehensive system of muscle testing (kinesiology) designed to reveal malfunctions in visceral organs through weakness in the related muscles (Goodheart, 1972–1977). More recently, chiropractors have begun to prescribe exercise and diet regimes and to include such healing modalities as acupuncture, massage, and homoeopathy in their practice.

History

D. D. Palmer, the founder of chiropractic, believed that there was a "universal intelligence" in all living matter that was responsible for its properties and actions and for maintaining its existence. He developed chiropractic as a science, art, and philosophy of health based on natural law, physiology, and anatomy. His original work was founded on the premise that the nervous system was physiologically the ultimate control mechanism of the human body. Palmer believed that if a way were discovered to insure the proper functioning of the nervous system, the restoration and maintenance of health would naturally follow.

Palmer felt that disease could result from excess or deficient neurological function and that interference with the normal transmission of nerve impulses was primarily due to the mechanical infringement of nervous tissue secondary to a subluxation. A common definition of a subluxation is "a condition in which one of the vertebrae has lost its juxtaposition with the one above or below to an extent less than a luxation (a severe misalignment of the joint) that occludes an opening, impinges on nerves, and interferes with normal neurological function." (Stephenson, 1948).

Palmer performed his first adjustment in September 1895. The patient, Harvey Lillard, had been deaf for seventeen years. In his writings, Palmer stated that "he [Lillard] could not hear the racket of a wagon in the street or the ticking of a watch" and that after a "specific adjustment" the man could "hear as before" (Palmer, 1910).

Subluxation and Chiropractic Analysis

Chiropractors utilize physical examination, X-ray, and laboratory procedures to evaluate their patients. Many include dietary advice, nutritional supplementation, discussion of exercise regimes, and counseling in their treatment and emphasize the importance of developing and maintaining a healthy life-style in practicing self-responsibility in health care. Still the cornerstone of the chiropractic treatment is examination of the spine and treatment of its subluxations.

The detection of vertebral subluxation is the first step in determining the need for chiropractic care in a given individual. Specific techniques for detecting vertebral subluxations include:

- *Static palpation.* Digital examination of the paravertebral tissues is used to detect muscular dystonia and gross mechanical misalignment. Anatomical variants also may be observed at this time. Areas of tenderness noted during this examination indicate possible areas of neurological involvement. The examination is usually conducted with the patient prone or seated (National Institute of Neurologic and Communicative Disorders and Stroke, 1975; Street, 1969).

- *Motion palpation.* In this procedure, the various vertebral motor units are taken through their ranges of motion by the examiner. The primary objective is to determine changes in ranges of motion. Changes are frequently associated with vertebral subluxation. Areas exhibiting aberrant motion may also indicate congenital abnormalities, anatomical variants, or pathological processes (National Institute of Neurologic and Communicative Disorders and Stroke, 1975; Street, 1969).

- *Spinal x-ray examination.* Specialized X-ray procedures are used to locate and measure spinal disrelationships associated with subluxation. Alterations of spinal curves, disc angulations, anatomical variants, congenital abnormalities, and spinal pathologies may be noted. Visual examination of the spine enables the chiropractor to tailor the adjustment to the needs of the patient and to determine possible contraindications to adjustment of a given area (Kent and Skibbe, 1976; Inman, 1973; Toftness, 1977; Palmer, 1938d).

- *Muscle testing.* Tests of specific muscle strength may be conducted to determine if the subluxation is interfering with normal muscular function. Weaknesses in specific muscles have been correlated to disrelationships in specific spinal segments. Instruments such as dynamometers may be used in evaluating muscle strength (Goodheart, 1972–1977).

- *Extremity length measurements.* Measurements of leg and arm length with the patient in the prone or supine position may demonstrate changes in paravertebral muscle tones and indicate possible subluxations. If the paravertebral muscles on one side of the spine are in a state of contraction while their counterparts on the opposite side are relaxed, one extremity may appear longer than the other. Such asymmetries are frequently associated with vertebral subluxation (Kent and Simons, 1979; Wells, 1955; Thompson, 1973; DeJarnette, 1976).

- *Postural analysis.* Evaluation of a patient's posture aids in evaluating spinal curves. Changes in posture have been noted in a wide variety of specific symptoms, conditions, and diseases. The use of plumb lines and other postural measurement instruments may be part of the chiropractic analysis (National Institute of Neurologic and Communicative Disorders and Stroke, 1975).

- *Skin temperature analysis.* Changes in skin temperature have been shown to indicate changes in the function of the autonomic nervous system. By measuring skin temperature differentials of the paravertebral area, changes in autonomic function may be evaluated. Such changes have been shown to result from vertebral subluxation (Korr, 1955, 1974; Kent and Daniels, 1974).

The pathophysiologic manifestations of vertebral subluxations that chiropractors are able to observe, palpate, or discern on radiologic examination are extensive and pervasive. By interfering with normal neurological function, vertebral subluxations may cause disease or disharmony anywhere in the organism. The specific malfunction that results will be determined by the organs and tissues innervated by the nerves affected by the subluxation and by the various environmental, inherited, nutritional, and traumatic stressors imposed on the organism.

There are thirty-one pairs of spinal nerves: eight cervical, twelve thoracic, five lumbar, five sacral, and usually one coccygeal. The first twenty-five pairs exit from mobile segments of the spine through foramina that protect the nerves and vessels against external influences while leaving room for vertebral column motion. Chiropractors believe that changes in the form and width of the foramina may impinge on the nerves that exit from them and thereby affect the function of the innervated structures.

According to this theory, subluxations may cause visceral dysfunction at all spinal levels. For example, subluxation at the level of the first cervical vertebra may produce such clinical symptoms as cephalgia, vestibular mechanism dysfunction (e.g., dizziness), or cerebellar system dysfunction (e.g., incoordination). Subluxations at the level of the second thoracic vertebra may cause functional heart conditions, thoracic pain, coronary artery involvement, and dysfunction of the glands innervated by the sympathetic nervous system (International Chiropractic Association, 1979b).

Vertebral subluxations represent channels of increased vulnerability to adverse environmental stressors. The greater the influence of these stressors, the more the balance is tipped toward disease. The subluxation apparently intensifies the effects of these stressors by interfering with the body's defense mechanisms—its ability to successfully adapt and establish a new state of dynamic equilibrium.

Chiropractors have been criticized by medical professionals, who argue that organs and tissues secrete, relax, and contract in the absence of direct nervous stimulation. Chiropractors would agree, contending only that the nervous system plays a central regulatory role in the establishment of normal body function and that even if the precise intermediary mechanisms are as yet unknown, neural dysfunction will inevitably disrupt bodily homeostasis.

The chiropractor integrates these clinical findings, rules out the possibility of specific contraindications to manipulation – fractures, etc. – and determines which, if any, vertebrae needs adjustment. The adjustment itself is tailored to the specific needs of the individual patient and is designed to correct the subluxation with the minimum necessary force. Scores of techniques, divided into two categories, have been developed to accomplish the adjustment. "Thrust adjustments" are characterized by the sudden quick application of force to the offending vertebrae using the bony processes as levers. "Low force adjustments" use sustained pressure on the vertebrae to enable the muscles of the body to readapt and correct the subluxation.

Research

Though there are countless anecdotal reports of chiropractic cures of physical and emotional disorders, there is little hard research and as yet no satisfactorily controlled clinical studies of, for instance, chiropractic versus medical care. In the past, chiropractic has been inhibited by the disinclination of clinicians to pursue research and by the lack of research funds for what is, after all, considered a "fringe profession." As chiropractic education becomes increasingly rigorous and as chiropractic becomes a more acceptable form of therapy, research will increase.

The first effort of the profession to formalize research was the establishment of the B. J. Palmer Research Clinic in 1937. Patients were diagnosed by medical physicians, given a chiropractic examination, and placed under chiropractic care. Hematologic, audiometric, electrocardiographic, and other physiological measures were made before and after a regimen of chiropractic care. Although these patients showed clinical and physiologic improvement (Palmer, 1938a, 1938b, 1938c), this kind of research yielded little knowledge of the specific mechanisms involved in the pathophysiology of the subluxation and its effects on organs and organ systems.

In 1970 the University of Colorado instituted a major research program into the biomechanical and neurophysiological basis of chiropractic. This work, cosponsored by the National Institutes of Health and the International Chiropractic Association, is concerned with elucidating the relationships between the nervous system and the spinal column and the effects of these relationships on health and disease. The head of the research team, Chung Ha Suh (1974), has been primarily interested in three-dimensional computer modeling of the spine and simulations of spinal motion. Other researchers have already demonstrated that spinal nerve roots are far more susceptible to compression blockage than peripheral nerves (Sharpless et al., 1975) and that nerves subjected to compression by ligation produce toxic protein substances (Luttges and Groswald, 1977).

This work suggests that the small anatomical changes of the subluxation prolonged over a period of time may produce substantial pathology and functional change in nervous tissue. It dovetails nicely with the osteopathic research of I. M. Korr (1955, 1974). Korr discovered that in subluxated segments of the spinal cord the anterior and lateral horn cells were hypersusceptible to stimuli and produced an increase in neural transmission. This increased rate of transmission in turn caused dystonia, exaggerated sympathetic activity, vasoconstriction, and ultimately altered visceral function. Examination of pathological tissue changes following artificial induction of vertebral subluxation in rabbits provides preliminary experimental confirmation of this process (Cleveland, 1965).

Chiropractic research is, however, still in its infancy and will not make major gains until there is some resolution of interprofessional rivalries. The first steps in this process were taken in February 1975 by the National Institute of Neurologic and Communicative Disorders and Stroke (NINCDS, 1975), which brought doctors of medicine, osteopathy, and chiropractic together to discuss the research status of spinal manipulative therapy. Though the meeting was marked by much interdisciplinary acrimony and ended with the workshop chairman (deputy director of NINCDS, Dr. Murray Goldstein) declaring that "specific conclusions cannot be derived from the scientific literature for or against either the efficacy of spinal manipulative therapy or the pathophysiological foundations from which it is derived" (Goldstein, 1976), it was nonetheless a beginning (Manber, 1978). More recently the chiropractic profession has reviewed the state of its own art at a conference in Anaheim, California, entitled "Modern Development and the Principles and Practices of Chiropractic" (International Chiropractic Association, 1979c).

Clinical Efficacy and Cost Effectiveness of Chiropractic Care

Studies so far published would seem to indicate that chiropractic care is a particularly effective and inexpensive treatment for many of the more than 3.5 million back injuries that each year afflict Americans (International Chiropractic Association, 1979a). Comparisons of the results of chiropractic and medical treatment of industrial injuries using data supplied by workmen's compensation commissions have demonstrated that people under chiropractic care show (1) reduced treatment costs, (2) reduced compensation costs, (3) reduced work time lost, and (4) reduced workers' disability and suffering (American Chiropractic Association, 1979). In one study sponsored by the medical director of the Workmen's Compensation Board of the State of Oregon, for example, 82 percent of the claimants treated only by chiropractors resumed work after a one-week time loss, while only 41 percent of the claimants with similar injuries with comparable diagnosis who were treated by M.D.'s were able to return to work in the same period (Martin, 1975). A second Oregon study—limited to back injury cases involving sprains and strains—found an average total cost (including physicians' and hospital fees as well as compensated time loss) of $298.52 under medical care as compared to $72.92 under chiropractic care. Similar findings have been made in the states of Florida (First Research Corporation, 1960), Kansas, and Iowa (American Chiropractic Association, 1979).

According to its patients and practitioners, chiropractic is also an acceptable form of primary health care. Chiropractors feel that by relieving the pressure of subluxation on spinal nerve roots that they are establishing the preconditions for the body to heal itself, that their treatment is a step toward homeostasis, and that it yields emotional as well as physical functioning (Dintenfass, 1975; Quigley, 1973; Homewood, 1962; Schwartz, 1973). Studies of chiropractic patients indicate that satisfaction with all aspects of their care is high; 96 percent of the chiropractic patients surveyed by the University of Wisconsin (Duffy, 1979) feel that their chiropractor is adequately trained as a primary health care provider.

The Present Status of Chiropractic

Since D. D. Palmer first established his College of Chiropractic in Davenport, Iowa, the professional and public acceptance of chiropractic has gradually grown. Today there are sixteen four-year chiropractic colleges, graduating some 1,700 students a year. Their curriculum resembles medical education in its attention to the basic sciences and clinical practice but differs in its emphasis on spinal analysis, chiropractic practice, nutrition, and its lack of attention to surgery and pharmacology. Currently there are more than 18,000 chiropractors in the United States. According to the American Chiropractic Association they provided care to some seven million people in 1974, an increase of 77 percent over the previous decade. Chiropractors are licensed in all states, the District of Columbia, and Puerto Rico, and their treatments are covered by Medicare, Medicaid, federally funded vocational rehabilitation programs, and an increasing number of union health plans. Since the passage of the National Health and Resources Development Act in 1974, their perspective has been integrated into the planning functions of health systems agencies.

Conclusion

Chiropractors, with their emphasis on hands-on contact and natural forms of therapy, are becoming more and more acceptable to Americans who are dissatisfied with surgical and pharmacological remedies and who want more informal and personal contact with their doctors. As chiropractors—and other health professionals—deepen their research efforts, as they begin to provide objective evidence of the effects that alteration in musculoskeletal structures may have on bodily functioning, it is entirely possible that manipulation of the spine and joints will once again become an integral part of a holistic approach to health and illness.

References

American Chiropractic Association. *Benefits of Chiropractic Inclusion in Your Health and Welfare Program.* Des Moines, Iowa: Author, 1979.

Cleveland, G. S. Researching the subluxation on the domestic rabbit: a pilot study research program. *Science Review of Chiropractic,* August 1965. **1 (4)**.

DeJarnette, J. *Sacro-Occipital Technique Notes.* Omaha, Nebr.: Author, 1976.

Dintenfass, Julius. *Chiropractic: A Modern Way to Health.* New York: Pyramid Books, 1975.

Duffy, D. Public attitude toward chiropractic and patient satisfaction with chiropractic in the State of Wisconsin. *Journal of Chiropractic,* February 1979. **16 (2)**, 19–24.

First Research Corporation. *A Study and Analysis of the Treatment of Sprain and Strain Injuries in Industrial Cases.* Davenport, Iowa: International Chiropractic Association, 1960.

Goldstein, Murray. NINCDS issues. *International Review of Chiropractic,* September 1976.

Goodheart, G. *Applied Kinesiology Notes.* Detroit, Mich.: Author, 1972–1977.

Homewood, A. E. *Neurodynamics of the Vertebral Subluxation.* Ontario, Canada: Chiropractic Publishers, 1962.

Inman, O. (Ed.). *Basic Chiropractic Procedural Manual.* Des Moines, Iowa: American Chiropractic Association, 1973.

International Chiropractic Association (Compiler). *Independent Studies of Industrial Back Injuries.* Davenport, Iowa: Author, 1979a.

International Chiropractic Association. *International Chiropractic Association Manual.* Davenport, Iowa: Author, 1979b.

International Chiropractic Association. *Modern Developments in the Principles and Practice of Chiropractic.* New York: Appleton-Century-Crofts, 1979c.

Kent, C., and Daniels, J. Chiropractic thermography. *International Review of Chiropractic,* December 1974.

Kent, C., and Simons, V. Electromyographic evaluation of vertebral challenge analysis. *Digest of Chiropractic Economics,* January–February 1979. **21 (4)**.

Kent, C., and Skibbe, R. Electrophotographic manifestations of neural dysfunction. *Digest of Chiropractic Economics,* July–August 1976.

Korr, I. M. Symposium of the functional implications of segmental facilitation. *Journal of the American Osteopathic Association,* January 1955.

Korr, I. M. The Andrew Taylor Still Memorial Lecture. *Journal of the American Osteopathic Association,* January 1974.

Luttges, Marvin, and Groswald, Douglas. *Peripheral Nerve Injury.* Presentation at the Eighth Annual Biomechanics Conference on the Spine, University of Colorado, Boulder, Colorado, December 3–4, 1977.

Maigne, Robert. *Orthopedic Medicine.* Springfield, Ill.: Charles C. Thomas, 1972.

Manber, Malcolm. Chiropractic—pushing for a place on the health care team. *Medical World News,* December 11, 1978.

Martin, R. A. A study of time loss back claims: workmen's compensation board (Medical directors' report, State of Oregon). *Archives of the California Chiropractic Association,* 1975. **4 (1)**.

National Institute of Neurologic and Communicative Disorders and Stroke. *The Research Status of Spinal Manipulative Therapy.* Washington, D.C.: Department of Health, Education, and Welfare; National Institutes of Health, 1975. (National Institute of Neurologic and Communicative Disorders and Stroke Monograph 15; NIH Publication 76-998.)

Palmer, B. J. *Hematological Changes under Specific Chiropractic.* Davenport, Iowa: Palmer School of Chiropractic, 1938a.

Palmer, B. J. *Electrocardiograph Changes under Specific Chiropractic.* Davenport, Iowa: Palmer School of Chiropractic, 1938b.

Palmer, B. J. *Audiometric Changes under Specific Chiropractic.* Davenport, Iowa: Palmer School of Chiropractic, 1938c.

Palmer, B. J. *Precise, Posture Constant Spinograph Comparative Graphs.* Davenport, Iowa: Palmer School of Chiropractic, 1938d.

Palmer, D. D. *The Science, Art, and Philosophy of Chiropractic.* Portland, Oreg.: Portland Printing House, 1910.

Quigley, W. H. Physiological psychology of chiropractic in mental disorders. In Herman S. Schwartz (Ed.), *Mental Health and Chiropractic.* New York: Sessions Publishers, 1973.

Schwartz, Herman. *Mental Health and Chiropractic.* New York: Sessions Publishers, 1973.

Sharpless, S. K.; MacGraegor, R. J.; and Luttges, M. V. A pressure vessel model for nerve compression. *Journal for Neurological Sciences,* 1975. **24**, 299–304.

Stephenson, R. W. *Chiropractic Textbook.* Davenport, Iowa: Palmer School of Chiropractic, 1948.

Street, G. *Correlative Chiropractic Technics.* Olney, Ill.: Author, 1969.

Suh, C. H. The fundamental of computer audio X-ray analysis of the spine. *Journal of Biomechanics,* 1974. **71**, 161–169.

Thompson, J. *Thompson Technique.* Davenport, Iowa: Author, December 1973.

Toftness, I. N. *A Look at Chiropractic Spinal Correction.* Cumberland, Wisc.: Author, 1977.

Wells, K. *Kinesiology.* Philadelphia: W. B. Saunders, 1955.

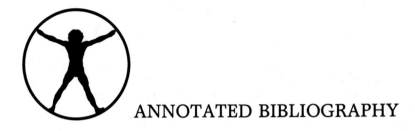

ANNOTATED BIBLIOGRAPHY

Readings

American Chiropractic Association/International Chiropractic Association. **Opportunities in a Chiropractic Career.** New York: Vocational Guidance Manuals, 1967.

> Written for the prospective chiropractic student, this short book contains information on education and career opportunities for the chiropractic profession.

Bach, Marcus. **The Chiropractic Story.** Los Angeles: DeVorss, 1968.

> The historical and philosophical roots of chiropractic are traced, and a discussion of spinal manipulation is included in this readable popular volume.

Baum, Allyn Z. **Who on earth goes to a chiropractor?** *Medical Economics,* July 1, 1971.

> Baum's article provides a general overview of chiropractic and of the kinds of people who consult chiropractors. It describes, through narrative and photographs, a patient's visit to a chiropractor.

Canadian Memorial College of Chiropractic. **The Archives: An Anthology of Literature Relative to the Science of Chiropractic** (2 vols.). Toronto, Canada: Author, 1974.

> An excellent source of reference, these two volumes contain abstracts of over 1,200 publications divided into three sections: Medicine and Basic Science, Chiropractic Literature, and Osteopathic Literature. There are indexes according to key word, title, and author which make these volumes an extremely convenient resource.

Dintenfass, Julius. **Chiropractic: A Modern Way to Health.** New York: Pyramid Books, 1975.

> Written for the layman, this book traces the history and development of chiropractic, describes education and research in chiropractic, and tells the reader what to expect on a visit to a chiropractor.

Duffy, D. **Public attitudes toward chiropractic and patient satisfaction with chiro-**

practic in the State of Wisconsin. *Journal of Chiropractic,* February 1979. **16** (2), 19–24.

The study discussed was conducted at the University of Wisconsin to measure public understanding and acceptance of the chiropractor as a health provider. It indicates a high degree of patient satisfaction with chiropractic care. Ninety-six percent of chiropractic patients surveyed felt that a chiropractor is adequately trained as a primary health care provider, and most (90 percent) thought a chiropractor should be allowed to admit patients to a hospital. Almost all patients felt that chiropractic treatment should be covered by health insurance. More than one-third of the Wisconsin public has utilized the services of a chiropractor (12.5 percent in the past two years).

International Chiropractic Association. **Modern Developments in the Principles and Practice of Chiropractic.** New York: Appleton-Century-Crofts, 1979.

A collection of papers presented at the Anaheim Conference of February 1979, this book includes reports on current research studies on the spine, visceral responses to somatic stimulation, low back pain syndromes, spinal X-ray evaluation and technique, physical and laboratory examination, adjusting methods, and sociological issues in chiropractic.

Klein, Lawrence, and Meyer, Sharon. **Chiropractic: An International Bibliography.** Des Moines, Iowa: Foundation for Chiropractic Education and Research, 1976.

A comprehensive listing of the world's literature on chiropractic and manipulative therapy that includes history, popular works, regional studies, government publications, theses, and books and articles on chiropractic and other forms of manipulative therapy.

National Institute of Neurologic and Communicative Disorders and Stroke. **The Research Status of Spinal Manipulative Therapy.** Washington, D.C.: Department of Health, Education, and Welfare; National Institutes of Health, 1975. (National Institute of Neurologic and Communicative Disorders and Stroke Monograph 15; National Institutes of Health publication no. 76-998.)

This collection of papers presented at the National Institute of Neurologic and Communicative Disorders and Stroke conference sponsored by the National Institutes of Health includes research from all branches of the healing arts and demonstrates a wide range of opinion as to the status and benefits of manipulation. Included are the evolution and history of spinal manipulative therapy; concepts and terminology used in chiropractic and osteopathy; discussions on the impact of spinal manipulation on the health care system; anatomical, biochemical, and neurological studies on spinal manipulation; pathophysiology; diagnoses of the subluxation; and studies on the therapeutic utility of spinal manipulation.

Palmer, D. D. **The Science, Art, and Philosophy of Chiropractic.** Portland, Oreg.: Portland Printing House Company, 1910.

An interesting and insightful history of chiropractic, this book (the original text) provides an in-depth examination of the practice through the eyes of its founder. Palmer discusses his basic theories of chiropractic; the anatomy, neurology, and chemistry he thought to be involved in the subluxation complex; and specific adjusting procedures.

Schafer, R. C. (Ed.). **Basic Chiropractic Procedural Manual.** Des Moines, Iowa: American Chiropractic Association, 1977.

Written for the chiropractor, this book includes information on orthopedic, neurological, and laboratory testing; X-ray; nutrition; physiotherapy; and other aspects of the clinical management of a chiropractic patient.

Schwartz, Herman (Ed.). **Mental Health and Chiropractic.** New York: Sessions Publishers, 1973.

René Dubos, Linus Pauling, and many chiropractors contributed to this interesting collection of articles on alternative approaches to mental health care. Contributions from scientists working in the fields of anthropology, biochemistry, education, psychology, and psychiatry add to this inquiry into the legitimacy of the chiropractic role in the field of mental health.

Thie, John. **Touch for Health.** Santa Monica, Calif.: DeVorss and Company, 1973.

Applied kinesiology is a system of chiropractic diagnosis based on testing muscle strength to determine certain body weaknesses; it correlates information from Chinese and Western medicine. The book was written for the layman and explains the methods of diagnosis and treatment in applied kinesiology, offering basic instruction in those methods.

Vogl, A. J. **It's time to take chiropractic seriously.** *Medical Economics,* December 9, 1974. 76–85.

This is a politically oriented article discussing chiropractic. It describes some of the changes in attitudes toward chiropractic and summarizes both the medical and chiropractic positions on the state-of-the-art.

Walters, David S. **Applied Kinesiology.** Pueblo, Colo.: Systems DC, n.d.

This book is written for the physician, particularly the chiropractor interested in utilizing applied kinesiology. It is a technical manual.

Journals

Digest of Chiropractic Economics. 1958–. 1–. Farmington Hills, Mich.: Author.

This journal represents a wide spectrum of opinion within the chiropractic profession. It publishes chiropractic research and other clinical information.

International Review of Chiropractic. July 1946–January 1969; mid-winter 1970–. 1–. Davenport, Iowa: International Chiropractic Association.

Journal of Chiropractic. 1964–. 1–. Des Moines, Iowa: American Chiropractic Association.

These are the monthly journals published by the respective professional organizations. They include articles on political and sociological issues concerning chiropractic, clinical procedures, current events, and some scientific and professional papers on the subject of chiropractic and manipulation.

16

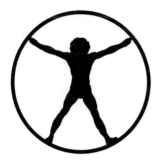

EASTERN SPIRITUAL AND PHYSICAL DISCIPLINES AND HEALTH: ANNOTATED BIBLIOGRAPHY

Arthur Hastings, Ph.D., James Fadiman, Ph.D., and James S. Gordon, M.D.

This annotated bibliography provides additional references to several Eastern and Far Eastern approaches to health, particularly ones that integrate spiritual and physical dimensions of the person. Related references will also be found in the following chapters in this volume: The Physical Disciplines and Health, by Donald B. Ardell; Chinese Medicine and Holistic Health, by David E. Bresler; and Alternative Forms of Diagnosis, by Arthur Hastings.

Cheng, Man-ch'ing, and Smith, Robert W. **Tai Chi.** Rutland, Vt.: Charles Tuttle, 1967.

Cheng, Man-ch'ing. **Tai Chi Chuan: A Simplified Method of Calesthenics for Health and Self Defense.** Washington, D.C.: Almega Institute, 1960.

> These books are the most comprehensive volumes on tai chi chuan. The edition by Professor Cheng is preferable to the abbreviated version by Cheng and Smith, in which the photos are difficult to follow and are mirror images of the correct positions.
>
> Professor Cheng, a traditional Chinese physician, was largely responsible for the dissemination of tai chi in the West. In his text he draws on forty years of teaching experience to explain clearly and concisely the philosophy and practices of the art. The pictures are superb illustrations of the correct postures of the tai chi form.
>
> Available only from the Almega Institute, 2316 18th Street, N.W., Washington, D.C.

Funderburk, James. **Science Studies Yoga: A Review of Physiological Data.** Honesdale, Pa.: Himalayan International Institute of Yoga Science and Philosophy, 1977.

One of the claims for yoga practices and techniques is that they have significant effects on the body and health. This book is a summary of more than one hundred studies testing the physiological effects of hatha yoga (the physical positions) and meditation. While it is uncritical in its stance, it is a useful compilation of the literature because some of the research is from medical and yoga journals published in India that are difficult to obtain in the United States. The other studies come from a broad range of physiological, medical, and psychological publications in Western literature.

The findings are organized into chapters on muscle tension and capabilities, circulation, respiration, endocrine functioning, and the nervous system, including EEG correlates of the postures and meditations. The studies generally confirm that yoga practices have important effects on the human system, some of which have medical potential (e.g., reduction of blood pressure and improvement of vital capacity in respiration).

Horwitz, Ten; Kimmelman, Susan; with Lui, H. H. **Tai Chi Chuan.** Chicago: Chicago Review Press, 1976.

This book is a good introduction to tai chi chuan. It contains an excellent history of the art along with a genealogical table tracing the major developments from its founding by Cheng Sab-feng approximately seven hundred years ago to the present. The authors present a section containing translations of works by tai chi masters covering a span of five hundred years.

Although this book is not useful for learning the tai chi form, it does explore the relationship of tai chi exercises to health maintenance and healing.

Ichazo, Oscar. **Arica Psychocalisthenics.** New York: Simon and Schuster, 1976.

As the name indicates, psychocalisthenics are active physical exercises designed to also affect the psyche—in terms of emotional stability, energy, resistance to stress, and mental balance. They are used in the Arica program, a human development and consciousness training system created by the author. Many of the exercises are original; some are taken from yoga and other exercise systems.

The exercises are made up of twenty-five illustrated and well-described movement patterns, some vigorous, some gentle. These movements exercise joints and limbs, move flexor and extensor muscles, and coordinate breathing with body movements. They may be done singly, or the entire sequence may be performed in about thirty minutes. The later sections of the book discuss selected exercises to use for relieving stress, getting quick energy, physical conditioning, spinal improvement, and for other special needs.

Iyengar, B.K.S., **Light on Yoga.** London: George Allen and Unwin, 1976.

The understanding of yoga is not easily transmitted in the form of the written word, and no book, no matter how good, can substitute for direct, live instruction. However, Iyengar's integrity, clarity, and his insistence on working from the very basics of yoga philosophy make this book least likely to be misinterpreted. He says, "My purpose is to describe as simply as possible, the asanas (postures) and pranayamas (breathing disciplines) in the light of our own era, its knowledge and requirements."

An extensive list of asanas are covered. They are presented in order of approach, are carefully described, and are illustrated. The use of the practices for health purposes is also indicated. Iyengar's approach to yoga is one of the most widely used today, and the book is authoritative.

Jiyu-Kennett, Roshi P.T.N.H., and MacPhillamy, Rev. Daizui. **The Book of Life.** Mt. Shasta, Calif.: Shasta Abbey Press, 1979.

From this Buddhist perspective, the law of karma is inevitable and inexorable, and physical and mental illness result from spiritual and karmic disturbances—the effects of unresolved experiences or traumas in past lives or present existence. The prevention of illness and the cure of the roots of symptoms thus require treatment of both the body and the spirit. Roshi Jiyu-Kennett, a Zen master born in the West and trained in Japan, is Abbess of Shasta Abbey in California, a seminary and monastery for Buddhist training. Rev. MacPhillamy is a clinical psychologist and ordained Zen priest at the abbey.

The first part of the book discusses the role of karma and Buddhist attitudes toward the act of conception, childbirth practices, causes of illness, prevention, visiting the sick and dying, and psychic forces, such as ghosts and visions. The second part of the book presents a series of mudras, which are postures and self-harmonizing positions for physical and emotional conditions, including spiritual cleansing, reverence, emotional protection, self-discovery, anger/compassion, joy/sadness, and energy balance. The positions involve placing the hands at various locations on the body and holding particular postures or arm and leg positions. The text explains the spiritual and emotional responses evoked by these mudras, usually over a long period of practice, and cautions that they are not a substitute for medical diagnosis and treatment.

The mudra points overlap acupuncture and acupressure points, but they are not organized in the same way. The authors provide a cross-correlation of their point locations with those of jin shin do, acupuncture, and g-jo (another acupressure system).

Regarding the source of this material, Roshi Jiyu-Kennett says, "*All* of what is written here is either spoken of, or depicted, openly, or described in somewhat flowery language, throughout the Buddhist Scriptures, so there is nothing 'invented' or 'imagined' in the pages that follow." This is one of the few books that takes up the spiritual dimension of health and healing, though with premises that are quite different from our current Western paradigm.

Radha, Swami Sivananda. **Kundalini: Yoga for the West.** Spokane, Wash.: Timeless Books, 1978.

Kundalini yoga postulates a psychic energy system with form and structure within the human body. This energy is called "kundalini" and moves through seven centers along the spinal column, beginning at the base of the spine and moving to the top of the head. Each of these centers, called "chakras," is associated with a particular sense organ, a mode of action, sensations, emotions, motivations, personal issues, and aspects of consciousness. It is a sophisticated system, and the practice of kundalini yoga is designed to focus consciousness at each of these levels and to understand and use its energy in appropriate ways. Swami Radha, a Western woman initiated into the Swami order by Indian yogi Sivananda, presents the traditional kundalini system as a practice for developing perception, emotions, mind, and spirit.

The kundalini chakra concept is comparable to Western theories of motivation or personality, but beyond the theory, this book provides exercises for self-questioning, meditation, and action based on each of the chakras to help individuals accept and clarify their development in that mode. The topics of these exercises include competition, sex, love, death, speech, using the mind, self-image, relationships with others, the ego, self-responsibility, and specific work on sensory modalities and action. Many of these exercises will be of interest to those in the helping professions for their work with clients, and the system itself is a useful conceptual tool for looking at personality and consciousness.

Rama, Swami; Ballentine, Rudolph; and Ajaya, Swami (Allan Weinstock). **Yoga and Psychotherapy: The Evolution of Consciousness.** Glenview, Ill.: Himalayan Institute, 1976.

The authors of this volume are an Indian Swami who has worked with the Menninger Foundation in Topeka, Kansas, a U.S. physician and psychoanalyst, and a U.S. clinical psychologist. The latter two studied yoga philosophy and psychology under Swami Rama. In this volume the authors explain concepts and techniques of yoga in relation to Western psychology and psychotherapy – with references to Freud, Jung, Assagioli, Reich, Klein, Sullivan, Maslow, and other Western clinicians and psychologists.

This is not a handbook for learning yoga practices but rather an explanation of yoga and its applications to mental health. The Raja Yoga and Vedanta systems are clearly described in understandable language. Yoga philosophy is related to the main Western streams of understanding. For example, biofeedback training is compared to the physical self-control techniques used by highly trained yogis. However, this is not to say that yoga is simply Western psychology in another form. It is a coherent system with a world view; it is a personality theory; and it is a set of specific self-development practices with spiritual dimension and purpose.

Chapters applicable to mental health discuss the structures of the mind, levels and functions of consciousness, and the development of discrimination. Other sections take up hatha yoga (the physical exercises), breath, meditation, the unconscious, psychosis, and mysticism. A clear explanation is given of the chakra system – energy centers identified with specific locations in the body, each relating to an aspect of personality and motivation, from security and sexual needs to intuition and insight. An appendix describes Weinstock's use of yoga principles in a psychotherapy program with mental patients (mostly child molesters and rapists!), starting with work on the body and proceeding through breathing and meditation, to enable them to gain control over impulsive behavior and interpersonal situations.

Experimental and clinical research on yoga is cited and references are given to relevant Hindu and Western literature. The book is valuable for its knowledgeable application of yoga principles to mental health.

Teeguarden, Iona. **Acupressure Way of Health: Jin Shin Do.** San Francisco: Japan Publications, 1978.

Derived from traditional Japanese acupressure and Taoist philosophy, "jin shin do" means "the way of the compassionate spirit." It is a system of thirty pressure points on the body, located from head to foot, that can be held to release tension, balance circulation, and improve the body's homeostatic balance of energy. The system was developed by Teeguarden from the study and practice of Oriental health arts, including "jin shin jitsu," an acupressure technique originating with Jiro Murai in Japan. Both jin shin do and jin shin jitsu are being taught in the United States, but this is the only book currently available on these similar systems.

Jin shin do is based on the concept of the Tao—the way of the universe, harmony, and balance, as expressed in the ideas of yin and yang. Body energies—muscle tensions, emotions, breathing, thinking, physiology—are affected by flows of "ki" energy (sometimes spelled "chi"). Pressure along the lines of these flows, or meridians, will help bring excessive or deficient energy back into balance.

The thirty main acupressure points are illustrated and described. They are principally along the "strange" meridians that control the balance of the organ meridians. The release techniques involve putting finger pressure on two points at a time and visualizing the flow of ki from the practitioner to the recipient. Instructions are given for full body releases and for specific releases for head and neck, back, shoulder, deep breathing, and emotional states (such as grief, anger, fear, and worry). The system can also be used for self-treatment.

Jin shin do is becoming more popular in the United States and this book is a useful, gentle introduction to finger pressure therapy.

Tohei, Koichi. **Aikido in Daily Life.** San Francisco: Japan Publications, 1966.

Aikido is descended from Japanese martial arts, and in addition to martial techniques it places emphasis on centering, personal development, and inner spiritual work. This book emphasizes the inner aspects of aikido rather than the external methods of self-defense. The principles of aikido are applied to getting up, working, sleeping, dealing with others, and many aspects of daily activities.

There are excellent chapters on breathing and on vital energy, called "ki," which is related to the Chinese concept of "chi." The author gives many exercises and tests to help the reader develop "centering." One technique, for example, is learning to consciously lower one's center of gravity to become more balanced and stable.

As a martial art, aikido is becoming more popular today, and many persons in Japan and the United States are using the basic approach of this book for their own personal growth.

Tohei, Koichi. **The Book of Ki: Coordinating Mind and Body in Daily Life.** San Francisco: Japan Publications, 1978.

This practical and inspirational book presents meditations, exercises, and breathing techniques for increasing and balancing "ki," the vital energy or life force. The topics covered include "how to overcome disease," "how to cure whiplash," and "how to remain calm in front of people." Tohei, an aikido master, draws on the principles and techniques of the art for ways of achieving physical and emotional balance.

Tulku, Tarthang. **Kum Nye Relaxation** (2 vols.). Berkeley, Calif.: Dharma Publishing, 1978.

Kum nye (pronounced "koom nyay") is a system of self-massage, physical positions, exercises, and related meditative techniques that originated in Tibet, where it was used as an adjunct to medical healing and in spiritual practice. In these two volumes,

Tarthang Tulku, a Tibetan lama, presents more than one hundred exercises intended to promote relaxation, balance, and awareness of one's physical and mental energies. Beyond the physical effects, kum nye is directed towards self-understanding; the positions, relaxation, and tension are likely to evoke emotional and psychological awareness of the practitioner.

The exercises are arranged in sequence and are carefully structured. They can be learned from the text and illustrations. The author says he has adapted the traditional (and unwritten) system to modern needs. There are similarities to Indian yoga and Chinese acupuncture, but the flavor is quite different. Volume 1 is titled *Theory, Preparation, Massage,* and volume 2 is called *Movement Exercises.*

Vishnudevananda, Swami. **The Complete Illustrated Book of Yoga.** New York: Bell Publishing, 1960.

This book focuses on hatha yoga—the system of postures, breathing, and physical practices—but it is not truly complete. It does, however, illustrate a variety of beginning and advanced exercises.

17

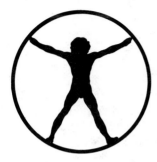

FOOD AND NUTRITION

James Fadiman, Ph.D.

One who tastes, knows.
    —Sufi saying

What is the correct diet for an individual to assure adequate or even optimum health? This question is at the center of so many controversies that it is necessary to open this section with a reminder that the answer will not be found here nor in the annotated bibliography that follows. There are as many well-considered opinions as there are brands of breakfast food and the followers of each opinion have data and research to bolster their claims and strengthen their polemic.

Nutritional research, while extensive, is vastly overshadowed by political, economic, and social influences on the growing, processing, distributing, and consumption of foods and food supplements. One result is that the quantity and quality of misinformation—or at least mutually contradictory information—is as likely to be found in the board room of General Mills as in a health food store in Southern California.

An additional cautionary note to keep in mind is that there are a number of very old, very vigorous, clear-eyed persons who, with their own teeth and senses fully intact, eat (and smoke) a diet almost universally condemned on all sides. That these persons thrive on a diet that renders laboratory animals sterile, quarrelsome, and tumor-ridden suggests that there are other factors not fully considered in any discussion of nutrition. Therefore you will not find here opinions with which to agree or disagree but rather an orientation to help reduce the ambiguity and confusion that so clearly dominate the field of nutritional research.

Food

Until this century there was little need for nutritional information since there was little that was done to food. It was grown only where it could grow without artificial aids. It was not shipped over long distances nor was it stored for long periods of time. It was eaten in season and in whatever quantities were available. It was dried, stored, or canned to preserve it. If we read the history of food and foodstuffs, there are recurrent periods of localized famines as well as times of relative surplus. There is little discussion of specific nutritional deficiencies since little was known and less could be done.

In the history of medical education in the United States, it is clear that almost no attention was paid to nutrition; it was not taught at all. Even now, it is neither required nor available in most medical schools. Perhaps this startling lack of interest was due to the fact that there were few choices about food when medical school curricula were being developed. As Robert Rodale has pointed out, there used to be only one kind of food, the kind we now call "health food"—not processed, grown without artificial fertilizers, containing few additives, and available only in season. Diets were standard, often within a cultural setting, and there appeared to be no point in adding the common knowledge about food to a specialized medical curriculum.

Now, with extensive food processing and preserving, the creation of new forms for foodstuffs, wider choices regardless of seasons, and our increased knowledge of nutritional needs, we are at a different point in understanding the nutritional values of food. Regardless of media claims about the taste and palatability of processed foods, the underlying drive for processing grew out of the need of food companies to extend the life of a product so that it might be transported, stored, and sold over long distances and over long periods of time. White flour simply stores longer without spoiling than whole grain flour. Butter with added salt stays saleable longer than butter without salt.

The prevention of spoilage is important for health reasons. It enables food to be available in all seasons, to be exported and imported to meet food shortages, and to be stockpiled for emergencies. However, this may result in nutritional problems. White flour loses important B vitamins in processing (some of which are added artificially to the finished product), salt added to butter and other foods may increase blood pressure levels, and nitrites for preserving meats are under investigation as carcinogens. Processing is a two-edged sword.

Once the initial goal of longer shelf life had been accomplished, there was a renewed interest in gaining a larger share of the market place for one variety of food over another. This battle led to questionable nutritional practices, such as the addition of sugar to everything from soup to nuts, including catsup, crackers, vegetables, and so on. More questionable was the introduction of various chemicals to already processed foods to improve their taste, smell, color, and texture, or to keep them soft or hard. While the evidence is certainly unclear, additive by additive, the fact is that there exist over 2,400 different additives in our foodstuffs. None of them had to pass the stringent criteria established by the FDA for medical preparations. The fact that some of them have been found to be unhealthy for laboratory animals (such as red dye no. 2, and artificial sweeteners) is not encouraging to those concerned with the purity of foodstuffs.

Unfortunately, despite labels of ingredients (listed in order of amount), lists of vitamins on the backs of cereal boxes, and media claims touting health, the nutritional needs of our foods have taken a back seat to the economic, production, processing, and marketing needs of the food suppliers. The person who eats the food has very little choice and almost no control over what is available. At least fifty years ago, if a consumer did not like one farmer's produce, he or she could go to another, and when you canned your own beans, you knew what went into the jar. Now, the nutritional quality of foodstuffs is protected, if at all, by the federal government – often against a laggard and reluctant food industry – and increasingly with the support of consumers, nutritional experts, and biochemists, who are recognizing the powerful contribution of nutrition to health.

Current Diet

It is axiomatic in the health food and nutritional literature to begin one's book or article with an exposé of the multiple and manifold deficiencies of the American diet. The criticism usually includes the following:

- excessive intake of processed foods
- inadequate intake of fiber (roughage)
- excessive intake of salt
- excessive intake of sugar
- excessive intake of preservatives and additives
- imbalance in ratios of fats, carbohydrates, and protein
- inadequate intake of vitamins and minerals due to all of the above.

The specific criticisms and their solutions vary from author to author, but there seems to be a universal agreement that many aspects of the current diet are medically unsound, and the problem has been getting progressively worse for some decades (Passwater, 1976).

The evidence for these criticisms comes from two kinds of reports. The first is from data on laboratory animals that, when given various components of the American diet, do not thrive. The other kind of data compares various populations whose diet differs from our own and considers the health and morbidity statistics in that culture in contrast to ours. For example, persons living in Japan have a lower incidence of cancer of the colon, and this has been attributed to the large amount of rice in the diet. Some of this data, however, conflict with widely accepted positions. For instance, the data suggest that some diets that are terrible by accepted health-food criteria (such as the blood and milk-products diet of the African Masai) do not lead to the illnesses predicted by laboratory studies and our nutritional knowledge. More acceptable studies are done on persons from one culture who later come to this country and adopt our diet. Indeed, colonic cancer does increase in Japanese who come to the United States and change their diet. The shift in kinds and amounts of illness forms a sound data base for correlating the changes of diet, culture, and health. What has emerged from these cross-cultural studies is the identity of "holistic nutrition" as a total set of inputs from the environment, including the quality of air, of water, of exercise, of meaningful work, of other noncaloric variables, and of food. While the American diet may have overall nutritional weaknesses, it is still necessary to evaluate the total nutritional input for a given individual before suggesting any change.

The Role of Government

More and more the federal government has begun to involve itself in the regulation of the food industry. The results to date are spotty. Government rules about the quality and sanitation of processed food are considered adequate, while the enforcement of these rules and the inspection of food processing facilities is deficient. The FDA is alternately praised and damned by the larger nutritional community. Still the trend is toward more–not less–control, more–not less–regulation, and more–not less–reliance on numerous agencies instead of consumer education.

A very different tone was set, however, by the publication of the McGovern report (Senate Select Committee on Nutrition and Human Needs, 1977), *Dietary Goals for the United States.* This Senate report may be the new guidepost to government regulation over the next decade. It suggests that the problem is best considered from a total nutritional program, and it phrases the issues in terms of promoting a more sound and sensible national eating pattern. As nutritional ideas become more commonplace it may become safe for political figures to propose nutritional policies without fearing that the major food lobbies will attack them.

Diets and Disease

Popular nutrition books and nutritional research literature alike agree that specific ailments and predispositions may be linked to diet. A disease or predisposing cause may be apparently diet-linked, as in the case of scurvy, which is caused by a deficiency in vitamin C, or pellagra, which is brought on by a deficiency in certain amino acids and niacinamide. More usually, some change in diet has been shown to alleviate the specific conditions in either laboratory studies or in clinical populations (Williams, 1977; Pfeiffer, 1975; Nutrition Search, 1979). For example, rickets can be alleviated by adding vitamin D to a diet that has adequate calcium and phosphrous.

The evidence for such linkages ranges from the impeccable to the nonexistent. There is a basic agreement that there are substantial links between specific conditions and specific changes in diets (Williams, 1973; Cheraskin, Ringsdorf, and Clark, 1977), but there still exist a multitude of confusing theories. What can be said is that it is simple prudence for anyone suffering from an ailment not responding easily to conventional treatment to supplement that treatment by modifying their diet along lines that seem valid or hopeful to them, based on clinical reports, nutritional experts, and the available research. In the case of diseases where conventional medical support is generally known not to lead to cures, including the so-called degenerative diseases, the attending physician should seriously explore the improvement of nutrition as part of the treatment, including the use of megadoses of supplements.

The burden for deciding on any given shift in nutrition in relation to a given set of health problems falls directly on the consumer and the physician, who are aided by the experts of their choice. One caution: if the expert of choice says that nutrition plays no part in this syndrome or its alleviation, verify that fact yourself by consulting the literature.

Diets—"I'll Start Tomorrow"

Atkins Schmatkins
Stillman, Schillman
Grapefruit, Shapefruit.
　　　　—Karen R., *That First Bite*

At the other end of the scale from the undernourished is the vast subgroup of the overweight. There seems to be a jungle of fads, fantasies, follies, deceptions, huckstering, and pandering to the misery of the overweight. To those who suffer from obesity it is an endless succession of changes, improvements, modifications, regimes, books, classes, and medical or nonmedical treatments for a recurring symptom (R., 1979).

For the overeater, changing the diet or the pattern of food consumption is far more difficult than almost any other specific intervention. The problem stems from the fact that a new food pattern must be:

- *Participative.* It doesn't just happen. The eater must be the agent in daily decision making and daily actions.

- *Active.* New food patterns imply new cooking patterns, new shopping habits, different ways of serving meals, and a different approach to eating itself.
- *Daily.* The new pattern is not temporary, not now and then; it is intended to last for years. It is not a quick fix but a fundamental shift in life-style.
- *Different.* It usually involves the restructuring or elimination of deeply ingrained habits and the actual opposition to ethnic, cultural, or personal patterns that have led to improper eating.
- *Complex.* Overeating is an interlocking effect of psychological additions, physiological predispositions, and cultural supports. They are so meshed that many of the failures so visible within the diet world can be traced simply to a denial of this underlying complexity. A case in point is to recognize that almost every holiday is celebrated by excessive food consumption, usually emphasizing snacks and foods high in calories, low in nutrition. The equation of love and food, symbolized by candy on Valentine's Day, pervades the culture. Food and pleasure are so linked that being "on a diet" is almost always associated with a limitation of pleasure in one's life.

What approach works for reducing excess weight? Education is the only way (other than fear) that has been used sufficiently to deserve mention. Education works most successfully, however, if embedded in a socially reinforcing context, such as Weight Watchers or the more powerful Overeaters Anonymous. In general, while any reducing diet will result in weight loss when followed, many diets are so nutritionally deficient that it is a toss-up whether the excess weight or the diet is worse for your health (Cheraskin, Ringsdorf, and Brecher, 1976.)

Keep in mind what Roger Williams calls biochemical individuality. The fact is that each of us is a unique individual with unique dietary needs, which may vary widely from any published norm and which vary within wide limits from day to day, season to season, and certainly from year to year. Carlton Fredricks said that any *printed* diet is wrong; a diet must be designed for a person, not for a magazine. The goal within the holistic model is not to come up with an ideal diet but to encourage persons to gain control over their eating so that they may make changes from time to time to meet their changing living pattern, health conditions, and social situation.

Vitamins and Minerals

The disagreements over the quality and adequacy of foodstuffs are mild and reasonable compared with the level of disagreements in the vitamin and mineral fields. However, it is universally agreed that vitamins and minerals are part of human nutritional needs and that some amounts of a wide range of these substances are critical to maintaining health (Goodhardt and Shils, 1973; Gerras et al., 1977; Stone, 1972). How much, in what form, in what dose, and for what conditions depends on what you read. Virtually ignored by the holistic researchers is the U.S. government Recommended Dietary Allowance (RDA). Almost no author, researcher, or company in the health-food field concurs with the government levels. They say that the level of RDA is only enough to stave off serious illness and is not enough to retain health. Nevertheless these standards are applied widely in the food processing industries, where labels state that a product has such-and-such percentage of your daily vitamin requirement.

What is a realistic daily supplemental intake of vitamins and minerals for a healthy adult? The list in Table 17.1 from Williams (1977) is regarded by many writers as sane, realistic, prudent, and well researched. It is a formulation widely available through various commercial firms. Note that the amounts in Table 17.1 are suggested only to maintain good health and are in the average range for most people. Factors mentioned by Williams that might cause a person to supplement this basic formulation include heart conditions, pregnancy, mental disease, alcoholism, or residing in a highly industrial setting. He suggests consultation with a physician or a nutritional expert to determine individual needs.

The trend of research in this area has led to adding substance after substance to the list of necessary aspects of nutrition and to adding condition after condition that seems to respond to supplements, both in animals and in people. The most recent change in emphasis, the use of megavitamins (the intake of vitamins in units hundreds of times higher than the ones listed here), is best known from the results obtained with vitamin C and vitamin E (Pauling, 1976; Passwater, 1976; Williams and Kalita, 1977). As long as we are living with and eating from the usual American diet with its manifold deficiencies, it is likely that we will continue to need and develop methods, models, and information to aid individuals in balancing their inner environment with supplements and special food choices.

Foods and Fads

Every year or two a new wonder food appears in the health food community, is stocked by health food stores, and is eaten by the faithful, who pronounce it the answer to piles, baldness, and inflation. Then it becomes a staple, eventually finding its way into conventional supermarkets, or it passes out of fashion. Foods that have made it into the mainstream include yogurt, sprouts, herbal teas, and peanut butter without additives. Foods that have languished include chia seeds, ginseng, rennetless cheeses, and ice cream made with honey rather than sugar. The health food industry is open to the same kinds of business practices that exist everywhere else. The final decision is still the consumer's. As James Thurber said, "Seeing isn't believing; eating is believing."

Table 17.1
Suggested Vitamin and Mineral Formulation for Nutritional Insurance

Nutrient	Recommended Amount		
Vitamins			
Vitamin A	7,500	units	
Vitamin D	400	units	
Vitamin E	40	units	
Vitamin K (Menedione)	2	mg	
Ascorbic acid (vitamin C)	250	mg	
Thiamin	2	mg	
Riboflavin	2	mg	
Vitamin B_6	3	mg	
Vitamin B_{12}	9	mcg	
Niacinamide	20	mg	
Pantothenic acid	15	mg	
Biotin	0.3	mg	
Folic acid	0.4	mg	
Choline	250	mg	
Inositol	250	mg	
P-aminobenzoic acid	30	mg	
Rutin	200	mg	
Minerals			
Calcium	250	mg	
Phosphate	750	mg	(equivalent to 250 mg phosphorus)
Magnesium	200	mg	
Iron	15	mg	
Zinc	15	mg	
Copper	2	mg	
Iodine	0.15	mg	
Manganese	5	mg	
Molybdenum	0.1	mg	
Chromium	1.0	mg	
Selenium	0.02	mg	
Cobalt	0.1	mg	

Conclusions

Nutrition is not a medical specialty; almost no foods are limited by prescription. However, there are a host of excellent information sources available to physicians and consumers in any community in the United States for improving one's personal diet and the diets of friends and patients. Any health professional who does not encourage his or her clients to consider the effects of diet on their mental and physical health does the client a disservice and may inhibit the effectiveness of the treatment involved.

If all we know about nutrition were applied to modern society, the result would be an enormous improvement in public health, at least equal to that which resulted when the germ theory of infectious disease was made the basis of public health and medical work.

—Frank G. Boudreau, M.D.

References

Cheraskin, E.; Ringsdorf, W. M., Jr.; and Brecher, Arline. *Psychodietetics*. New York: Bantam, 1976. (Originally published by Stein and Day, 1974).

Cheraskin, E.; Ringsdorf, W. M., Jr.; and Clark, J. W. *Diet and Disease*. New Canaan, Conn.: Keats, 1977.

Gerras, Charles, and the staff of *Prevention Magazine*. *The Complete Book of Vitamins*. Emmaus, Pa.: Rodale Press, 1977.

Goodhardt, Robert, and Shils, Maurice (Eds.). *Modern Nutrition in Health and Disease* (5th ed.). Philadelphia: Lea and Febiger, 1973.

Nutrition Search, Inc. *Nutrition Almanac* (2nd ed.). New York: McGraw-Hill, 1979.

Passwater, Richard A. *Supernutrition*. New York: Pocket Books, 1976.

Pauling, Linus. *Vitamin C, The Common Cold and the Flu*. San Francisco: W. H. Freeman, 1976.

Pfeiffer, Carl. *Mental and Elemental Nutrients: A Physician's Guide to Nutrition and Health Care*. New Canaan, Conn.: Keats, 1975.

R., Karen. *That First Bite: Journal of a Compulsive Overeater*. New York: Pomerica, 1979.

Senate Select Committee on Nutrition and Human Needs. George McGovern, Chairperson. *Dietary Goals for the United States*. Washington, D.C.: U.S. Government Printing Office, 1977. (Publication no. 052-070-03913-2.)

Stone, Irwin. *The Healing Factor: Vitamin C Against Disease*. New York: Grosset and Dunlap, 1972.

Williams, Roger. *Nutrition Against Disease*. New York: Bantam, 1973. (Originally published by Pitman, 1971.)

Williams, Roger. *The Wonderful World Within You: Your Inner Nutritional Environment*. New York: Bantam, 1977.

Williams, Roger, and Kalita, Dwight (Eds.). *A Physician's Handbook on Orthomolecular Medicine*. Elmsford, N.Y.: Pergamon Press, 1977.

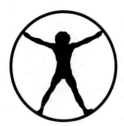 ANNOTATED BIBLIOGRAPHY

The following books were chosen as representative samples of the books available in this field. In this area, especially, let the reader beware. The claims for food and nutrition systems are greater than the generally accepted results. Conversely, the low level of nutritional information taught within the general medical community has placed its skepticism on shaky scientific grounds.

Airola, Paavo. **Dr. Airola's Handbook of Natural Healing: How To Get Well.** Phoenix, Ariz.: Health Plus Publishers, 1974.

This is a hard book to review. On the one hand it has all the earmarks of the dogmatic, anticonventional, treatment-for-everything health-food fanatic. The author is pushy, offers no apologies, and nothing seems to be unproved or unsure. This book's tone will upset people used to the timid, scrupulous medical literature. On the other hand it is a lucid and complete description of nutritional supplements for everything from acne to worms. For each condition, Airola lists a series of suggestions backed by his own clinical experience and the experiences of physicians who have worked with him.

Many of these recommendations are clearly sound and are in accord with nutritional research, while others appear plausible or possible. Still others seem to be without any other research support beyond the author's. This book presents a complete range of nutritional interventions and demands that the reader learn to exercise judgment before attempting self-medication.

Cheraskin, E.; Ringsdorf, W. M., Jr.; and Brecher, Arline. **Psychodietetics.** New York: Bantam, 1976. (Originally published by Stein and Day, 1974.)

While many books in this field focus on physical illness, this one suggests that many, if not most, mental diseases are linked to metabolic problems and incorrect diets. Through case histories and a review of the relevant data, the authors describe the possible links between incorrect eating and alcoholism, schizophrenia, hypoglycemia, drug-induced illness (side effects of medication), and neurotic symptoms. The authors propose that by improving one's diet and by learning about one's individual nutritional needs, many mental problems may be reduced or alleviated.

The book takes a hard look at the psychological and the psychiatric professions that ignore the physical symptoms, the medical history, and the nutritional regimes of their clients. It suggests that such treatment, common as it is, should be called "malpractice." Although it espouses an extreme position, this book is a valid and useful approach to expanding the horizons of people working in mental health settings.

Cheraskin, E.; Ringsdorf, W. M., Jr.; and Clark, J. W. **Diet and Disease.** New Canaan, Conn.: Keats, 1977.

If you want to own one book in this area, this is the one to get. It is technical but not unreadable and includes charts, data, exhaustive references, and a minimum of chatter. It covers the rise of various diseases in the United States and the possible dietary links and describes fully the known relationships between diet (including fats, protein, vitamins, and minerals) and selected conditions, including infertility, obstetrical complications, congenital defects, mental retardation, psychological disorders, cancer, and heart disease. In each section the authors clearly distinguish between correlational findings and therapeutic findings as well as the differences between animal and human results. This approach is such an improvement over the one used in most popular books in the field that it alone makes the book valuable.

Cleve, T. L. **The Saccharine Disease.** New Canaan, Conn.: Keats, 1975.

This book is an indictment of the presence of excessive sugar and the lack of fiber in the modern diet. The subtitle on the cover is "The Master Disease of Our Time"; the subtitle on the inside is "Conditions Caused by the Taking of Refined Carbohydrates Such as Sugar and White Flour." Cleve describes how the rise of diabetes, tooth decay, ulcers, heart disease, and circulatory conditions have paralleled the rise in refined food products. He makes a case for these health problems being linked to the change in diet. He cites evidence that the reversal of these dietary habits results in very noticeable improvements in the incidence of these and other diseases.

There are other more strident antisugar books on the market. Cleve's is more technical than most and probably more balanced. The author overdoes the single-cause-for-a-host-of-ills point of view, but the information is sound.

Dong, Collin H., and Banks, Jane. **New Hope for the Arthritic.** New York: Ballantine Books, 1975.

This book revolves around Dr. Dong's diet, which prohibits meat, fruit, dairy products, vinegar, pepper, spices, chocolate, alcoholic beverages, and soft drinks as well as all additives. The book is evenly divided between a discussion of the relationship of arthritis to diet and the mechanics of the diet itself plus recipes, meal plans, and so forth. The food plan is a generally healthy one and relates to many other disease-specific diets. For those who have tried it and found their arthritic pain sharply reduced (and I know several) this book has been an invaluable supplement to their medical treatment. For those who question this kind of book and this kind of diet, the volume is an excellent example of the genre. It is honest in its intention, does not push a particular product, and does put the reader through a personal examination of what he eats. If a person has not been helped by less extreme or more conventional methods, there appear to be few if any risks associated with the procedures suggested here.

Gerras, Charles, and the staff of *Prevention Magazine*. **The Complete Book of Vitamins.** Emmaus, Pa.: Rodale Press, 1977.

This large (814 pp.) volume is three separate books linked by the common thread of vitamins and nutrition. The first book is a short, basic overview of the role of vitamins in daily life. It covers likely areas of deficiencies, how to choose supplements, government regulations, medical information, and other general topics. The second book is a description of the various major vitamins and some of their effects both in animals and in man. Each short article deals in depth with a single aspect of a single vitamin. For example, there is one article on vitamin C and blood cholesterol among eighteen separate articles on vitamin C. The third book, titled "Vitamin Therapy for Disease," looks at specific conditions (such as arthritis, hay fever, kidney stones, acne, and varicose veins) and describes vitamin regimes that seem to have been helpful for those conditions.

The articles apparently originated in *Prevention Magazine* and have been re-edited here for consistency. The writing style is breezy, critical of nonnutritional medicine, and easy to understand. A minimum of jargon balanced with a considerable amount of research data makes this an instructive overview of the position in favor of vitamins and supplements.

Goodhardt, Robert, and Shils, Maurice (Eds.). **Modern Nutrition in Health and Disease** (5th ed.). Philadelphia: Lea and Febiger, 1973.

A massive (1,153 pp.), extensive (seventy-five contributors), fully referenced handbook on clinical nutrition. This is among the standard textbooks in the field. It is useful for medical specialists who wish to review the research in the field or to look more closely at a specific nutrient or at an area of clinical specialization. The book is divided into six sections: Foundations of Nutrition, Safety and Adequacy of the Food Supply, Interrelations of Nutrients and Metabolism, Malnutrition, Nutrition during "Physiologic" Stress, and Nutrition in the Prevention and Treatment of Disease. This is a mainline medical text and does not agree with or even consider many of the current issues raised by people in the natural foods movement, in nutrition therapy, or in the megavitamin research areas.

Nutrition Search, Inc. **Nutrition Almanac** (2nd ed.). New York: McGraw-Hill, 1979.

A remarkably balanced, extensive reference book on foods, vitamins, and minerals. It reports the basic findings on each separate element in the diet, the ways nutrients blend or supplement each other's actions, and the relationship of foods to specific conditions. It carefully suggests how to achieve a more balanced diet without recourse to any special fad and fancy within the health food camp. It is a reference book that must be studied and worked with to gain familiarity. It is an unusually sane balance of information and convenience in this emotionally charged and swiftly changing field.

Passwater, Richard A. **Supernutrition.** New York: Pocket Books, 1976.

In spite of the hype on the cover ("In just 10 weeks you can have the kind of energy and vibrant health you never dreamed possible"), the book is a realistic account of the data and ideas that have led to sharply revised suggestions for vitamin intake.

Passwater suggests that medical supervision of any plan to add supplements to your diet is wise. However, he writes about various vitamins in a way that might cause readers to dose themselves. Passwater clearly and elaborately debunks the simple-minded connections between cholesterol and heart disease, suggesting that to treat one aspect of the body in isolation is poor medicine and worse nutrition. He details the current positive thinking about vitamin E, the work of Pauling and others on vitamin C, plus a section on vitamin supplements as part of cancer therapy. This is a popular book, undoubtedly open to criticism by the orthodox medical establishment, yet it does not seem to go beyond the available data and appears to be realistic in its suggestions. It would probably be useful as a book to get people looking seriously at their whole food intake.

Pauling, Linus. **Vitamin C, The Common Cold and the Flu.** San Francisco: W. H. Freeman, 1976.

This is an update of Pauling's earlier book, *Vitamin C and the Common Cold.* It contains an additional six years of studies that support Pauling's position. The conclusion of the book is an excellent and accurate summary. "Most people suffer from regular bouts with the common cold and occasional attacks of the influenza. I believe that the application of a simple form of orthomolecular medicine, the use of ascorbic acid, can be effective in averting and ameliorating the common cold and influenza, and can contribute significantly to the control also of other diseases." The book spells out the history, biochemistry, uses, and side effects of vitamin C. There is also a chapter on the medical establishment and Pauling's jousts with it. This is an informative volume written for the educated layperson. It is not as exciting or as inflamatory as one might expect, but it is a sober, well-reasoned description of an issue of considerable concern.

Pfeiffer, Carl. **Mental and Elemental Nutrients: A Physician's Guide to Nutrition and Health Care.** New Canaan, Conn.: Keats Publishing, 1975.

A cheerful, skillfully written volume about food, vitamins, and minerals. Pfeiffer takes the position that the standard U.S. diet is dangerous and inadequate for most of us. He details the problems associated with various foods and presents the possible consequences (both mental and physical) for diets that are lacking in specific minerals or vitamins.

The chapters on minerals are especially clear; the data are carefully examined and the conclusions are explicit. It is a useful book for introducing the vitamin-mineral literature to patients or to professionals. The author has strong opinions and a good grasp of the kinds of research that have led him to state these opinions. The preface indicates that the book is most useful to persons or institutions dealing with mental disease; however, the general public has become more knowledgeable, and this book should be useful to a wider audience.

R., Karen. **That First Bite: Journal of a Compulsive Overeater.** New York: Pomerica, 1979.

An honest, funny, and tragic look at people who are seriously overweight. It is the firsthand account of the endless succession of diets, doctors, friends, lovers, and others who both help and prevent Karen from gaining control of her own weight. It is a useful book both for health professionals and for those millions who hope that tomorrow will bring a better diet and the end to their preoccupation with their weight. Her eventual work with Overeaters Anonymous suggests that the spiritual dimension, neglected in both medical and nutritional circles, must be taken into account.

Senate Select Committee on Nutrition and Human Needs. George McGovern, Chairperson. **Dietary Goals for the United States.** Washington, D.C.: U.S. Government Printing Office, 1977. Pub. no. 052-070-03913-2.

An explanation of the dietary goals, reasons for dietary change, and additional information about the food habits of Americans. The publication of this report generated responses—even criticisms—from the AMA, the National Dairy Council, the Cattlemen's Association, and of course the sugar companies. The major recommendations are to reduce the amount of fats, cholesterol, sugar, and salt and to increase the amount of complex carbohydrates. No change in the amount of protein is recommended. The report is highly conservative from the holistic perspective, yet it is a first step toward accepting the current nutritional level as a national problem.

Silverman, Milton, and Lee, Philip. **Pills, Profits, and Politics.** Berkeley, Calif.: University of California Press, 1976.

Not a book about food or nutrition, this volume is a sharp critique of the current and past ways in which drugs are marketed, sold, and used in conventional medicine. The book details the unusual pricing and profits of the major drug companies, the problems with drug efficacy and drug quality, the drawbacks to over-the-counter medications, the adverse effects of widely used medications, and a critical evaluation of the physician, "Healer or Health Hazard?" The book is fully referenced and draws heavily from government hearings into the ethics of pharmaceutical operations. It is a disturbing book that should make health officials more aware of their personal responsibilities regarding drug use by patients and should encourage the health industry to clean up some outstanding problems and inequities. The book has the facts upon which so many rumors are founded in the popular and health food press.

This book is included here to bring to mind that the most widely considered alternative to nutritional approaches is medication. The holistically oriented practitioner will be in a better position to evaluate drug information and promotion after reading this book.

Stone, Irwin. **The Healing Factor: Vitamin C Against Disease.** New York: Grosset and Dunlap, 1972.

Vitamins and minerals seem destined to be spotlighted in books devoted solely to a single nutrient and the research associated with it. The quality of the writing and the extensiveness of the research covered in such books varies widely. This book is done by a man who has taken the time to cull the world medical literature in order to clarify the applications of megavitamin doses of ascorbic acid. Stone corrects the public impression that Pauling and the others "created" a new area of research. Indeed it draws on fifty years of data in a number of countries, which curiously enough has received little notice within the U.S. research community. It is a volume with a clear position—that this substance can and does improve a wide variety of physical ailments. The author avoids polemics and sticks to turning the data into usable information. He clarifies the distinction adroitly in his introduction: "The number 382436 is just plain data, but 38-24-36, that is information." I wish the other one-vitamin books were this well balanced and well written.

Williams, Roger. **Nutrition in a Nutshell.** New York: Doubleday, 1962.

This is a simple, direct, and unusually sensible book on nutrition. Williams introduces the issues involved in shifts in food habits with just enough charm to keep you reading. It is one of the few books in this area that you can read without feeling guilty, defensive, or self-righteous about your own eating. It is probably the best book available to orient people to their own need for nutritional awareness.

Williams, Roger. **Nutrition Against Disease.** New York: Bantam, 1973. (Originally published by Pitman in 1971.)

What Williams's earlier (1962) book does for health this one does for the major degenerative diseases. Most books on nutrition and disease are filled with specific formulas and descriptions of cures that amazed the bumbling physician. Williams recognizes that each person has different nutritional requirements and that each person, with professional help as needed, must come to his own dietary conclusions. It is a fair and balanced book, replete with research indicating that changes in diet can and do improve outstanding physical conditions. Throughout, he gently debunks the more popular kinds of books. He asks, for example, "Why is calorie counting often ineffective? One reason is that it cannot be accurate enough. If someone were consistently to count all the calories he consumed, but missed his count by leaving out the equivalent of three peanuts each day, his mistake could theoretically result in a gain of eighty-eight pounds in twenty years. . . . Any individual who wished to make optimum use of the chart would have to know his own specific and unique nutritional requirements. And that, of course, is something that modern medical science should be able to—but in fact cannot—tell him."

Williams, Roger. **The Wonderful World Within You: Your Inner Nutritional Environment.** New York: Bantam, 1977.

Roger Williams—discoverer of pantothenic acid, first biochemist to be elected president of the American Chemical Society, and author of more technical publications than any dozen other researchers—has written a technically up-to-date, deliberately popular book on nutritional enrichment or improvement. Williams starts the book by discussing the nutritional needs of the cells themselves. From this vantage point he explains the various requirements of a healthy cellular environment.

In a chapter on choosing your own nourishment, he uses a series of diagrams that allow a quick and easy comparison of foods in terms of all their vitamin and mineral contents. Given the lengthy and impossible-to-use food charts that supplement many books in this field, this one innovation is worth the price of the book. Williams has retained his capacity to gently upgrade the quality of a person's diet and knowledge without resorting to fear or intimidation.

Williams, Roger, and Kalita, Dwight (Eds.). **A Physician's Handbook on Orthomolecular Medicine.** Elmsford, N.Y.: Pergamon, 1977.

"Orthomolecular Medicine is essentially the treatment and prevention of disease by the expert adjustment of the natural chemical constituents of our bodies. It places its reliance on these agents in preference to chemicals and drugs which are foreign to healthy metabolism."

This book was a surprise. It is expensive, large, and the title warns nonphysicians to stay away. Yet the book is a fine collection of papers drawn from all levels of the literature, written for physicians and the educated public by the major figures in the orthomolecular field. It is a review of the state-of-the-art, written by researchers whose primary desire is to communicate clearly their findings and the implications of these findings. Beyond the expected sections on nutrition, orthomolecular medicine, and orthomolecular psychiatry, there are selections on ecological considerations. They include an excellent chapter on vision by John Ott, comments on the problems faced by this expanding field in the courts (and with the insurance companies), and an extensive review article of the available literature.

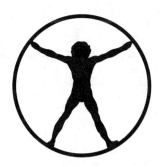

THE THERAPEUTIC USE OF PLANTS

Leslie J. Kaslof

Introduction

The history of plants used in medicine is virtually the history of medicine itself. They have figured prominently in the healing practices of every recorded culture. In North America, Native Americans used an enormous variety of plant substances, and their significant contribution to the materia medica of the United States is reflected in the fact that over two hundred of these herbs were adopted in the *Pharmacopoeia of the United States* in its first edition in 1820 and later into the first *National Formulary* in 1888 (Vogel, 1970). In addition, thousands of unofficial references were made to these plant substances, and hundreds of physicians based their practices mainly on their use.

In the colonial era, there were few professionally schooled physicians. Consequently, anyone with the slightest knowledge or experience in tending the sick was in great demand. The school-graduated doctors relied primarily on bloodletting, blistering, mercury, and antimony, whereas the "uneducated" practitioners mainly used roots, barks, flowers, and leaves for their remedies. Sometimes these unschooled herbalists made major and widely recognized contributions. For example, Samuel Thompson, who was born in Alstead, New Hampshire, in 1769, successfully treated a number of diseases including a severe local epidemic of yellow fever with herbs.

However, many of these pioneers' successes were obscured by the proliferation of quacks and charlatans, as this was the era of "medicine shows" and "patent medicines." By the end of the nineteenth century, these opportunists had discouraged many Americans from the use of their native remedies. Interest in the use of medicinal plants and folk medicine declined, and greater emphasis was placed on synthetic drugs and the school-graduated doctors who prescribed them. Then, in the middle of the twentieth century, interest in medicinal plant use began to revive, stimulated by the known effectiveness of plant substances such as curare, quinine, cocaine, and digitalis.

Current interest in the uses of plants in healing is continuing to increase, as reflected in the large number of practitioners, publications, and researchers now engaged in the field. The specific uses of plant substances in health and healing can best be learned from references such as those in the annotated bibliography to this chapter, along with training from an experienced practitioner. This chapter will introduce some of the principles relevant to the medical uses of plants and plant substances.

"Active Principles" versus Whole Plant Substances

During recent decades the pharmaceutical companies have spent huge sums of money exploring and developing new substances from plants. Unfortunately, in preparing these substances many drug companies isolate the "active principles" from the whole plant. Though this process of separation and isolation (S and I) may be attractive to a reductionist scientist, it may be a serious error. In addition to the so-called active principles, there exist within whole plant substances inactive ingredients and unique organizing principles, many of which have yet to be recognized or understood. These subtler substances, while seemingly unimportant, appear to be necessary to catalyze and balance the effect of the active principles in the plant as well as in the human who ingests it.

Additionally, though it has not been demonstrated experimentally, it may be that the long-term consumption of nutritional supplements that contain only separated and isolated elements (e.g., vitamin K as opposed to alfalfa in supplement form) may not only have a cumulative effect but may diminish the body's ability to extract these elements from food, eventually creating a dependency. Whole plant substances, on the other hand, not only contain nutritional elements but by virtue of their whole form stimulate and nourish the body's process of elemental extraction, a process equally as important as obtaining the elements themselves.

Dr. Norman R. Farnsworth (1978), dean of the School of Pharmacology and Pharmacognosy at the University Of Illinois Medical Center, Chicago, states:

Those physicians who do treat congestive heart failure with whole-leaf Digitalis purpurea, rather than purified [i.e., S and I] cardiac glycoside digitoxin (or digoxin from

D. lanata) cite a more easily reproducible activity, better stability, and greater ease in controlling blood levels. . . . Such subtle differences are difficult to measure; therefore, comparative studies in the published literature are rare.

In the United States today, a substantial portion of prescriptions sold through pharmacies contain pure separated and isolated plant substances as their active ingredients. These medicines range from the well-known digitalis and reserpine to the relatively new and highly potent antitumor drugs vincristine and vinblastine. At the same time there are a large number of prescriptions that are composed entirely or partially of the extracts from whole plants. In other countries—most notably the People's Republic of China—this number is far greater. In a visit to the People's Republic of China in 1974, the American Herbal Pharmacology Delegation (1975) observed that the Chinese people consume considerable quantities of herbal remedies, many of which are in use in hospitals throughout China. The Chinese make little effort to isolate "active principles," but they direct major efforts toward making these remedies more stable and palatable.

Variability of Plant Constituents

Certain plants of the same species will only survive in a particular type of environment; however, many do grow in a variety of environments. Research has shown that even though these plants may be of the same species, the percent and quality of composition—and thus their therapeutic applicability—may vary greatly according to certain factors, some of which are soil conditions and climate. In addition, and in some cases as a result of these factors, a transformation of plant constituents may occur during the year. In a specific season all or part of a particular constituent may be absent, inactive, relatively low, or in the midst of change. *Taraxacum officinale* (WEBER), dandelion root, which varies widely in its composition in different seasons, is a good example:

> The chief constituents of Dandelion roots are Taraxacin (of which the yield varies at different seasons) and Taraxacerin, an acrid resin, with Inulin, gluten, gum, and potash. The root contains no starch, but early in the year contains much uncrystallizable sugar and levulin. This diminishes in quantity during summer and becomes Inulin in the autumn (Grieve, 1970).

In general, maximum activity takes place in the roots of plants during spring and fall, in the stems and leaves during spring to summer, in the leaves and flowers during summer to fall, in the berries in the late summer and early fall, and in the seed during early to late fall.

In many ethnoindigenous systems of medicine, a great deal of attention is paid to other characteristics of plants and the context in which they are used, the conditions under which they are raised, and the season in which they are picked.

For example, there are plants that have not only medicinal but also sensorial properties (hot and cold) ascribed to them. This factor is often used to determine their seasonal use. *Mentha piperita*—peppermint (considered a "cool" herb)—would be used for its sudorific properties in summer fever, whereas *Capsicum minimum* (ROXB.)—cayenne (a "hot" herb)—would be chosen for its sudorific properties in winter fever.

Preparation

The use of nontoxic fresh plants is in most cases superior to the use of dried material, as there are important substances not present in the dry plant that are still active in the fresh. In general, spring is the best time for making use of fresh plants. Many that have a low toxicity at this time develop greater toxicity as the season progresses. For example, *Phytolacca decandra* (LINN.), poke, which may be used in salad in the spring, becomes quite toxic by late summer. Drying and boiling reduces the toxicity of some but not all toxic plants. Some of them must be boiled and the water changed two or three times before they become palatable or the water becomes safe to drink.

The combining of herbal substances in formulation was first introduced in ancient China as an art. Through the centuries it has developed into an exacting and comprehensive system. The safest and easiest system for formulation divides the herbs into two categories. Category 1 combines one to three herbs relating to a specific problem. Category 2 combines an herb having a demulcent or emollient action (to alleviate any irritability in the recipient's system and to counteract any possible gastrointestinal irritation resulting from the action of the herbs themselves) with an herb having an aromatic-carminative action (to promote an agreeable taste and prevent cramping) and another that functions as a laxative or eliminative (i.e., diaphoretic or diuretic) depending on the particular circumstances. A sample formula appears in Table 18.1.

Table 18.1
Formula For Mucous Accumulation in the Upper Bronchial System

Category	Herb	Proportion	Function
1 (Active)	Elecampane	5 parts	expectorant
	Horehound	4 parts	expectorant
	Coltsfoot	3 parts	expectorant
2 (Adjunct)	Peppermint	2 parts	aromatic-carminative
	Marshmallow	2 parts	emollient
	Cascara	1 part	laxative

Whenever possible, plants included in Category 2 should have similar properties or action to those included in Category 1. For example, both marshmallow and peppermint have a specific affinity for the upper bronchial system and therefore act synergistically with the herbs included in Category 1 in addition to performing their function as an emollient and aromatic-carminative.

Administration

Plant substances may be introduced into the body by placing them in contact with or rubbing them into the skin as ointments, lotions, oils, poultices (the ground herb made into a paste by adding water), fomentation (cloth soaked in preparation), through the respiratory tract by inhalation of vapors, atomized fluids, or powders, or rectally in solution as an enema. Most often, however, they are administered by mouth.

An oral agent may be administered in one of two ways: by placing the substance under the tongue, so it can be absorbed quickly into the system through the mucosa, or by swallowing, so it can be absorbed through the gastrointestinal tract. Most substances should be given on an empty stomach so they may diffuse rapidly into the blood; if administered during digestion, the acid gastric juice and the starch of the food may alter the chemical composition and weaken their action. Exceptions to this, however, are substances that may have a tendency to irritate the stomach lining. These should be given directly with food.

"Subtle" Energies and Plants

There is an enormous variety of systems for using plants in their whole form and as extracts, including systems of inhalation or aromatherapy, in which oils and essenses are inhaled; and osmotic therapy, a system in which herbal baths are administered and oils applied (McGarey, 1970). There are also systems that base their theory on "emanations" from plants to bring about changes in physical and emotional states. Though there is no "hard" research on the effectiveness of these systems, impressive anecdotal documentation is available on some. One of these systems, the Bach Flower Remedies, has recently aroused considerable interest in the United States and abroad.

Repelled by the discovery that many of the drugs he administered to his patients seemed to do more harm than good, Dr. Edward Bach, a young physician, gave up his successful Harley Street practice in London in the spring of 1930 to search for remedies in nature that would be neither harmful nor unpleasant. In the Welsh countryside Bach found wildflowers that would later make up his thirty-eight flower remedies. Experimenting on himself, he discovered that certain plants would cause specific responses in his body. "If he held a petal or bloom in the palm of his hand or placed it on his tongue he could feel in his body the effects of the properties within that plant" (Weeks, 1977). Bach later experimented and found that the early morning dew that collected on these flowers after exposure to the sun's rays contained particularly potent healing energies. Because collecting dew from each flower head proved to be a lengthy process, he decided to pick them and place the plants in the sun in a glass bowl filled with spring water to extract the healing properties. Like Paracelsus, Bach believed that various moods and negative states of mind could lead to disturbances or disease in the physical body. He chose his thirty-eight remedies for their ability to positively affect twelve negative states of mind. These included: fear, indecision, indifference, self-distrust, and pride or aloofness.

Through subsequent research and use Bach concluded that all patients who were subject to one particular state of mind would react to the proper remedy in a similar manner and that whatever disease affected them would in turn dissipate. These remedies have been employed by physicians and lay people extensively in England, Europe, and the United States with good results, particularly with emotional problems. Though the theory of action is obscure, presumably relying on some as yet undiscovered "subtle energy" present in plants and humans, the anecdotal reports of success seem to justify further investigation and controlled studies.

Prospects for the Future

Current research continues to reveal medicinal properties in a variety of common plants. Compounds from daffodils have been tested with positive results in treating myasthenia gravis and multiple sclerosis; the common sweet pea has been found to contain a neuroactive factor, which is now being tested on animals; lady's slipper has lowered high blood pressure; and buttercup juice has been proved to stop the growth of anthrax, pneumococci, staph, strep, and tubercle bacillus. In fact, the U.S. Department of Agriculture has found an extraordinary variety of plants that have antibiotic properties (Krieg, 1964).

Equal attention has been given to *Sanguinaria canadensis,* bloodroot, which has been used by Native Americans for generations to treat cancerous diseases as well as warts and nasal polyps. Recent scientific investigation by Stickl (Lewis and Elvin-Lewis, 1977) has corroborated its effectiveness as an antitumor agent and has found that the alkaloids sanguinarine and chelerythrine exert a distinct therapeutic action on Ehrlich carcinoma in mice. Likewise, Sher et al. have reported that these alkaloids had a significant necrotizing effect on sarcoma 37 in mice (Lewis and Elvin-Lewis, 1977).

The current disillusionment with the side effects of synthetic drugs and of processed food will in the years to come undoubtedly stimulate a good deal more research into the nutritional and medicinal effectiveness of plant substances, particularly of their use in whole form. It is reasonable to expect that their preparation and use will once again become widespread, that in addition to offering us specific healing tools they may help us re-establish a connection with the environment and our own nature that we have too long neglected.

References

American Herbal Pharmacology Delegation. *Herbal Pharmacology in the People's Republic of China.* Washington, D.C.: National Academy of Sciences, 1975.

Farnsworth, Norman R. Pharmacognosy in wholistic medicine. In Leslie J. Kaslof (Ed.), *Wholistic Dimensions in Healing.* New York: Doubleday, 1978.

Grieve, Maude. *A Modern Herbal* (2 vols.). Darien, Conn.: Hafner, 1970. (Originally published in 1931.) Also, New York: Dover, 1971.

Krieg, Margaret B. *Green Medicine.* New York: Rand McNally, 1964.

Lewis, Walter H., and Elvin-Lewis, Memory P. F. *Medical Botany: Plants Affecting Man's Health.* New York: Wiley-Interscience, 1977.

McGarey, William A. *Edgar Cayce and the Palma Christi.* Virginia Beach, Va.: Edgar Cayce Foundation, 1970.

Vogel, Virgil J. *American Indian Medicine.* Norman, Okla.: University of Oklahoma Press, 1970.

Weeks, Nora. *The Medical Discoveries of Edward Bach, Physician: What the Flowers Do for the Human Body.* London: C. W. Daniel, 1977. (Originally published in 1940.)

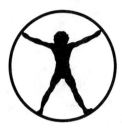

ANNOTATED BIBLIOGRAPHY

If one were to compile a full list of all the possible references related to plant use in medicine, the task would prove endless and would have to include such diverse fields as economic botany, pharmacognosy, ethnopharmacology, folk medicine, medical anthropology, and hundreds of others. The following references have been chosen as a general starting point for the clinician or researcher interested in the use of plants for healing.

General Reading

Bach, Edward. **The Twelve Healers and Other Remedies.** London: C. W. Daniel, 1979. (Originally published in 1933.)

    This excellent introduction provides descriptions of various emotional states and the appropriate Bach flower remedies.

Bach, Edward. **Heal Thyself.** London: C. W. Daniel, 1978. (Originally published in 1931.)

    A poetic presentation of "the vital principles which will guide medicine in the near future and are indeed guiding some of the more advanced members of the profession today."

British Herbal Pharmacopoeia. London: British Herbal Medicine Association, 1971.

    Published by the British Herbal Medicine Association's Scientific Committee, this text lists herbal substances by their botanical names and includes information about their country of origin, their appearance, their therapeutic action and indications for use, their combination with other botanicals, and their preparation and dosage. The text is loose leaf and unnumbered for easy addition and deletion of information.

Christopher, John R. **School of Natural Healing.** Provo, Utah: BiWorld, 1976.

    This text is mostly culled from a variety of literary works on herbal medicine as well as from the author's personal experience. Individual listings of herbs by common name are followed by species and Latin name, identifying characteristics, parts used, therapeutic action, formulas, preparation, dosage, and uses. Other sections include descriptions of medicinal properties, diet and recipes, formulations, vehicles of application, collecting and drying, and storing. The book is well indexed and easy to read.

Clymer, R. Swineburn. **Nature's Healing Agents.** Philadelphia: Dorrance, 1963. (Originally published in 1905.)

This is a classic reference written by a physician who for many years practiced the Thomsonian System of herbal medicine, which he later renamed and developed into the Natura System. The text begins with basic principles and practices of these systems and proceeds to listings of common herbs with descriptions of their indications and use. It offers an excellent therapeutic basis for the application and use of herbal substances.

Ellingwood, Finley, and Lloyd, John Uri. **Materia Medica and Therapeutics.** Chicago: Medical Times, 1905.

Ellingwood, Finley, and Lloyd, John Uri. **New American Materia Medica Therapeutics and Pharmacognosy.** Evanston, Ill.: Ellingwood Therapeutist, 1919.

These classic but hard-to-locate works contain the clinical experiences of noted physicians of the day and include sections on the definition of and types of preparations, therapeutic activities of nontoxic plants, and therapeutic methods and classification of remedies by organ system. They are highly recommended.

Grieve, Maude. **A Modern Herbal** (2 vols.). Darien, Conn.: Hafner, 1970. (Originally published in 1931.) Also, New York: Dover, 1971.

Meticulously researched, this encyclopedic work is extremely well written and easy to read. It covers the medicinal, culinary, cosmetic properties, and the folklore attributed to over 2,400 plants, trees, fungi, shrubs, and grasses. Each plant's common and botanical name is given as well as its history, the parts used, its habitat, cultivation, constituents, medicinal action, and use. Over two hundred beautifully rendered line drawings in half-tones are also included. It is highly recommended.

Harper-Shove, Lt. Col. F. **Prescriber and Clinical Repertory of Medicinal Herbs.** Devon, England: Health Science Press, 1972. (Originally published in 1938.)

A unique reference work presented in classic homoeopathic style listing sections according to various bodily parts and systems. The information is then subreferenced by symptom and indication and specific herb. For example: HEAD, Eye, inflammation—granular, purulent, sclerotic of, etc. Well indexed with definitions of terms, notes on prescribing and dosage, and contraindications.

Hutchens, Alma R. **Indian Herbology of North America.** Kumbakonam, South India: Homoeopathy Press, 1969.

This volume offers an interesting compilation of folklore and clinical information. Each listing includes a field description, the part of the plant used, its physiological activity, and occasionally its homoeopathic uses. A fairly extensive annotated bibliography on Russian and English sources of herbal research is included.

Kaslof, Leslie J. **The Herb and Ailment Cross-Reference Chart.** Woodmere, N.Y.: United Communications, 1972. (30" x 40")

Hand-lettered and bordered with flowering herbs, the chart includes an extensive section cross-referencing the use of more than 160 herbs for various common ailments. Additional information includes the astrological signs governing herbs, the parts used, the medicinal properties and definitions of medicinal terms, directions for preparing all types of herbal material, and the vitamin and mineral content of many of the herbs listed.

Kaslof, Leslie J. (Ed.). **Wholistic Dimensions in Healing.** New York: Doubleday, 1978.

This volume provides in its section on herbs a comprehensive list of herbal sources — botanical museums, journals, and services.

Kloss, Jethro. **Back to Eden.** Coalmont, Tenn.: Longview, 1968. (Originally published in 1939.)

One of the most popular contemporary books on the healing virtues of herbs, it incorporates extensive though general information on many aspects of family and personal health maintenance. Kloss includes descriptions of the healing virtues of hundreds of herbs and trees, definitions of the medicinal properties of plants and their applications to various disorders, directions for preparation and use, formulas, and chapters on exercise, fasting, and diet. It is a good reference if one can pick through the generalities and certain obvious inaccuracies.

Krieg, Margaret B. **Green Medicine.** New York: Rand McNally, 1964.

This popular book includes interviews with some of the most important physicians and scientists in medical botany both in the United States and overseas. Though written as a novel, it contains much valuable information that is unobtainable from other sources. Out of print but recommended.

Lewis, Walter H., and Elvin-Lewis, Memory P. F. **Medical Botany: Plants Affecting Man's Health.** New York: Wiley-Interscience, 1977.

Clinically oriented, this volume is of special interest to the physician and professional practitioner who wishes to learn more about the use of botanicals in medicine. It is divided into three sections: "Injurious Plants," "Remedial Plants," and "Psychoactive Plants." These sections are then subcategorized. Extensive research and bibliographic references on the clinical, laboratory, and folklore use of plants are also presented. Highly recommended.

Mausert, Otto. **Herbs.** Eugene, Oreg.: Elaine M. Muhr, 375 Carolyn Drive, 1974. (Originally published by the author under the name *Herbs for Health* in 1932.)

An easy-to-read introduction to the use of herbal substances for healing. The text contains a section on symptoms, their causes and suggested remedies, and an excellent cross-index on herbal formulas. Other sections include a materia medica and information on the cultivation of herbs and the vitamins they contain.

Morton, Julia F. **Major Medicinal Plants.** Springfield, Ill.: Charles C. Thomas, 1977.

Extremely well researched, this volume provides an illustrated scientific reference to the major natural sources of drugs currently used in medicine. The comprehensive bibliography, composed of more than six hundred international research reports, will be of particular use to the serious student of medicinal plants.

Pelikan, Wilhelm. *Heilpflanzenkunde Der Mensch Und Die Heilpflanzen.* Dornach, Switzerland: Philosophisch-Anthroposophischer Verlag, 1958. Parts 1 and 2 have been reprinted in English under the title of *Healing Plants.* London: Rudolf Steiner, 1976.

Fascinating collection of information on the deeper nature of plants and their relationship to other living things. Individual chapters include such titles as "Disease Process and Medicinal Plants" and "The Labiatae," of which the herb *Salvia officinalis* (sage) is a member. Rudolf Steiner draws particular attention to the importance of the tannin from sage in the treatment of asthma. Highly recommended.

Shepherd, Dorothy. **A Physician's Posy.** Devon, England: Health Science, 1969.

In a compelling and sensitive account, Dr. Shepherd shares her many experiences in healing the sick with herbal and homoeopathic preparations, with whole chapters devoted to individual plants. Other books by Dorothy Shepherd include *The Magic of the Minimum Dose* (1973) and *More Magic of the Minimum Dose* (1974), both published by Health Science Press.

Shook, Edward E. **Advanced Treatise on Herbology.** Mokelumne Hill, Calif.: Health Research, 1974. (Reprint.)

This is a rare classic and an inspiration to many early herbalists and practitioners. Each chapter describes an individual herb, its habitat, use, chemical constituents, and physiological activity. Despite some of the text's scientific speculation, misspellings, and occasional pharmacological inaccuracies, it is a fascinating and valuable work. A companion text by the same author entitled *Elementary Treatise in Herbology* was published in 1974 by Trinity Center Press, Beaumont, California.

Tompkins, Peter, and Bird, Christopher. **The Secret Life of Plants.** New York: Harper and Row, 1973.

This recent popular volume contains interesting and controversial information on paranormal research and experiments on the relationship between plants and humans and the environment. It includes studies on the use of plants as lie detectors, Soviet research with plants, and the potential for communication between plants and human beings. Though it is somewhat sensationalistic, it is a fascinating and thought-provoking account.

United States Dispensatory (5th–25th ed.). Philadelphia: Lippincott, 1880s–1960.

These voluminous works (from 1,500 to 2,377 pp.) contain extensive information on preparation of extracts and tinctures, medicinal properties, and their pharmacological description and physiological activity. Botanicals listed include those listed in the U.S. pharmacopoeia of the day and those not listed in the *USP* but still used widely in practice. The 25th edition (1960) was the last *United States Dispensatory* to contain a "natural products" section.

Indigenous Plant Medicine

American Herbal Pharmacology Delegation. **Herbal Pharmacology in the People's Republic of China.** Washington, D.C.: National Academy of Sciences, 1975.

> This is a report of the American Herbal Pharmacology Delegation, a group of physicians and scientists who visited China in the early 1970s to determine the extent of herbal and pharmacological knowledge there. It includes information on the clinical use of herbal medicines, a Chinese pharmacology, laboratory research, and the evidence for validating claims of traditional Chinese medicines. Highly recommended.

Chopra, Sir R. N. and I. C.; Handa, K. L.; and Kapur, L. D. **Chopra's Indigenous Drugs of India** (2nd ed.). Calcutta: U. N. Dhur and Sons, 1958.

> This important work lists the chemical, pharmacological, and clinical application of plant drugs indigenous to India. It includes sections on "History of Indian Materia Medica" and "Medical and Economic Aspects of Indian Indigenous Drugs." Also included are chapters on various plant constituents and their associated species.

John E. Fogarty International Center for Advanced Study in the Health Sciences (Trans). **The Barefoot Doctor's Manual.** Bethesda, Md.: National Institutes of Health, 1974 (Department of Health, Education, and Welfare, publication no. (NIH) 75–695). Also published by Running Press, Philadelphia, 1977.

> This text for primary health care practitioners in the People's Republic of China combines useful basic knowledge derived from Chinese and Western health care systems. It includes chapters on understanding the human system according to Chinese theory and practice, occupational health, diagnosis, hygiene, acupuncture, contraception, first aid, and a long section on Chinese medicinal plants.

Keyes, John D. **Chinese Herbs.** Rutland, Vt.: Charles Tuttle, 1976.

> An illustrated, well-referenced text, listing about 250 Chinese herbs and their medical and botanical uses. Chapters describe areas of distribution and some medicinal information and dosage. Other sections include a glossary of terms, table of toxic herbs, and drugs of animal origin.

Vogel, Virgil J. **American Indian Medicine.** Norman, Okla.: University of Oklahoma Press, 1970.

> Well written and informative, this account contains sections on the early observation

of Native American medicinal practices, detailed descriptions of Native American medicine men treating settlers, an account of the influence of native medicine on the materia medica, and an extremely comprehensive and well-researched bibliography on Native American medicine as a whole.

Watt, John Mitchell, and Breyer-Brandwijk, Maria Gerdina. **Medicinal and Poisonous Plants of Southern and Eastern Africa** (2nd ed.). New York: Churchill Livingston, 1962.

This voluminous work references the indigenous medicinal uses of plants among natives and other groups of Africa. Chemical composition, pharmacological effects, and human and veterinary toxicology of the flora are meticulously researched and presented here. It includes many photographs and line drawings of plants (some in color) and their European and vernacular names.

Journals

British Homoeopathic Journal. Ashford, Kent, England: Headley Bros. Invicta Press.

Homoeopathic remedies and medicinal herbs.

Chemical and Pharmaceutical Bulletin. Tokyo: Pharmaceutical Society of Japan.

Pharmacological and chemical properties of plants.

Economic Botany. New York: Society for Economic Botany and the New York Botanical Gardens.

Medicinal and economic uses of plants.

Ethno Medicine. Hamburg, West Germany: Helmut Buske.

Medicinal and pharmacological properties of plants, mostly in German.

The Homeopathic Digest. Ossining, N.Y.: Box 667.

Homeotherapy. San Francisco: Box 31100.

Homoeopathic remedies.

Journal of the American Institute for Homeopathy. Falls Church, Va.: 6231 Leesburg Pike, Suite 506.

Homoeopathic remedies.

Journal of Ethnopharmacology. Lausanne, Switzerland: Elsevier Sequoia, S.A., P.O. Box 851.

Journal of Pharmaceutical Sciences. Washington, D.C.: 2215 Constitution Avenue.

Pharmacological and chemical properties.

Lloydia: The Journal of Natural Products. Cincinnati, Ohio: The Lloyd Library and Museum and the American Society of Pharmacognosy. 917 Plum Street.

Pharmacological and chemical properties.

Medicina Traditional. Mexico 12, D.F.: IMEPLAM, Luz Savinon 214.

Medicinal and folklore uses of plants.

Planta Medica. Stuttgart, West Germany: Hippokrates-Verlag GMBH., Neckarstr, 121, Postfach 593.
Medicinal, folklore, and pharmacological aspects of plants.

Plantes Medicinales et Phytotherapy. Angers, France: Centre d'Etudes des Plantes Medicinales.

Medicinal and pharmacological aspects of plants (in French).

Quarterly Journal of Crude Drug Research. Lisse, The Netherlands: Swets Publishing Co.

Pharmacology, folklore and medicinal plants.

Editors' note: The word homeopathy/homoeopathy has been spelled according to the original reference.

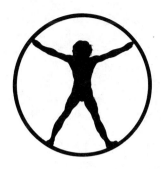

MUSIC AND SOUND IN HEALTH

Helen L. Bonny, Ph.D.

Sound is so much a part of life from birth to death that man accepts it, uses it, enjoys it, but seldom questions it. Its presence is like the background music of a moving picture, largely unnoticed but leaving overtones of feeling (Knapp, 1953). Silence, or cessation of all sound, is experienced only by the deaf or in specifically prepared sound-deprivation areas. But even in soundproof rooms the individual hears—perhaps for the first time—the noises of his internal viscera, a vast complex of unceasing sound waves ordinarily masked by conflicting environmental noise.

The process of hearing sounds involves a complexity of phenomena: the morphology of the ear, the neuronal connection with the brain, the reactions of the autonomic nervous system to sound signals. These all result in emotional and physiological reactions to sound (Wagner, 1977). The feelings aroused by sound are instantaneous but variable; each of us may react differently at any moment.

Music

Music is defined as organized sound made up of varying relationships of sound and silence and perceived as continuity. Tones do not move; they occur and they are gone, but we hear motion. We can say that the experience of hearing music, then, is in both the physical and nonphysical, subjective world. "Hearing music does not mean hearing tones, but hearing, in the tones and through them, the places where they sound in the seven-tone system" (Zuckerkandl, 1956). From the Gestalt point of view musical tones are events in a dynamic field; they are conveyors of forces, and hearing music means hearing an action of forces. Zuckerkandl points out that each tone is an element of a key and therefore carries within itself a relation to a larger whole. It is a system in which the whole is present and operative in each individual locus, and each individual locus "knows" its position in the whole.

Anthropologists have found musical instruments to be essential in emerging cultures (Merriam, 1964), and the dynamics of musical sound have contributed throughout human history to the therapeutic use of sound. Ancients knew the hypnagogic effects of sustained vocal tones (Sachs, 1943), and the Greeks used music in the preparation and actuation of healing rituals (Meier, 1964). In the development of Western cultures, music has been a controlling and influencing measure in human institutions. Liturgical music in worship, martial music to inspire courage and shared emotions in military ventures, and the educational use of singing by rote have long been known to be efficacious in modifying attitudes and emotions.

In recent decades there has been an organized effort through the discipline of music therapy to document functional uses of music as they affect physiology and behavior (Eagle, 1976; Gaston, 1968; *Journal of Music Therapy,* 1964–present.) Music therapy is defined as the systematic application of music, as directed by the music therapist, to bring about changes in the emotional or physical health of the person. A variety of musical activities and modes are employed with institutional and private clients (National Association for Music Therapy, 1978). Undergraduate and graduate programs in music therapy combine academic and clinical training toward registration as a music therapist (R.M.T.).

Music has a number of capabilities that contribute to its psychotherapeutic use. It opens avenues of nonverbal emotional communication and has been called the language of the emotions (Farnsworth, 1969), which implies the communication of both generalized and specific meanings to the hearer beyond those intended by the composer (Sessions, 1971). Music can evoke and sustain emotional affect. Pratt (1952) wrote, "Music sounds the way emotions feel." A theory called "depth provocation" explains that "music because of its abstract nature detours around the ego and intellectual controls and, contacting the lower centers directly, stirs up latent conflicts and emotions which may be expressed and re-enacted through music" (Taylor and Paperte, 1958). Langer (1942) describes music as the "formulation and representation of emotions, mood, mental tensions, and resolutions."

Another capability has been systematized by Bonny and Savary (1973), who use music with relaxation-concentration exercises to explore imagery in altered states of consciousness. Based on studies at the Maryland Psychiatric Research Center (Bonny and Pahnke, 1972), this innovative approach, called "guided imagery and music" (GIM), encourages a response to music in the form of kinesthetic, visual, and feeling imagery. The music is chosen to provide the appropriate mood and structure for exploration of conflicted areas of the self but does not limit the flow or access to a wide variety of other experiences—such as positive, oceanic, and religious imagery that may have life-changing properties for the individual (Bonny, 1978). Transpersonal aspects of sound are explored by Halpern (1978), who has studied its effect in evoking states of meditation and physiological indices of relaxation.

It was once categorically stated that music could markedly affect bodily processes. However, research to date is limited and largely dependent on that done by Diserens and Fine (1939) with some modifications (Farnsworth, 1969; Eagle, 1976). Of recent interest and possible application is the work on brain anatomy and hemispheric differentiation in response to music stimuli (Critchley and Henson, 1977; Bogen, 1969; Ferguson, 1978; McKee et al., 1973). Three neurophysiological processes may be activated by musical material. Because it is nonverbal, music can move through the auditory cortex directly to the center of emotional responses; verbalization tends to be reductionist and resistance-creating. Also it may be able to activate the flow of stored memory material across the corpus callosum so that right and left hemispheres of the brain work in unity rather than in conflict. Further, calming, quieting music may well help produce the large molecules called peptides that relieve pain by acting on specific receptors in the brain.

Research in the physics of sound make it clear that there can be damaging as well as therapeutic processes at work. Sound is usually thought of as purposeful and organized. But in our culture there is often a high decibel input of purposeless and disorganized sound designated as noise or auditory pollution. For instance, rock music played at its usual high volume output can be physically damaging, while classical music, which depends more on melodic line and contrapuntal construction, shows much less auditory damage even at its loudest decibel peaks (Kryter, 1970). An essential skill in the therapeutic use of music is a knowledge of which music is damaging and which music serves a healing purpose. Specialized training in music as well as in psychology is essential. Training of this type is provided in formal and internship programs at the Institute for Consciousness and Music (1978) and at many universities and colleges.

For those who are seeking to develop new and effective modes of healing, it appears that research and development in the skillful use of sound through music may hold promise for the healing of people in the future even more effectively than the ancient and traditional patterns of the past. New insights may allow greater differentiation and control of purposeless noise that pollutes body and mind and may promote the sensitive and healing use of sounds that we call music.

Present Practices in Music Therapy

In small and large groups and in individual sessions, music therapy is used to effectively promote healing and changed behavior in a variety of patient group categories. These include the institutionally mentally ill, mentally retarded, physically impaired, and socially ostracized persons in our society who as a group require specialized interventions. In recent years therapy clients have increasingly been persons seeking not only to solve personal problems but also to explore their human potential (*Music Therapy as a Career*, n.d.).

Music therapists are trained to identify goals for treatment, which may be increased self-esteem, emotional change, personal gratification, communication skills, improved environment, and physical healing. Music therapy may accomplish several goals at once. For example, the use of music with senior citizens in nursing homes, hospitals, and day centers creates a climate for reliving meaningful past life experiences through singing hymns or popular songs of their era. It encourages the expression of feelings as an antidote to isolation, and through the playing of rhythmic instruments, music therapy promotes muscular coordination and stimulates mental concentration (Bright, 1972).

Musical improvization in the hands of a skilled therapist becomes an effective bridge of communication to the autistic child, leading to the joy of shared musical experience. The pentatonic Orff instruments allow the mentally retarded child or adult access to immediate gratification on those beautifully tuned, easily mastered instruments (Bitcon, 1975). For the emotionally disturbed child developmental music therapy is a positive reinforcement to enhance learning in four basic areas: socialization, behavior, communication, and academics (Purvis and Samet, 1976). Learning for persons who are visually or auditorily handicapped can be enriched by the introduction into their lives of various sound stimuli (Michel, 1976). Increasingly, the music educator and the special education teacher are turning to the music therapist as a primary aide in meeting the needs inherent in mainstreaming handicapped children in the public schools.

In private psychiatric practice guided imagery and music (GIM) is becoming known as a gentle way to help release blocked areas of the personality, to bring about insight into why the problems have arisen, and to suggest modes of action to correct and sustain growth. In GIM sessions, movement, action, and change can occur with the working-through process of internal imagery.

References

Bitcon, C. H. *Alike and Different: The Clinical and Educational Use of Orff-Schulwerk.* Santa Ana, Calif.: Rosha Press, 1975.

Bogen, J. E. The other side of the brain: an appositional mind. *Bulletin of the Los Angeles Neurological Societies,* July 1969. **34 (3)**, 135–162.

Bonny, H. L. *Facilitating GIM Sessions.* Baltimore: Institute for Consciousness and Music, 1978.

Bonny, H. L., and Pahnke, W. N. The use of music in psychedelic (LSD) psychotherapy. *Journal of Music Therapy,* 1972. **9 (2)**, 64–87.

Bonny, H. L., and Savary, L. M. *Music and Your Mind: Listening with a New Conscious-ness.* New York: Harper and Row, 1973.

Bright, E. *Music in Geriatric Care.* New York: St. Martin's Press, 1972.

Critchley, M., and Henson, R. A. (Eds.). *Music and the Brain: Studies in the Neurology of Music.* London: William Heinemann Medical Books, 1977.

Diserens, C. M., and Fine, H. *A Psychology of Music.* Cincinnati, Ohio: Authors, 1939.

Eagle, C. T. (Ed.). *Music Therapy Index.* Lawrence, Kans.: National Association for Musical Therapy, 1976.

Farnsworth, Paul R. *The Social Psychology of Music.* Ames, Iowa: Iowa State University Press, 1969.

Ferguson, M. Music and rhythm: in harmony with the brain? *Brain/Mind Bulletin,* August 1978. **3 (18),** 1–2.

Gaston, E. Thayer (Ed.). *Music in Therapy.* New York: Macmillan Press, 1968.

Halpern, S. *Tuning the Human Instrument.* Palo Alto, Calif.: Spectrum Research Institute, 1978.

Institute for Consciousness and Music. *Newsletter.* Baltimore: Author, Summer 1978.

Journal of Music Therapy. Lawrence, Kans.: National Association for Music Therapy. 1964–.

Knapp, P. H. The ear: listening and hearing. *Journal of American Psychoanalysis,* 1953. **1,** 672–689.

Kryter, K. D. *The Effects of Noise on Man.* New York: Academic Press, 1970.

Langer, S. *Philosophy in a New Key.* New York: Penguin, 1942.

McKee, G.; Humphrey, B.; and McAdam, D. W. Scaled lateralization of alpha activity during linguistic and musical tasks. *Psychophysiology,* July 1973. **10 (4),** 441–442.

Meier, C. A. *Ancient Incubation and Modern Psychotherapy.* Evanston, Ill.: Northwestern University Press, 1964.

Merriam, A. P. *Anthropology of Music.* Evanston, Ill.: Northwestern University Press, 1964.

Michel, D. E. *Music Therapy.* Springfield, Ill.: Charles C. Thomas, 1976.

Music Therapy as a Career. Lawrence, Kans.: National Association for Music Therapy. n.d.

National Association for Music Therapy. *Newsletters.* Lawrence, Kans.: Author, 1978.

Pratt, C. C. *Music and the Language of Emotion.* Washington, D.C.: Library of Congress, 1952.

Purvis, J. P., and Samet, S. *Music in Developmental Therapy.* Baltimore: University Park Press, 1976.

Sachs, C. *The Rise of Music in the Ancient World, East and West.* New York: W. W. Norton, 1943.

Sessions, R. *The Musical Experience of Composer, Performer, and Listener.* Princeton, N.J.: Princeton University Press, 1971.

Taylor, I. A., and Paperte, F. Current theory and research in the effects of music on be-havior. *Journal of Aesthetics,* 1958. **17 (2),** 251–258.

Wagner, M. J. *Introductory Musical Acoustics.* Raleigh, N.C.: Contemporary Publishing, 1977.

Zuckerkandl, Victor. *Sound and Symbol: Music and the External World.* Princeton, N.J.: Princeton University Press, 1956.

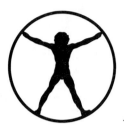 ANNOTATED BIBLIOGRAPHY

Bonny, H. L., and Savary, L. M. **Music and Your Mind: Listening with a New Consciousness.** New York: Harper and Row, 1973.

Bonny and Savary have provided structure for the age-old approach of listening to music as a means of exploring the many dimensions of the mind. Concentration/relaxation exercises are presented for use with carefully prepared music materials to evoke altered states of consciousness leading to feeling and imagery states that are life-changing in scope. The book presents theory, practice, and appendixes of appropriate "how-to-do-it" data on mood choice and recorded music. A trade book of simple application that, for the serious practitioner, should be complemented with more recently published materials from the Institute for Consciousness and Music (204 S. Athol St., Baltimore, Maryland).

Clynes, Manfred. **Sentics: The Touch of the Emotions.** Garden City, N.Y.: Anchor Press/Doubleday, 1978.

Clynes presents the concepts of his newly developed field of science—sentics. His basic theory postulates that each emotion (of his sentic cycle) and its expression has a specific brain-wave pattern associated with it. This substantiates a basis for universal communication of emotions among humans, since each person elicits a similar pattern in expressing any particular emotion. Clynes generalizes this principle to include emotional expression in music. He explains that "the composer translates the neurophysiological engram of his basic temperamental nature into musical notation," and the listener responds as the result of the activation of his similar engram. The concepts of sentics should be of interest to those in fields such as therapy, biofeedback, imagery, and the arts.

Critchley, M., and Henson, R. A. (Eds.). **Music and the Brain: Studies in the Neurology of Music.** London: William Heinemann Medical Books, 1977.

In twenty-four chapters, the authors illustrate different aspects of music and neurology. Music is discussed genetically, psychologically, and physiologically. Illnesses related to music such as amusia and deafness are also described. The final chapter discusses the role and types of musical therapy. The book is valuable to anyone interested in music and its effects. It summarizes many of the studies of music that have been done outside the field of music therapy and is therefore an important contribution to the field. The chapter dealing with musical therapy is well done but should not be thought of as an overview of the field.

Eagle, C. T. (Ed.). **Music Therapy Index.** Lawrence, Kans.: National Association for Music Therapy, 1976.

An interdisciplinary index to literature of the psychology, psychophysiology, psychophysics, and sociology of music, designed as a resource for scholars, researchers, and practitioners concerned with the influence of sound, specifically music, on human behavior. Titles of pertinent articles published internationally between 1960 and 1975 are covered, based on a computer-assisted information-retrieval system. An excellent resource for the researcher in music.

Farnsworth, Paul R. **The Social Psychology of Music.** Ames, Iowa: Iowa State University Press, 1969.

Farnsworth presents full coverage of major phenomena associated with the psychology of music from a sociopsychological orientation. Ten chapters cover concepts of music, musical abilities, musical taste, and the applications of music to industry and therapy. Extensive footnotes, bibliography, and research reports place this book in the valuable resource category.

Gaston, E. Thayer. (Ed.). **Music in Therapy.** New York: Macmillan, 1968.

This is a comprehensive survey of theory, research, techniques, and clinical practice that is designed to serve as a basic text for students of music therapy. In thirty-nine chapters grouped under ten parts, the sixty contributors—each writing in areas in which they are most expert—provide a complete discussion of all aspects of music therapy. Bibliography, notes, and indexes are included.

Unfortunately the book is dated, for in the twelve years since it was written many new and effective practices have replaced previous techniques, but until a new edition is published the basic information presented provides a good foundation for music therapy practice.

Kayser, H. **Akroasis: The Theory of World Harmonics.** Boston: Plowshares Press, 1964.

"Akroasis" (Greek for "hearing") is the rediscovered Pythagorean theory of harmonics in which the law of numbers and form inherent in the world can be translated into the sphere of hearing. Kayser's explanation of harmonics is not the theory of a musical system of chords, but rather what he perceives as "a metaphysical reality which can be related directly to the animate universe whereby the ear becomes the transmitter of a new understanding of the world." This book presents a possible holistically oriented, nonreductionist theoretical scheme as a focus for creative thinking.

McKee, G.; Humphrey, B.; and McAdam, D. W. **Scaled lateralization of alpha activity during linguistic and musical tasks.** *Psychophysiology,* July 1973. **10** (4), 441–442.

This is a brief report of a study of brain waves recorded during musical and linguistic tasks. The authors' results confirm previous studies and substantiate the finding that left hemisphere/right hemisphere alpha rhythm ratios are highest for musical tasks and diminish with increasingly difficult linguistic tasks. (Alpha activity seems to indicate that a hemisphere is idling.) This concise report adds to the evidence for lateralization of different functions in the brain.

Nordoff, Paul, and Robbins, Clive. **Music Therapy in Special Education.** New York: John Day, 1971.

The authors' first book, *Music Therapy for Handicapped Children* (1971, now out of print), which was based on their own experience, is followed by this concise "how-to-do-it" package of techniques, resource material, case studies, and valuable insights for working with the child whose development is affected by mental, physical, or emotional dysfunction. Six chapters cover singing, resonator bells, instrumental activities, plays with music, "Pif-Paf-Poltrie," case studies, and anecdotes. Four appendixes deal with group instrumental activities for physically disabled children, rhythmic patterns and speech phrases in classroom work, a music therapy bibliography, and a list of suppliers of special instruments. There are ample photographs. Although the book was written for use with children in special education settings, it should be useful in a variety of clinical situations where specialized music procedures are indicated.

Priestley, Mary. **Music Therapy in Action.** London: Constable, 1975.

Priestley gives an overview of "analytical music therapy," an approach developed and currently prevalent in England. Analytical music therapy is a "way of exploring the unconscious with an analytical music therapist by means of sound expression." Releasing and synthesizing the clients' bound-up energy is facilitated by techniques such as guided imagery and music, improvization, music listening, and relaxation to music. The importance of music as a nonverbal means of communication and expression and the relationship of client and therapist are stressed in helping the clients achieve their full human potential.

Priestley also discusses the use of instruments and music repertoire in therapy, training and qualifications for therapists, and different populations that could benefit from analytical music therapy. She presents her concepts simply (usually through case studies) and with obvious enthusiasm, making this book one of the most informative and enjoyable on the subject of music therapy.

Zuckerkandl, Victor. **Sound and Symbol: Music and the External World.** Princeton, N.J.: Princeton University Press, 1969.

Zuckerkandl expresses his philosophy of the musical concept of the external world. Music, composed of tones, is discussed as "the purely dynamic transcending the physical, space without distinction of places, time in which past and future coexist with the present, and the external and the inward interpenetrating." He makes an in-depth comparison of the physical world and that of purely dynamic events (tones) in terms of motion, time, and space. The book is primarily a discussion of the existence of music and its relation to the physical world. It is difficult to read, and a knowledge of musical concepts will be helpful in understanding it.

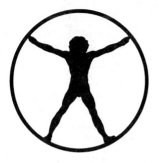

20

THE USE OF LIGHT AND COLOR IN HEALTH

Philip C. Hughes, Ph.D.

The physical environment is an object of increasing concern, not only to environmental scientists but also to health practitioners. The destruction of our natural environment through air, noise, and water pollution is now recognized as a major undesirable effect of our ever accelerating technological development. However, the need for concern over the nature of our indoor illuminated or lighted environment in contrast to our natural sunlighted environment has only recently come to the attention of environmentally oriented specialists.

The Effects of Sunlight

The dawn of human history saw humanity developing and adapting to a specific sunlight, adjusting and timing its internal physiology and activities to the sun and the sky's unique range of radiation and colors. Near optimum environmental conditions existed in the regions where humankind had their greatest sociocultural beginnings. The fertile crescent – the regions of Egypt, the land of Abraham, and the Tigris/Euphrates river basin where ancient Babylon and Nineveh had their start – had ideal climatic conditions that persist even today, with abundant sunlight and a seventy-degree isotherm. The sun confers high levels of the kind of ultraviolet (UV) light that promotes general health.

Ecological pressures forced people to migrate from their place of origin. A high price was paid, for when people moved from optimal environmental conditions to suboptimal, their general life span was drastically shortened. Exposure to "healthy" sunlight was greatly reduced, as were the associated benefits derived from sunlight. Some authorities set the average life span of the Nordic prehistoric man at sixteen to eighteen years. It is only in the last century with the rapid advances in medicine and science that humanity has climbed back up the road to longer life.

Along with food, air, and water, sunlight is a most important survival factor in human life. It is literally a nutrient to the body, allowing it to grow properly with a minimum of disease. For example, one of the best known biological effects of sunlight is the production of vitamin D in the skin. This vitamin, really a hormone, is essential for normal intestinal absorption of calcium and phosphorus from the diet and for normal mineralization of bone. It is vital to infants for the growth of a strong bone structure. It is important to the young for the full development of their immunological defenses against disease and hence beneficial to general health. And it is essential to the elderly for maintaining a healthy skeletal structure by preventing the common posture deformities of age and the fragility of brittle bones. Solar radiation activates other important biochemical events in our bodies involved in endocrine control, timing of our biological clocks, entrainment of circadian rhythms, immunologic responsiveness, sexual growth and development, regulation of stress and fatigue, control of viral and cold infections, and dampening of functional disorders of the nervous system (Wurtman, 1975).

These beneficial effects of sunlight were, and still are, dependent upon the full range of solar radiation, including both the ultraviolet and visible regions of the spectrum. Various physiological functions are dependent upon specific regions of the solar spectrum with all spectral parts playing some vital role in human functioning. It is important to realize that solar radiation can be specifically defined and that, whether direct or diffuse, it is rather stable in the proportion of radiation emitted in the near ultraviolet (320–380 nanometers— nm) and visible (380–750 nm) regions, whereas the middle ultraviolet (290–320 nm) region varies with sun angle. Global radiation, the radiation from the sun and sky, ranges in correlated color temperature from about 5,500 K (Kelvin) to 6,800 K, with 5,500 K representing the color temperature of global radiation when the sun is at ninety degrees from the horizon in a clear sky. Natural outdoor sunlight refers to such global radiation having a correlated color temperature of 5,500 K and a color rendering index (CRI) of 100. It was global radiation at 5,500 K that existed in the natural environments of the fertile-crescent cultures.

Indoor Illumination

Indoor illumination, and the quality of its spectral power distribution, has become an important consideration in designing living space. As people moved indoors to escape the elements of nature, they were forced to give up the benefits of natural sunlight and replace it with the fire and candle. Associated with the move to indoor living were often ill health, infection, and rampant diseases. Windows were considered a luxury and in England from 1696 to 1851 the government actually taxed window area (Collins, 1961).

The early period of the industrial revolution saw many people live out most of their lives indoors in inadequately lighted facilities. In fact, the outdoor environment was little better due to pollution. Loomis (1960) reports that rickets was quite common in England at the time of the industrial revolution. Rickets "in smoky cities was the first air-pollution disease." It resulted from a lack of sunlight, with smoke and smog putting up an umbrella against the healthy transmission of sunlight, which makes vitamin D synthesis possible in the body.

Fortunately, light is one environmental input that is modifiable. Better ways of lighting the indoor environment became essential as scientific investigations began to discover the effects of light on the human body. Technology was able to provide artificial light sources that made possible the efficient illumination of an indoor space. Light's relative environmental importance to the worker is seen in the recent study of Hardy (1974) in which 900 office workers rated the importance for their work of twelve environmental factors. Good lighting ranked first in importance followed by good ventilation, comfortable temperature, and plenty of space.

There are various approaches to creating and designing an indoor illumination for a space. Many of the approaches are overly simplistic in that they call for installing a specific number of light sources to provide illumination without giving any consideration to the many needs of the individuals using the space. Environmental lighting design must take into consideration not only light level but also human factors, task requirements, and architectural design parameters. A variety of light sources have been used to achieve these objectives, but the emphasis has too often been centered on meeting only the visual needs of the individual. Thus special attention is given to the application problems involved in visual performance, such as excessive brightness differences, discomfort glare, and veiling reflections.

These strictly visual approaches to illumination neglect the fact that light, especially sunlight, has important biological properties that affect human health. Light is able to influence the individual both by virture of its energy (photobiological effect) and as a source of information about the world (visual stimulus). For example, the neuroendocrine system receives significant light mediating inputs known to modify or affect sexual development, reproduction, metabolism, body temperature, activity, sleep-wakefulness, and many rhythmic endocrine functions (Neer et al., 1971; Wurtman and Weisel 1969; Wurtman 1975). The object of indoor illumination is to maximize both the visual and biological environments for optimum human functioning. To achieve this effectively the spectral power distribution of the light source must be considered.

The Spectral Power Distribution of Light

The amount of power from a lamp in each spectral region (color band) is termed the spectral power distribution (SPD). The importance of the relative spectral power distribution of the light source for maximum vision, comfort, and health is evident in recent research (Aston and Bellchambers, 1969; Lemaigre-Voreaux, 1970; Loomis, 1960; and Thorington, Parascandola, and Cunningham, 1971). Light sources can vary greatly in their SPD. The familiar incandescent filament lamps, in use since the turn of the century, all have basically the same spectral power distribution. Most of their visible energy from the hot filament is emitted in the red end of the spectrum with virtually no ultraviolet emission. Spectrally, the incandescent is quite similar to fire and candlelight, having a low correlated color temperature (2,850 K). It is perceived visually as a relatively warm light source. The lower the color temperature of a light source the warmer—that is, redder—its apparent color. A color temperature of 5,000 K to 5,500 K is considered neutral white with higher temperatures appearing cooler and bluer.

Fluorescent lamps are more recent in origin, dating from the 1930s. They generate visible energy by a nonthermal excitation of phosphors coating the inner wall surface of the fluorescent tube. The relative SPD of fluorescent lamps varies greatly depending upon the phosphors being utilized on the tube wall (see Figure 20.1). The most commonly encountered fluorescent lamp in office, industry, and schools is the standard "cool-white" lamp. The SPD of the standard cool-white fluorescent lamp was developed to maximize achromatic visibility (Ivey, 1963) but at the cost of differing greatly from natural sunlight in both the ultraviolet and visible spectrums. By concentrating as much of the lamp's energy output as possible in the yellow-green region of the spectrum, illuminating engineers were able to increase the lumen output of the lamp. This does not mean that more radiant energy is emitted by the lamp. It means only that the radiant output is being shifted into the yellow-green region, where the eye is more sensitive to brightness, rather than being distributed more evenly throughout the regions of the visible spectrum, as in natural sunlight.

One shortcoming of restricted SPDs is that they poorly render the colors in the environment (Thorington, 1973). It was because of the importance of color in the environment that the color rendering index (CRI) was developed for lamps. The CRI became a standard in 1965 (Nickerson and Jerome, 1965). The CRI is a rating of the degree to which a colorimetric shift of a test object occurs under one lamp when compared to its color under a reference source of the same correlated color temperature (Judd, MacAdam, and Wyszecki, 1964).

The cool-white fluorescent lamp has a CRI of 68 and natural daylight a CRI of 100. Thus, significant distortions and colorimetric shifts can occur when the environment is illuminated by the cool-white fluorescent as compared with natural daylight. Other fluorescent lamps vary in their CRI, and it is now possible to obtain a full-spectrum fluorescent light source (sold as Vita-Lite) that closely duplicates natural daylight in both the ultraviolet and visible regions of the spectrum with a CRI of 91 (see Figure 20.1).

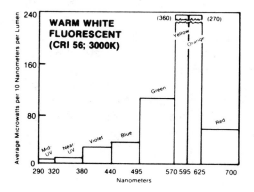

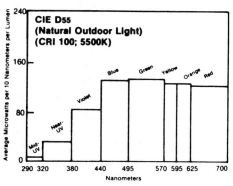

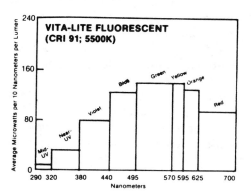

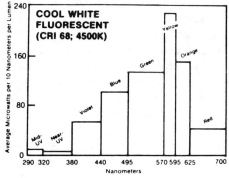

SPECIAL POWER DISTRIBUTION CHARTS compare "color ingredients" of the international standard CIE D55 for this phase of natural light versus Vita-Lite, Cool White fluorescent and Warm White fluorescent.

Figure 20.1

Color distortion can also be avoided by using the conventional incandescent lamp with its continuous spectrum and high CRI. However, the incandescent SPD is not balanced in relation to natural sunlight. It is visually a much warmer source and emits virtually no ultraviolet radiation, an essential spectral component for proper health. Moreover, it is energy inefficient with respect to producing light.

The lighting specialist still has a number of options open when optimizing the space for maximum well-being, health, and quality of life. Starting with the assumption that proper lighting means employing light that simulates natural sunlight with its balanced SPD and high CRI, one can utilize several methods. One approach is to use fluorescent light sources that match global solar radiation in both the visible and ultraviolet regions of the spectrum. For an artificial light source to truly simulate natural outdoor sunlight (direct or diffuse) it must admit substantially the same quantity of total ultraviolet radiation per lumen of visible light as found in natural sunlight at 5,500 K. Moreover, the ratio of near ultraviolet to middle ultraviolet radiation must be substantially the same as found in natural sunlight—that is, a ratio of at least eight.

It is important to note that nearly all light sources emit some energy in the ultraviolet regions of the spectrum, but unless specially designed, they do so in an unbalanced way when compared to natural global radiation. It is important to have substantially more energy emitted in the near ultraviolet than in the middle ultraviolet region. This can be achieved only by carefully choosing the phosphors and restricting the tolerance of the thickness of the glass tube wall of the fluorescent lamp. At present, the only commercially available fluorescent light source that simulates global radiation in both the ultraviolet and visible spectrum is the full-spectrum Vita-Lite brand lamp.

Other alternative or conjunctive approaches are the use of large window areas, solariums, atriums, courtyards, and skylights that expose the individual to natural sunlight for significantly long periods of time during their workday. If done appropriately, such approaches can also be energy saving. If plastic windows are used one must be sure to employ ultraviolet transmitting plastics.

Visual Clarity

The significance of using a high-CRI full-spectrum light source for illuminating work and living areas (as opposed to using a conventional cool-white source with a low CRI) has been examined by a number of researchers. Lemons and Robinson (1976) stress that high-CRI lamps produce a subjective visual clarity that is significantly greater than can be achieved by conventional cool-white lamps. They state that based on visual-clarity studies, the most widely used fluorescent lamps in the United States have CRIs less than the CRI of 85 that is recommended in Europe for lighting (Boyce, 1977).

Additionally, the English researchers Aston and Bellchambers (1969) have demonstrated that a higher-CRI lamp will give a greater apparent clarity to an environment than the lower-CRI cool-white lamp. They call this effect "visual clarity." Lemaigre-Voreaux (1970) in France has observed the same effect and found that about 60 footcandles of a high-CRI lamp provided the same visual clarity and satisfaction as 100 footcandles of a cool-white source. This research has been replicated by others (Boyce, 1977).

The differences between fluorescent light sources are indeed great. For example, for equal luminous flux the cool-white fluorescent lamp has about 29 percent more spectral power in the yellow-green region (i.e., 560–600 nm) than does natural sunlight and its full-spectrum simulation. Similarly, in the red region, between 630–700 nm, natural sunlight and the full-spectrum lamp have approximately three times more power than does cool white. This imbalance in the SPD of the cool-white fluorescent lamp is reflected in health effects as well as the visual appearance of objects and environments.

Light and Health

Much of the work on the biological effects of light has pointed to the importance of full-spectrum sunlight-simulating radiation in the indoor environment, strongly suggesting that increased amounts of sunlight, or its indoor full-spectrum equivalent, have wide implications for the designing of environmental spaces for prophylactic purposes and health enhancement. The use of such lighting appears to minimize environmental stress and to maximize biological functioning.

A recent study at Cornell University by Maas, Jayson, and Kleiber (1974) demonstrates that exposure to high-CRI full-spectrum sunlight-simulating fluorescent light sources can have a positive impact on an individual's general well-being. They found that students studying for four hours under two different fluorescent light sources exhibited significantly better visual acuity and less physiological fatigue at the end of the work period when the space was illuminated with sunlight-simulating full-spectrum Vita-Lite than with conventional cool white. No significant differences between the groups were found at the start of the period.

One of the important features of a full-spectrum source is its simulation of sunlight in the near ultraviolet (UV). Earlier work by Zamkova and Krivitskaya (1966) has shown "a shorter reaction time to light and sound, a lower fatigability of the visual receptors and improved working capacity" for individuals receiving additional UV along with their normal lighting as compared with those who did not.

The early work of Allen and Cureton (1945) reported a reduction in colds following UV treatments. They also reported that significant improvement in physical fitness resulted from suberythemal doses of sun exposure, that is levels below those needed to produce minimal reddening of the skin. Moreover, they cited an increase in motor and cardiovascular fitness as well as a trend toward decreased pulse rate and lowered systolic blood pressure. These effects are due, at least in part, to the many metabolic and neuroendocrine effects of light. Such metabolic and endocrine effects may play a major role in shaping the growth pattern of various organs. For example, Wurtman and Weisel (1969) have demonstrated that the gonads of rats maintained under the conventional cool-white fluorescent grow more slowly than the gonads of rats maintained under full-spectrum fluorescent lighting.

Work with school children has shown that such lighting reduces the incidence of colds and viral infections and is especially effective among individuals recuperating from illness. Zamkova and Krivitskaya (1966) report that children under full-spectrum lighting had a lower fatigability, significantly improved working capacity, and improved academic performance. Such research findings have led the Soviet Union to mandate such lighting in many of its indoor work environments (Volkova, 1967). Their researchers and health specialists have documented that the body's tolerance to environmental pollutants is increased by full-spectrum light, which also increases the effectiveness of immunization procedures (Dantsig et al., 1967; Kolomiytseva et al., 1972). Conversely, the West German government restricts the use of the cool-white fluorescent lamp from public buildings because of its distorted spectral output.

One of the effects of sunlight is to promote the synthesis of vitamin D in the body. Such effects are important for proper calcium absorption. Thus, Sharon et al. (1971) report that golden hamsters exposed to full-spectrum fluorescent light, which simulated both the visible and UV spectra of natural sunlight, had one-fifth as many dental caries as animals exposed to conventional fluorescent light. Moreover, the severity of the decay was ten times greater under the cool white. Additional support for the Wurtman and Weisel (1969) results was gained in the findings that indicated the total body, gonad, and submandibular gland weights were greater for the animals raised under the simulated sunlight. The researchers also note that microscopic examination of histologic sections from the testes of animals exposed to full-spectrum fluorescents showed active spermatogenesis and increased mitotic activity in the primary germ cell layer of the seminiferous tubules that was not found in the control animals. These findings strongly suggest that the spectral quality of the illuminant is a major determinant of its effects on mammalian growth and development.

Neer et al. (1971) have shown that the same calcium effect exists for people. They examined changes in the calcium absorption of institutionalized elderly people and found that those exposed to full-spectrum fluorescent light significantly increased the efficiency of their intestinal calcium absorption over those exposed to conventional cool-white lighting.

The Role of Color

Plack and Schick (1974) summarize the effect of color on nonvisual processes in humans. The effects include changes in mood and emotional state, psychomotor performance, muscular activity, rate of breathing, pulse rate, and blood measure. Gerard's (1958) dissertation research is probably the most detailed examination of the differential effects of colored light on psychophysiological functions. His study investigates the effect of different colors on psychophysiological measures indicative of emotional changes. Blue, red, and white lights of equal brightness were each projected for ten minutes on a screen in front of twenty-four normal adult males. The autonomic nervous system and visual cortex were found to be significantly less aroused during blue than during red or white illumination. The colors also elicited significantly different feelings, with blue being associated with increased relaxation, less anxiety, and less hostility and red illumination being associated with increased tension and excitement. Manifest anxiety level was significantly correlated with increased physiological activation and subjective disturbance during red stimulation. He found responses in the opposite direction of quiescence and relief during blue illumination. The work of Aaronson (1971) reports much the same effect of specific colors on activation and arousal.

The implications of these findings for designing appropriate color and light sources in environments to minimize chronic tension and anxiety need study. Further work will be needed to determine specific ways in which various SPDs may selectively affect the total environment. If color and the SPDs can be used to maximize appropriate psychological and physical effects, then they are important tools for the health care professional and the environmental designer.

Therapeutic Uses of Light

A number of skin diseases can be treated by including photosensitization reactions on the surface of the body. For example, psoriasis can now be treated by exposing the skin area to radiation from special lamps that emit strongly in the near ultraviolet region when patients are orally administered the photosensitizing agent methoxysoralen.

Another phototherapeutic use of light is the treatment of premature infants for hyperbilirubinemia. If bilirubin is allowed to build up it could result in the clinical syndrome kernicterus, which can end in brain damage and even death. Exposure to light breaks down the potentially dangerous levels of bilirubin in the blood so that the infant's physiologically immature liver can mature sufficiently to take over the function (Lucey, 1972).

Conclusion

The artificial indoor environment is a reality that humankind must face. Fortunately, there are alternatives that can allow us to spend much of our time indoors, at work and play, and yet simulate natural sunlight by means of skylighting and artificial full-spectrum lighting. These alternatives must be utilized if humankind is to continue its process of maximizing the environment for optimum human functioning.

References

Aaronson, B. S. Color perception and affect. *American Journal of Clinical Hypnosis*, 1971. **14**, 38–42.

Allen, R. M., and Cureton, T. K. Effect of ultraviolet radiation on physical fitness. *Archives of Physical Medicine and Rehabilitation*, 1945. **26**, 641–644.

Aston, S. M., and Bellchambers, H. E. Illumination, colour rendering and visual clarity. *Lighting Research and Technology*, 1969. **1**, 259–261.

Boyce, P. R. Investigations of the subjective balance between illuminance and lamp colour properties. *Lighting Research and Technology*, 1977. **9**, 11–24.

Collins, John S. *The World of Light.* New York: Horizon, 1961.

Dantsig, N. M.; Lazarev, D. N.; and Sokolov, M. V. Ultraviolet installations of beneficial action. *CIE* (Commission Internationale de l'Eclairage) *Publication*, 1967. **20**, 67.

Gerard, R. M. *Differential Effects of Colored Lights on Psychophysiological Functions.* Unpublished doctoral dissertation, University of California at Los Angeles, 1958.

Hardy, A. C. A case for reduced window areas. *International Lighting Review*, 1974. **25**, 90–92.

Ivey, H. F. Color and efficiency of luminescent light sources. *Journal of the Optical Society of America*, 1963. **53**, 1185–1198.

Judd, D. B.; MacAdam, D. L.; and Wyszecki, G. Spectral distribution of typical daylight as a function of correlated color temperature. *Journal of the Optical Society of America*, 1964. **54**, 1031.

Kolomiytseva, M. G.; Voznesenskaya, E. A.; Isayeva, E. A.; and Generalov, A. A. Role of ultraviolet radiation in increasing natural resistance of the animal organism when associated with different amounts of copper and manganese in the daily ration. *Journal of Hygiene, Epidemiology, Microbiology and Immunology*, 1972. **16**, 240–246.

Lemaigre-Voreaux, P. In favor of "de luxe" fluorescent lamps. *Lux*, 1970. **60**, 564–565.

Lemons, T. M., and Robinson, A. V. Does visual clarity have meaning for IES illumination recommendations for task lighting? *Lighting, Design, and Applications*, 1976. **6**, 24–28.

Loomis, W. F. Rickets. *Scientific American*, 1960. **223** (6), 77–91.

Lucey, Jerold F. Neonatal jaundice and phototherapy. *Pediatric Clinics of North America*, 1972. **19** (4), 1–7.

Maas, J. B.; Jayson, J. K.; and Kleiber, D. A. Effects of spectral difference in illumination on fatigue. *Journal of Applied Psychology*, 1974. **59**, 524–526.

Neer, R. M.; David, T.R.A.; Walcott, A.; Koski, S.; Schapis, P.; Taylor, I.; Thorington, L.; and Wurtman, R. J. Stimulation by artificial lighting of calcium absorption in elderly human subjects. *Nature*, 1971. **229**, 225. (Also unpublished observations.)

Nickerson, D., and Jerome, C. W. Color rendering of light sources: CIE method of specification and its application. *Illuminating Engineering*, 1965. **60**, 253.

Plack, J. J., and Schick, J. The effects of color on human behavior. *Journal of the Association for Study in Perception*, 1974. **9**, 4–16.

Sharon, I. M.; Feller, R. P.; and Burney, S. W. The effects of lights of different spectra on caries incidence in the golden hamster. *Archives of Oral Biology,* 1971. **16 (12)**, 1427–1431.

Thorington, L. Light, biology, and people. *Lighting Design and Application,* 1973. **3**, 19–23; 31–36.

Thorington, L.; Parascandola, L.; and Cunningham, L. Visual and biologic aspects of an artificial sunlight illuminant. *Journal of the Illuminating Engineering Society,* 1971. **1**, 33–41.

Volkova, N. V. Experience in the use of erythemic radiation in the general lighting system of a machine shop. *Gigiena i Sanitariia,* 1967. **32**, 109–111.

Wurtman, R. J. The effects of light on man and other mammals. *Annual Review of Physiology,* 1975. **37**, 467–483.

Wurtman, R. J., and Weisel, J. Environmental lighting and neuroendocrine function: relationship between spectrum of light source and gonadal growth. *Endrocrinology,* 1969. **85 (6)**, 1218–1221.

Zamkova, M. A., and Krivitskaya, E. I. Effect of irradiation by ultraviolet erythema lamps on the working ability of school children. *Gigiena i Sanitariia,* 1966. **31**, 41–44.

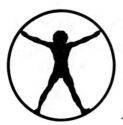

ANNOTATED BIBLIOGRAPHY

Aaronson, B. S. **Color perception and affect.** *American Journal of Clinical Hypnosis,* 1971. **14,** 38–42.

> The results of Aaronson's study using posthypnotic hallucination of colors for a twenty-four–hour period suggest that there exists a general association between color and arousal, going from warm activating colors (such as red) to cooler colors (such as blue, with purple being intermediate). Except for black, which was depressing, the achromatic tones appear to have little effect.
>
> The subjects' individual responses to specific colors appear influenced by the associations evoked by the specific colors.

Aston, S. M., and Bellchambers, H. E. **Illumination, colour rendering and visual clarity.** *Lighting Research and Technology,* 1969. **1,** 259–261.

> The article discusses the attractiveness of an interior space as being a function of the pattern of color, area, lightness, and brightness of each part. Hue, value, and chroma must be balanced against shape, form, and proportions, but this balance can be easily destroyed if a carefully selected indoor environment is distorted by lighting that has an unbalanced spectral power distribution.
>
> A comparison of the spectral power distribution of a number of light sources demonstrated that the same degree of visual satisfaction for the light space was provided by the high color-rendering lamp at levels of illumination significantly lower than the comparison levels with high efficiency, low color-rendering lamps.

Birren, Faber, **Color Psychology and Therapy.** Secaucus, N.J.: University Books, 1961.

> A survey and description of how people have used and responded to color, including applications to medical treatment, health, and design. Occult and mystical traditions are reviewed as well as the "chromopathic" color healers, who prescribed colored lights for various illnesses. Some scientific research is cited for biological effects and psychological and therapeutic reactions. Applications to functional design are suggested for reduced eyestrain and psychological effects.
>
> There is a good bibliography for occult, mystical, and "color healing" references, but there is inadequate coverage of scientific literature.

Gerard, R. M. **Differential Effects of Colored Lights on Psychophysiological Functions.** Unpublished doctoral dissertation, University of California at Los Angeles, 1958.

This study still represents the most detailed treatment on the subject of color effects. The earlier literature is carefully reviewed and then the study investigates the effect of different colors on psychophysiological measures indicative of emotional changes. Blue, red, and white lights of equal brightness were each projected for ten minutes on a screen in front of twenty-four normal adult males. The autonomic nervous system and visual cortex were significantly less aroused during blue than during red or white illumination. Different colors also elicited significantly different feelings: for instance, greater relaxation and less anxiety and hostility during blue, more tension and excitement during red illumination. Manifest anxiety level was significantly correlated with increased physiological activation and subjective disturbance during red stimulation. Findings for blue in the opposite direction of quiescence and relief suggested that blue illumination may benefit individuals with chronic tension and anxiety. Implications of the results for Rorschach theory, psychodiagnosis, and color therapy are discussed.

Himmelfarb, P.; Scott, A.; and Thayer, P. S. **Bactericidal activity of a broad-spectrum illumination source.** *Applied Microbiology,* 1970. **19**, 1013–1014.

This reports a comparative test of the bactericidal effects of full-spectrum (Vita-Lite) and cool-white fluorescent lamps on *staphylococcus aureus.* The results showed that an eight-hour exposure to the full-spectrum light source had an effective killing rate (approximately 90 percent), whereas the standard cool-white fluorescent lamp produced little effect.

Hughes, P. C., and Neer, R. M. **Lighting for the elderly: a psychobiological approach to lighting.** *Human Factors,* 1979 (in press).

The article reviews the role of illumination in shaping the indoor environment of the elderly person. The approach is that lighting has a two-fold impact on the individual: as a source of information about the environment (i.e., visual) and photobiologically through the skin or photoreceptor.

Research on the visually lighted environment is reviewed, looking first at the physiological changes that occur during the aging process, then at the effect of aging on visual performance, and finally at the importance of qualitative factors in assessing the adequacy of an illuminated environment for the elderly. Special attention is given to application problems in lighting for the elderly (i.e., excessive brightness differences, discomfort, glare, veiling reflections, and the importance of color and spectral power distribution of the light source). The advantages of a full-spectrum light source that simulates natural sunlight for indoor illumination is discussed with regard to recent research.

The biologically lighted environment is also reviewed in terms of the potential role that indoor illumination can play in regulating important biochemical processes in the elderly population (such as neuroendocrine control, vitamin D_3 synthesis, immunologic mechanisms, and cardiovascular regulation).

Loomis, W. F. **Rickets.** *Scientific American,* 1970. **223** (6), 77–91.

The article indicates that while rickets is still regarded as a dietary deficiency disease resulting from a lack of vitamin D, it is caused in fact from a lack of sunlight. In smoky cities it was the earliest air-pollution disease because solar ultraviolet was significantly blocked by industrial smog.

Indoor living is cited as having a marked effect on incidence of rickets in several countries, including India. A higher incidence is found among the wealthy, well-fed Moslems whose married women enter purdah and whose infants remain indoors. A lower incidence is found among well-to-do Hindus whose children are outdoors more and among poor Hindus who have bad diets but who work outdoors and whose young play outdoors.

Maas, J. B.; Jayson, J. K.; and Kleiber, D. A. **Effects of spectral differences in illumination on fatigue.** *Journal of Applied Psychology,* 1974. **59**, 524–526.

This study tested the effects of different fluorescent lamp spectra of environmental illumination on fatigue and visual acuity after a period of perceptual studying in a university conference classroom. The results indicated that full-spectrum illumination closely approximating the spectral quality of natural sunlight produced less perceptual fatigue and increased visual acuity when compared to standard cool-white fluorescent illumination.

Neer, R. M.; Davis, T.R.A.; Walcott, A.; Koski, S.; Schapis, P.; Taylor, I.; Thorington, L.; and Wurtman, R. J. **Stimulation by artifical lighting of calcium absorption in elderly human subjects.** *Nature,* January 22, 1971. **229**, 225–257.

Vitamin D is important in the prevention of bone disease in the elderly. Also, it cures or prevents rickets by its conversion in the liver to 25-hydroxvitamin D, which then allows mineral absorption by the intestines. These absorbed minerals then go to the bones and increase their strength. When one is exposed to natural or artificial ultraviolet, vitamin D is formed in the skin. The study shows that full-spectrum (sunlight simulation) fluorescent lamps emitting ultraviolet radiation significantly increase calcium absorption in the elderly when compared to conventional cool-white fluorescent lamps.

Ott, John. **Health and Light.** Old Greenwich, Conn.: Devin-Adair, 1973.

An interesting popularized account of recent work on the effects of light on plants, animals, and man. The author brings together both anecdotal and published findings, presenting them in a forceful and convincing style. The major premise of the work is that the full spectrum of natural sunlight – including both visible and ultraviolet radiation – under which life on earth evolved is essential to humankind's optimal physical and mental health. A bibliography of seventy-one references is included.

Sharon, I. M.; Feller, R. P.; and Burney, S. W. **The effects of lights of different spectra on caries incidence in the golden hamster.** *Archives of Oral Biology,* 1971. **16** (12), 1427–1431.

Golden hamsters exposed to full-spectrum fluorescent light that simulates natural sunlight in both the visible and the ultraviolet ranges had one-fifth as many caries as animals exposed to conventional cool-white fluorescent lamps. The total body, gonad, and submandibular gland weights were greater for the animals raised under the simulated natural light. Differences in gonad and submandibular gland development were histologically demonstrated with haematoxylon and eosin sections. The conclusion is that light affects caries incidence, submandibular gland development, and sexual maturity.

Sharpe, Deborah T. **The Psychology of Color and Design.** Totowa, N.J.: Littlefield, Adams, 1975.

A review of research on color, with suggestions on using color in design. The review focuses principally on scientific and psychological studies of color preferences in relation to age, personality, culture, and psychological pathology, and to a lesser extent on the effects of color on people. There are extensive footnotes but no bibliography.

Part Four

APPLICATIONS THROUGHOUT THE LIFE CYCLE

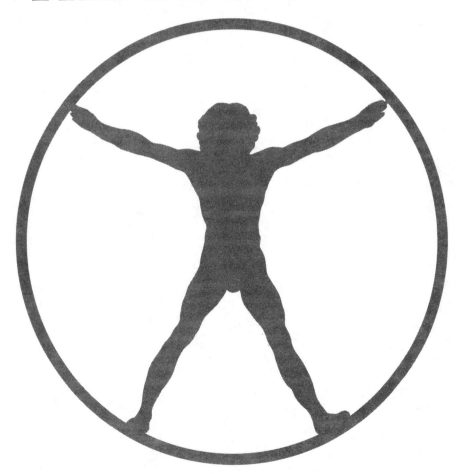

21

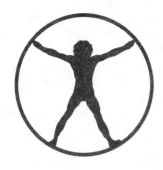

ALTERNATIVES IN CHILDBIRTH

James S. Gordon, M.D., and Doris B. Haire

In the last century in the United States, childbirth has been transformed from a normal physiological process to a medical procedure and a pathological event. This distortion may be seen as an overreaction to the dangers of some births, resulting in the application to all children and mothers of a biomedical model and technologies that may save some few endangered babies. The current movement for alternative birthing practices is a reaction against the dehumanizing and dangerous effects of excessive technological management, an attempt to restore the experience of childbirth to women and their families, and an effort to synthesize humanistic practice and scientific precision.

History

Through much of the nineteenth century American mothers gave birth to their children in their homes, surrounded and supported by people who knew and cared about them, assisted in their delivery by empirically trained midwives. As immigration, migration, and urbanization eroded stable communities of women, as a medical belief in an active interventionist approach to all aspects of health and illness—including childbirth—came into prominence, midwives began to disappear, and doctors—some far less experienced than the midwives—began to

303

assume control of childbirth (Wertz and Wertz, 1977).

Not long afterward, the fear of complications that might be forestalled by physicians, the availability of anesthesia and analgesia, the presence of full-time paid auxiliary helpers, and a larger cultural tendency to institutionalize and centralize functions combined to change the scene of birth. In 1900, less than 5 percent of all women delivered in hospitals, by 1939 half of all births and 75 percent of those in urban areas took place there, and by 1970 more than 95 percent of all American children were being born in hospital delivery rooms.

The medicalization of childbirth and the application of emerging technologies to the detection and treatment of pathological conditions was in many ways a great advance. By the early part of the century, doctors could diagnose and treat such dangerous conditions as eclampsia and maternal syphilis. Advances in surgical techniques and in anesthesia made it possible for them to perform safe Caesarean sections when placenta previa, cephalopelvic disproportion, or fetal distress occurred. Subsequently, physicians were able to use intrauterine transfusions to treat, and high-titer anti-Rh gamma globulin to prevent, Rh incompatibility and to enable mothers with heart disease, diabetes, and other serious illnesses to have the children they wanted.

Unfortunately, their training in detecting and treating pathology and the impressiveness of some of their technological interventions, combined with a degree of self-interest, tended to narrow the perspective of many physicians. Specialists in obstetrics, as in other areas of medicine, were unable to appreciate fully the overriding importance of factors unrelated to medical care – economic well-being, good nutrition and prenatal care, the broader acceptance of contraception and abortion (which tended to decrease parity and lead to an earlier cessation of child bearing) – in improving maternal and infant mortality statistics. Increasingly, physicians began to feel that safe childbirth demanded continual medical intervention, even in situations where there was no reason to expect risk or abnormality. By 1920 Dr. Joseph DeLee (1920) was successfully advocating routine use of forceps and episiotomy in all deliveries. He believed, and was apparently able to convince his colleagues, that labor was "a decidedly pathologic process," that the physician's job was not to attend or to assist in it, but to "improve on" its natural course.

The Critique of Medically Managed Childbirth

Only in the last two decades have there been attempts to examine critically the routine procedures and surgical and pharmacological interventions that have been introduced in childbirth in the last seventy years. The results of the studies that are beginning to appear raise serious questions about the efficacy – and indeed the safety – of virtually every modern "improvement" in the course and conduct of labor and delivery.

Although confining the laboring woman to bed may be convenient for the hospital staff and necessary for a sick woman, the practice has been shown to prolong a healthy woman's labor, increase the need for such further interventions as epidural anesthesia and forceps delivery, and diminish the Apgar scores of their babies (Flynn et al., 1978). Though it is important to shave the pubic hair of louse-ridden women, this unpleasant procedure does not reduce sepsis in others who come for delivery (Burchell, 1964; Kantor et al., 1965). Amniotomy (artificial rupture of the fetal membranes) to induce labor produces immediate danger of prolapse and compression of the umbilical cord and may lead to long-term damage by increasing intracranial pressure and causing misalignment of the cranial bones (Althabe et al., 1969; Caldeyro-Barcia et al., 1974). The lithotomy position (in which the woman has her legs spread wide apart above her head in stirrups) that Louis XIV introduced because he wished to watch his mistresses give birth (Arms, 1977) may be convenient for obstetricians but it is unnatural and dangerous as well as inhibiting and degrading to women. Virtually unknown outside of Western society, this position diminishes blood flow to the placenta, causing a drop in fetal heart rate during each uterine contraction, and stretches the perineum, thereby making episiotomy more likely (Caldeyro-Barcia, 1978).

Analgesia, sedatives, anesthetics, and labor-stimulating drugs—though sometimes necessary in high-risk deliveries and in emergencies—are decidedly counterproductive in low-risk births. With rare exceptions these drugs cross the placenta and may produce profound changes in the physiology of mother and child and long-term adverse effects on the child's physical and cognitive development (Aleksandrowicz, 1974; Brackbill and Broman, 1979; Brazelton et al., 1979; Brown et al., 1972; Hoult et al., 1977; Kron et al., 1966; Myers and Myers, 1979; Ralston and Shnider, 1978; Turner and MacFarlane, 1978). We are now discovering that the incidence of Caesarean section—which is accompanied by the morbidity and mortality of general anesthesia and major abdominal surgery—is increasing at a rate that apparently far exceeds its life-saving utility. From 1968–1976 the rate of Caesarean sections more than doubled to 11.4 percent (Marieskind, in press). Finally, some of the most recent advances in the technology of childbirth—including the expensive and widely touted electronic fetal monitors—may prove to have limited application in high-risk deliveries and to be counterproductive in the ordinary experience of birth. The Congressional Office of Technology Assessment (Banta and Thacker, 1979) concluded that widespread use of electronic fetal monitoring was premature and as yet unjustified, and Haverkamp et al. (1979), who had been staunch proponents of electronic monitoring, demonstrated in two controlled studies of high-risk mothers that there was no difference in infant outcome between those who were monitored and those who were not.

This information about the physical dangers of medically managed childbirth has been augmented in the last decade by studies describing the emotional and interpersonal disturbances that routine hospital birth procedures may cause. Drs. Marshall Klaus and John Kennell (1976) at Case Western Reserve Medical School have observed a specific bonding ritual between the human mother and her newborn infant that is frustrated and shortcircuited by technological birth and the routine separation of the infant from its mother after birth. According to Klaus and Kennell the bonding process involves intense and direct eye-to-eye contact, extensive holding and touching, maternal soothing and crooning sounds, and mutual smiling, and it appears to be crucial in orienting infants to their surroundings and in establishing an intimacy with those who will care for them.

Klaus and Kennell's work shows that the technological approach to childbirth and the hospital procedures that accompany it traumatize both mother and child and make them less available for bonding. In a matched controlled study, Klaus found that mothers who were allowed sixteen hours of extra contact with their infants at birth were more reluctant to leave their infants with someone else when the children were one month and one year old, that they "usually stood and watched during the [routine physical] exams, showed significantly greater soothing behavior and engaged in significantly more eye-to-eye contact and fondling." Norma Ringler's five-year follow-up study (1975) of Klaus and Kennell's work indicates that infants who have more intimate contact with their mothers during the hours and days postpartum achieve developmental milestones significantly earlier than those who were separated by standard hospital procedures. Ringler found that at age five the I.Q.'s as well as speech and language comprehension of these children were significantly superior to those of the control group, with groups matched and controlled for drugs.

Some preliminary follow-up studies of Frederick Leboyer's work provide tentative confirming evidence. French infants born by Leboyer's "method" – into a warm, quiet, dimly lit delivery room, whose umbilical cords are left intact, who are given a warm bath at birth, and who are allowed virtually continuous contact with their mothers – appear calmer, more responsive, and more relaxed than those born among the bright lights, sharp noises, and cold surfaces of the ordinary hospital delivery room. In a multiyear follow-up study (controlled for drugs) of 120 babies born to women randomly assigned to conventional and Leboyer-type delivery rooms, standardized psychomotor examinations, clinical observations, and parental interviews have indicated that the "Leboyer" children are exceptionally adroit with both hands, that they begin to talk at an earlier age, and display less difficulty in toilet training and self-feeding than the control group. In addition, it appears that their fathers may take a greater interest in them (as a far greater number come to follow-up visits) than those of the control group (Trotter, 1977).

The Alternative Birth Movement

Even before the information about the dangers and counterproductivity of medicalized childbirth became available, some parents and some physicians were seeking alternatives to procedures they regarded as mechanical and alienating. In the 1930s Grantly Dick-Read's *Childbirth Without Fear,* now revised (1970), helped give many women and their husbands the courage to take a more active role in childbirth. In the late 1950s Fernand Lamaze's (Karmel, 1959) adaptation of Pavlovian breathing techniques, massage, and muscular contraction offered them specific techniques for assuming this control. And in the 1960s Robert A. Bradley's *Husband-Coached Childbirth* (1974) showed how parents and physicians could cooperate in restoring the familial context of childbirth while decreasing the need for anesthetics and analgesics.

In the 1960s these reforms in obstetrical practice were enlarged on predominantly by educated, middleclass women who began in consciousness-raising groups to discuss their health, to study their anatomy and physiology, and to examine their bodies. Soon they were questioning the treatment they had received at the hands of mostly male physicians. The movement for alternative births began as part of this more general movement by women to reclaim control over their own bodies. While some established mutual help groups, feminist therapy collectives, and women's clinics, even larger numbers began to look for alternatives to hospital births. They searched for hospital-based obstetricians who could be counted on to refrain from using analgesics, anesthetics, oxytocin, forceps, and episiotomies; for other women—physicians, nurse-midwives, and lay-midwives—who would provide extensive emotional support as well as technical care during pregnancy and delivery; and for homelike settings that would permit the father, siblings, and friends to participate in the birth of their child.

The alternative birth movement that has evolved from this search is as diverse as the women and men who seek alternatives to the present system, as the variety of birth attendants who are willing to assist them, and as the places they have created for birth to take place. A number of programs like New York's Maternity Center Associates (Lubic and Ernest, 1978) rely on nurse-midwives (nurses with postgraduate training in midwifery) backed up by obstetricians to provide all routine prenatal care and to attend deliveries in homelike birth centers. Others, like the Berkeley Family Health Center and Maternity Center Associates in Bethesda, Maryland, are staffed by physicians and nurse-midwives who attend births at home. Still others—including the Santa Cruz Midwives and the Midwifery Program of the Farm (Gaskin, 1978), an agricultural and spiritual commune in rural Tennessee—rely on lay midwives (women and men without nursing training who have learned how to attend births from obstetricians and other midwives) backed up by physicians for primary care and home delivery. Hospitals, too, began to create alternatives: Denver's Mercy Hospital leased space to nurse-midwives who run the independent Denver Birthing Center, and—long before most other hospitals had one—Mt. Zion Hospital in San Francisco and San Francisco General Hospital had developed homelike in-hospital environments for birth.

Though prenatal regimens, techniques of labor and delivery, the settings in which births take place, and the professional identities of the birth attendants vary widely, there are certain approaches and attitudes that characterize the alternative birth movement as a whole. Some have their counterparts in holistic medical care, and many have, in one form or another, always been part of sound obstetrical practice. Among the approaches and attitudes are:

- A conviction that each birth should be tailored to the personal, familial, cultural as well as the medical needs of the participants. There should be a willingness to include others—fathers, siblings, and close friends—in prenatal discussions, in planning for childbirth, and in the experience of birth itself.
- A belief that there should be a variety of options in the place of delivery and in the person and profession of birth attendants available to each woman.
- An emphasis on the importance of the personal qualities—patience, kindness, and wisdom—as well as on the technical skills of the birth attendant.
- An intimate and flexible relationship between birth attendant, the pregnant woman, and her family that encourages the discussion of interpersonal as well as physiological concerns.
- A team approach to pregnancy, labor, and delivery in which highly trained obstetricians provide initial screening, medical back-up, and active involvement in potential high-risk deliveries but assume a secondary role in normal pregnancies and deliveries.
- An increased emphasis on the role of trained midwives in providing primary care for pregnant women and their families and in attending births.
- An emphasis on a process of education and self-care for families as well as expectant mothers throughout pregnancy rather than on treatment and medical prescription.
- A conviction that mothers and members of their families can take primary responsibility for the conduct of labor and delivery.
- Avoidance, except in cases of clear medical necessity, of all prenatal and intrapartum medication.
- Minimal use of invasive diagnostic procedures, including pelvic examinations, during pregnancy and delivery, and of technological and surgical intervention during delivery.
- Careful attention to diet and exercise before, during, and after pregnancy.
- Encouragement of bonding between mother—and, where desired, father, siblings, and close friends—and the newborn.
- The creation of a warm and welcoming emotional and physical space for each newborn.
- A conviction that the newborn is a conscious being capable of cognition and of emotional reaction.

- An appreciation of the physiological and psychological value of breast feeding.
- Active involvement by past clients in shaping and delivering an institution's services.

Midwives and Obstetricians, Home and Hospital Birth

As the alternative birth movement has attracted more adherents, it has drawn considerable criticism from obstetricians who sharply question the abilities of midwives and the safety of nonhospital births. Though the American College of Obstetricians and Gynecologists (1978a) recognizes that "the certified nurse-midwife . . . may assume responsibility for the complete management of the uncomplicated pregnant woman," she (or he) is expected to do so only under the "direction" of a "qualified obstetrician-gynecologist." This subordination of midwives to physicians may yield good results—a clinical study of this team approach by Gatewood and Stewart (1975) indicated high patient satisfaction with the supervised midwives—but it does tend to prevent the midwives from being considered "the expert" in the care of the healthy, pregnant mother, and it does force their practice to conform to a medical model and to a technology that may well be dangerous to mother and child.

The necessity for subordinating nurse-midwives to doctors is not justified by evidence. In some countries with far lower infant mortality rates than ours, including The Netherlands and Sweden, midwives attend virtually all low-risk births and have status as independent professionals. Though matched controlled studies of the performance of physicians and midwives have not been done, the data we do have seem to indicate that for low-risk women midwives are as effective here as they are abroad. More than forty years ago a survey by the New York Academy of Medicine revealed that midwives had a maternal mortality rate of 1.4 per thousand, while general practitioners' patients died at the rate of 2.2 per thousand. The Frontier Nursing Service, founded in 1925 by Mary Breckinridge, has successfully delivered the children of poor and poorly nourished Appalachian women for fifty years. Midwives at Kings County Hospital in New York City, where the clients are 95 percent nonwhite, have helped that institution to reduce its infant mortality to less than half the national average for teaching hospitals of its size (Arms, 1977). At the University of Mississippi Medical Center (Slome et al., 1976; Thiede, 1971) the outcome for deliveries with nurse-midwives was as good as with the medical housestaff, and in underserved Madera County, California (Levy et al., 1971), two nurse-midwives were able in three years to diminish the incidence of prematurity by 50 percent and to reduce neonatal mortality from 23.9 per thousand to only 10.2 per thousand. Two years after the pilot program had been disbanded neonatal mortality climbed to 32.1 per thousand.

Though lay midwives without adequate training are obviously dangerous, well-trained lay midwives, backed up by physicians, may be able to obtain at least as successful an outcome as physicians and nurse-midwives who work in a hospital setting. Lewis Mehl's study (performed without a control group) of 289 births attended by the lay midwives of the Santa Cruz Birth Center (Arms and Arms, 1973; Mehl, 1976) revealed a perinatal mortality of 3.2 per thousand during a period when the figure for the United States as a whole was 27.1. The Apgar scores of the babies delivered by these midwives averaged 9.4 at one minute and 9.7 at five minutes (Arms, 1977). Lay midwives at the Farm in Summertown, Tennessee, have in the last seven years attended some 722 births (Gaskin, 1978). There have been only fifteen perinatal deaths, seven of which occurred during hospital births (undertaken because the midwives judged the mothers to be high risk) and eight in the course of home births. Of the 683 deliveries by midwives in maternal homes, the perinatal mortality was 11.7 per thousand, approximately half that of the United States as a whole. Only 1 percent of the mothers received Caesarian sections.

The American College of Obstetricians and Gynecologists (ACOG) recognizes the utility of nurse-midwives. Though it also "supports actions and programs that encourage family-centered maternity care" (1978a), it is far less favorably inclined to out-of-hospital births. According to the ACOG, family-centered, maternity care must "continue to provide the mother and her infant with the accepted standards of safety available only in a hospital setting." To buttress its position the ACOG cites statistics that show far higher perinatal mortality rates for babies delivered at home than in the hospital (1978b). These figures include a preponderance of women who had little or no prenatal care and who were attended by untrained persons. In Oregon (Oregon State Health Division, 1977), for example, 40 percent of the babies born outside of the hospital "were delivered by attendants without any kind of health or professional license." These figures do not have much bearing on the outcome of home births for mothers who deliver after good prenatal care and under the supervision of competent midwives or physicians.

Studies that do attempt to compare home and birthing center births with hospital births are still very preliminary. Though the early ones are subject to some methodological criticisms, they are nevertheless suggestive. For example, Louis Mehl's and Robert Mendelsohn's (1976) retrospective matched study of 1,046 home and 1,046 hospital births (in which there was no advanced indication of special risk) revealed certain facts. There were thirty significant birth-related injuries among hospital births, none in home births; fifty-two infants required resuscitation in the hospital while only fourteen did so in the home; there were six diagnoses of neurological damage to children born in the hospital and only one such diagnosis among those born in the home. A second study by Mehl (1976) comparing planned home births with hospital deliveries performed by one of the groups of physicians involved in home births revealed "no significant differences in risk with home delivery versus hospital delivery."

The Future of the Alternative Birth Movement

As the critique of medically managed hospital birth for low-risk mothers grows more convincing, the trends toward out-of-hospital birth, toward the use of birth attendants other than obstetricians, and toward a more humanistic and holistic approach to birth are becoming stronger. Suzanne Arms (Gordon, n.d.) estimates that the percentage of babies born at home in Sonoma County, California, has increased from less than 1 percent five years ago to 10 percent in 1978, while statistics kept by the State of Oregon (Oregon State Health Division, 1977) indicate that the percentage of total registered births outside of the hospital had risen from 0.5 percent in 1963 to 2.7 percent in 1976. David Stewart, Director of the National Association of Parents and Professionals for Safe Alternatives in Child Birth (NAPPSAC), estimates that between 1 and 2 percent of all births nationwide are home births (Gordon, n.d.).

The number of births in birthing centers, within and outside of hospitals, has increased even more precipitously than the percentage of out-of-hospital births. In 1972 there was one nonhospital birth center. A year ago the NAPPSAC *Directory of Alternative Birth Services and Consumers' Guide* (Simkin, 1978) listed fifty birth centers around the country, and today there are at least twice as many already operating or about to open. Some are staffed primarily by obstetricians or by nurse-midwives, while others integrate childbirth educators, social workers, and health aides into a comprehensive system of care and education. Virtually all programs include fathers as active participants and offer classes in natural childbirth, breast feeding, and child development and give detailed advice on nutrition and exercise. Some, like the Berkeley Family Health Center and the Santa Cruz Midwives, emphasize the importance of marital counseling and of home visits, and others, like the Denver Birth Center, offer special programs for the newborn's siblings (Gordon, 1978).

At a time when birthrates and obstetrical revenues are declining, hospitals have also been responding to consumer demands for alternatives. All but unheard of five years ago, hospital birth rooms have been proliferating at an accelerating rate. A recent issue of *Medicial Tribune* (*Brain Mind Bulletin*, 1979) reported that "90 per cent of New York State's hospitals either have installed homelike birthing centers or plan to do so in the next several months," while David Stewart estimates that across the country several hundred are already in operation. Programs like the one at Hennepin County Hospital in Minneapolis and Mt. Zion in San Francisco have in many ways come to resemble out-of-hospital birth centers. They are indeed homelike and do offer genuinely "family centered birth" in comfortable rooms with beds large enough for mother, father, and infant in a setting free from unnecessary intravenous drips, medications, stirrups, pubic preps, etc. Unfortunately, a number retain the technology and attitude of medicalized childbirth and are different only in appearance.

In the last several years proponents of birth alternatives have created a number of national and local organizations to provide information to parents, to promote communication among those who are attending births, and to stimulate research on the comparative safety and effectiveness of the various birth alternatives. NAPPSAC, which has been instrumental in this nationwide organizational movement, holds a yearly conference—last year close to 1,500 people attended—publishes research findings and commentaries, is catalyzing a dialogue between the alternative birth movement and the American College of Obstetricians and Gynecologists, and provides parents and professionals with a directory of alternative birth services (Simkin, 1978).

All of this activity is having an effect on people who several years ago would have been terrified of an out-of-hospital or indeed an unanesthetized birth. An increasingly large number of prospective mothers and fathers of all social classes are well informed and concerned about the long-term deleterious effects of pharmacological, technological, and surgical interventions. They are beginning to want and expect ongoing intimate relationships with those who will deliver their babies, a more natural family centered childbirth, and are actively seeking out programs to meet their needs. There is little doubt that in the future alternatives to routine hospital birth will become more—rather than less—important.

Conclusion and Recommendations

The bulk of this chapter has dealt with the critique of medically managed birth and the development, among a small group of educated middle- and upper-middle-class women, of alternative methods of childbirth. It seems important, in conclusion, to put these alternatives into a broader context, to suggest ways in which the most valuable aspects of the alternative model may be elaborated to address the needs of all women, to lower our still shamefully high infant mortality rate, and to provide a satisfying birth experience for all families. What follows is an outline of some elements that might be part of a comprehensive program to improve the experience—and the outcome—of birth.

1. *Improvement of the nutritional status and the physical well-being of school girls whose ill health and poor nourishment are responsible for many premature and low-birth-weight infants.* At a minimum this would involve ongoing instruction in health promotion, regular rigorous exercise, and the elimination of most processed foods in school cafeterias and vending machines.

2. *Adequate sexual education for all young people, including education about childbirth, child rearing, and contraception.*

3. *Prenatal support and care to all mothers.* This should begin with checkups and screening, nutritional advice, exercise programs, and education about fetal and infant development and maternal-infant bonding. It should include information about the effects of drugs (including obstetrical drugs), smoking, and alcohol on the pregnant woman and her child; discussions of the various birth alternatives; adequate counseling services for young women and their husbands (or

male partners or boy friends) to help them deal with the questions or conflicts that pregnancy may stimulate; support groups for prospective parents; and small residences where women who have nowhere else to go can live during pregnancy and during the first weeks after delivery. These programs would be undertaken jointly by midwives and "maternity aides" and would include consultation with obstetricians where appropriate.

4. *Creation of a new health care professional, the maternity aide.* In Holland maternity aides working with midwives make regular visits to discuss concerns with the family throughout pregnancy, are present at delivery, and help out in the days after birth. Their educational and practical homemaking services could be made universally available by encouraging some women in each neighborhood to inform pregnant women of their existence. Something like this exists in Cuba, where local neighborhood groups (the Committees for the Defense of the Revolution) talk to pregnant women and encourage them to come to prenatal clinics.

5. *The creation of a variety of safe alternatives, including home birth, birthing-center birth, and hospital birth.* Early in pregnancy each mother would, in consultation with a midwife and a physician, choose a location for birth that is appropriate for her and her family. In all cases, arrangements would be made so that the full panoply of technological intervention could be used if necessary. In a home birth this might involve making sure adequate facilities for delivery and resuscitation were available at home, determining how long it took to go from the mother's home to the hospital, and arranging for emergency back-up from the same physician who had examined the mother during pregnancy.

6. *Facilitation of maximal participation by family (and friends if desired) in the experience of birth and in bonding in the hours after birth.* This would happen naturally at home or in the birth center. It could be encouraged in the hospital by providing labor lounges (comfortable living rooms for couples in labor) to which they could retreat and stay during labor and delivery with beds large enough for fathers as well as mothers. Rooming-in would be the rule rather than the exception.

7. *The creation of an independent profession of midwifery, of schools to train midwives, and of licensing procedures specifically for them.* These schools would follow the World Health Organization's recommendation for three years of formal training, including at least one year of nursing, or three years of training in nursing and one in midwifery. In choosing students the schools would seek out people thoughtful enough to anticipate risks, sensitive enough to provide emotional as well as technical support to pregnant women and their families, self-critical and modest enough to know when it is necessary to refer endangered patients to obstetricians, and patient enough to sit calmly through long hours of labor.

8. *A system of prepaid care including pre- and postnatal care by maternity aides.* This system would be designed to eliminate financial incentives for unnecessary medical intervention on the one hand and for unwise retention of patients by midwives on the other. Thus, for example, physicians would make no more

money if their patients received a Caesarian section than if they had a vaginal delivery, and midwives would be paid fully even if they felt it necessary to refer a patient to an obstetrician.

9. *Adequate postnatal care and support for mother and child.* The presence of a maternity aide to help with child care and housework in the week after birth would provide the mother with an opportunity for intimacy with her newborn child as well as a chance to rest and recuperate after delivery. The aide would offer ongoing instruction in child care and would help the family to deal with the stresses of the postpartum period. Thus, the aide would help reduce the need for expensive hospital care by eliminating one of the major reasons that mothers have babies in hospitals—their desire to have a respite from the responsibilities at home.

10. *A refinement of the role of the obstetrician.* The obstetrician is a highly skilled medical professional, trained to identify and whenever possible remedy medically any deviation from the normal progress of labor and delivery. Unless obstetricians are willing to emulate the midwife in managing the obstetric care of normal birth, their role should be limited to these medical functions and to the training of midwives and physicians.

11. *An assumption that technological, pharmacological, and surgical interventions are potentially damaging and are necessary only in exceptional instances.* This assumption would lead to the creation of committees in each hospital to evaluate carefully the drugs given (including general and local anesthesia, labor stimulating drugs, and analgesics) prenatally and intrapartum, the techniques employed (including forceps, lithotomy position, amniotomy, and electronic fetal monitoring), and the surgical procedures used (Caesarian sections and episiotomies, etc.). Such committees would contribute substantially to limiting these interventions to appropriate situations.

12. *Active solicitation of questions and criticisms about the care they receive from current and former consumers.* This would be part of the ongoing interaction between all members of the health care team—midwife, obstetrician, maternity aide—the pregnant woman, and her family. Consumers should be involved in the committees evaluating medical intervention and in planning for future services.

The alternative birth movement was created in reaction to excesses of technological management and to provide a few women with a more natural approach to childbirth. It is possible that it may catalyze the creation of an entirely new approach to childbirth in which modern science serves the human function of childbearing, in which each birth is tailored to meet the specific needs of participants, and in which comprehensive public health measures are tempered and shaped by democratic participation. Perhaps it is not unrealistic to hope that such a synthesis will reduce our rates of infant mortality, improve relationships between parents and children, and reduce the cost of childbirth and of caring for those who are damaged in the course of pregnancy and in the process of birth.

References

Aleksandrowicz, M. The effect of pain relieving drugs during labor and delivery on the behavior of the newborn: a review. *Merrill Palmer Quarterly,* April 1974. **20 (2),** 121–141.

Althabe, O.; Aramburu, G.; Schwarcz, R.; and Caldeyro-Barcia, R. Influence of the rupture of membranes on compression of the fetal head during labor. In R. Caldeyro-Barcia (Ed.), *Perinatal Factors Affecting Human Development.* Washington, D.C.: Pan American Health Organization, 1969. 143–160. (Scientific Publication no. 185.)

American College of Obstetricians and Gynecologists. *Health Department Data Shows Danger of Home Births.* Chicago: Author, January 4, 1978a.

American College of Obstetricians and Gynecologists. *The Responsibilities of the Health Team in Maternity Care.* Chicago: Author, April 1978b.

Arms, Suzanne. *Immaculate Deception: A New Look at Women and Childbirth in America.* New York: Bantam, 1977.

Arms, Suzanne, and Arms, John. *A Season to Be Born.* New York: Harper and Row, 1973.

Banta, H. D., and Thacker, S. The costs and benefits of electronic fetal monitoring. *Obstetrics and Gynecology Survey, Supplement,* August 1979.

Brackbill, Yvonne, and Broman, Sarah. *Obstetrical Medication and Development in the First Year of Life.* Bethesda, Md.: Office of Scientific and Health Supports, National Institute of Neurologic and Communicative Disease Disorders and Stroke, National Institutes of Health, 1979.

Bradley, Robert A. *Husband-Coached Childbirth* (Revised ed.). New York: Harper and Row, 1974.

Brain Mind Bulletin. Boom in birth centers. February, 7, 1979. **4.**

Brazelton, T. B.; Tryphonopoulou, Y.; and Lester, B. A comparative study of the behavior of Greek neonates. *Pediatrics,* 1979. **63,** 279–285.

Brown, Walter A. et al. Relationship of antenatal and perinatal psychologic variables to the use of drops during labor. *Psychosomatic Medicine,* 1972. **34,** 119–127.

Burchell, R. C. Predelivery removal of pubic hair. *Obstetrics and Gynecology,* 1964. **24,** 272–273.

Caldeyro-Barcia, R. The influence of the maternal position during the second stage of labor. In P. Simkin (Ed.), *Kaleidoscope of Childbearing.* Seattle: Pennypress, 1978.

Caldeyro-Barcia, R. et al. Adverse perinatal effects of early amniotomy during labor. In L. Gluck (Ed.), *Modern Perinatal Medicine.* Chicago: Yearbook Medical Publications, 1974.

DeLee, Joseph. The prophylactic forceps operation. *American Journal of Obstetrics and Gynecology,* 1920. **1,** 34–44.

Dick-Read, Grantly. *Childbirth Without Fear* (2nd revised ed.). New York: Harper and Row/Perennial Library, 1970.

Flynn, A.; Kelly, J.; Hollins, C.; and Lynch, P. Ambulation during labour. *British Medical Journal,* August 26, 1978. **6137,** 591–593.

Gaskin, Ina May. *Spiritual Midwifery* (Revised ed.). Summertown, Tenn.: Book Publishing, 1978.

Gatewood, T. Schley, and Stewart, Richard B. Obstetricians and nurse midwives: the team approach in private practice. *American Journal of Obstetrics and Gynecology,* September 1, 1975. **123 (1),** 35–40.

Gordon, James S. Special study on alternative mental health services. *Report to the Presi-*

dent's Commission on Mental Health. Washington, D.C.: U.S. Government Printing Office, 1978.

Gordon, James S. Personal communication, n.d.

Haverkamp, Albert et al. The evaluation of continuous fetal heart rate monitoring in high risk pregnancy. *American Journal of Obstetrics and Gynecology,* June 1, 1979. **125,** 310–320.

Hoult, I.; MacLennon, A.; and Carrie, L. *Lumbar epidural analgesia in labour—relation to fetal malposition and instrumental delivery. British Medical Journal,* January 1, 1977. **6052,** 14–16.

Kantor, H. et al. Value of shaving the pudendal-perineal area in delivery preparation. *Obstetrics and Gynecology,* 1965. **25,** 509–512.

Karmel, Marjorie. *Thank You, Dr. Lamaze: A Mother's Experience in Painless Childbirth.* Philadelphia: Lippincott, 1959.

Klaus, M., and Kennell, J. *Maternal and Infant Bonding.* St. Louis: C. V. Mosby, 1976.

Kron, R.; Stein, M.; and Goddard, K. Newborn sucking behavior affected by obstetric sedation. *Pediatrics,* 1966. **37,** 1012–1016.

Levy, B.; Wilkinson, F.; and Marine, W. Reducing neonatal mortality rate with nurse-midwives. *American Journal of Obstetrics and Gynecology,* 1971. **109,** 50–58.

Lubic, Ruth Watson, and Ernest, Eunice K. N. The child-bearing center: an alternative to conventional care. *Nursing Outlook,* December 1978. **26 (12),** 754–760.

Marieskind, Helen. *An Evaluation of Caesarian Section in the United States of America.* Washington, D.C.: Office of Planning and Evaluation, Department of Health, Education and Welfare, in press.

Mehl, Lewis E. Statistical outcomes of home births in the United States, current status. In David Stewart and Lee Stewart (Eds.), *Safe Alternatives in Childbirth.* Chapel Hill, N.C.: National Association of Parents and Professionals for Safe Alternatives in Childbirth, 1976.

Mehl, Lewis E., and Mendelsohn, Robert. *Home Birth vs. Hospital Birth: Comparisons of Outcomes of Matched Populations.* A paper presented at the annual meeting of the American Public Health Association, Miami, Florida, 1976. Paper available from Dr. Lewis E. Mehl, Center for Research on Birth and Human Development, 2340 Ward St., Room 105, Berkeley, California 94705.

Myers, R., and Myers, S. Use of sedative, analgesic, and anesthetic drugs during labor and delivery: bane or boon? *American Journal of Obstetrics and Gynecology,* 1979. **133,** 83–104.

Oregon State Health Division. *Bulletin of the Oregon State Health Division,* October 1977. **55 (1).**

Ralston, D., and Shnider, S. The fetal and neonatal effects of regional anesthesia in obstetrics. *Anesthesiology,* 1978. **48,** 34–61.

Ringler, Norma E. *Mothers' Language to Young Children and the Effects of Early and Extended Contact on the Speech and Language Comprehension at Five.* A paper presented at the annual conference of the National Association for the Education of Young Children, Dallas, Texas, November 1975.

Simkin, P. *NAPPSAC Directory of Alternative Birth Services and Consumers' Guide.* Marble Hill, Mo.: National Association of Parents and Professionals for Safe Alternatives in Childbirth, 1978.

Slome, C. et al. Effectiveness of certified nurse midwives: a perspective evaluation study. *American Journal of Obstetrics and Gynecology,* January 15, 1976. **124 (2),** 177–182.

Thiede, Henry A. A presumptuous experiment and role, maternal and child care. *American Journal of Obstetrics and Gynecology,* November 1, 1971. **111** (5), 736–742.

Trotter, Robert J. Leboyer's babies. *Science News,* January 22, 1977. **111** (4), 59.

Turner, S., and MacFarlane, A. Localization of human speech by the newborn baby and the effects of pethidine (meperidine). *Developmental Medicine and Child Neurology,* 1978. **20**, 727–734.

Wertz, Richard W., and Wertz, Dorothy C. *Lying In: A History of Childbirth in America.* New York: The Free Press, 1977.

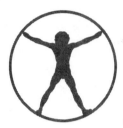

ANNOTATED BIBLIOGRAPHY

Aleksandrowicz, M. **The effect of pain relieving drugs during labor and delivery on the behavior of the newborn: a review.** *Merrill Palmer Quarterly,* April 1974. **20 (2),** 121–141.

An especially clear review of the literature that describes the inhibiting effects of commonly employed obstetric drugs on human development during the early months and years of life. The paper is particularly suitable for psychologists who are working with learning disabled and brain impaired children but who do not have a sufficient knowledge as to how obstetric drugs influence brain function in the fetus, the newborn infant, and the child's subsequent development.

Althabe, O.; Aramburu, G.; Schwarcz, R.; and Caldeyro-Barcia, R. **Influence of the rupture of membranes on compression of the fetal head during labor.** In R. Caldeyro-Barcia (Ed.), *Perinatal Factors Affecting Human Development.* Washington, D.C.: Pan American Health Organization, 1969. 143–160. (Scientific Publication no. 185.)

This paper describes the risks to the fetal brain of artificially rupturing the membranes (bag of water) in order to induce labor. The authors carefully explain by diagram how the artificial rupture of membranes increases the risks of (a) prolapse and compression of the umbilical cord, which can diminish or pinch off the supply of oxygenated blood to the fetal brain and other tissues; (b) increased intracranial pressure; and (c) marked misalignment of the cranial bones, which in turn increases the likelihood of tears and hemorrhage in the membranes that cover the brain.

American Academy of Pediatrics Committee on Drugs. **Effect of medication during labor and delivery on infant outcome.** *Pediatrics.* 1978. **62,** 402–403.

The Committee on Drugs has cautioned in the past (*Pediatrics,* 1973, **51,** 297) that no drug has been proved safe for the unborn child. The committee now takes the position that the physician has an obligation to advise the expectant mother of the known adverse effects and potential benefits of the drugs offered to her during pregnancy, labor, delivery, and lactation. It is interesting to note that the committee does not mention that the physician is obligated to advise the expectant mother of the potential *risks.* Since no drug has been proved safe, there is a possibility that the drugs administered to pregnant or parturient women may result in long-term adverse effects that cannot be determined at this time and therefore that women have a right to know of these risks.

American College of Obstetricians and Gynecologists. **Informed consent.** In American College of Obstetricians and Gynecologists, *Standards for Obstetric-Gynecologic Services.* Chicago: Author, 1974. 66–67.

This section on informed consent carefully spells out the physician's legal obligation to inform the obstetric patient of the risks, hazards, and alternatives to any proposed drug or procedure the physician plans to employ in caring for the obstetric patient during pregnancy, labor, and delivery. The section is particularly clear in discussing those excuses that *cannot* be used by the physician to justify failure to inform.

Annas, G. **The Rights of Hospital Patients: The Basic ACLU Guide to a Hospital Patient's Rights.** New York: Avon Books, 1975.

Many of the frustrations and disappointments obstetric patients experience in the hospital would be diminished if they had a better sense of their rights while in the hospital. This book, part of a series by the American Civil Liberties Union (ACLU), offers information that will, at least to some degree, keep the obstetric patient from feeling victimized by the system. The book describes how the hospital is organized, the rules the hospital must follow, the typical admission and discharge procedures, informed consent, the right to refuse treatment, the rules of human experimentation, access to hospital records, the names of various organizations working for patient's rights, and so on.

Arms, Suzanne. **Immaculate Deception: A New Look at Women and Childbirth in America.** New York: Bantam, 1977.

This is an angry and articulate polemic against the medical domination and distortion of childbirth in twentieth-century U.S. hospitals. Arms is a photo-journalist who began work on this project in part because she felt robbed of her own experience in childbirth. She is stunningly effective in exposing the arrogance of current obstetrical practice and its deleterious physical and psychological effects on birthing mothers, their children, and their families. She combines, with considerable skill, summaries of relevant research on the hazards of technological intervention, the importance of early maternal-infant bonding, etc., with personal accounts and photographs of mothers, their children, and those who attend their births. The last half of the book provides an excellent overview of the effective alternatives to hospital births that have been developed—particularly by lay midwives in the United States—and of the political, medical, and legal controversy that surrounds them.

Banta, H. D., and Thacker, S. **The costs and benefits of electronic fetal monitoring.** *Obstetrics and Gynecology Survey, Supplement,* August 1979.

This review of the research carried out on electronic fetal monitoring (EFM) stresses that widespread use of EFM, a widely used technology of uncertain benefit associated with definite risks and financial costs, is premature and, as yet, unjustified. The authors (Dr. David Banta, Health Program Manager, Office of Technology Assessment, Congress of the United States; and Dr. Stephen Thacker, Chief, Consolidated Surveillance and Communication Activity, Bureau of Epidemiology, Center for Disease Control) suggest the need for changes in public and private policies toward evaluation and control of medical technologies.

Brackbill, Yvonne, and Broman, Sarah. **Obstetrical Medication and Development in the First Year of Life.** Bethesda, Md.: Office of Scientific and Health Supports, National Institute of Neurologic and Communicative Disease Disorders and Stroke, National Institutes of Health, 1979.

A follow-up of 3,528 full-term singleton infants born to healthy mothers with uneventful pregnancies, labors, and deliveries demonstrated a strong relationship between obstetric drugs and neurologic dysfunction in the first year of life. Subsequent follow-up indicates that in many cases neurologic dysfunction persisted throughout the seven-year testing period. It is important to note that the criteria set in 1966 by NIH for inclusion of infants in the sample group (the elimination of normal mothers who had demonstrated abnormal responses to the drugs administered to them during labor and delivery) tended to reduce the numbers of children who would be affected adversely by drugs. Thus, the pervasiveness of neurological damage to newborns is probably far greater than indicated even by this alarming study.

Brazelton, T. B.; Tryphonopoulou, Y.; and Lester, B. **A comparative study of the behavior of Greek neonates.** *Pediatrics,* 1979. **63,** 279–285.

The investigators evaluated interactive processes, motor processes, the "ability to regulate" state, and the physiologic organization of three groups of full-term normal-sized infants who developed no indication of jaundice or neurologic signs during the neonatal period. All of the mothers of the three groups of infants were classified as having had healthy, uneventful pregnancies and normal labors. Infants in Group A were born to unmarried mothers of lower social class, who suffered self-inflicted semistarvation to hide their condition during the first seven months of their pregnancies, who received little or no drugs during their pregnancies and during labor and birth, and who subsequently gave up their infants for adoption (these infants were subsequently bottlefed on a four-hour schedule). Infants in Group B were born to married mothers of the same lower social class who were adequately nourished during pregnancy, who received no drugs during labor and birth, who kept their babies and breastfed them on demand. The infants in Group C were born to middle-class married mothers who were adequately nourished during pregnancy, who kept their babies, who were administered both predelivery medication and spinal or local anesthesia for birth.

In almost all physical and behavioral parameters infants in Group B scored significantly better than the infants in Group C and in Group A. The investigators postulate that the reason for the differences between Group B and Group C may well be the drugs administered to the mothers of the infants in Group C. Infants in Group C, the middle-class group, had the worst physiologic scores and were similar to the Group-A babies in having depressed interactic motor and state behaviors. There was no indication in the report that Group A and Group C caught up to Group B during the ten-day test period.

The implications of this finding for maternal attachment, child abuse, subsequent social adjustment, and cognitive functioning in the offspring can only be determined by subsequent research.

Brewer, G., and Brewer, T. **What Every Pregnant Woman Should Know: The Truth About Diets and Drugs in Pregnancy.** New York: Random House, 1977.

The authors discuss the fallacy of using diuretics and a salt-free diet to control the edema and toxemia of pregnancy. Their emphasis is on good nutrition, the need for protein, and an adequate diet in assuring the well-being of the pregnant woman and the outcome of her pregnancy.

Brown, Walter A.; Manning, Tracey; and Grodin, Jay. **Relationship of antenatal and perinatal psychologic variables to the use of drugs during labor.** *Psychosomatic Medicine,* 1972. **34**, 119–127.

The investigation by Brown and his colleagues indicates that it is not the mother's expression of discomfort or pain at the time of labor and birth that determines the amount and kind of drugs she will receive during this time, but the physician's opinion of the mother's condition and the attitude that the physician formed weeks before the mother's labor began.

Burchell, R. C. **Predelivery removal of pubic hair.** *Obstetrics and Gynecology,* 1964. **24**, 272–273.

This follow-up study of 7,600 patients who were not shaved in preparation for birth points to the unnecessary nature of this uncomfortable and humiliating practice.

Caldeyro-Barcia, R. **The influence of the maternal position during the second stage of labor.** In P. Simkin (Ed.), *Kaleidoscope of Childbearing.* Seattle: Pennypress, 1978.

Those who have long thought the lithotomy position for childbirth was not only degrading but unscientific will take heart from this learned but concise discussion of the disadvantages of the lithotomy position by the current president of the International Federation of Obstetricians and Gynecologists. Dr. Caldeyro-Barcia presents these facts: in normal spontaneous labor the vertical position (walking, standing, or sitting) facilitates the progress of labor, shortens its duration, and reduces maternal discomfort and pain. The author then explains the mechanics that make this true.

This book is available from the International Childbirth Education Assocation, Book Division, P.O. Box 70258, Seattle, Washington 98107.

Caldeyro-Barcia, R. et al. **Adverse perinatal effects of early amniotomy during labor.** In L. Gluck (Ed.), *Modern Perinatal Medicine.* Chicago: The Yearbook Medical Publications, 1974.

The investigators describe the adverse effects on the fetus of amniotomy, the artificial rupture of the "bag of waters." Amniotomy disturbs the normal balance of pressure on the uterine contents (fetus, placenta, and umbilical cord) during uterine contractions and bearing down efforts, which in turn creates uneven compression and deformation of the fetal head and occlusion of umbilical vessels. The resulting malalignment of the cranial bones increases the risk of tears (and subsequent hemorrhage) in the membranes that separate and support portions of the brain. The resulting cord compression causes marked alterations in the pattern of fetal heart rate.

Chard, T., and Richards, M. (Eds.). **Benefits and Hazards of the New Obstetrics.** Philadelphia: J. B. Lippincott Company, 1977.

This book compiles the work of several experts in the field of maternal and child health and deals with the continuing public controversy in the United States over increased obstetric intervention and its effect on both the mother and her child. The chapter by Ian Chalmers and Martin Richards, entitled "Intervention and Casual Interference in Obstetric Practice," is of particular interest to those who question the wisdom of routine induction of labor, medication, chemical stimulation of labor, forceps extraction, etc.

Collins, U. B. **Some legal problems that often confront physicians.** In R. C. Benson (Ed.), *Current Obstetric and Gynecological Diagnosis and Treatment* (2nd ed.). Los Altos, Calif.: Lange Medical Publishers, 1978.

Many women who are angry about the obstetric care they have received express a desire to bring a legal action against their physician or other health care providers involved in their case. This chapter helps to define when an obstetric patient does or does not have grounds to bring a legal action.

Dick-Read, Grantly. **Childbirth Without Fear** (2nd revised ed.). New York: Harper and Row/Perennial Library, 1970.

Though Dick-Read's book may seem antifeminist or overly romantic today, it was—when published in England in the 1930s—the major force in launching the movement for "natural childbirth." Dick-Read, a practicing obstetrician, believed that "science has been carried away by its enthusiasm," that the "best and safest anesthetic [for a laboring woman] is an educated and controlled mind," and that "the privilege of attending women in childbirth is far greater than we were taught to realize." He felt that if women could be helped to relax, to enjoy the "spiritually uplifting aspects of childbirth" they could overcome the "fear-tension-pain-syndrome" that debilitated them. He insisted that restoring the control of childbirth to women and to sympathetic "others" (preferably the woman's husband) would be instrumental in this process. The book provides instructions for prenatal care, labor and delivery, and postnatal care, including breast feeding.

Doering, S., and Entwisle, D. **Preparation during pregnancy and the ability to cope with labor and delivery.** *American Journal of Orthopsychiatry,* 1975. **45,** 825–837.

The title of this paper does not disclose an important finding of the investigators—that the higher the level of the mother's awareness of the physical as well as emotional sensations of birth the more positive her response to her child. The investigators compared the reactions toward their newborn infants of three groups of mothers. Group A received little or no drugs during labor and birth and were therefore fully aware of the physical as well as the emotional sensations of birth. Group B received regional anesthesia (epidural, saddle, caudal, etc.) that obliterated or significantly diminished the sensations of birth but left them mentally aware. Group C were completely anesthetized and therefore unconscious during the birth of their infants.

The investigators found that in general the strongest indications of affectional attachment occurred among those mothers in Group A who were completely awake and physically aware of the sensations of birth, and that a painful experience did not adversely affect the more positive attitudes shown toward their infants. The mothers comprising Group B tended to score significantly lower in their affectional attachment to their infants. The poorest attachment occurred among the women in Group C, who were unconscious during the birth of their infants.

Enkin, M. et al. **A prospective randomized clinical trial of the Leboyer approach to childbirth.** *Birth and the Family Journal,* in press.

Enkin and his colleagues evaluated the labors, births, and infant outcome of three groups of women. Group A was insistent on having a Leboyer-type birth, while Group B was randomly assigned at thirty-seven weeks gestation to a Leboyer-type birth. Group C was assigned to a "gentle birth" group. Group A had an average labor of twelve hours, Group B had an average labor of seven hours, and Group C had an average labor of fourteen hours. There was no significant difference in the infants' various assessment scores. The investigators postulate that the reason the Leboyer *assigned* group had such significantly shorter labors than even the Leboyer *insistent* group is that the Leboyer assigned group felt assured that the physician and nurses caring for them in the obstetric unit would do everything possible to see that they had a good birth experience, whereas the women who were insistent on having a Leboyer birth may have had a certain amount of distrust and therefore were less relaxed during their labors.

Fitzgerald, Dorothy et al. **Home Oriented Maternity Experience: A Comprehensive Guide to Home Births.** Tacoma Park, Md.: Home Oriented Maternity Experience, 1976.

This primer is invaluable for all those considering a home birth. It is practical and comprehensive. Information on everything from equipment required for a home birth to breast feeding, from psychological aspects of home birth to the use of herbs is included in this brief, readable account.

Home Oriented Maternity Experience is located at 511 New York Avenue, Tacoma Park, Maryland 20012.

Flynn, A.; Kelly, J.; Hollins, C.; and Lynch, P. **Ambulation during labour.** *British Medical Journal,* August 26, 1978. **6137**, 591–593.

This is the first study to measure the effects of ambulation in labor using continuous monitoring by radiotelemetry (presenting part electrode and intrauterine pressure catheter). In this prospective study of sixty-eight women, half of the women were assigned to an ambulant group, the other half were confined to bed during labor. Women in the ambulant group, who were encouraged to walk about during labor, had shorter labors (by more than two hours), less or no need for analgesia or epidurnal anesthesia, fewer but more efficient contractions, and five times less need for a forceps-assisted delivery than did those mothers confined to bed during labor. The infants also benefitted by their mothers' ambulation during labor. They demonstrated more normal heart-rate patterns during labor and better Apgar scores at one minute and five minutes after birth than did those infants born to mothers who were confined to bed during labor.

Gaskin, Ina May. **Spiritual Midwifery** (Revised ed.). Summertown, Tenn.: Book Publishing, 1978.

The Farm is a 1,200-person, 1,000-acre agricultural and spiritual commune in rural Tennessee founded by Stephen Gaskin. In this book Ina May Gaskin offers a compendium of the Farm's "amazing birthing tales," counsels prospective parents, and presents detailed, well-illustrated instructions for midwives and midwives-in-training. The overall effect is remarkable. The book she has produced, like the midwives she has trained, manages somehow to combine exuberance with common sense and professionalism. Do not be put off by the "hippie" language or some repetition in the "amazing tales." Ina May and the Farm people have much to teach us, not only about what they call the "sacrament of birth" but also about proper obstetrical care.

Gold, Edwin. **Pelvic drive in obstetrics: an X-ray study of 100 cases.** *American Journal of Obstetrics and Gynecology*, 1950. **55**, 890–896.

A series of X-rays taken to evaluate the pelvic outlet demonstrated that the outlet is increased when the mother is allowed to assume a normal squatting position.

Gots, R., and Gots, B. **Caring for Your Unborn Child.** New York: Stein and Day, 1977.

This popular and easy-to-read book by a physician-couple discusses the unborn child's vulnerability to insult from maternal disease, environmental hazards, and over-the-counter as well as prescription drugs in a way that will be interesting even to those who don't like "baby books."

Haire, D. **Instructions for Nursing Your Baby.** Milwaukee, Wisc.: International Childbirth Education Association, n.d.

An inexpensive six-page information leaflet that concisely covers a great deal of information that a mother needs in order to successfully initiate and continue breast feeding. The information has been approved by the American Academy of Pediatrics Committee on Fetus and Newborn. The International Childbirth Education Association also publishes a companion leaflet by the same author, entitled "How the Breast Functions," which is as informative to most health professionals as it is to the mother.

Haire, D. **The Cultural Warping of Childbirth.** Rochester, N.Y.: International Childbirth Education Association Publication Center, 1972. Reprinted in a special issue of *Environmental Child Health*, 1973. **19**, 171–191.

This extensively documented analysis of obstetric care inthe United States and abroad demonstrates that many of the drugs and procedures employed in U.S. obstetric care are potentially damaging to both mother and child. The information on how the Food and Drug Administration currently rates the "safety" of obstetric drugs is of particular interest. The author makes the point that there is no drug that when taken by or administered to a childbearing woman has been proven safe for the unborn child. The monograph has been updated several times.

Haire, D. **The Pregnant Patient's Bill of Rights.** Milwaukee, Wisc.: International Childbirth Education Association, 1976.

This four-page pamphlet defines the legal and moral rights of the pregnant woman – the right to be told of the risks as well as the benefits of various obstetric drugs and procedures commonly employed in the care of women during pregnancy, labor, and delivery. The pamphlet also includes an excerpt on informed consent from the American College of Obstetricians and Gynecologists' *Standards for Obstetric-Gynecologic Services* (above).

A complimentary copy of the pamphlet will be sent on receipt of a stamped, self-addressed, business-sized envelope mailed to P.P.B.R., Box 1900, New York, New York 10001.

Haire, D. **Obstetric medication: better for whom?** In P. Simkin (Ed.), *Kaleidoscope of Childbearing.* Seattle: Pennypress, 1978.

The author discusses the fact that many times the administration of drugs to women during labor is the result of misguided kindness and, not infrequently, because a health professional in training needs the experience.

This book is available from the International Childbirth Education Association, Book Division, P.O. Box 70258, Seattle, Washington 98107.

Haverkamp, Albert et al. **The evaluation of continuous fetal heart rate monitoring in high risk pregnancy.** *American Journal of Obstetrics and Gynecology,* June 1, 1979. **125,** 310–320.

A prospective randomized study of the 483 high-risk obstetric patients in labor was carried out in which the effectiveness of electronic fetal monitoring was compared with nurse auscultation of fetal heart tone. The infant outcome was measured by neonatal death, Apgar scores, cord blood gasses, and neonatal nursery morbidity. There were no differences in infant outcomes in any measured category between the electronically monitored group and the auscultated group. The Caesarian section rate was 16.5 percent in the electronically monitored group and 6.8 percent in the auscultated group.

Hazell, Lester D. **A study of 300 elective home births.** *Birth and the Family Journal,* 1975. **2,** 11–18.

This is an anthropological study of some three hundred families in the San Francisco area who elected to have home births. Hazell discovered that 90 percent of them lived as nuclear families, that they were distinguished from their neighbors only by a somewhat stronger interest in nutrition, health foods, ecology, and humanistic psychology. Though it was not a controlled study and though virtually all the parents were low risk, the success of home birth was particularly striking. The infant mortality rate was only 3.3 per 1,000 and neither forceps nor episiotomy was used in any of the three hundred deliveries. The majority of births were attended by the father of the baby and by lay midwives.

Hicks, J.; Levenson, G.; and Shnider, S. **Obstetric anesthesia training centers in the U.S.A.: 1975.** *Anesthesia and Analgesia,* 1976. **55**, 839–845.

An examination of the information women are given regarding the risks, hazards, and alternatives to obstetric related drugs indicates that the vast majority of women do not receive sufficient information on which to base decisions as to whether to accept or decline the drugs offered to them during labor and delivery.

Hoult, I.; MacLennon, A.; and Carrie, L. **Lumbar epidural analgesia in labour — relation to fetal malposition and instrumental delivery.** *British Medical Journal,* January 1, 1977. **6052**, 14–16.

The investigators found the rate of forceps extraction to be five times greater (70 percent in first-time mothers with 59 percent overall) and the rate of malposition of the fetal head to be three times greater (21 percent overall) when the woman in labor was administered an epidural block with 0.05 percent bupivacaine (brand name Marcaine). When sensation was allowed to return to all levels in the second stage, the overall incidence of forceps extraction was decreased but was still high (39 percent overall). However, the rate of malposition of the fetal head remained about the same (20 percent).

Kantor, H. et al. **Value of shaving the pudendal-perineal area in delivery preparation.** *Obstetrics and Gynecology,* 1965. **25**, 509–512.

The investigators compared the growth of bacteria in the perineal area of fifty mothers whose pudendal-perineal area was shaved in preparation for birth to that of fifty mothers who remained unshaven. Bacterial growth was found to occur in both groups. No advantage was shown to result from perineal sterilization or from shaving the perineal area.

Karmel, Marjorie. **Thank You, Dr. Lamaze: A Mother's Experience in Painless Childbirth.** Philadelphia: Lippincott, 1959.

Karmel, an American who lived in Paris in the 1950s, was instrumental in introducing "the Lamaze method" of natural childbirth to the United States. This combination of exercise, muscle control, massage, and breathing is based on "Pavlovian theory" and the woman's capacity to control her own labor and reduce its pain by a variety of conditioning techniques. Though this technique encourages the autonomy of laboring women, many feel that its mechanistic approach removes them from the intimate emotional experience of birth.

Kitzinger, S., and David, J. **The Place of Birth.** New York: Oxford University Press, 1978.

Experts in the various areas of maternal and child health discuss the validity of requiring all births to occur in the hospital. The statistical data supporting positions both for and against out-of-hospital births is presented. Those who are interested in knowing how the Dutch system of domicillary (home) obstetrics is organized will appreciate the chapter on the subject by G. J. Kloosterman, professor and chair, Department of Obstetrics and Gynecology, University of Amsterdam.

Klaus, M., and Kennel, J. **Maternal and Infant Bonding.** St. Louis: C. V. Mosby, 1976.

The lasting impact of early mother-infant contact immediately following birth is the subject of this book. The authors, both pediatricians, discuss how early mother-infant attachment can be facilitated by the health professionals who care for them in institutional settings. The authors also discuss the home-birth movement and the value of being able to study mother-infant interaction in a home setting in order to avoid the influences of a hospital environment.

Kron, R.; Stein, M.; and Goddard, K. **Newborn sucking behavior affected by obstetric sedation.** *Pediatrics,* 1966. **37**, 1012–1016.

Sedatives containing barbiturates administered to the mother during labor were shown by Kron to adversely affect the infant's suckling reflexes for the first four or five days following birth. The investigators discuss the significance of a drug effect like this one, which causes a basic "survival" reflex to dysfunction.

Lang, Raven. **Birth Book.** Cupertino, Calif.: Genesis Press, 1972.

This is an attractive, well-illustrated guide to home birth by one of the Santa Cruz lay midwives. Lang describes the equipment necessary for home delivery, discusses the use of natural remedies, and presents a brief history of childbirth. Though other works are more detailed and more scholarly, Lang's is particularly valuable as a portrait of the home-birth movement of the early 1970s.

Levy, B.; Wilkinson, F.; and Marine, W. **Reducing neonatal mortality rate with nurse-midwives.** *American Journal of Obstetrics and Gynecology,* 1971. **109**, 50–58.

By now it is well recognized that the utilization of nurse-midwives in the care of medically indigent women can improve the outcome of their pregnancies. This study shows very clearly that the mortality rate among women who had no prenatal care at all dropped significantly during the two years that midwives were assigned to provide care to women during labor and delivery. The high rate of infant mortality among women with no prenatal care resumed after the discontinuance of the nurse-midwifery program.

Lipnack, Jessica. **Birth: You've come a long way, baby!** *New Age Journal,* October, 1977.

In this "special section" of the *New Age Journal,* Jessica Lipnack provides a useful overview of women's efforts to reclaim the process of birth for themselves and their families. Lipnack, who couples the alternative birth movement with the holistic health movement, also includes interviews with Suzanne Arms and Ina May Gaskin, a personal account of "Birth in the Redwoods" by Karen Schultz, and reviews of several birthing books.

Lubic, Ruth Watson, and Ernest, Eunice K. N. **The child-bearing center: an alternative to conventional care.** *Nursing Outlook,* December 1978. **26 (12)**, 754–760.

This paper, by the general director of the Maternity Center Association in New York City and a consultant to that center, summarizes the childbearing center's three years of operation. Included are brief descriptions of the program's content (education for childbirth, medical screening, labor and delivery, post partum care, etc.), statistics on the program's first three years of operation, and discussion of the "nine principles" that underlie the development of a successful childbearing center. The authors emphasize the importance of using certified nurse-midwives (who are trained to regard birth as a normal process and yet have the skills to recognize and deal with pathological processes in mother, infant, and other family members), the need to involve parents actively in their own education as well as in childbirth, and the cost effectiveness of the program.

Marieskind, Helen. **An Evaluation of Caesarian Section in the United States of America.** Washington, D.C.: Office of Planning and Evaluation, Department of Health, Education, and Welfare, in press.

In this as yet unpublished study, Marieskind reports on her survey of the incidence and causes of Caesarian section in approximately one-hundred departments of obstetrics and gynecology. She concludes that the increased incidences of Caesarian sections—11.4 percent of births in 1976, up 128 percent from 1968—has multiple causes, among them the fear of malpractice suits, the policy of "routine repeat" on women who have had previous Caesarian sections, fetal distress secondary to induction of labor, inefficient use or absence of "maternal mortality committees," the advanced medical treatments that make births possible for women with complicated medical conditions (such as lupus erythematosis and diabetes), and the impatience of obstetricians.

Mead, M., and Newton, N. **Cultural patterning of perinatal behavior.** In S. Richardson and Alan Guttmacher (Eds.), *Childbearing: Its Social and Psychological Aspects.* Baltimore: Williams and Wilkins, 1967.

This cross-cultural look at birth and the rituals surrounding that event is one of the basic papers in the field. The authors' description of the many cultural differences in the practices employed in the care of women during pregnancy, labor, and birth has served as a catalyst to others who were beginning to question the wisdom of "modern" obstetric practices in the late 1960s and 1970s.

Montagu, Ashley. **Life Before Birth.** New York: Signet, 1965.

First published in 1961, this sensitive well-written book has inspired many in the field of maternal and child health to question the wisdom of exposing the unborn child directly and indirectly to the many drugs and interventions that comprise traditional "modern" U.S. obstetric practices. It should be required reading for everyone who is going to have a child or is concerned professionally with childbirth.

Myers, R., and Myers, S. **Use of sedative, analgesic, and anesthestic drugs during labor and delivery: bane or boon?** *American Journal of Obstetrics and Gynecology,* 1979. **133**, 83–104.

This extensive review of the literature describes the many studies carried out in monkeys that demonstrate that when a wild monkey, experiencing contractions, is purposely frightened and inflicted with pain, the adrenal medulla of the wild monkey produces an excess of catecholamines (adrenalin and similar compounds), which in turn cause uterine blood vessels to constrict, causing hypoxia (oxygen deprivation) in the fetus. The authors are careful to point out that this relationship has not been demonstrated in humans or in sheep. Unfortunately, the authors do not mention that this relationship also has not been shown in tame monkeys accustomed to human contact.

Those who are anxious to justify the administration of drugs to low-risk women during labor and birth may try to use this data to justify their position. The cautious reader will discern that the discomfort and pain of normal labor and birth have *not* been shown to cause an increase in maternal catecholamines nor a sympathetic nerve reaction sufficient to cause fetal hypoxia.

The Myers's review also points out that the addition of glucose to the intravenous infusion solution routinely administered to most women during labor increases the likelihood of brain damage if the infant is born hypoxic.

New York State Public Health Law. **New York State Health Code,** 1978. Section 2503.

A new law, which became effective September 1, 1978, and which has become part of the New York State Health Code, reads as follows:

> Drug Information to be Furnished Expectant Mothers. The physician or nurse-midwife to be in attendance at the birth of a child shall inform the expectant mother, in advance of the birth, of the drugs that such physician or nurse-midwife expects to employ during pregnancy and of the obstetrical and other drugs that such physician or nurse-midwife expects to employ at birth and of the possible effects of such drugs on the child and mother.

Nilsson, Lennart. **A Child is Born.** New York: Dell Books, 1966.

This is a gorgeous step-by-step photographic account of human development from conception to birth. Though it is particularly valuable for children anticipating the birth of a sibling, it can make embryological development a living reality for readers of any age.

Ralston, D., and Shnider, S. **The fetal and neonatal effects of regional anesthesia in obstetrics.** *Anesthesiology,* 1978. **48**, 34–61.

The volume of scientific literature discussed by the authors, both anesthesiologists, leaves no doubt that obstetric drugs administered or taken—by injection, perfusion, infusion, suppository, mouth, or nose—all have the potential for changing the fetal environment and directly or indirectly adversely affecting maternal and fetal physiology. It is ironic that after many pages of discussing the adverse reactions experienced by mothers, fetuses, and newborns, the authors conclude that properly administered drugs are not likely to have long-term adverse sequelae—a contention the authors do not support with properly controlled follow-up evaluation and documentation.

Simkin, P. **NAPPSAC Directory of Alternative Birth Services and Consumers' Guide.** Marble Hill, Mo.: National Association of Parents and Professionals for Safe Alternatives in Childbirth, 1978.

> The directory describes various alternative birth centers in the United States and Canada and offers guidelines for locating individuals, both lay and professional, who are sympathetic to the alternative birth movement. It also provides listings of publications on birth alternatives and of organizations concerned with publicizing them.
> NAPPSAC is located at P.O. Box 267, Marble Hill, Missouri 63764.

Stewart, David, and Stewart, Lee (Eds.). **Safe Alternatives in Childbirth.** Chapel Hill, N.C.: National Association of Parents and Professionals for Safe Alternatives in Childbirth, 1976.

> This collection of papers from the first national conference on "Safe Alternatives in Childbirth" received one of the *American Journal of Nursing* Books of the Year Award in 1976. The essays included provide an excellent overview of the alternative birthing movement. Among them are "Childbearing and Maternity Centers–Alternatives to Home Birth and Hospital Care," Dr. Lewis Mehl's study of outcomes of home births versus hospital births, Nancy Mills's personal article on "The Lay Midwife," and a discussion by George J. Annas on "Legal Aspects of Home Births and Other Childbirth Alternatives."
> NAPPSAC is now located at P.O. Box 267, Marble Hill, Missouri 63764.

Stewart, David, and Stewart, Lee. **Twenty-first Century Obstetrics Now** (volumes I and II). Chapel Hill, N.C.: National Association of Parents and Professionals for Safe Alternatives in Childbirth, 1977.

> This collection, which is more than twice as long as *Safe Alternatives in Childbirth,* is based on NAPPSAC's 1977 conference. It contains the beginning of a dialogue between those who favor nonhospital births for uncomplicated, no-risk delivery and official and skeptical representatives of the American College of Obstetricians and Gynecologists. The rest of the collection is approximately equally divided between historical and scientific critiques of modern obstetrical care and accounts of the birthing practices that are developing outside of hospitals. Some of the articles are overly rhetorical (perhaps because they were originally speeches), but taken together they provide both an overview (i.e., Lewis Mehl's "Research on Alternatives in Childbirth: What Can It Tell Us About Hospital Practice?") and detailed portraits of a variety of different kinds of home-birth programs.

Tarnopol, L., and Tarnopol, M. **Reading Disabilities and International Perspective.** Baltimore: University Park Press, 1976.

> As the title implies, this compilation of studies by experts in the field of learning disabilities provides comparative data from several countries. It is particularly interesting to note that the incidence of learning disability in The Netherlands, where

almost half of the children are still delivered by a midwife in the mother's own home, is substantially less than in Belgium, an adjacent demographically similar country where the approach to obstetric care is almost identical to that of the United States.

Turner, S., and MacFarlane, A. **Localization of human speech by the newborn baby and the effects of pethidine (meperidine).** *Developmental Medicine and Child Neurology,* 1978. **20**, 727–734.

The influence of pethidine (known as Demerol in the United States) was evaluated on a group of infants. Eight newborn babies were tested to see whether they could make discriminating head turn responses to the sound of a nine-second recording of a human voice coming 15 degrees, 30 degrees, and 80 degrees from midline and from both the right and left side. Pethidine given to the mother during labor had a significantly negative effect, both on the degree of response and on the babies' ability to localize sound.

U.S. Senate Subcommittee on Health and Scientific Research of the Committee on Human Resources. **Proceedings of the Hearing on Obstetrical Practices in the United States.** Washington, D.C.: U.S. Government Printing Office, 1978.

This hearing examined obstetrical practices such as the use of fetal monitoring, the increasing rate of Caesarian sections, elective induction of labor, the artificial rupture of membranes, and the use of drugs in pregnancy, labor, and delivery. The expert witnesses who testified were, among others: Dr. Roberto Caldeyro-Barcia, president, International Federation of Gynecologists and Obstetricians; Doris Haire, president, American Foundation of Maternal and Child Health, Inc., New York, New York; Dr. Arnold D. Haverkamp, Denver General Hospital, Denver, Colorado; Dr. Ronald R. Rindfuss, department of sociology, University of North Carolina.

Ward, Charlotte, and Ward, Fred. **The Home Birth Book.** New York: Doubleday, 1977.

This is an extremely useful account in words and pictures (by a former White House photographer) of the Ward family's home birth. Though this is a decidedly personal book, it explores the historical, medical, psychological, and sociological aspects of home birth in a thoughtful and even-handed way.

Wertz, Richard W., and Wertz, Dorothy C. **Lying In: A History of Childbirth in America.** New York: Free Press, 1977.

This clearly written, understated history carefully charts the economic, social, and ideological currents that swept childbirth from its familial and communal moorings in the colonial era into the male-dominated hospital in the latter part of the nineteenth century. The book, which draws on fascinating primary sources to make its points, is particularly strong in documenting the usurpation of childbirth first by the untrained male midwife and later by the hospital-based medical-school graduate. The light it casts reveals as much about the evolving professionalization and disease-orientation of health care as it does about our changing attitudes toward childbirth. This is an extraordinarily valuable and readable book.

White, G. **Emergency Childbirth.** Franklin Park, Ill.: Police Training Foundation, 1975.

The clearly presented information in this training manual for police officers is based on experience gained by a physician who has assisted several hundred women giving birth at home in the Chicago area. The information is especially reassuring to the couple who is concerned that it lives too far from the hospital and is trying to decide whether or not to accept the risk of an induced birth. (The U.S. Food and Drug Administration does not consider distance from a hospital to be a valid medical indication for the induction of labor.)

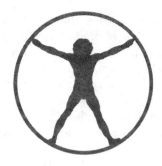

22

HOLISTIC APPROACHES TO ORAL HEALTH AND DENTISTRY

Leo Wollman, M.D., Erwin DiCyan, Ph.D., George Goldberg, D.D.S., and Arthur Hastings, Ph.D.

Dentistry can be viewed as a specialized aspect of internal medicine in that it ministers to an organ group or specialized body area. This is similar to another specialty, dermatology, which ministers to the largest organ of the human body, the skin.

Just as signs of internal disease are often reflected in the skin—the pallor of anemia, the jaundice of gall bladder dysfunction—so metabolic and other disorders of the *milieu interieur* are frequently reflected or previewed in mucous membranes of the mouth, on the tongue, and in the condition of the teeth. The signs of leukemia or diabetes mellitus often appear in the mouth before they are diagnosed by the usual laboratory or clinical methods. Diseases such as lichen planus or some forms of oral cancer may be detected early by an examination of the mouth before they develop systemic repercussions. Thus, as the oral cavity is a part of the overall body, it is not surprising that it would reflect the state of health of the person, in mind and body.

Oral health is inextricably interrelated with the person's environment, with his or her life-style, and with internal and external functioning. This chapter reviews some of the health factors that are contributing to the emerging holistic attitude in dentistry and oral health.

Nutritional Factors in Oral Health

In addition to mirroring some of the patient's internal conditions, the mouth can have specific dysfunctions due to nutritional imbalances and deficiencies. Susceptability to caries is increased by large quantities of refined carbohydrates (sugar) and by deficiencies in vitamins A, C, and D, calcium, and phosphorus (Shaw and Sweeney, 1973). Deficiencies in vitamin C also contribute to poor gum condition, causing bleeding gums or "pink toothbrush." General poor nutrition can also result in periodontal disease in which the teeth may be healthy but the framework in which they are set, the gums, will not support them. It is, of course, axiomatic that a sufficient and balanced diet creates general good health, and hence good oral health. Conversely, a high proportion of "junk foods," highly processed, refined, and bland-textured foods, refined carbohydrates, and sugar intake all contribute to poor oral health, caries, and mouth diseases.

A nutritionally adequate diet acts as a preventive measure for healthy teeth and gums, enables teeth to develop initially, and promotes health in mature teeth. The use of nutritional supplements of vitamins and minerals may be useful to prevent diseases of deficiency. Additionally, there are reports that large doses of vitamin E reduce the deposits of exogenous tartar on teeth (Bertrand, 1975) and that megadoses of vitamin C can heal canker sores in the mouth (Pauling, 1976).

However, in the field of dental nutrition we have vast areas of ignorance, even according to the standard establishment criteria. While we justifiably enrich certain foods with vitamins, our research on minerals—which in many instances act to enable the metabolism of vitamins—is regrettably lacking. "Eat a good diet" is the advice—but what is a good diet for most people (see Chapter 17, Food and Nutrition)? The picture is further obscured by the promoters of putative health foods. Nevertheless, nutritional factors clearly play an important role in oral health, enhancing health and preventing disease as well as being a therapy for certain disorders.

Oral Health and Mental Health

Life-style and psychological factors are also related to dental health. Perhaps the most familiar expression of this is that gingivitis (trench mouth) increases sharply in dental clinics at universities and colleges during high-stress periods—the weeks of final examinations. Vogel et al. (1977) found a clear relationship between psychic stress and periodontal disease. In addition, they found a correlation between introversion and the severity of the disease.

Two other problems frequently seen by dentists can be brought on by mental and emotional conditions of stress. Temporomandibular joint dysfunction (the TMJ syndrome) of jaw aches, tension, and even bite problems can be caused by social stresses, according to Dr. Nathan A. Shore, New York School of Dentistry, whose research on 2,800 patients prompted this observation. Thomas et al. (1973) conducted an experiment with ten TMJ patients and ten matched-control patients. They subjected each group of patients to mild electric shocks (to produce anxiety) and a frustrating problem (to produce anger or irritation). The TMJ patients reacted to both shocks and frustration with high tension in the jaw muscles, while the control patients showed comparatively little jaw muscle reaction. The TMJ patients reacted more strongly to the frustration than to the anxiety situation. This research suggests that attention to muscle-relaxation techniques and ways of changing a patient's reactions to life situations may become an aspect of treatment for the TMJ syndrome.

Bruxism (grinding the teeth) and clenching also appear to be tension related. Laskin (1977) found nocturnal bruxism to be related to life stress, while Zeldow (1976) reports that he has had success in treating clenching and bruxism in a majority of his patients by teaching them to relax the frontalis (forehead), tongue, and masseter muscles. He also instructs patients to give themselves bedtime instructions to relax their jaw muscles if they begin to clench while they are asleep.

Life-style and personality affect oral health in more general ways as well. Conventional oral health practices (such as brushing, flossing, and checkups) must be regular and habitual to be maximally effective. When a person's life activities or mental states are disorganized, stressed, or distractable, checkups and flossing are the first to go and brushing is not far behind.

Oral problems may also affect general physical health. Malocclusion and bite problems may cause aches and pain and result in uncomfortable shifts in the muscles of the head and neck. Fonder (1976) calls this the dental distress syndrome (DDS) and reports that it often causes or contributes to breathing and respiratory problems, sinusitus, postnasal drip, hearing problems, and postural changes. Correction of the faulty malocclusion relieves the problems.

Preventive Oral Health

More than most other medical specialties, dentistry has emphasized, promoted, and institutionalized preventive health practices. Good dental habits (such as regular brushing, flossing, and gum massage) are taught by dentists and hygienists, are presented in schools, and promoted through public service advertising. Recent popular books such as *The Tooth Trip* by McGuire (1972) have cheerfully explained how to care for one's teeth and have unraveled the mysteries of dental treatment to an increasingly interested audience of adults (Himber, 1977).

In professional practice, dentists urge patients to have regular cleaning of plaque and tartar from teeth along with checkups. This significantly reduces oral health problems and catches disease in its early stages. At the level of corrective treatment, orthodontics—especially with children—reduces later problems through correcting malocclusion and bite problems, reducing tooth crowding, and in effect creating a more comfortable mouth for the person.

In the area of environment and ecology, preventive dentistry has encouraged fluoridation to strengthen tooth enamel—either through treatment of the water supply or through direct application of fluoride to the teeth. With regard to nutrition, patients are encouraged to avoid sugars and high-carbohydrate foods and to eat crisp and raw snacks rather than soft foods that stick to the teeth (Shaw and Sweeney, 1973). More can be done along nutritional lines to ensure a more than minimal intake of vitamins A, C, and D and minerals such as calcium and phosphorus.

Other ecological factors that deserve attention are sunlight and the spectrum of artificial illumination. Natural sunlight causes the production of vitamin D by the body, which is essential for calcium absorption. For this to occur, apparently the full spectrum of sunlight must be present, including the ultraviolet range. Artificial indoor lighting, such as standard cool-white fluorescents and regular incandescent lamps, are deficient in the UV range. Prolonged exposure to them in place of natural sunlight or full-spectrum lamps appears to increase caries and reduce calcium absorption (Mayron et al., 1975; Sharon, Feller, and Burney, 1971; Neer et al., 1971). Particularly in urban, industrialized, or business settings, persons could be encouraged to be in the sunlight and use adequate full-spectrum fluorescent lamps (e.g., commercial brands such as Vita-Lite) to ensure adequate vitamin D synthesis.

The dental profession has developed a sophisticated and high technology for repair and restorative work, and it is greatly to the credit of the dental professionals that they are equally concerned with preventive dentistry.

Patient Anxiety and Pain

As most patients and dentists realize, anxiety is the most frequent emotional reaction to dental work (Firestein, 1976). Patients have a fear of pain and discomfort, not always unjustified, that is frequently a carry-over from childhood experiences, from their parents' fears, or from other dental patients' stories. Then, too, the mouth is an area that evokes emotional concern. The mouth and teeth are an essential part of a person's smile and appearance, involved in the intimacy of kissing and close contact. They are also essential organs for nutrition. No wonder that work on the mouth is a source of concern. In addition, the patient in the chair feels defenseless and vulnerable. The physical position, the state of anxiety, and the physical trauma may produce a feeling of helplessness in which the patient cannot easily trust the dentist.

What the dentist can do is to recognize the patient's need for support and assurance. It is wise and will save time to take several minutes to talk, preferably in an office separate from the treatment room or operatory. Take time to relax the patient and acknowledge the anxiety when it is appropriate. For some patients premedication of aspirin or Valium may be indicated. Explaining the stages of the procedure ahead of time is often a valuable reassurance; it informs the patient what will happen and assures him or her that there will be an end to it.

Dealing with pain is perhaps the most difficult task in dentistry, especially because many dentists themselves are uncomfortable about causing pain, even in the service of oral health. Patients may not realize this, of course, with the result that each covertly resents the other. This does not mean that the dentist has to apologize, but certainly some shared communication on the need for discomfort is advisable, and the dentist should do what he or she can to handle discomfort and to employ effective anesthetics or other procedures.

Pain is subjective as well as objective, and the psychological and emotional state of the patients alters the level of reported pain. Talking with the anxious patients and allowing time for them to begin to relax will often be helpful. (Of course, some patients will want to get right on with it to get it over with as soon as possible.) Aspirin or a tranquilizer can also reduce the sensitivity to pain, as can soft music in the background or in headphones.

Hypnosis and relaxation techniques have also proven to be highly successful in reducing and even eliminating pain sensations (Hilgard and Hilgard, 1975). Hypnosis has been used for pain control with extractions, pulpectomies, periodontal surgery, and other operations. It is effective in promoting relaxation and hence in relieving anxiety for fearful patients. In addition, hypnosis (or self-hypnosis) can be used to control bleeding during dental work. It has been used to promote circulation in alveoalgia (dry socket) and to control bleeding in regular patients and hemophiliacs (Thompson, 1963; Lucas et al., 1962). Hypnosis for dental use can be learned through special workshops and training programs, in conjunction with the literature and reports by practitioners (Hilgard and Hilgard, 1975; Moss, 1977).

Anxiety in patients is best relieved by developing a supportive relationship between the dentist and the patient. Treating patients as persons rather than as accessories to their teeth takes more time and more personal involvement on the part of the dentist or hygienist, but it promotes better understanding and long-term improvements in oral health.

Dentists and Their Own Health

One of the principles emerging in holistic approaches to health is that the practitioners are beginning to pay attention to their own health. Doctors in all areas of the medical professions have often been remiss in this—booking themselves into overwork, getting little exercise, and failing to obtain medical treatment when they should. In dentistry this inattention to self-responsibility is fairly common. At a recent American Dental Association meeting, a test of 856 dentists showed that their blood pressure averaged significantly higher than the national norms—27 percent had diastolic pressures over 90 mm Hg and 22 percent had systolic pressures over 140 mm Hg—high enough to be classed as hypertension (Cutright et al., 1977).

Regarding nutrition, a study of 1,086 dentists and their wives showed that a significant number of the dental couples consumed suboptimal amounts of vitamin C, even according to the low recommended dietary allowances (RDA) set by the Food and Nutrition Board, and a study of dentists, wives, and staff attending two recent dental conferences indicated that from one-third to one-half of the subjects had poor tissue vitamin C levels (Cheraskin and Ringsdorf, 1977). Dentists may often be in poor mental health as well. Gutwirth (1976) reports that in a Newark, New Jersey, clinic, 42 percent of the dentists were in an anxiety and exhaustion state (compared with 12 percent of the patients), and the condition was more frequent in younger dentists, those between ages thirty and fifty.

Dental practice, despite its rewards in service, knowledge, and income, is a stressful occupation. The major source of stress for most dentists is probably time pressure. In a study of thirty-three Canadian dentists, 60 percent stated they were either occasionally or continually behind their patient schedule. The situation is exacerbated by patients who miss appointments or who require emergency treatments as well as by complications that require additional time during a regular appointment (Howard et al., 1976). Important causes of stress listed by west coast dentists are: falling behind schedule, patient overload, difficult or nervous patients (including children), causing pain, and difficult procedures. Hygienists, in a similar survey, listed their major problems as being behind schedule (with the result that they do not have enough time to do a good job), and patients who are nervous, sensitive, or otherwise difficult. Dentists and hygienists both reported having tense muscles, headaches, worrying, anxiety, and irritability as a result of their work (Hastings, 1979).

Unfortunately, for many dentists the problem arises because of high patient demand for their services and a desire to schedule as many patients as possible (Howard et al., 1976). Working shorter hours, using more assistants, and booking fewer patients can reduce the tension of practice, but such tactics also reduce incomes. On the other hand, allowing more time for patients and between patients, taking time to relax and release tense muscles, and getting regular exercise will improve the dental professional's health, extend life expectancy, and probably also improve his or her work with patients. In the Canadian study, dentists who made a specific attempt to get a minimum amount of exercise each week had fewer symptoms of stress than their nonexercising colleagues. Exercise worked off the tensions of the job and improved their physical condition as well.

Holistic Dentistry and Holistic Medicine

Holistic medicine strives to encompass all areas of human health, though much information is still lacking. It is well documented that the frustrations of tensions, boredom, emotional conflicts, and lack of a goal and its pursuit can produce illness that may manifest itself in physical as well as mental symptoms. The need to love and to have a satisfying loving relationship is part of the design of wellness – in contradistinction to illness. Unfulfilled needs produce frustration, and frustrations are illness-producing.

The holistically oriented dentist inquires about his patient's dietary habits, emotional states, and life habits. To ignore the societal and emotional components of dental problems is a myopic attitude. This is *not* psychiatric treatment but rather a human ministration on the part of the dentist.

A holistic approach also recognizes the need for satisfying the spirit. In fact, the word in German that denotes mental disturbance is *Geisteskrankheit,* disease of the spirit. The doctor who is holistically oriented may help the patient with this attitude as well so that the need may be satisfied in a fashion that the individual finds comforting. With some, it is a return to religion; with others, it may be alternative spiritual growth.

Further, the dentist can consider other methods of healing without necessarily renouncing the present standard medical models. Holistic medicine includes a plea for open-mindedness – including the use of acupuncture, hypnosis, psychic healing, and other alternatives – without demanding that necessary medication and surgery be renounced. Holistic dentistry, as the name implies, considers that there are many facets to oral health – including the nutritional, emotional, mental, sexual, familial, physical, spiritual, and psychological aspects of healing and health.

References

Bertrand, F. R. Vitamin E benefits. *Journal of the American Dental Association,* 1975. **91**, 1136–1137.

Cheraskin, E., and Ringsdorf, W. M. Dentists need more Vitamin C? *Journal of the Tennessee Dental Association,* 1977. **57 (4)**, 177–178.

Cutright, D. E.; Carpenter, W. A.; Tsaknis, P. G.; and Lyon, T. C. Survey of blood pressures of 856 dentists. *Journal of the American Dental Association,* 1977. **94**, 918–919.

Firestein, S. K. Patient anxiety and dental practice. *Journal of the American Dental Association,* 1976. **93**, 1180.

Fonder, A. C. Dental stress and distress. In F. J. McGuigan (Ed.), *Tension Control: Proceedings of the Second Meeting of the American Association for the Advancement of Tension Control.* Blacksburg, Va.: University Publications, 1976.

Gutwirth, S. W. The application of scientific tension control in dental practice. In F. J. McGuigan (Ed.), *Tension Control: Proceedings of the Second Meeting of the American Association for the Advancement of Tension Control.* Blacksburg, Va.: University Publications, 1976.

Hastings, Arthur. Unpublished research data, 1979.

Hilgard, Ernest R., and Hilgard, Josephine R. *Hypnosis in the Relief of Pain.* Los Altos, Calif.: William Kaufmann, 1975.

Himber, Jacob. *The Complete Family Guide to Dental Health.* New York: McGraw-Hill, 1977.

Howard, J. H.; Cunningham, D. A.; Rechnitzer, P. A.; and Goode, R. C. Stress in the job and career of a dentist. *Journal of the American Dental Association,* 1976. **93**, 630.

Laskin, Daniel M. Stress-related oral activities during sleep. *Journal of the American Medical Association,* 1977. **238**, 895.

Lucas, O. N.; Finkelman, A.; and Tocantius, L. M. Management of tooth extractions in hemophiliacs by the combined use of hypnosis, protective splint, and packing of sockets. *Journal of Oral Surgery, Anesthesia, and Hospital Dental Service,* 1962. **20**, 188–200.

Mayron, L. W. et al. Light, radiation and dental caries. *Academic Therapy,* 1975. **10**, 441–448.

McGuire, Thomas. *The Tooth Trip.* New York: Random House, 1972.

Moss, Aaron A. Hypnodontics: hypnosis in dentistry. In William Kroger, *Experimental and Clinical Hypnosis.* Philadelphia: J. B. Lippincott, 1977.

Neer, R. M.; Davis, T.R.A.; Walcott, A.; Koski, S.; Schepis, P.; Taylor, I.; Thorington, L.; and Wurtman, R. J. Stimulation by artificial lighting of calcium absorption in elderly human subjects. *Nature,* 1971. **229**, 255–256.

Pauling, Linus. *Vitamin C, The Common Cold, and the Flu.* San Francisco: W. H. Freeman Company, 1976.

Sharon, I. M.; Feller, R. P.; and Burney, S. W. The effects of lights of different spectra on caries incidence in the golden hamster. *Archives of Oral Biology,* 1971. **16**, 1427–1431.

Shaw, James H., and Sweeney, Edward A. Nutrition in relation to dental medicine. In Robert S. Goodhart and Maurice E. Shils. *Modern Nutrition in Health and Disease.* Philadelphia: Lea and Febiger, 1973.

Thomas, L. J.; Tiber, N.; and Shireson, S. The effects of anxiety and frustration on muscular tension related to the temporomandibular joint syndrome. *Oral Surgery,* 1973. **36**, 763–768.

Thompson, K. F. A rationale for suggestion in dentistry. *American Journal of Clinical Hypnosis,* 1963. **5**, 181–186.

Vogel, Richard et al. Relationship of personality traits and periodontal disease. *Psychosomatics,* 1977. **18**, 21.

Zeldow, Leonard L. Treating clenching and bruxing by habit change. *Journal of the American Dental Association,* 1976. **93**, 31.

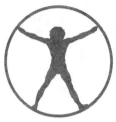

ANNOTATED BIBLIOGRAPHY

Leo Wollman, M.D., and Arthur Hastings, Ph.D.

Firestein, S. K. **Patient anxiety and dental practice.** *Journal of the American Dental Association.* 1976. **93**, 1180.

> The author describes some of the fears patients often have regarding dental treatment – physical, emotional, and psychological – and the results, such as lateness, cancelled appointments, anxiety, nervousness, and, of course, poor oral health. He explains approaches to building trust between the patient and the dentist, including the use of explanations, making procedures predictable, talking with children and adults before operations, and care in the use of language.

Fonder, A. C. **Dental stress and distress.** In F. J. McGuigan, *Tension Control: Proceedings of the Second Meeting of the American Association for the Advancement of Tension Control.* Blacksburg, Va.: University Publications, 1976.

> The "dental distress syndrome" occurs when an extreme malocclusion of the teeth creates stress throughout the rest of the body. Fonder reports cases where this has resulted in hearing loss, imbalance of neck and shoulder muscles, postural changes, and breathing and respiratory problems, including sinusitis and severe headaches. Correction of the faulty occlusion relieved the concomitant problems.

Hilgard, Ernest R., and Hilgard, Josephine R. **Hypnosis in the Relief of Pain.** Los Altos, Calif.: William Kaufmann, 1975.

> This book contains a thorough review of the literature on the use of hypnosis for pain relief in dentistry along with applications for preventing gagging, reducing bruxism, control of bleeding, and other dental needs. The chapter on hypnodontics is not a guide for learning hypnosis. It covers the uses very thoroughly with a careful appraisal of effectiveness by these leading scientific researchers. It will guide the practitioner to clinical reports and techniques for specific topics.

Himber, Jacob. **The Complete Family Guide to Dental Health.** New York: McGraw-Hill, 1977.

> The keynotes to dental health, says the author, are to prevent, cure, preserve, and restore. The book lucidly and easily explains and motivates the reader to do his or her

part toward excellent oral health. Straightforward chapters explain choosing a dentist, brushing and flossing, children's teeth, repairs and restorations, oral health problems, and the questions of payment, insurance, and what to do about improper dentistry. The advice appears quite sound and is appropriately qualified where necessary. This book can be recommended to both patients and their dentists; it will improve patient's health and the communication between patient and doctor.

Howard, J. H.; Cunningham, D. A.; Rechnitzer, P. A.; and Goode, R. C. **Stress in the job and career of a dentist.** *Journal of the American Dental Association,* 1976. **93**, 630.

Studying thirty-three dentists in a Canadian education program, the authors found that stress levels are higher for dentists who work longer hours, who are occasionally or usually behind schedule, who take less time for lunch, and who use fewer assistants. They are also less physically fit and have higher incomes. The more a dentist attempted to get at least a minimum of exercise, the fewer stress symptoms he had. Lower stress levels were also associated with higher job satisfaction. The authors include a diagram of factors in dental work that lead to stress and reduced health levels.

Jacoby, James D. **Practical suggestions for dentists working with the patient in a trance.** *American Journal of Clinical Hypnosis,* 1967. **10** (1), 39–43.

A valuable listing and explanation of several dozen ideas and techniques with practical advice for dentists (and other dental professionals) who use hypnosis or suggestion in their practice. These include ways of inducing relaxation and trance states; producing anesthesia; reducing fear and anxiety; maintaining the trance; supporting the patient's confidence in the procedure, his reactions, and the dentist; and ways of awakening the patient with positive suggestions. The author is especially sensitive to creating a good relationship with the person undergoing treatment. The article will benefit any dentist who is using hypnosis or relaxation techniques.

McGuire, Thomas. **The Tooth Trip.** New York: Random House, 1972.

One of the first books on oral health written for a popular audience, this book is hip in style, cheerfully written, very motivating, and contains a wealth of sound advice for persons on brushing, flossing, flushing, and other aspects of tooth self-care. In addition, dental procedures are explained as to when they are needed and why. Suggestions for choosing a dentist and how to relate to him or her are given, with some emphasis on "consumer" protection. The author even gives recipes for making toothpaste and powder (one of which unfortunately includes honey as a sweetener). The point is clearly made that good oral health will save teeth and that the dentist and the patient should work together.

Moss, Aaron A. **Hypnodontics: hypnosis in dentistry.** In William Kroger, *Experimental and Clinical Hypnosis.* Philadelphia: J. B. Lippincott, 1977.

This chapter describes how to apply hypnotic techniques in dental practice for relaxation, removal of fears, dealing with discomfort, and changing poor dental habits. Moss, a dentist, explains one hypnotic induction technique to use with patients and gives a detailed procedure for using hypnosis to prevent gagging. However, there is no discussion of specific procedures for hypnoanalgesia, the use of hypnosis for operations, or of the more advanced applications.

Shaw, James H., and Sweeney, Edward A. **Nutrition in relation to dental medicine.** In Robert S. Goodhardt and Maurice E. Shils, *Modern Nutrition in Health and Disease* (5th ed.). Philadelphia: Lea and Febiger, 1973.

The authors summarize and review the research on nutrition in oral health, including the role of vitamins, carbohydrates, fluorides, and general foodstuffs. Much of the research is focused on nutritional deficiencies, but increasingly there is concern with the preventive role of food and supplements. The authors conclude that the best selection of foods for dental health is one where as many of the foods as possible are purchased in their natural state without excessive refining and where the cooking procedures conserve the maximum nutritive value.

Spiegelford, Morton B. **Psychosomatic disturbances and dental health.** *Journal of the American Society of Psychosomatic Dentistry and Medicine,* 1979. **26**, (in press).

Spiegelford, a dentist, reviews findings on relations between mental health and oral health. Personality traits such as introversion affect oral health, emotional stress is associated with specific periodontal disease, and stress factors and dental caries have positive correlations with each other.

23

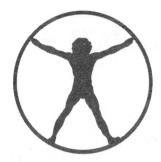

STRESS: THE NEW ETIOLOGY

Thomas H. Holmes, M.D.

The studies discussed in this chapter are concerned with the "new etiology" of disease. The research and theory establish a dimension of clinical science that permits an understanding not only of cause but also of the probable bodily mechanisms of many signs and symptoms heretofore considered to be without explanation. These clinical and laboratory experiments make meaningless the dualism of functional, hysterical, psychosomatic illness used as the antithesis of organic disease.

Harold G. Wolff ushered in this new etiology in the preface to *Life Stress and Bodily Disease* in 1950 (1):

> This symposium was oriented about the view that adaptive and protective capabilities are limited, that the response to a variety of noxious agents in any given man may be similar, that the form of this reaction depends more upon the individual's nature and experience than upon the particular noxious agent evoking it. Also, that man, constituted as he is, is as capable of reacting to symbols of danger as to actual assault. Since, further, he is a tribal animal with a long period of development and dependence, jeopardized as well as supported by his fellows, he may feel more threatened by cultural and individual human pressures than by other forces. Hence, conspicuous

---

References in this chapter are indicated by numbers in the text because of the large number of citations for some topics.

in such a symposium must be consideration of the effects of man upon man especially as they are relevant to disease.

In keeping with the dictum of Alexander Pope that "the proper study of mankind is man," the point of departure in all the work discussed here is the human subject, the patient. In this context, Wolff and his students were interested in the interrelationship of three open-ended scientific disciplines: the biological, the psychological, and the sociological. The life chart invented by Adolf Meyer (2) provided a format for demonstrating the relationship by organizing the data from the medical history as a biography. The life chart provided the opportunity to document not only the life situation in which an illness had its onset but also the background dynamics of the growth, development, and maturation of the patient that brought him or her to this stage.

Studies of individual patients using this format revealed that many disorders occurred in a life situation that provoked conflict and a variety of emotions (see special reference section for this chapter). Laboratory experiments on selected patients documented disease onset under these conditions. While monitoring the physiologic function of a given organ or tissue in a patient, the critical event determined from the life chart was introduced as the noxious stimulus and the correlated psychological (verbal report) and physiological responses were identified. This stimulus-response experimental design provided data about the etiology of disease that conformed to the requisites of Koch's postulates for cause in infectious diseases. Such experiments have been conducted on many bodily systems (3–42), and they reveal the occurrence of tissue damage and disease or of functional changes that increase susceptibility to disease. These experiments represent some of the rare occasions when the development of a disease in human subjects has been observed directly.

The word "stress" (as its meaning has evolved since the 1940s) has now come to encompass the new etiology and to identify a universe of discourse that is a subset of pathology – the scientific discipline concerned with the parameters of cause and host response. This new dimension of pathology provides for a more complete understanding of the natural history of many diseases than has previously existed.

Another important dimension of the new etiology has been the contribution of Graham and his coworkers (43–46) to the question of specificity. Again the point of departure was the Meyer life chart. Graham and his colleagues analyzed systematically the verbal reports made by patients as they responded psychologically with affect or emotion to a stimulus situation or life event (see Table 23.1). His formulation that specific attitudes and physiological patterns constitute two dimensions of a disease is one of the most salient discoveries of the past quarter century.

Hinkle et al. (47–50), using the life chart, documented the frequency and variety of diseases in different populations. His data indicated that disease patterns are well established by adulthood, occur predominantly in a small segment

Table 23.1
Verbal Statements of Attitudes

Disease	Attitude
Metabolic Edema	This person feels he is carrying a heavy load and wants somebody else to carry all or part of it. He has too much on his shoulders, has too much responsibility; he wants others to take their share of it.
Hypertension	This person feels threatened with harm and has to be ready for anything. He feels in danger; anything could happen at any time from any side. He has to be prepared to meet all possible threats; he has to be on guard.
Regional Enteritis	This person feels he has received something harmful and wants to get rid of it. He has been given or has received something damaged or inferior. He feels he has been poisoned. He wants the situation to be finished, over and done with, disposed of.
Raynaud's Disease	This person wants to take hostile physical action. He wants to hit or strangle; he wants to take action of any kind. He has to do something.
Hives	This person feels he is taking a beating and is helpless to do anything about it. He is being knocked around, hammered on; he is being mistreated or unfairly treated.
Nausea and Vomiting	This person feels something wrong has happened and probably feels responsible. He wishes it had not happened, is sorry it happened, and wishes he could undo it. He wishes things were the way they were before. He wishes he had not done it.
Acne	This person feels he is being picked on and wants to be left alone. He is being nagged.
Hyperthyroidism	This person feels he might lose somebody or something he loves and takes care of and is trying to prevent the loss. He is trying to hold on to a loved one who is being taken away.
Psoriasis	This person feels something constantly gnawing at him that he has to put up with it.

Table 23.1 (continued)

Disease	Attitude
Asthma	This person feels left out in the cold and wants to shut the person or situation out. He feels unloved, rejected, disapproved of, shut out, and he wishes not to deal with the person or situation. He wishes to blot it or him out and not to have anything to do with it or him.
Eczema	This person feels he is being frustrated and can do nothing about it. He feels interferred with, blocked, prevented from doing something; he feels unable to make himself understood.
Constipation	This person feels he is in a situation from which nothing good could come but keeps on with it grimly. He feels things will never get any better but has to stick with it.
Multiple Sclerosis	This person feels forced to undertake some kind of physical activity and does not want to. He has to work without help, has to support himself and usually others. He does not want to and wishes help or support.
Ulcerative Colitis	This person feels he is being injured and degraded and wishes he could get rid of the responsible agent. He is being humiliated; he wants the situation to be finished, over and done with, disposed of.
Backache	This person wants to run away. He wants to walk out of there, to get out.
Migraine	This person feels something has to be achieved and relaxes after the effort. He has to accomplish something, is driving himself, striving. He has to get things done. A goal has to be reached. Then he lets down, stops the driving.

Table 23.1 (continued)

Disease	Attitude
Duodenal Ulcer	This person feels deprived of what is due him and wants to get even. He does not get what he should, is owed, or promised. He wants to do to some other person what the other person has done to him.
Rheumatoid Arthritis	This person feels tied down and wants to get free. He feels restrained, restricted, confined, and wants to be able to move around.
Hernia	This person feels like exploding. His focus of attention is on controlling feelings of anger, not on the feeling itself or the object of the anger.
Heartburn	This person is getting what he wants.
Tuberculosis	Despite a valiant effort this person feels overwhelmed by circumstances.
Paroxysmal Auricular Tachycardia	This person feels that things are not proceeding according to schedule and that they should be speeded up. Typical statements: "Let's get going; let's get things started."
Diabetes	This person is starving to death in the midst of plenty. He is surrounded by most of the things that have meaning but his perception is that none is available to him.
Diarrhea	This person sees himself faced with a meaningful task and wishes it were over, finished, or done with. He wishes impending events were behind him.

Source: David T. Graham, William J. Grace, and Thomas H. Holmes. See Graham, D. T., and Graham, F. K. Specific Relations of Attitude to Physiological Change. Progress report. Madison: University of Wisconsin School of Medicine, 1961.

Table 23.2
The Social Readjustment Rating Scale

Life Event	Mean Value
1. Death of spouse	100
2. Divorce	73
3. Marital separation from mate	65
4. Detention in jail or other institution	63
5. Death of a close family member	63
6. Major personal injury or illness	53
7. Marriage	50
8. Being fired at work	47
9. Marital reconciliation with mate	45
10. Retirement from work	45
11. Major change in the health or behavior of a family member	44
12. Pregnancy	40
13. Sexual difficulties	39
14. Gaining a new family member (e.g., through birth, adoption, oldster moving in, etc.)	39
15. Major business readjustment (e.g., merger, reorganization, bankruptcy, etc.)	39
16. Major change in financial state (e.g., a lot worse off or a a lot better off than usual)	38
17. Death of a close friend	37
18. Changing to a different line of work	36
19. Major change in the number of arguments with spouse (e.g., either a lot more or a lot less than usual regarding childrearing, personal habits, etc.)	35
20. Taking on a mortgage greater than $10,000 (e.g., purchasing a home, business, etc.)	31
21. Foreclosure on a mortgage or loan	30
22. Major change in responsibilities at work (e.g., promotion, demotion, lateral transfer)	29
23. Son or daughter leaving home (e.g., marriage, attending college, etc.)	29
24. In-law troubles	29
25. Outstanding personal achievement	28
26. Wife beginning or ceasing work outside the home	26
27. Beginning or ceasing formal schooling	26
28. Major change in living conditions (e.g., building a new home, remodeling, deterioration of home or neighborhood)	25
29. Revision of personal habits (dress, manners, associations, etc.)	24
30. Troubles with the boss	23
31. Major change in working hours or conditions	20
32. Change in residence	20
33. Changing to a new school	20
34. Major change in usual type and/or amount of recreation	19

Table 23.2 (continued)

Life Event	Mean Value
35. Major change in church activities (e.g., a lot more or a lot less than usual)	19
36. Major change in social activities (e.g., clubs, dancing, movies, visiting, etc.)	18
37. Taking on a mortgage or loan less than $10,000 (e.g., purchasing a car, TV, freezer, etc.)	17
38. Major change in sleeping habits (a lot more or a lot less sleep, or change in part of day when asleep)	16
39. Major change in number of family get-togethers (e.g., a lot more or a lot less than usual)	15
40. Major change in eating habits (a lot more or a lot less food intake, or very different meal hours or surroundings)	15
41. Vacation	13
42. Christmas	12
43. Minor violations of the law (e.g., traffic tickets, jaywalking, disturbing the peace, etc.)	11

Source: Holmes, T. H., and Rahe, R. H. The Social Readjustment Rating Scale. *Journal of Psychosomatic Research*, 1967. **11** 213–218.

of the population, and involve multiple bodily systems, the most common of which is the system of thought, feeling, and behavior. Hinkle and his coworkers also demonstrated that illnesses are not randomly distributed throughout people's lives but occur in clusters or chains. Disorders of various types follow each other in rapid succession, with intervals free from illness intervening before the next cluster begins.

The development of the Social Readjustment Rating Scale (SRRS) was begun in 1949 with a systematic study of the life-event items observed empirically to occur in the setting in which disease developed. Again the point of departure was the application of the life-chart format to a single disease, pulmonary tuberculosis. This case-history method suggested that the disease had its onset in a life situation of acute downward social mobility characterized by the ocurrence of many undesirable life events. Prospective studies of hospitalized patients revealed that the occurrence of new tuberculosis, exacerbation of the old disease, or failure of the existing disease to improve was strongly associated with the occurrence of a life crisis, a reaction of the patient with depression and with feelings of being overwhelmed, and a dramatic decrease of the urinary excretion of 17-ketosteroids that were used as an index of resistance to infection.

The salience of events was established by using a method derived from psychophysics that generates a ratio scale (see Table 23.2). The scale has been validated by cross-cultural studies that indicate a universal consensus about the rank order and relative magnitude of the amount of readjustment required by each life event. The scale provides a quantitative measure for the risk of onset of both serious and minor disease in relation to events in the patient's life (51–54).

Since a major dimension of the natural history of disease is psychological, it is understandable that psychological therapeutic techniques have a powerful impact on favorably modifying the course of a disease once it gets started (see Table 23.3). The outcome is also strongly influenced by the quality and quantity of psychological and social assets that the patient brings to the doctor-patient equation.

Finally, preliminary experiments in prevention, using the new etiology as a point of departure, hold great promise influencing life-style so that resistance to disease is enhanced (see Table 23.4).

Table 23.3
Therapeutic Procedures

Procedure Used	Cases[a]
Reassurance and emotional support	309
Free expression of conflicts and feelings	304
Advice regarding attitudes, habits, and activities	173
Explanation of psychophysiologic processes	140
Symptomatic drug therapy	123
Intravenous use of sodium amytal	112
Ruling out neoplastic and infectious disease	112
Dealing with other members of the family	101
Development of insight	99
Analysis of emotional development	91
Atempts to modify situation	71
Dream analysis	52
Help from Social Service Department	39

[a]Number of cases in which procedures were used successfully: N = 690.
Source: Ripley, H. S.; Wolf, S.; and Wolff, H. G. Treatment in a psychosomatic clinic. *Journal of the American Medical Association*, 1948. **138**, 949–951.

Table 23.4
Preventive Measures

The following suggestions are for using the Social Readjustment Rating Scale for the maintenance of your health and prevention of illness.

1. Become familiar with the life events and the amount of change they require.

2. Put the scale where you and the family can see it easily several times a day.

3. With practice you can recognize when a life event happens.

4. Think about the meaning of the event for you and try to identify some of the feelings you experience.

5. Think about the different ways you might best adjust to the event.

6. Take your time in arriving at decisions.

7. If possible, anticipate life changes and plan for them well in advance.

8. Pace yourself. It can be done even if you are in a hurry.

9. Look at the accomplishment of a task as a part of daily living and avoid looking at such an achievement as a "stopping point" or a time for letting down.

10. *Remember*, the more change you have, the more likely you are to get sick. Of those people with more than 300 Life Change Units for the past year, almost 80 percent get sick in the near future; with 150 to 299 Life Change Units, about 50 percent get sick in the near future; and with less than 150 Life Change Units, only about 30 percent get sick in the near future. Thus, the higher your Life Change Score, the harder you should work to stay well.

References

1. Wolff, H. G.; Wolf, Stewart G., Jr.; and Hare, Clarence C. (Eds.). *Life Stress and Bodily Disease* (Research Publications, Association for Research in Nervous and Mental Diseases, vol. 29). Baltimore: Williams and Wilkins, 1950.

2. Lief, A. (Ed.). *The Commonsense Psychiatry of Dr. Adolf Meyer.* New York: McGraw-Hill, 1948.

3. Stevenson, I. P.; Duncan, C. H.; Wolf, S.; Ripley, H. S.; and Wolff, H. G. Life situations, emotions, and extrasystoles. *Psychosomatic Medicine,* 1949. **11**, 257–272.

4. Stevenson, I. P.; Duncan, C. H.; and Wolff, H. G. Circulatory dynamics before and after exercise in subjects with and without structural heart disease during anxiety and relaxation. *Journal of Clinical Investigation,* 1949. **28**, 1534–1543.

5. Stevenson, I. P., and Duncan, C. H. Alterations in cardiac function and circulatory efficiency during periods of life stress as shown by changes in the rate, rhythm, electrocardiographic pattern, and output of the heart in those with cardiovascular disease. *Research Publications, Association for Research in Nervous and Mental Disease,* 1950. **29**, 799–817.

6. Duncan, C. H.; Stevenson, I. P.; and Ripley, H. S. Life situations, and paroxysmal auricular arrhythmias. *Psychosomatic Medicine,* 1950. **12**, 23–37.

7. Wolff, H. G. Life stress and cardiovascular disorders. *Circulation,* 1950. **1**, 187–203.

8. Schneider, R. A. The relation of stress to clotting time, relative viscosity and certain other biophysical alterations of the blood in normotensive and hypertensive subjects. *Research Publications, Association for Research in Nervous and Mental Disease,* 1950. **29**, 818–831.

9. Stevenson, I. P.; Duncan, C. H.; Wolf, S.; and Wolff, H. G. The relation of life stress to cardiovascular symptoms and disease. *Medical Clinics of North America,* 1950. **34**, 817–831.

10. Stevenson, I. P.; Duncan, C. H.; and Ripley, H. S. Variations in the electrocardiogram during changes in emotional state. *Geriatrics,* 1951. **6**, 164–178.

11. Wolf, S.; Cardon, P. V.; Shepard, E. J.; and Wolff, H. G. *Life Stress and Essential Hypertension: A Study of Circulatory Adjustments in Man.* Baltimore: Williams and Wilkins, 1955.

12. Graham, D. T.; Kabler, J. D.; and Lunsford, L. Vasovagal fainting: a diphasic response. *Psychosomatic Medicine,* 1942. **23**, 493–507.

13. Mittlemann, B., and Wolff, H. G. Emotions and gastroduodenal function: experimental studies on patients with gastritis, duodenitis, and peptic ulcer. *Psychosomatic Medicine,* 1942. **4**, 5–61.

14. Engel, G. L.; Reichsman, F.; and Segal, H. L. A study of an infant with a gastric fistula. I. Behavior and the rate of total hydrochloric acid secretion. *Psychosomatic Medicine,* 1956. **18**, 374–398.

15. Engel, G. L., and Reichsman, F. Spontaneous and experimentally induced depressions in an infant with a gastric fistula. A contribution to the problem of depression. *Journal of the American Psychoanalytic Association,* 1956. **4**, 428–452.

16. Schottstaedt, W. W.; Grace, W. J.; and Wolff, H. G. Life situations, behavior patterns, and renal excretion of fluid and electrolytes. *Journal of the American Medical Association,* 1955. **157**, 1485–1488.

17. Schottstaedt, W. W.; Grace, W. J.; and Wolff, H. G. Life situations, behaviour, attitudes, emotions, and renal excretion of fluid and electrolytes. I. Method of study. *Journal of Psychosomatic Research,* 1956. **1**, 75–83.

18. Schottstaedt, W. W.; Grace, W. J.; and Wolff, H. G. Life situations, behaviour, attitudes, emotions, and renal excretion of fluid and electrolytes. II. Retention of water and sodium; diuresis of water. *Journal of Psychosomatic Research,* 1956. **1**, 147–159.

19. Schottstaedt, W. W.; Grace, W. J.; and Wolff, H. G. Life situations, behaviour, attitudes, emotions, and renal excretion of fluid and electrolytes. III. Diuresis of fluid and electrolytes. *Journal of Psychosomatic Research,* 1956. **1**, 203–211.

20. Schottstaedt, W. W.; Grace, W. J.; and Wolff, H. G. Life situations, behaviour, attitudes, emotions, and renal excretion of fluid and electrolytes. IV. Situations associated with retention of water, sodium, and potassium. *Journal of Psychosomatic Research,* 1956. **1**, 287–291.

21. Schottstaedt, W. W.; Grace, W. J.; and Wolff, H.G. Life situations, behaviour, attitudes, emotions, and renal excretion of fluid and electrolytes. V. Variations in excretion of endogenous creatinine. *Journal of Psychosomatic Research,* 1956. **1** 292–298.

22. Hinkle, L. E., Jr., and Wolf, S. Experimental study of life situations, emotions, and

the occurrence of acidosis in a juvenile diabetic. *American Journal of Medical Sciences,* 1949. **217**, 130–135.

23. Hinkle, L. E., Jr.; Conger, G. B.; and Wolf, S. Studies on diabetes mellitus: the relation of stressful life situations to the concentration of ketone bodies in the blood of diabetic and non-diabetic humans. *Journal of Clinical Investigation,* 1950. **29**, 754–769.

24. Hinkle, L. E., Jr., and Wolf, S. Studies in diabetes mellitus: changes in glucose, ketone, and water metabolism during stress. *Research Publications, Association for Research in Nervous and Mental Disease,* 1950. **29**, 338–389.

25. Hinkle, L. E., Jr.; Edwards, C. J.; and Wolf, S. Studies in diabetes mellitus, II. The occurrence of a diuresis in diabetic persons exposed to stressful life situations, with experimental observations on its relation to the concentration of glucose in blood and urine. *Journal of Clinical Investigation,* 1951. **30**, 818–837.

26. Hinkle, L. E., Jr.; Evans, F. M.; and Wolf, S. Studies in diabetes mellitus, III. Life history of three persons with labile diabetes and relation of significant experiences in their lives to the onset and course of the disease. *Psychosomatic Medicine,* 1951. **13**, 160–183.

27. Hinkle, L. E., Jr.; Evans, F. M.; and Wolf, S. Studies in diabetes mellitus, IV. Life history of three persons with relatively mild, stable diabetes, and relation of significant experiences in their lives to the onset and course of the disease. *Psychosomatic Medicine,* 1951. **13**, 184–202.

28. Hinkle, L. E., Jr., and Wolf, S. Importance of life stress in course and management of diabetes mellitus. *Journal of the American Medical Association,* 1952. **148**, 513–520.

29. Hinkle, L. E., Jr., and Wolf, S. A summary of experimental evidence relating life stress to diabetes mellitus. *Journal of the Mount Sinai Hospital,* 1952. **19**, 537–570.

30. Hinkle, L. E., Jr., and Wolf, S. The effects of stressful life situations on the concentration of blood glucose in diabetic and nondiabetic humans. *Diabetes,* 1952. **1**, 383–392.

31. Schottstaedt, W. W.; Pinsky R. H.; Mackler, D.; and Wolf, S. Sociologic, psychologic, and metabolic observations on patients in the community of a metabolic ward. *American Journal of Medicine,* 1958. **25**, 248–257.

32. Graham, D. T. The pathogenesis of hives: experimental study of life situations, emotions, and cutaneous vascular reactions. *Research Publications, Association for Research in Nervous and Mental Disease,* 1950. **29**, 987–1009.

33. Wolff, H. G.; Lorenz, T. H.; and Graham, D. T. Stress, emotions, and human sebum: their relevance to acne vulgaris. *Transactions of the Association of American Physicians,* 1951. **64**, 435–444.

34. Graham, D. T., and Wolf, S. The relation of eczema to attitude and to vascular reactions of the human skin. *Journal of Laboratory and Clinical Medicine,* 1953. **42**, 238–254.

35. Lorenz, T. H.; Graham, D. T.; and Wolf, S. The relation of life stress and emotions to human sebum secretion and to the mechanism of acne vulgaris. *Journal of Laboratory and Clinical Medicine,* 1953. **41**, 11–28.

36. Graham, D. T. The relation of psoriasis to attitude and to vascular reactions of the human skin. *Journal of Investigative Dermatology,* 1954. **22**, 379–388.

37. Graham, D. T. Cutaneous vascular reactions in Raynaud's disease and in states of hostility, anxiety, and depression. *Psychosomatic Medicine,* 1955. **17**, 200–207.

38. Clarke, E. R.; Zahn, D. W.; and Holmes, T. H. The relationship of stress, adrenocorti-

cal function, and tuberculosis. *American Review of Tuberculosis,* 1954. **69**, 351–369.

39. Ripley, H. S., and Wolff, H. G. Life situations, emotions, and glaucoma. *Psychosomatic Medicine,* 1950. **12**, 215–224.

40. Ripley, H. S. Life situations, emotions, and glaucoma. *Research Publications, Association for Research in Nervous and Mental Disease,* 1950. **29**, 523–536.

41. Holmes, T. H., and Wolff, H. G. Life situations, emotions, and backache. *Research Publications, Association for Research in Nervous and Mental Disease,* 1950. **29**, 750–772. Also in *Psychosomatic Medicine,* 1952. **14**, 18–33.

42. Dorpat, T. L., and Holmes, T. H. Mechanisms of skeletal muscle pain and fatigue. *Archives of Neurology and Psychiatry,* 1955. **74**, 628–640.

43. Graham, D. T.; Stern, J. A.; and Winokur, G. Experimental investigation of the specificity of attitude hypothesis of psychosomatic disease. *Psychosomatic Medicine,* 1958. **20**, 446–457.

44. Graham, D. T.; Stern, J. A.; and Winokur, G. The concept of a different specific set of physiological changes in each emotion. *Psychiatric Research Reports #12,* January 1960. 8–15.

45. Stern, J. A.; Winokur, G.; Graham, D. T.; and Graham, F. K. Alterations in physiological measures during experimentally induced attitudes. *Journal of Psychosomatic Research,* 1961. **5**, 73–82.

46. Graham, D. T.; Lundy, R. M.; Benjamin, L. S.; Kabler, J. D.; Lewis, W. C.; Kunish, N. O.; and Graham, F. K. Specific attitudes in initial interviews with patients having different "psychosomatic" diseases. *Psychosomatic Medicine,* 1962. **24**, 257–266.

47. Hinkle, L. E., Jr.; Pinsky, R. H.; Bross, I.D.J.; and Plummer, N. The distribution of sickness disability in a homogeneous group of healthy adult men. *American Journal of Hygiene,* 1956. **64**, 220–242.

48. Hinkle, L. E., Jr., and Wolff, H. G. The nature of man's adaptation to his total environment and the relation of this to illness. *Archives of Internal Medicine,* 1957. **99**, 442–460.

49. Hinkle, L. E., Jr.; Christenson, W. W.; Kane, F. D.; Ostfeld, A.; Thetford, W. N.; and Wolff, H. G. An investigation of the relation between life experience, personality characteristics, and general susceptibility to illness. *Psychosomatic Medicine,* 1958. **20**, 278–295.

50. Hinkle, L. E., Jr.; Redmont, R.; Plummer, N.; and Wolff, H. G. An examination of the relation between symptoms, disability, and serious illness in two homogeneous groups of men and women. *American Journal of Public Health,* 1960. **50**, 1327–1366.

51. Masuda, M., and Holmes, T. H. Magnitude estimations of social readjustments. *Journal of Psychosomatic Research,* 1967. **11**, 219–225.

52. Wyler, A. R.; Masuda, M.; and Holmes, T. H. Seriousness of Illness Rating Scale. *Journal of Psychosomatic Research,* 1967. **11**, 363–374.

53. Bramwell, S. T.; Masuda, M.; Wagner, N. N.; and Holmes, T. H. Psychosocial factors in athletic injuries: development and application of the Social and Athletic Readjustment Rating Scale (SARRS). *Journal of Human Stress,* 1975. **1** (2), 6–20.

54. Wyler, A. R., Masuda, M., and Holmes, T. H. Magnitude of life events and seriousness of illness. *Psychosomatic Medicine.* 1971. **33**, 115–122.

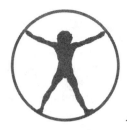

ANNOTATED BIBLIOGRAPHY

The following annotated bibliography departs from the standard, alphabetized form established by the editors. These references have been arranged in a historical and conceptual perspective that parallels the presentation of ideas in the chapter itself.

Wolff, Harold G.; Wolf, Stewart G., Jr.; and Hare, Clarence C. (Eds.). **Life Stress and Bodily Disease** (Research Publications, Association for Research in Nervous and Mental Diseases, vol. 29). Baltimore: Williams and Wilkins, 1950.

> This volume is a monument to the genius of Harold G. Wolff, its senior editor. It contains the proceedings of the annual meeting of the Association for Research in Nervous and Mental Diseases and in many ways is the "bible" of research in psychosomatic medicine. Published in 1950, the book includes the early work of such currently prominent researchers as Stewart Wolf, Hans Selye, Franz Alexander, Thomas Almy, Meyer Friedman, David Graham, Roy Grinker, Lawrence Hinkle, Thomas Holmes, Theodore Lidz, Dane Prugh, Morton Reiser, Herbert Ripley, and Ian Stevenson.
>
> Experimental evidence is presented about the genesis of many diseases and their signs and symptoms, which involve most body systems. The evidence reveals significant new dimensions of many familiar illnesses (such as heart disease, hay fever, diabetes, ulcerative colitis, and peptic ulcer), and the data provide insight into the bodily mechanisms of signs and symptoms heretofore considered vague and difficult to classify.

Hinkle, Lawrence E., Jr., and Plummer, Norman. **Life stress and industrial absenteeism—the concentration of illness and absenteeism in one segment of a working population.** *Industrial Medicine and Surgery*, 1952. **21**, 365–373.

Plummer, Norman, and Hinkle, Lawrence E., Jr. **Medical significance of illness and absence in an industrial population.** *Annals of Internal Medicine*, 1953. **39**, 103–115.

> These studies initiate the "new epidemiology" generated by research on the relationship of life stress and disease. Illness, sickness, disease, accidents, injury, and ab-

senteeism are not randomly distributed throughout the general population but are concentrated in a relatively small segment of the people. In addition to the high frequency of illness, this segment of illness-prone people has multiple diseases—often serious—involving multiple body systems. Quite striking was the finding that disorders of thought, feeling, and behavior were by far the most commonly occurring diseases and often coexisted with diseases of other bodily systems. This pattern of illness is well established by early adulthood and persists as a life-style for at least the next twenty or thirty years. Psychologically these people are tense and dissatisfied, and they react vigorously to salient life situations. They are often upwardly mobile people who strive toward unrealistic goals and seldom find a resting point of satisfaction.

Wolff, Harold G. **Headache and Other Head Pain** (2nd ed.). New York: Oxford University Press, 1963. (See also 3rd ed., Donald J. Delassio, Ed. New York: Oxford University Press, 1972.)

This book is a masterpiece of clinical science in the tradition of the famous English clinician Sir Thomas Lewis. Wolff, using direct and usually simple techniques of observation and measurement on human subjects, generated data on the nature of pain, pain sensitive structures in the head, and mechanisms for the genesis of pain from these structures. Pain was clearly demonstrated to be a sensation, subserved by a unique neural apparatus, initiated by a high-energy stimulus producing tissue damage (often of low magnitude). Like other sensations (vision, hearing, etc.), pain has a threshold and a range of intensity from the threshold to the ceiling (or maximum).

Laboratory experiments were designed to identify the pain-sensitive structures of the head and to study mechanisms by which these structures produced pain. Commonly acknowledged sources of headache were the eyes, ears, teeth and other oral structures, nasal and paranasal structures, skin, and muscles. By far the most ingenious experiments dealt with the pain generated by the cranial vasculature in major arteries and venous sinuses. Dilation (migraine), traction or displacement (space occupying lesions), and inflamation are the critical events responsible for the sensation.

The only reservation possible about this work is a result of its quality—it is so well done and illuminating that it may well retard further research in this area of clinical medicine for another century.

Holmes, Thomas H.; Goodell, Helen; Wolf, Stewart; and Wolff, Harold G. **The Nose: An Experimental Study of Reactions Within the Nose in Human Subjects During Varying Life Experiences.** Springfield, Ill.: Charles C. Thomas, 1950.

This book, along with those on the stomach and colon, is one of a trilogy of studies of mucous membranes. It is an experimental study of reactions within the nose in human subjects during varying life experiences. The mucous membranes of the nose react with hyperemia, hypersecretion, swelling, and obstruction to breathing due to a variety of noxious environmental and naturally occurring stimuli. This reaction to particulate matter and chemical fumes protects deeper respiratory tissues by shutting out, neutralizing, and washing away the noxious substances. The same reaction to cold ambient temperature, by dramatically warming the inspired air, protects deeper tissues from frostbite. This mucous membrane hyperfunction is defined as a biologically appropriate protective reaction pattern, since the reaction has relevance and pertinence for adapting or coping with the assault on the nose by the noxious stimulus.

Experimental application of noxious pressure to the head produces headache and hyperfunction of the nasal mucous membranes. This reaction is defined as a biologically inappropriate protective reaction pattern. The nasal reaction does not protect the body from the assault. Similar reactions to symbols of threat such as an unsympathetic spouse or mother-in-law are also biologically inappropriate, since they fail to protect. The nasal reaction to symbols of threat, when coupled with conflict and feelings of helplessness and "being left out in the cold," can be intense and sustained. The by-product or epiphenomenon of this reaction is tissue damage and disease. When such stimuli engendered by interpersonal and social situations are combined with other noxious stimuli (such as pollen), the nasal hyperfunction, tissue damage, and disease are apt to be of greater intensity and duration.

Wolf, Stewart, and Wolff, Harold G. **Human Gastric Function: An Experimental Study of a Man and His Stomach** (2nd ed.). New York: Oxford University Press, 1943.

This book reports on numerous observations and experiments on Tom, who had lived with a gastric fistula from childhood to his middle years when these studies began (1940s). Unlike the stomach of his famous fistulous predecessor, Alexis St. Martin—who over one hundred years ago provided an opportunity to apply the new scientific techniques of biochemistry to the process of digestion—Tom's stomach provided the opportunity to apply the developing technique of Pavlovian psychology to the study of life situations, emotions, and gastric function.

Mucous membrane blood flow, motility, acid-pepsin secretion, and mucous production were measured from the exposed stomach lumen and correlated with numerous naturally occurring and experimentally induced life situations. Observations were made on the effects of drugs on gastric function in a variety of psychophysiological states. For example, ipecac, accompanied by the author's suggestion of benefit, brought about relief of gastric hypofunction and nausea, the opposite of ipecac's usual effects. Gastric sensation was also evaluated and the mechanism of nausea and pain demonstrated. For the first time in the history of clinical science, a peptic ulcer was produced experimentally in man. The study explains many abdominal signs and symptoms often considered vague and without a basis in human biology.

Grace, William J.; Wolf, Stewart; and Wolff, Harold G. **The Human Colon.** New York: Harper and Row (Hoeber), 1951.

This book details the relationship of life situations, emotions, and human colon function. The substance of the book is provided by four adult male subjects with colonic fistulae, supported by various other subjects whose intact colons were studied by more conventional techniques of indwelling ballons, proctoscopy, X-ray, fluoroscopy, and chemistry of the colonic content.

The data document the role of life events in provoking disorders of function of the colon: diarrhea occurs as a consequence of colonic hyperfunction and appears to be an exaggerated process of normal defecation; constipation is associated with the colonic hypofunction and appears to be an exaggeration of colonic inactivity, which accompanies vigorous bodily action.

As with the studies on Tom's stomach, (Wolf and Wolff, 1943, above) Dr. Grace and his colleagues were able to "cause" the onset of ulcerative colitis in his fistulous subjects by introducing sensitive topics for discussion. As the subject reacted with strong feeling, the exposed colonic mucous membrane became turgid, engorged, and red, as blood flow increased. Motility was exaggerated and on occasion a vigorous contraction was followed by the appearance of petechiae. The fragility of mucous membrane was further demonstrated when, at the peak of the emotional reaction, the hyperfunctioning mucosa was lightly stimulated with a glass rod. A trail of minute hemorrhages followed the path of the stimulus.

Some implications for treatment may be derived from the fact that replacement of the sensitive topic with neutral topics and the communication to the subject of warmth, reassurance, and emotional support brought about a resolution of the colonic hyperfunction and the hemorrhagic process in the mucous membrane.

Dudley, Donald L.; in collaboration with Martin, C. J.; Masuda, Minoru; Ripley, Herbert S.; and Holmes, Thomas H. **Psychophysiology of Respiration in Health and Disease.** New York: Appleton-Century-Croft, 1969.

This book focuses on the relationship of feeling states, patterns of behavior, and such parameters of respiratory function as movement of air in the system, gas concentration and exchange in the lungs, metabolism, and content in the blood of oxygen and carbon dioxide. Two patterns of behavior were identified as relevant to health and disease in both normal subjects and subjects with chronic obstructive pulmonary diseases (COPD). Action-oriented behavior, which includes such states as anxiety and anger, was associated with respiratory and metabolic *hyper*function Nonaction-oriented behavior, which includes such states as depression, withdrawal, and hibernation, were associated with respiratory and metabolic *hypo*function. Both behavior patterns were associated with dyspnea. In the presence of advanced COPD both these patterns had ominous consequences for the patient, i.e. acidosis and death.

Prospective studies of patients with advanced COPD revealed that the high mortality rate was strongly associated with limited psychosocial assets. Often death occurred shortly after the patient decided the time had come to die. Both physiologically and psychologically the behavior resembled hibernation, and these patients were relatively comfortable and satisfied as death approached. The final event appeared to be a dramatic fall in blood pH generated by progressive acidosis.

Holmes, Thomas H.; Hawkins, Norman G.; Bowerman, Charles E.; Clarke, Edmund R., Jr.; and Joffe, Joy R. **Psychosocial and psychophysiologic studies of tuberculosis.** *Psychosomatic Medicine*, 1957. **19**, 134–143.

Holmes, Thomas H. **Infectious diseases and human ecology.** *Journal of Indian Medical Profession*, 1964. **10**, 4825–4829.

These studies, completed in the 1950s just as the antibiotics for the treatment of tuberculosis were introduced, and discussed in these two articles, are the last major epidemiologic investigations of this infectious disease in the United States. Case-finding methods made it possible to study most of the known, live cases of active tuberculosis in a metropolitan area in the northwest United States.

Tuberculosis is a cohort disease with most cases in the United States being derived from that population born in 1900, plus or minus twenty years. It is predominantly a disease of socially and economically marginal males of minority status who are skid-row or city-center residents of rural or foreign origin. In addition to frequent physical diseases in the past, the tuberculous patients have high frequencies of prison records or mental illness.

The disease commonly has its onset in a crisis situation that terminates a highly mobile, peripatetic life-style of frequent divorces and job and residential changes. In this setting of stressful events, the patients react by feeling overwhelmed, accompanied by a dramatic reduction in parameters of biological resistance to infection. With these intimate bodily changes, the germ, which has probably been present for years in the pulmonary mast cells, initiates the tissue reaction. Prognosis depends not only on appropriate chemotherapy and regulation of behavior but also on the quality and quantity of psychosocial assets present in the patient as well.

The epidemic of tuberculosis in the Western Hemisphere began with the establishment of the factory and the replacement of the rural-agrarian life-style with the urban-industrial way of life. As the latter has become the mode for the Western world and as biological and social evolution have progressed, the factors responsible for tuberculosis have largely disappeared. The epidemic that at one time threatened the survival of the Western world has gone out of fashion.

Grace, William J., and Graham, David T. **Relationship of specific attitudes and emotions to certain bodily diseases.** *Psychosomatic Medicine,* 1952. **14**, 243–251.

This publication is now considered a classic in the medical literature and represents a major achievement in the field of psychosomatic medicine. The research defines specific *attitudes* associated with specific diseases. Using the clinical interview as a method for discovery, the authors examined the cognitive state of patients whose disease had its onset in response to a life crisis or stressful life situation. An attitude was defined as the patient's perception of the precipitating life event, its meaning for the patient, how it made him feel, and what – if anything – the patient did or felt like doing about the situation. Attitudes were defined for twelve common diseases: urticaria, eczema, Raynaud's disease, vasomotor rhinitis, asthma, diarrhea, constipation, nausea and vomiting, duodenal ulcer, migraine headache, arterial hypertension, and low back pain. For example, in duodenal ulcer, the attitude of the subject was one of seeking revenge and injury of the person who had injured him; in nausea and vomiting, the subject was preoccupied with something he wished had never happened.

The conclusions are that a disease can be defined in physiological terms (peptic ulcer crater) and in psychological terms (wishing for revenge). The two dimensions together define the pathophysiology and the psychopathology of peptic ulcer. This research clearly establishes "emotion" as a response to a life-event stimulus and not a cause of the bodily response.

Holmes, Thomas H., and Rahe, Richard H. **The Social Readjustment Rating Scale.** *Journal of Psychosomatic Research,* 1967. **11**, 213–218.

This study, which produced a major breakthrough in the discourse of the new etiology, provides a quantitative value for life events that "cause" and account for the time of onset of disease. The method used in quantifying this value is derived from psychophysics, the branch of psychology that is concerned with man's ability to make subjective magnitude estimations of certain of his experiences (i.e., brightness of light or loudness of sound). A ratio scale is generated when this method is applied to the assessment of the amount of adjustment required by forty-three life events empirically observed to occur before the onset of illness. Of the events listed, death of a spouse requires the most change in adjustment by people, and minor violations of the law and the Christmas season the least. Put in other words, death of a spouse requires twice as much change in adjustment as marriage, over three times as much as in-law trouble, and ten times as much as a traffic ticket. The rank order agreement about the magnitude of change in adjustment is usually very high (coefficient of correlation above 0.90) between discrete samples of subjects from most demographic categories.

This method allows for a quantitative definition of the life situation in which disease has its onset to complement the qualitative report of the same events. It also makes possible a quantitative base for the prediction of the population with high risk for the development of disease and a base for evaluating the outcome of preventive intervention.

Holmes, Thomas H., and Masuda, Minoru. **Life change and illness susceptibility.** In J. P. Scott and E. C. Senay (Eds.), *Symposium on Separation and Depression.* Washington, D.C.: American Association for the Advancement of Science, 1973. 161–186. (AAAS Publication no. 94.)

This paper summarizes the results generated by applying the Social Readjustment Rating Scale to a variety of clinical situations. The items from the scale (with the omission of Christmas) are incorporated into a paper-and-pencil test (Schedule of Recent Experience – SRE), which allows the respondent to indicate the frequency of occurrence of the items within a specified time interval. When the frequency of the items multiplied by their scale values are summed for the time intervals, the result is the number of Life Change Units. The association of this life-change magnitude with illness onset, studied both retrospectively and prospectively, shows a dramatic coincidence. The greater the magnitude of change units, the greater the probability of illness onset. This relationship holds for a range of time. A one- to two-year life-change base predicts the onset of serious disease for the next two years, a six-month base predicts onset of moderately serious disease for the next six months, and daily life-change magnitude predicts for that day the occurrence of the signs and symptoms of illness. Also, the higher the life-change magnitude the greater the probability that if a disease does occur in the near future it will be a serious one.

Ripley, Herbert S.; Wolf, Stewart; and Wolff, Harold G. **Treatment in a psychosomatic clinic.** *Journal of the American Medical Association,* 1948. **138,** 949–951.

This vignette is a tour de force about the doctor's treatment techniques and their impact on patients and their diseases. It is not surprising that the most salient and frequently used methods are psychological: providing reassurance and emotional support, encouraging the free expression of conflicts and feelings; and offering advice regarding attitudes, habits, and activities. When combined with the powerful impact of examination of the patient by the doctor, the use of laboratory tests in ruling out infection and cancer, and drug therapy for relief of symptoms, the outcome for the majority of patients is improvement. The key to this therapeutic achievement is the doctor whose transaction with the patient is free from moral judgments and conveys warmth, interest, and understanding to the patient.

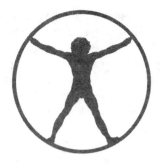

24

HOLISTIC APPROACHES TO HEALTHY AGING AND PROGRAMS FOR THE ELDERLY

Ken Dychtwald, Ph.D.

There are few processes more natural and inevitable than aging. As soon as we are born, aging begins, and unless early death interferes we will all, regardless of our sex, race, or socioeconomic status, become older people. Yet at present we live in an era in which youth is the hero and old age is something to be resisted, postponed, and denied. Aging is seen as a disease, and the elderly are frequently viewed with uneasiness. In a culture where so much emphasis is placed on youthful vigor, economic productiveness, and sexual/social competition, it is not surprising that older people are often pushed aside and denied a dignified and truly meaningful role.

However, the emphasis on youth and the young is shifting. In the past few decades, aging in the United States has begun to take on new shapes and meanings as our society quite literally "grows up." We are shifting gradually from being a culture of young people to being one in which the fastest growing segment of the population is elderly. Since the turn of the century, the total U.S. population has nearly tripled, while the number of those sixty-five or older has increased an astounding eight times (National Council on Aging, 1977). There are approximately 23 million Americans over the age of sixty-five, representing roughly 12 percent of the total U.S. population. With each passing day, 3,000 people die and 4,000 enter into the ranks of "senior citizenry" (Hendricks and Hendricks 1977). As the "aging of America" continues we can expect that by the year 2,000 nearly one-fourth of the population will be over sixty-five years old (Kuhn and Hessel, 1977).

As more Americans experience the pains and pleasures of aging we will have a growing opportunity to learn about the attitudes, preparations, and experiences that are most conducive to a full and healthy life. Never before have there been so many elders alive on our planet. Yet, sadly, many people remain unwilling to acknowledge the passing of youth and the natural progression toward an old age that in many cultures is considered the most special and revered time of one's life—a time for self-awareness, continued health, wisdom, adventure, and deep personal sharing.

As more has been learned about the biological, psychological, and sociological dimensions of aging, it has become increasingly clear that not only are we living longer than we did several decades ago but we are also aging and dying from different causes. Dramatic advances in health care and environmental sanitation have extended the average life span from approximately 45 years at the turn of the century to roughly 70.4 years in 1970. Yet very few Americans are living to 120, the age that many researchers believe to be our more natural biological end point (Hendricks and Hendricks, 1977). Certainly, explorations into the life-styles of special communities (such as the Hunza) suggest that there is yet a long way to go toward eliminating the causes of sickness and "premature" aging.

As we have become more "civilized" and industrialized, we have nearly eliminated many infectious diseases, but we have done very poorly at initiating and maintaining the kinds of healthy life-styles, nutritional habits, interpersonal relationships, and exercise activities that would reduce the wear and tear of stress and tension and fortify us against the often debilitating influence of modern living. We can no longer blame germs or doctors alone for the stress-related ailments—cardiovascular disorders, cancer, respiratory diseases, and arthritis—that cause up to 80 percent of the disease in our aging culture, nor can we expect that these environmental and life-style related diseases will be eliminated with drugs or symptomatic medical intervention. Instead, these particular aging and "diseasing" patterns suggest that the problems of "aging" in the United States are very much connected to the nature of "living" in this country, that the solution to these problems lies in some measure in a large-scale restructuring of the images, beliefs, values, and practices that surround the way we live, care for ourselves and each other, and age.

In the United States, old age is often viewed as a life stage somehow separate from the rest of one's life—a time of decreased social worth and involvement, a period of loss and decline and accompanying loss of beauty and health (Butler, 1975). These negative images serve to severely hamper and limit our natural growth and development. They suggest that the later years are not times of intimacy, wisdom, pleasure, awareness, joy, and love. Aging, rather, is seen as a never-ending battle against the forces of loss, anxiety, dependency, loneliness, and sickness.

These negative images and attitudes affect all of us, for they instill in us the fearful notion that when we lose our youth, physical potency, and economic productiveness we will be neglected, worthless, and eventually discarded. For example, a study conducted by the National Council on Aging (1977) discovered that only 29 percent of the public eighteen to sixty-four years of age viewed the older persons as "very bright and alert." In addition, only 19 percent viewed older persons as "very open-minded and adaptable" and 35 percent believed that older persons were "very good at getting things done."

Historically, images about aging and attitudes toward the elderly have emerged and developed through direct personal experience with elders. Until recently the family was set up so that each person had ample opportunity to interact with his or her parents, grandparents, aunts, uncles, neighbors, and the older relatives of friends. The older people, having been around the longest, were well known to the community, and knowledgeable about the various processes and procedures of life. Today, changes in familial, work, and social patterns have radically changed this configuration. Because many people get married later in life, their children never get to meet their grandparents. Younger people move away from home to attend college, get married, or "find themselves," thus disengaging themselves from active involvement in the lives of their parents and grandparents.

Rapid life-style change and an imbalance of natural experience and formal education among the generations have served to disrupt the traditional social mechanisms for mixed-age interaction, while mandatory retirement, assembly line factories, and large stores and businesses have eliminated many of the small shops, working teams, and apprenticeship models that once provided a great deal of intergenerational involvement and support. Finally, with the advent of retirement communities, many elders have chosen to isolate themselves from young people. As a result, large numbers of Americans find they have no occasion for direct and ongoing personal involvement with elders.

With the growing absence of direct and meaningful involvement with healthy elders, many people learn about aging and old age second hand or through the media. For their part, the media tend to disregard the thoughts, contributions, concerns, needs and pursuits of the elderly. For example, advertisements—particularly for products designed to enhance romance, sexuality, or self-worth—seldom portray older people in a positive light. Even magazines and shows designed specifically for older people frequently use young people in the advertisements and commercials. The message is that the elderly are not worth writing about nor are they interesting, healthy, beautiful, or loving.

The impact of cultural priorities on our image of aging also affects and influences the shaping of our physical environments. Most environments seem tailored to people with a standard size and a specific range of mental and neurological abilities. Our contemporary cities are like monstrous cookie cutters shaped to exclude people who cannot function within certain limited physical parameters. Many older people cannot ride buses because the steps are too high; they cannot attend public events because the transportation is inappropriate, the walkways too slippery, the rooms too dark, or the lettering on the signs too small. There are often no elevators and the bathrooms are too hazardous. When one tries to perceive the world through the mind and body of an elderly person, it becomes immediately obvious that as one ages, environments that were once comfortable and supportive become transformed into dark, slippery, crime-ridden, scarcely navigable obstacle courses. Perhaps we see fewer and fewer older people around town because we have built our towns to exclude them.

Unfortunately, too many older people do not realize that we have collectively created a world into which they do not comfortably fit. Instead, they internalize the message that they do not belong in the world. Where outrage would be an appropriate and reasonable response, we too often see resignation, sickness, low self-esteem, and anomie. In time, continued interaction with these negative images and structures directly translates into frustration, tension, unhappiness, loneliness, stress, and a decreased will to live (Curtin, 1972).

However, as we learn more about the process of aging and the impact of culture and environment on it, it becomes apparent that the right preparation, attitude, attention, and meaningful involvement can transform aging into a full and thoroughly rewarding maturation process—not unlike the ripening of a fine wine or musical instrument. The later years of life can hold within them a unique freedom from economic competition, social striving, child-rearing burdens and responsibilities, and worrisome jobs. In many ways, the "golden years" of life are the perfect time to develop self-awareness, cultivate special interests and skills, begin and enjoy new hobbies and leisure activities, enter into new professional relationships, and expand and deepen friendships. Old age provides an extended period to reflect on the trials and joys of a lifetime, to develop and articulate a special kind of wisdom and knowledge, self-knowledge, and sensitivity that can come only at the end of a life (Ellison, 1978; Dangott and Kalish, 1979).

Paradoxically, these possibilities are often stymied by the fact that most medical, counseling, and recreational services for the elderly are *not* focused on eliciting health, joy, and vitality but instead deal primarily with problem-oriented treatment, therapy, chemical prescription, and pass-time activities. Instead of being offered programs and practices for preventive health care, personal growth, continuing education, and community involvement, all too often the older person is encouraged, at most, to simply "maintain."

The holistic approach to health is an important antidote to this perspective and the illness-oriented treatment it dictates. Rooted in a deep appreciation of the unity of mind and body, it emphasizes preventive education, health promotion, and the realization that growth, exercise, self-responsibility, and meaningful interpersonal involvement are necessary ingredients in the healthy lifestyle. It is thus an effective guide to consideration of the ways we can facilitate psychological and physical health throughout the entire aging process—and especially in the later years. A holistic approach to health care for the elderly will include considerations of the social and psychological components of aging in addition to the various clinical practices, techniques, and procedures available for enhancing physical health and well-being.

Increasingly, this perspective seems to be taking root. In recent years a trend toward a more holistic approach to health care for the elderly has been emerging from medical, counseling, fitness, political advocacy, and religious interest groups. Without changing the need for acute or chronic medical care and its methods, a variety of individual practitioners and programs have begun to shift their focus away from reductionistic and mechanistic "problem centered" health programs and "pass-time" activities toward more creative, humanistic, and holistic approaches to aging and the elderly. Intergenerational living and exchange programs, nutritional guidance, vitalizing and stress-reducing exercises, interesting and meaningful social programs, and health-promotion education have all been employed to enrich the lives of older adults by improving self-esteem, health, and overall well-being. As these programs help to support connections between and within the generations, they strengthen the resistance of the entire cultural fabric to stress and psychosomatic breakdown. In addition, in recent years many alternatives to traditional medicine and counseling have emerged. Techniques such as biofeedback, autogenic training, yoga, relaxation training, meditation, art and dance therapy, and various types of "growth" groups for elders have met with a strong and positive response from elders and health practitioners who prefer preventive and holistic approaches to health.

In the rest of this chapter I want to present sketches – and the addresses – of a variety of programs for the elderly that successfully model a multidimensional and holistic approach to physical and psychological health care. While these programs are in many ways different from each other and few if any deal with all aspects of growing old in the United States, they do embody the kind of social concern, clinical sensitivity, and program ingenuity that may help us to understand and experience the process of aging in a new and more positive way.

The *Bridge Project* of Fairhaven College in Bellingham, Washington, was the first attempt to bring older people completely into college life. This is a program for elderly people who attend classes with regular students and receive credits and degrees while they live in a remodeled dormitory, eat in the college dining hall, and participate in all the extracurricular events the college has to offer. Since its inception in 1973, the Bridge Project has included approximately thirty older students per term. In addition to the regular curriculum, Fairhaven has also begun to offer courses of particular interest to "Bridgers" – like "post-retirement potential," "life-history writing," "death and dying," "exercise," "body awareness," and "older women in America." Most recently, the Bridgers have created a day-care center at the college for four-year-olds. Bridgers have consistently described the benefits of friendship and stimulation during their involvement with the program, while younger Fairhaven students report that the opportunity for involvement with the Bridge elders has provided an atmosphere of excitement and warmth unmatched in their other activities.

> The Bridge
> Fairhaven College
> Bellingham, Washington 98225

The *Seniors Health Program* of Augustana Hospital in Chicago, Illinois, was created in 1975 to help combat the overuse and abuse of drugs among the older population. This program is designed to provide older people with helpful information about medications, their uses and effects, and to sensitize medical professionals to the emotional and physical needs of the elderly.

The Seniors Health Program sends trained staff people into the community to hot-lunch programs, churches, Y's, public libraries, and other programs where seniors congregate. At these locations, staff meet and talk with elders about their health, the drugs they take, and the methods and techniques for health promotion that may help them to reduce dosages or diminish unnecessary drugs altogether. Recently, the program extended its resources to include experiential activities, such as gentle bending, breathing, and stretching exercises, progressive relaxation, and massage. Over the years, the Seniors Health Program has been very well received by consumers and health professionals throughout the Chicago area. It now includes training materials, workshops, lectures, and a variety of health manuals.

> Seniors Health Program
> Augustana Hospital
> 411 West Dickens Avenue
> Chicago, Illinois 60614

The *SAGE* (Senior Actualization and Growth Explorations) *Project* in Berkeley, California, is the first program to effectively create a holistic approach to health and self-development to meet the demand for positively oriented gerontological programs and services. Since its inception in 1974, SAGE has been attempting to generate positive images of aging by demonstrating that people over sixty can grow and transcend the often negative expectations of our culture. Staffed by twenty psychologists, physicians, and breathing, movement, and art therapists, SAGE work is eclectic in technique. It draws on Western therapeutic practices, such as co-counseling, biofeedback, autogenic and relaxation training, and psychodrama as well as such Eastern disciplines as yoga, meditation, and tai chi. The SAGE approach focuses on the individual as a whole person.

Each year the SAGE Project continues to grow and expand. It has already successfully extended its resources into local nursing homes, community centers, hospitals, universities, medical centers, growth centers, and health clinics and has provided a model for a number of programs across the nation. In almost every case, the SAGE process has produced considerable subjective improvement in the overall health and well-being of the elderly participants. Quantitative measurements of this physical and psychological growth are currently being undertaken.

> SAGE
> 114 Montecito Avenue
> Oakland, California 94610

The *Senior Health Source* (SHS) was created in 1976 in Albuquerque, New Mexico, as an informal "health club" for elders. Since its inception, the program has expanded to twenty locations (four housing sites, fifteen meal sites, and a senior citizens' center) and will soon include a senior day-care center. Groups of elders meet weekly with SHS staff members at these sites for sessions that focus on a topic related to health and well-being. Some of the topics that have been especially well received are: therapeutic touch, memory, healing herbs, meditation, relaxation, sleep and dreaming, nutrition, and skin care.

Members of the original SHS groups graduate from these classes and move on to become instructors and leaders at other senior locations. The SHS also makes active use of the skills, facilities, and support of existing community groups, such as the Red Cross, local hospitals, the university, etc. Recently, as an outgrowth of the SHS program, a hospice for the terminally ill patient was set up in the Albuquerque area. At the hospice, the staff is dedicated to creating a humanistic alternative to the dying process that allows the dying person, his or her family, and close friends a chance to experience death with a sense of grace and dignity. The SHS program is thus an excellent example of a successful and comprehensive community-based holistic health program for elders.

> Senior Health Source
> 1024 Washington Street
> Albuquerque, New Mexico 87108

The *Elvirita Lewis Foundation* in Santa Cruz, California, believes that elders should be actively involved in helping others as well as themselves and that this in turn will enable them to feel more proud and hopeful about themselves. In association with other existing community agencies, the foundation has organized a series of free dental clinics, made possible the distribution of free produce to elders, and published an area-wide Resource Directory for Elders. The foundation's Senior Companion Program matches able with impaired elders in a peer support program and is planning to create an elder services center in the near future. In addition, elderly participants in the foundation's activities have created and staffed the Intergenerational Child Care Center, which has become a vital focus for community participation and social activity. Residents of local nursing homes are encouraged to drop by the center to help out with the children and to perform various organizational tasks.

> The Elvirita Lewis Foundation
> 230 Third Avenue
> Santa Cruz, California 95062

The *Nursing Home Residents' Advisory Council* (NHRAC) is an independent nonprofit organization run primarily by and for residents of nursing and boarding-care homes in Minnesota. Based in Minneapolis, this organization was originally organized in 1972 with residents of three facilities as an attempt to encourage residents of nursing homes to become more responsible for themselves, their health, and their living environment. At present, the NHRAC has already expanded to include more than 4,000 members in forty different homes throughout the state. The huge success of the NHRAC may be attributed to the opportunity for responsible activity and meaningful involvement that it has provided for the elderly residents of these homes.

As an offshoot of this project, the NHRAC elders decided to create the *Nursing Home Residents Advocates,* which provides advocacy services to prospective and long-term–care consumers. These elderly advocates both research and bring together information from various sources for use by those needing a nursing-home placement. When special problems arise, the advocates also provide peer counseling and services to current nursing-home residents.

By demonstrating that the institutionalized elderly can respond positively to opportunities for self-improvement and self-governance, the Nursing Home Residents' Advisory Council has already had a dramatic impact on institutions for the elderly throughout the country.

> Nursing Home Residents' Advisory Council
> 111 East Franklin, Suite 210
> Minneapolis, Minnesota 55404

The *Association for Humanistic Gerontology* (AHG) was founded in 1977 as an offshoot of the SAGE Project in Berkeley, California, in response to the need for propagating positive images of aging and increasing holistic services for the elderly. The association serves simultaneously as a professional association, an international resource-sharing network, and an information clearinghouse. Since its inception, AHG has already attracted members from forty-five states, four Canadian provinces, and several European countries. The quickly growing AHG membership represents a broad and comprehensive assortment of people, programs, and innovative ideas related to humanistic and holistic approaches to aging and programs for the elderly. To further research and disseminate information and support, AHG has thirty-five regional coordinators located in key geographic locations.

The Association for Humanistic Gerontology publishes a quarterly newsmagazine that lists workshops, lectures, training seminars, conferences, publications, and bibliographic material of direct personal and professional value. In addition, each newsmagazine presents illuminating profiles of AHG members involved in pioneer efforts and model projects in the fields of gerontology, health care, and psychology. The association also publishes a comprehensive members' catalog and sponsors conferences throughout the country. A book on holistic approaches to working with the elderly is forthcoming.

> Association for Humanistic Gerontology
> 1711 Solano Avenue
> Berkeley, California 94707

The *Gray Panthers* is a national coalition of old, young, and middle-aged activists that has become an outspoken national movement. The Panthers emphasize the relationship between personal growth, self-development, holistic health, and such larger cultural goals as self-determination and liberation from negative stereotyping, especially of the elderly. This group of "radical elders" is openly committed to the creation of a society in which self-actualization, health, and human values receive the highest priority.

Since their inception in 1970, the Gray Panthers have attracted more than 10,000 active members from throughout the United States. They have undertaken a wide range of tasks and programs related to social change and life-style improvement for the elderly. In the beginning, the Gray Panthers focused a great deal of energy on nursing home reform and elderly consumer affairs. In the past few years they have extended their activities to include lectures, demonstrations, workshops, publications, media watches, and political advocacy with regard to health care, mandatory retirement, and social security. They have been active in monitoring the policies of courts, banks, and municipal agencies, such as planning commissions and zoning boards, whose decisions affect the elderly and the programs that serve them.

As consumers of health care for the elderly, the Gray Panthers have been instrumental in facilitating healthy and positive images of aging among professionals as well as in promoting the kind of values, information, and experience that support a holistic approach to health care.

> The Gray Panthers
> 3700 Chestnut Street
> Philadelphia, Pennsylvania 19104

Other examples of successful holistic health programs for the elderly are senior exercise classes, foster grandparent programs, oral history projects, adopt-a-grandparent programs, elder hostels, emeritus college programs, RSVP (Retired Senior Volunteer Program) activities, involvement in the creative arts (such as music and painting), peer discussion groups, co-counseling programs, public lectures, continuing education programs, consciousness-raising activities at Y's and churches, intergenerational communes, and the effective use of media, such as the television show "Over Easy."

Although no one method or technique will effectively remedy all of the problems of our older population, it is urgent that we focus more of our time, energy, and money on pursing those activities, programs, and methodologies that support a multidimensional holistic approach to healthy aging and services for the elderly.

References

Butler, Robert N. *Why Survive? Being Old in America*. New York: Harper and Row, 1975.
Curtin, Sharon R. *Nobody Ever Died of Old Age*. Boston: Little, Brown, 1972.

Dangott, Lillian, and Kalish, Richard A. *A Time to Enjoy: The Pleasures of Aging.* Englewood Cliffs, N.J.: Prentice Hall/Spectrum, 1979.

Ellison, Jerome. *Life's Second Half: The Pleasures of Aging.* Old Greenwich, Conn.: Devin-Adair Company, 1978.

Hendricks, Jon, and Hendricks, C. Davis. *Aging in Mass Society: Myths and Realities.* Cambridge, Mass.: Winthrop, 1977.

Kuhn, Maggie, and Hessel, Dieter. *Maggie Kuhn on Aging.* Philadelphia: Westminster Press, 1977.

National Council on Aging. *Facts and Myths About Aging.* Washington, D.C.: Author, 1977.

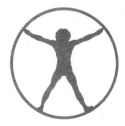 ANNOTATED BIBLIOGRAPHY

It is extremely difficult to present a list of books relating to holistic health and aging simply because there are very few books of this nature. Books about aging have tended to follow a fairly traditional biomedical approach, whereas most books about holistic approaches to health seem to leave out the needs and potentials of the older adult.

In this annotated list, I have chosen to combine the best and most essential readers in the field of aging with the few available books on holistic health and the elderly. While this assortment of literature will surely aim the health practitioner in the appropriate direction, a more comprehensive examination of holistic health and the elderly will have to wait until more research, articles, books, and programs have successfully emerged.

The following three books are considered the classic reference sources in gerontology. They are expensive, intelligently designed, brilliantly researched, and extraordinarily comprehensive in their presentation of information. They are unquestionably valuable as resources and reference books for the serious student of aging and the elderly.

Binstock, Robert H., and Shanas, Ethel. **Handbook of Aging and the Social Sciences.** New York: Van Nostrand Reinhold, 1976.

Birren, James E., and Schaie, K. Warner. **Handbook of the Psychology of Aging.** New York: Van Nostrand Reinhold, 1977.

Finch, Caleb E., and Hayflick, Leonard. **Handbook of the Biology of Aging,** New York: Van Nostrand Reinhold, 1977.

Atchley, Robert. **The Social Forces in Later Life: An Introduction to Social Gerontology.** Belmont, Calif.: Wadsworth, 1972.

> This is probably the best general text available on the social aspects of aging. It is well researched, efficiently organized, intelligently documented, and easy to read.

Butler, Robert N. **Why Survive? Being Old in America.** New York: Harper and Row, 1975.

> This sensitive and thoughtful Pulitzer Prize–winning book is probably the best available resource in the field of aging. Leaning heavily on the social policy aspects of aging, Butler provides immense amounts of data and research regarding all aspects of aging and the needs of the elderly, including the need for strong advocacy on their behalf. An outstanding piece of work.

Christianson, Alice, and Rankin, David. **Easy Does It Yoga for Older People.** New York: Harper and Row, 1979. (Originally published as *Easy Does It Yoga for People over Sixty.* Cleveland: Light on Yoga Society, 1977.)

> This is the best book for older people on yoga and yoga-related activities including breathing, meditation, and relaxation. It makes a suitable guide for health practitioners as well as an ideal handbook for elderly people who would like to revitalize themselves through the regular and mindful practice of gentle effective exercise. This book is extremely well illustrated and is thoughtfully printed in easy-to-read large bold type.

Comfort, Alex. **A Good Age.** Avenel, N.J.: Crown Publishers, 1976.

> Written for the older person as well as for the health professional, this book is one of the most attractive, informative, interesting, and readable volumes on aging. Dr. Comfort supports the idea that much of the effects of aging are due not so much to biological as to psychological, social, and political causes. His skillful assertion of the negative impact of agism is complemented by useful information on topics such as: bereavement, dignity, exercise, leisure, diet, religion, and nursing homes. An essential book for those who want to understand the kind of context within which natural aging may occur.

Curtin, Sharon R. **Nobody Ever Died of Old Age.** Boston: Little, Brown, 1972.

> This extremely compelling book deals in a striking fashion with the way the United States treats its elderly. Ms. Curtin shares her own respect for elderly family members and for the elderly she cared for and learned from in California and New York City. This book, which is extremely effective in illuminating the needs and possibilities of the later years, is superb reading for elders and health professionals alike.

Dangott, Lillian, and Kalish, Richard A. **A Time to Enjoy: The Pleasures of Aging.** Englewood Cliffs, N.J.: Prentice Hall/Spectrum, 1979.

> This easy-to-read upbeat book emphasizes the social and psychological dimensions of aging and health for both the elderly and health professionals. Key themes are: positive approaches to health, a review of aging research, taking responsibility for one's life, and the pleasures and benefits of growing older.

de Beauvoir, Simone. **The Coming of Age.** New York: Warner Publications, 1973.

> In this book, Simone de Beauvoir presents a comprehensive discussion of the ways aging has been viewed by numerous cultures throughout history. She examines the in-

dividual, psychological, and social dynamics of aging, presents a moving argument on the predicament of old people, and suggests numerous alternatives to a negative view and experience of aging. This book is vast in scope and can be read cover-to-cover or simply used as a cross-cultural reference source for a deeper understanding of the historical context of aging.

Dychtwald, Ken. **Bodymind.** New York: Jove, 1978.

The holistic health and human potential fields have given birth to a variety of techniques and philosophies that suggest direct and integrated relationships between the mind and body. In this comprehensive and easy-to-read book, Dr. Dychtwald presents an overview of many techniques for bodymind development and explains ways in which the life of the mind—feelings, thoughts, and attitudes—directly influence and shape the forms and patterns the body opts for as it ages. This book serves as an effective introduction to many dimensions of holistic health, alternative health care practices, and bodywork methods.

Ellison, Jerome. **Life's Second Half: The Pleasures of Aging.** Old Greenwich, Conn.: Devin-Adair, 1978.

Jerome Ellison is the founder of the Phoenix Society, which is a rapidly growing national society of elders who meet in small groups for purposes of discussion, reflection, and personal growth. A former editor of *Life* and *Reader's Digest,* Ellison, himself in his seventies, proposes a positive program for making the best of the later years. Written in a very practical and up-beat fashion, *Life's Second Half* covers a variety of topics, such as "Later Life Fulfillment," "Victory over Rage," "Do you Run your Body or Does it Run You?" and "Our Connection with the Infinite." This book makes an excellent resource for elders and for health professionals interested in exploring some of the most significant physical, psychological, and social issues that older people face today.

Erikson, Erik H. **Adulthood.** New York: W. W. Norton, 1978.

Erik Erikson is one of the great elder philosophers and thinkers of our time. In this stimulating book, he draws together a fascinating collection of essays on a wide range of issues related to aging and adulthood. In one chapter he summarizes the discussion of the life stages that he presented in *Childhood and Society* (New York: W. W. Norton, 1963). In addition, this book presents an international perspective on aging. Chapters include: Searching for Adulthood in America, The Promise of Adulthood in Japanese Spiritualism, Christian Adulthood, and The Confucian Perception of Adulthood. A highly provocative and well-edited reader, *Adulthood* should prove invaluable to anyone interested in exploring cross-cultural perspectives on aging.

Geba, Bruno. **Breathe Away Your Tension.** New York: Random House/Bookworks, 1973.

Breathing can be an effective tool for relaxation, stress reduction, and the general physical and mental stimulation that comes with increased oxygenation. In this simple, easy-to-follow guidebook, Dr. Geba presents a practical course in breathing instruction that will be useful to both health practitioners and elders.

Geba, Bruno. **Vitality Training for Older Adults.** New York: Random House/ Bookworks, 1974.

> Dr. Geba believes that an optimistic vital attitude toward life combined with the regular practice of relaxation, stretching, and vitalizing exercises will help promote health and well-being in the older adult. This book serves as a practical guide for clinicians who are interested in creating such a program. At times simplistic, it does provide good suggestions for developing a supportive relationship between the "teacher" and "student," teaching massage, breathing, and movement exercises, and encouraging the older "student" to assume greater responsibility for his or her life.

Harris, Raymond, and Frankel, Lawrence. **Guide to Fitness After 50.** New York: Plenum Press, 1978.

> Unquestionably the best book on fitness for the older adult, this comprehensive and research-oriented anthology intelligently covers such topics as fitness and the aging process, public health and fitness, exercises for the elderly, and the organization of exercise programs. It is an extremely valuable resource and reference book for most issues related to elderly exercise and fitness, which in addition explains, demonstrates, and illustrates several well-tested exercise programs.

Hendricks, Jon, and Hendricks, C. Davis. **Aging in Mass Society: Myths and Realities.** Cambridge, Mass.: Winthrop, 1977.

> This intelligently researched and comprehensive book deals with aging in historical context, demography and aging, theories of social gerontology, family relations in later life, and the elderly of tomorrow. While it is probably not appropriate for introductory work in gerontology, the book does provide an extremely sophisticated analysis of the social and psychological aspects of aging for the more advanced student or professional.

The Humanist, September/October, 1977. **47 (5).**

> This issue of *The Humanist* is devoted entirely to topics related to aging and the elderly. It is well conceived and easy to read. Themes covered include: the revolution of age, fulfillments in the later years, environments for older persons, and the economic status of the elderly. Highly recommended as a practical resource issue.

Jung, Carl G., with Jaffe, Aniela. **Memories, Dreams, Reflections.** New York: Vintage Books, 1965.

> Carl Jung was one of the most creative and influential thinkers, philosophers, and psychotherapists of our time. His work departed from the Freudian school partly because of his insistence that the spiritual life of the individual be included within the therapeutic context. Drawn from notes, letters, and journal entries, this book presents a fascinating glimpse into the personal life and mind of this remarkable man. In it, Jung shares his deepest feelings about life, relationships, love, God, aging, and death. Its treatment of the psychological and spiritual possibilities of the second half of life make it particularly enlightening for both elderly people and health professionals.

Kalish, Richard A. **Later Life: Applying Social Gerontology.** Monterey, Calif.: Brooks/Cole, 1977.

An excellent and highly informative reader in the area of social gerontology. Instead of addressing only the limitation and pathology frequently associated with aging, Dr. Kalish focuses on the physical, psychological, and social potentials inherent in the aging process. Including the work of an impressive assortment of contributors, this book covers a wide range of significant topics and themes that include demography, health, ethnicity, the family, and the criminal victimization of the elderly. An essential book for understanding the social context of aging.

Kuhn, Maggie, and Hessel, Dieter. **Maggie Kuhn on Aging**. Philadelphia: Westminster Press, 1977.

Maggie Kuhn is cofounder and chief spokesperson for the Gray Panthers, a national coalition of old and young people whose aim is to root out and eliminate agism in America. This radical group, now numbering 10,000 active members, has gone a long way to raise this country's consciousness about various issues related to aging, including mandatory retirement, myths of aging, sexuality, health care, life design, political advocacy, and intergenerational living. This book offers a stimulating and at times brilliant collection of Ms. Kuhn's lectures and workshops on these topics. Its passion and sensitivity provide a good balance to some of the more academic research-oriented texts on aging. Excellent for lay people and professionals.

Luce, Gay. **Your Second Life.** New York: Seymour Lawrence/Delacorte, 1979.

Dr. Luce is the founder of SAGE, the holistic health project for the elderly in Berkeley, California. *Your Second Life* presents an overview of the various clinical, theoretical, and philosophical aspects of this model project. A comprehensive assortment of experiential techniques (such as meditation, relaxation training, autogenics, group leadership, biofeedback, art therapy, and visualization) are effectively presented and demonstrated. An excellent resource for health practitioners interested in applying holistic health practices and techniques to the needs and potentials of the elderly.

New Age Journal, February 1978. **3.**

This issue of *New Age Journal* deals entirely with the new images of aging. As a sign that things have changed and as a source of information about these changes it makes for interesting reading for elders and health professionals alike. Topics covered include the elder within, liberating aging, innovative programs for the elderly, and "An Old Guy Who Feels Good."

Pelletier, Kenneth R. **Mind as Healer, Mind as Slayer: A Holistic Approach to Preventing Stress Disorders.** New York: Delta, 1977.

Perhaps the most practical and intelligent book available on the relationship between life-style, stress, and disease. In this book, Dr. Pelletier reviews the case for a holistic approach to health care. He bases this appeal on the beliefs that all states of health and disease are in some degree psychosomatic; that treating anyone involves treating the unique interaction of mind, body, and spirit in that person; that the patient and healer share responsibility for the healing process; that health care is not the exclusive province of medicine; and that healers must know and use themselves as human beings in the healing relation. In addition, this book includes easy-to-follow explanations of several holistic health methods such as meditation, autogenic training, and visualization. An essential book for any holistic health practitioner.

Samuels, Michael, and Samuels, Nancy. **Seeing with the Mind's Eye.** New York: Random House/Bookworks, 1973.

Visualization can be an effective clinical tool in working with the elderly, to facilitate relaxation, deepen breathing, expand creativity, and vitalize the mind. This is unquestionably the best book available on nearly every aspect of visualization. It is well constructed, easy to follow, and extremely comprehensive. Although it was not written specifically for the older person, it is nevertheless an invaluable resource.

25

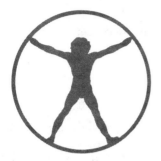

DYING AND DEATH

Charles A. Garfield, Ph.D.

Introduction

People have thought about life and death since Neanderthal times. The fact that "Living with Death" was a cover story of *Newsweek* (May 1, 1978) and that *Time* (June 5, 1978) did a feature story on "A Better Way of Dying" indicates the extent to which dying and death have become concerns to the lay public as well as the health professionals—a surprising development for a culture so often described as death denying. There are a number of reasons for this increasing awareness. Recent advances in innovative medical technology are significantly altering the nature of dying, often compelling the terminally ill to confront years of chronic illness before the actual moment of death. In addition, many postindustrial Americans are alienated from traditional family, religious, and community supports. The results are increased loneliness, anxiety, and self-doubt. Feifel (1977) observes that it is a historic phenomenon that consciousness of death becomes more acute during periods of social disorganization, when individual choice tends to replace automatic conformity to consensual social values. He states:

> With the advent of the H-bomb, physical science has presently made it possible for us all to share a common epitaph. Not only descendance in social immortality but history as well is being menaced. Time along with space can now be annihilated. Even celebration of the tragic will be beyond our power. Death is becoming a wall.

379

Death also has become more difficult to deal with because of its expulsion from daily life. Dying and death are now the responsibility of the "professional" (i.e., physician, nurse, clergyman, and funeral director). Unfortunately, many of us use our technical expertise as a defense against our own death-related anxieties.

Care of the Dying

As physicians, nurses, and allied professionals perfect their skill at providing care and support for the terminally ill, we must continually be aware of the enormity of the emotional trauma confronting our dying patients and their families. It is interesting to realize the word "care" derives from the Gothic *kara*, which means "to lament, to grieve, to experience sorrow, to cry out with." Nouwen (1974) notes that "we tend to look at caring as an attitude of the strong toward the weak, of the powerful toward the powerless, the haves toward the have nots." We often experience great discomfort when we are invited to enter into someone's pain before we have done something about it. But distant concern appears strangely antithetical to the basic component of caring, namely, empathy— the more expressive German translation of which is "einfuhlung," meaning "to feel oneself into." Nouwen continues with the observation that

> when we honestly ask ourselves which persons in our lives mean the most to us, we often find that it is those who instead of giving much advice, solutions, or cures, have chosen rather to share our pain and touch our wounds with a gentle and tender hand. The friend who can be silent with us in a moment of despair or confusion, who can stay with us in an hour of grief and bereavement, who can tolerate not knowing, not curing, not healing and face with us the reality of our powerlessness, that is the friend who cares.

In as emotionally charged an environment as exists in most of our contact with seriously ill patients and their families, attempts at decreased emotional involvement are frequently experienced by patients as painful abandonment. These attempts to remain objective are born of the notion that to become emotionally accessible to one's patients implies a loss of scientific objectivity, a compromising of rational judgment, and a decrease in the time-effective management of one's caseload. When communicated to our students and younger practitioners, this bias serves largely to disallow authentic human communication between helper and patient and prevents the next generation of health providers from mastering the art as well as the science of patient care.

To understand the nature of effective support for dying patients and their families, as health providers we must:

- Realize that role models appropriate to laboratory science are largely inappropriate to the effective emotional support of patients and families facing life-threatening illness. That is, we *are* emotionally involved with our patients and we need to be able to discuss this involvement with our patients and our colleagues in order to maximize the supportive nature of these basically interdependent relationships.

- Recognize that the psychosocial aspects of patient care require a great deal more than "hand holding." Almost without exception, physicians who take the psychological and social issues surrounding life-threatening illness seriously can develop a real mastery of this increasingly important aspect of patient care.
- Examine carefully our own attitudes concerning death and the dying patient and realize that when it comes to a subjective understanding of the nature of the dying process, most patients know a great deal more than those who care for them.

As health professionals, we are often involved in situations in which we are like lifeguards watching our patients flounder in the water several hundred yards off shore. Perhaps the distressed person does not know how to swim or, knowing how, simply does not have enough strength to make it to shore.

Our professional lifeguards, it seems, do not know how to swim themselves. To be sure, they have been given extensive training in many life-saving techniques, all of which they have tested in the children's pool. The know how to row a boat; they know how to throw out a ring buoy; they know how to give artificial respiration. But they do not know how to swim themselves. They cannot save another because, given the same circumstances, they could not save themselves (Carkhuff and Berenson, 1967).

Many of our attempts to understand the emotional realities of dying patients and their families are doomed to failure because we base our approaches on a set of faulty operational assumptions:

- We rely on summary information about the patient's emotional world, that is, notes in the chart or brief word-of-mouth explanations.
- Our values as health professionals are most often firmly rooted in middle-class thinking, making it difficult to comprehend cross-cultural variation in value systems.
- We are unable to effectively incorporate or interpret experiential and behavioral extremes in a meaningful fashion.
- We have great difficulty in dealing with emotional expression (for example, extreme anger, long-term depression, etc.). The somewhat presumptuous yet frequently invoked assessment of the patient's chosen form of expression as "inappropriate affect" is often a signal of our own inability to cope.
- We attempt to deal reasonably with what is most often – from the patient's perspective – an unreasonable life situation.

Our efforts to ignore or disqualify emotional expression, make decisions on the basis of cursory and most often superficial data, and eliminate extremes from the dying patient's emotional life are usually perfectly reasonable yet superficial. Our effectiveness will increase in direct proportion to our capacity to acknowledge the great range of quite normal emotional responses to life-threatening illness and the complexities of psychological functioning and assessment. Increased effectiveness results when we continue to be present to our patients in spite of the fact that the greater portion of their psychological functioning remains a mystery to us.

Feelings about death and the process of dying, like feelings about human sexuality, are very intimate concerns that most people are unwilling to share with those constrained by the scientific rigors of a tightly designed research protocol. As one elderly man dying of lung cancer stated, "I'll be damned if I share my feelings about dying and death with anyone who makes two-minute U-turns at the foot of my bed." To date, no research or systematic clinical observation has verified any preprogramed set of stages in the dying process; that is, researchers and practitioners have not empirically identified any set of linear, unidirectional, and invariant stages. Certainly, many patients who are dying exhibit denial, anger, bargaining, depression, and occasionally acceptance (Kübler-Ross, 1969), but it is inaccurate to suppose that all individuals, regardless of belief system, age, race, culture, and historical period, die in a uniform sequence. It is more likely that existing theoretical frameworks become self-fulfilling prophecies, imposed by health professionals who may coerce the dying person into conforming with a powerfully suggestive typology. All too frequently I have heard health professionals talk about "forcing a patient to move from stage three (bargaining) to stage four (depression) because the patient's condition was deteriorating so fast that he or she might not have time to reach stage five (acceptance)." To needlessly add one more ponderous agenda to a patient's already heavily burdened psyche is an injustice to all concerned. Out of respect and appreciation for Elisabeth Kübler-Ross and her work, I must note that she has made this point many times herself. With regard to all our theoretical models, I am reminded of Aristotle's observation: "Dear is Plato, but dearer still is truth."

In my own research, the major issues identified by the dying patient are (1) that he will become quietly isolated because of a decrease in communication resulting from the unwillingness of those responsible for his care to maintain the openness and emotional support essential for him to live out his life with some hope and participation in meaningful relationships; (2) that he will be subjected to painful, uncomfortable, and demanding procedures that might prolong existence without prolonging a desirable quality of life, and that the disease will force him to endure intense, chronic pain seemingly without end; and (3) that loss of control of bodily, interpersonal, and cognitive functions will compel him to confront a terrifying and alien set of experiences, stripped of all decision-making powers.

I have found the following outline useful in determining and meeting the psychosocial needs of terminal patients.

- With the assistance of the patient, define the major areas of emotional distress.
- Respond to the patient's requests for information with an honest, complete, and accurate presentation of the major aspects of illness and treatment.
- Inform the patient's family of the status of his health so that family members can assume their rightful status as members of the treatment team.
- Make it possible for the patient to be aware of staff expectations concerning treatment, patient-staff relationships, etc., and conversely for the staff to be aware of patient expectations.
- Always compare your perceptions of the patient and his situation with those of your colleagues. It is hazardous to make unilateral judgments about another person's emotional reality.
- Remember that psychosocial evaluation, like medical appraisal, is a continuous process. Two innovations that have proven successful in maintaining ongoing evaluation are (1) the institution of interdisciplinary psychosocial rounds, the specific purpose of which is to evaluate staff success in meeting the emotional needs of all patients (the option of inviting patients to talk to staff about how best to care for them has been a successful aspect of these rounds); and (2) the use of a psychosocial log in which all health providers may record their feelings and thoughts on various aspects of working with seriously ill patients. This log can serve as a catalyst for discussion during psychosocial rounds.

Hospice and Counseling Programs

Two important and creative responses to the needs of dying patients and their families have been the development of the hospice concept and volunteer counseling programs modeled after the SHANTI Project in the San Francisco Bay area. Pioneered successfully throughout England and other European countries, the hospice is seen by some as a major medical innovation in the United States and Canada. SHANTI Project volunteers currently number more than one hundred and are donating nearly 50,000 hours of counseling time per year.

In its most general sense, the hospice is a program that provides palliative and supportive care for terminally ill patients and their families. Originally a medieval name for a way station where pilgrims and travelers could be replenished and cared for, hospice in its current usage denotes a more humane philosophy of care and an organized program of support for dying patients and their families.

Liegner (1974) notes that the key principle of hospice care is reduction of pain; by pain he means not only physical pain but also psychic pain. The reduction of pain in a hospice is effected through several strategies:

- Polypharmacy — the practice of administering medication in doses adequate to keep the patient's pain always below the pain threshold
- Humane treatment and environment
- Psychological and pastoral counseling
- Special attention at the moment of death
- Social services for the bereaved

Ideally, hospices rely on a core of dedicated staff and volunteers. All health providers, physicians, nurses, and auxiliary staff are encouraged to listen carefully to the patient and to share their observations with other staff in the hope of more successfully meeting the physical and emotional needs of the patient.

Projects modeled after the SHANTI Project, often referred to as volunteer hospice programs, are appearing in many parts of the United States and abroad. Requests for volunteer counseling, companionship, and emotional support come from patients, family members, survivors of a death, and members of the health professions. Volunteers provide services to clients free of charge with primary allegiance to the client rather than to any single institutional setting. The project is committed to providing continuity of care for all clients; thus, volunteers continue to work with their clients in the home, general hospital, or extended care facility. After a rigorous screening and selection process, SHANTI Project volunteers go through a comprehensive training program and make a commitment to work at least one year with the project for a period of eight to ten hours per week. A training film for physicians and nurses, "Counseling the Terminally Ill," focusing largely on the work of the SHANTI Project, has been produced under the sponsorship of the National Institute of Mental Health.

National Hospice Organization
765 Prospect Street
New Haven, Connecticut 06511

SHANTI Project
106 Evergreen Lane
Berkeley, California 94705

Near-Death Experiences

A man is dying and, as he reaches the point of greatest physical distress, he hears himself pronounced dead by his doctor. He begins to hear an uncomfortable noise, a loud ringing or buzzing, and at the same time feels himself moving very rapidly through a long dark tunnel. After this he suddenly finds himself outside his own physical body but still in the immediate physical environment, and he sees his own body from a distance, as though he is a spectator. He watches the resuscitation attempt from this unusual vantage point and is in a state of emotional upheaval.

After a while, he collects himself and becomes more accustomed to his odd condition. He notices that he still has a body, but one of a very different nature and with very different powers from the physical body he has left behind. Soon other things begin to happen. Others come to meet and help him. He glimpses the spirits of relatives and friends who have already died, and a loving, warm spirit of a kind he has never encountered before—a being of light—appears before him. This being asks him a question, nonverbally, to make him evaluate his life, and helps him along by showing him a panoramic, instantaneous play back of the major events of his life.

At some point he finds himself approaching some sort of barrier or border, apparently representing the limit between earthly life and the next life. Yet, he finds that he must go back to the earth, that the time for his death has not yet come. At this point he resists, for by now he is taken up with his experiences in the afterlife and does not want to return. He is overwhelmed by intense feelings of joy, love, and peace. Despite his attitude, he somehow reunites with his physical body and lives (Goleman, 1977).

Raymond Moody, Jr., distilled the "normative" near-death experience described above from the 150 anecdotal reports published in his book, *Life After Life* (1975). Moody's composite contains the experiential elements most frequently reported by people in his sample who "had either been resuscitated after being pronounced dead, faced imminent death through injury or illness, or been with individuals who relayed their own experiences as they were dying" (Goleman, 1977). Most fascinating is his observation that these experiences occurred independently of both the individual differences among patients and the events and circumstances that resulted in their brush with death. From his analysis of the data, Moody concluded that the near-death experience profoundly alters a person's consciousness.

Karlis Osis and Erlender Haraldsson (1977) compiled the death-bed observations doctors and nurses in the United States and India made of nearly five hundred dying patients. The most common experience reported by dying patients in this sample had visions of a religious figure or a deceased loved one who came to escort the dying person to another realm.

The near-death experiences reported in the medical and psychological literatures do not appear to be "positive proof of life after death" but rather altered-state experiences not at all specific to the dying process. I have received several letters from women who, in natural childbirth, had very similar experiences. I believe that the near-death experiences described by Moody, Osis and Haraldsson, and others are a subclass of a larger group of altered-state experiences attainable through a variety of techniques and circumstances. In the past two years, I have worked with 173 cancer patients who have subsequently died. I spent an average of three to four hours per week with them for a period ranging from several weeks to almost two years. Among the 21 percent who told me of their altered-state experiences, four groups emerged.

The first group experienced a powerful white light and celestial music (as in Moody's accounts) as well as an encounter with a religious figure or deceased relative (similar to that reported by Osis and Haraldsson). The patients described these as "incredibly real, peaceful, and beautiful." A second group experienced demonic figures, nightmarish images of great lucidity. A third reported dream-like images, sometimes "blissful," sometimes "terrifying," sometimes alternating. The images were not nearly so lucid as those related by the first two groups. However, they appeared to have as great a variation in content. The fourth group experienced the void or a tunnel or both. That is, the patients reported drifting endlessly in outer space or being encapsulated in a limited environment with obvious spatial constraints. A common theme in their accounts was the contrast between maximal freedom and maximal constraint with, in some cases, fluctuation from one to the other.

My work has included interviews with individuals who have had near-death experiences or who have been pronounced clinically dead and then revived. In an effort to evaluate the anectodal reports of Moody, Kübler-Ross, and others, I conducted in-depth interviews with seventy-two intensive-care or coronary-care patients. Since my primary function is to provide basic emotional support, I was often the first person to interact with the patient for an appreciable length of time after his brush with death. My contact occurred anywhere from three hours to two days after the incident. Thirty-six patients reported no memory of the event at all. Their last memory before losing consciousness was of being in their hospital room and when they awoke they were either in the ICU or CCU "hooked up to the hardware." Fourteen reported experiences similar to those collected by Moody, Kübler-Ross, and Osis, including seeing a bright light, hearing "celestial" music, and meeting religious figures or deceased relatives. Eight reported lucid visions of a demonic or nightmarish nature. Eight reported having dreamlike images, four of which were entirely positive and the other four alternating between positive and negative. Six patients reported drifting endlessly in outer space among the planets, cut loose as if thrown from a space ship. No significant changes in content were expressed by any of the patients in three interviews conducted at weekly intervals after the event.

In light of this research, three main observations seem important. First, it appears that not everyone dies a blissful, accepting death. Recently my friend died. Her tortuous, labored breathing during the final twenty-four hours hardly appeared blissful. I hope those who suggest that she was really "feeling no pain" thanks to the "immunity" of the comatose state or because she was really "out of her body" are correct. However, almost as many of the dying patients I interviewed reported negative visions (encounters with demonic figures, etc.) as reported blissful experiences.

Second, Pelletier and Garfield (1976) note that context is a powerful variable in such altered-state experiences as the hypnotic, meditative, psychedelic, and schizophrenic. In keeping with the early LSD research, we might very well find that a caring environment including supportive family, friends, and staff is an important factor in maximizing the likelihood of a positive altered-state experience for the dying. Certainly helping dying patients relate to their experiences in a constructive fashion rather than imposing psychiatric judgment is the more supportive stance. Whatever they represent, those experiences were very important to the dying patients who had them. We need to examine more carefully the impact of context on the dying process, including the quality of advocacy and nonjudgmental caring offered by family and staff. Contextual as well as psychobiological factors may significantly influence the altered-state experiences of the dying patient.

The third observation is, as Kastenbaum (1977) notes:

> The happily, happily theme threatens to draw attention away from the actual situations of the dying person, their loved ones and their care givers over the days, weeks, and months preceding death. What happens up to the point of that fabulous transition from life to death recedes into the background. This could not be more unfortunate.

Will our aversion to death take yet another form and leave us prey to promises of life after death that we cannot integrate emotionally? It is certainly feasible that we run the risk of once again denying death and perhaps biasing our level of care to those who are dying. Will our "knowledge of life after death" leave us in a position to "abandon life-saving efforts for some people, try less hard to save lives at critical moments" (Kastenbaum, 1977)?

Conclusion

> It is hard to have patience with people who say "There is no death" or "death doesn't matter." There is death, and whatever happens has consequences, and it and they are irrevocable and irreversible. You might as well say that birth doesn't matter. I look up at the night sky. Is anything more certain than that in all those vast times and spaces, if I were allowed to search them, I should nowhere find her face, her voice, her touch? She died. She is dead. Is the word so difficult to learn (Lewis, 1963)?

C. S. Lewis astutely observes that whether we view death as annihilation or transition it is a real and often monumental event, an emotional blow associated with a change of form. Those I love in the form I love no longer exist. Those having near-death experiences exuberantly extol the virtues of loving and caring for one's fellow man. So let us have the courage to realize that death often will be a bitter pill to swallow. Our pain will almost always accompany the deaths of those we most love. Our wish will almost always be that help and caring are available.

> Real care is not ambiguous. Real care excludes indifference and is the opposite of apathy. The word "care" finds its roots in the Gothic "kara," which means "to lament." The basic meaning of care is: to grieve, to experience sorrow, to cry out with. I am very much struck by this background of the word care, because we tend to look at caring as an attitude of the strong toward the weak, of the powerful toward the powerless, of the haves toward the have-nots. And, in fact, we feel quite uncomfortable with

an invitation to enter into someone's pain before doing something about it. . . . Still, when we honestly ask ourselves which persons in our lives mean the most to us, we often find that it is those who, instead of giving much advice, solutions, or cures, have chosen rather to share our pain and touch our wounds with a gentle and tender hand. The friend who can be silent with us in a moment of despair or confusion, who can tolerate not knowing, not curing, not healing and face with us the reality of our powerlessness, that is the friend who cares. . . . Our tendency is to run away from the painful realities or to try to change them as soon as possible. But cure without care makes us into rulers, controllers, manipulators, and prevents a real community from taking shape. Cure without care makes us preoccupied with quick changes, impatient and unwilling to share each other's burden. And so cure can often become offending instead of liberating. It is therefore not so strange that cure is not seldom refused by people in need. . . . Those who can sit in silence with their fellow man not knowing what to say but knowing that they should be there, can bring new life in a dying heart. Those who are not afraid to hold a hand in gratitude, to shed tears in grief, and to let a sigh of distress arise straight from the heart can break through paralyzing boundaries and witness the birth of a new fellowship, the fellowship of the broken (Nouwen, 1974).

References

Carkhuff, R., and Berenson, B. *Beyond the Counseling and Therapy.* New York: Holt, Rinehart and Winston, 1967.

Feifel, Herman. *New Meanings of Death.* New York: McGraw-Hill, 1977

Goleman, D. Back from the brink. *Psychology Today,* April 1977. **10**, 56–59.

Kastenbaum, Robert. Temptations from the ever after. *Human Behavior,* 1977. **6** (1), 28–33.

Kübler-Ross, Elisabeth. *On Death and Dying.* New York: Macmillan, 1969.

Lewis, C. S. *A Grief Observed.* New York: Seabury Press, 1963.

Liegner, L. St. Christopher's hospice, care of the dying patient. *Journal of the American Medical Association,* 1974. **234**, 1047–1048.

Moody, Raymond. *Life After Life.* Atlanta: Mockingbird Books, 1975.

Nouwen, Henri. *Out of Solitude.* Notre Dame, Ind.: Ave Maria Press, 1974.

Osis, Karlis, and Haraldsson, Erlender. *At the Hour of Death.* New York: Avon Books, 1977.

Pelletier, Kenneth R., and Garfield, Charles. *Consciousness East and West.* New York: Harper and Row, 1976.

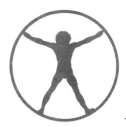 ANNOTATED BIBLIOGRAPHY

Becker, Ernest. **The Denial of Death.** New York: The Free Press, 1973.

In the first three chapters of this Pulitzer Prize–winning work, the author develops the thesis that man's innate fear of death is a principal source of his activity. In brilliant fashion, he develops the notion that the suppression of our innate vulnerability provides our major source of energy. Although the remainder of the book covers such topics as mental illness and especially the psychoanalytic theories of Otto Rank, the initial section is one of the best analyses of the relationship among dying, death, and the human condition.

de Beauvoir, Simone. **A Very Easy Death.** Harmondsworth: Penguin Books, 1969.

An insightful and moving account of her mother's death. I recommend it for its accurate description of the inexorable humiliation of a proud woman during a dying process that was far more tortuous than easy. The daughter's conflicting experiences of anger and affection in the face of her mother's death are superb and constitute an exposition of some of the experiences of a prototypic survivor.

Feifel, Herman (Ed.). **New Meanings of Death.** New York: McGraw-Hill, 1977.

This anthology is an update of the editor's influential work, *The Meaning of Death*, published in 1959. It examines the historical, sociological, psychological, developmental, and clinical aspects of death and dying. Some of the leaders in the field examine such topics as death and development through the life span, meanings of death to children, death and the physician, nurses and the human experience of dying, preparation for death, death education, and the relationship of death to immortality, the law, and poetry. This is an interesting collection of papers suitable for students, academicians, and clinicians.

Garfield, Charles A. **Psychosocial Care of the Dying Patient.** New York: McGraw-Hill, 1978.

This anthology is directed specifically at all physicians, nurses, and allied health professionals who work with dying patients and their families. It is intended as a resource text for clinicians to assist in identifying the emotional needs of the dying patient and family and to suggest helpful ways of providing the necessary support. A more ambitious intent is to identify the entire area of basic emotional support for patients and families as a legitimate and vital concern for any fully competent health professional. Topics covered include guidelines for terminal patient care, patients and families facing life-threatening illness, doctor-patient relationships, psychological needs of the terminally ill, counseling the patient's family, bioethical issues, the development of the SHANTI Project and the hospice movement.

Garfield, Charles A. **Stress and Survival: The Emotional Realities of Life-Threatening Illness.** St. Louis: Mosby, 1979.

This anthology is intended for physicians, nurses, and allied health professionals who provide support for patients and families facing life-threatening illness. A basic premise of the book is that one or more such supportive presences can markedly influence the patient's level of stress, will to live, and possibility of survival. The primary purposes of the book are: (1) in the words of Terrence Des Pres in his book *The Survivor,* "To understand the capacity of men and women to live beneath the pressure of protracted crisis, to sustain terrible damage in mind and body, and yet be there, sane, alive, still human"; (2) to offer insights into the ways that emotional support may be instrumental in promoting quality of life, longevity, and, at times, survival; and (3) to examine closely the optimal ways of providing emotional support to patients and families facing life-threatening illness. The topics include psychosocial elements of survival, the relation of social and psychological factors to illness, new dimensions in the alleviation of stress, emotional impact on health professional and patient, personal encounters with life-threatening illness, the chronically ill child, understanding pain and suffering, and care of the dying patient.

Glaser, Barney, and Strauss, Anselm. **Awareness of Dying.** Chicago: Aldine, 1965.

The best of the sociological studies available on the subject of dying. The data gathered for this book came from considerable field work in a variety of hospital settings. Perhaps the most important theoretical concept is that of varying contexts of awareness of death that exist in the hospital social system. This book will be of interest to hospital clinicians interested in understanding the impact of the hospital itself on staff, patients, and families.

Kastenbaum, Robert, and Aisenberg, Ruth. **The Psychology of Death.** New York: Springer Publishing, 1972.

This book is one of the most informative and interesting on the psychology of death. It is a scholarly work that combines original thought and the best research and thinking available. It contains enlightening analyses of historical, cultural, societal, developmental, and clinical issues involved in understanding the psychological aspects of dying and death.

Kübler-Ross, Elisabeth. **On Death and Dying.** New York: Macmillan, 1969.

This popular work has had more circulation than any other book in the field. It is a caring and humane analysis of the needs of the dying patient with practical advice for all those who provide care. Although Dr. Kübler-Ross's "five stage" model has been repudiated by most major thinkers in the field, this book should be regarded as a helpful and compassionate guide for clinicians.

Lewis, C. S. **A Grief Observed.** New York: Seabury Press, 1963.

"No one ever told me that grief felt so much like fear." So begins an extraordinarily honest and revealing exposé of the grief of this well-known writer-philosopher. Originally written as a self-therapy journal without plans for publication, this powerful little book provides a superb first-hand account of the existential and emotional plight of an individual who has lost the most important person in his world. I highly recommend this book as a resource in providing a humane balance to the more clinical literature on grief and bereavement.

Lund, Doris. **Eric.** Philadelphia: J. B. Lippincott, 1974.

This book is the product of a mother's ardous task of writing about the death of her seventeen-year-old son from acute leukemia. It is an inspiring and lovingly written story of a boy who challenged his illness and its insidious effects by living powerfully and creatively in the face of death. It will be of assistance to those clinicians who need to understand the plight of the parent in life-threatening illness and also provides a balance to the more detached clinical literature.

Parkes, Colin Murray. **Bereavement.** New York: Penguin, 1972.

This work is the result of a comprehensive study of adult grief and its impact. It is a scholarly work of use to those interested in more than a clinical distillation of grief reactions and their symptoms. Included are suggestions for helping the bereaved and understanding the psychological processes involved in coping with the loss of a loved one.

Rosenthal, Ted. **How Could I Not Be Among You?** New York: Braziller, 1973.

This is a collection of some extremely moving poetry and prose from Ted Rosenthal, a Berkeley poet, who discovered at the age of thirty that he was dying of acute leukemia. He powerfully shares the emotional realities confronting the dying patient by examining his life in general. At rock bottom, he becomes aware of the psychic outrageousness of "ceasing to be" and the emotionally unfathomable question, "How could I not be among you?" This book is highly recommended for anyone attempting to understand the existential drama confronting the dying patient.

Shneidman, Edwin. **Deaths of Man.** New York: Quadrangle/New York Times, 1973.

An extremely well-written analysis of death including some innovative ideas of considerable interest. This is a psychologically sophisticated work of interest to scholars and others interested in the impact and the implications of death for the human psyche. The author includes some of his own concepts such as survivor-victims and their assistance by postvention, subintentioned death, and the effects of megadeath.

Weisman, Avery. **On Dying and Denying.** New York: Behavioral Publications, 1972.

This scholarly work, based on some of the best research available, concentrates on the central role of denial in the dying process. The book contains some excellent clinical case material and is best suited for those with more than an elementary understanding of psychological processes.

Part Five

ALTERNATIVE MEDICAL PERSPECTIVES

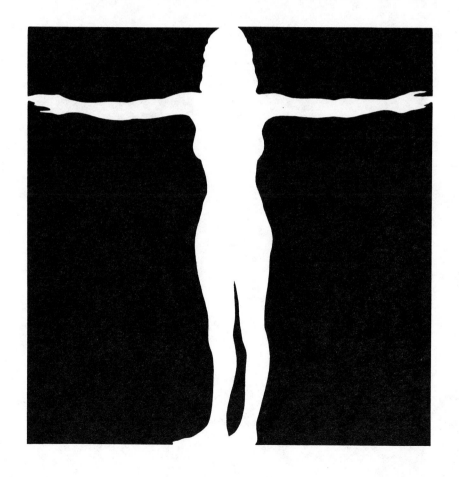

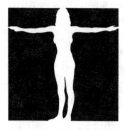

HOMOEOPATHIC MEDICINE

Harris L. Coulter, Ph.D.

Homoeopathy is a holistic form of pharmacological therapeutics developed in the early 1800s by the German physician Samuel Hahnemann (1755–1843). Although it was the culmination of the empirical[1] (holistic) tradition in Western medical thought, homoeopathy represents an original formulation of this tradition and deserves consideration as such.

When homoeopathy was first introduced into medicine by Hahnemann in the early nineteenth century, the pronounced doctrinal contrast with conventional medicine gave rise to the opinion that homoeopathy was "unscientific" and, in fact, quackery. Medicine in the United States from the mid-nineteenth to the early twentieth century saw an intense conflict between the allopaths, represented by the American Medical Association, and the homoeopaths, represented by the American Institute of Homoeopathy. Any physician deciding to accept homoeopathic practice was expelled from his local medical society and from the AMA, and the latter's code of ethics forbade any professional relations between homoeopaths and allopaths. In spite of this opposition, throughout the nineteenth century homoeopathy gained strength until, by 1900, about 10 percent of the medical profession called itself homoeopathic. In 1903 the AMA did revise its code of ethics to permit homoeopaths to become members. Thereafter this movement declined as the allopathic physicians, adopting the reforms introduced and popularized by homoeopathy, humanized themselves and became more acceptable to the patient.

The last ten years have seen a true resurgence of homoeopathy in the United States, due primarily to the public's dissatisfaction with conventional medicine and its desire for an alternative. Conditions today, in fact, resemble those of the 1830s when homoeopathy was first introduced into this country, and the nineteenth-century history of homoeopathy may serve as a blueprint for the immediate future of homoeopathy today.

Hahnemann's discovery of the principles of homoeopathy was the consequence of his dissatisfaction with the existing system of practice. Physicians in his day (as those of today) thought they possessed the capacity to isolate the disease "cause" inside the body and then to annihilate it by applying a medicine of "contrary" quality (like the modern antibiotic). In his numerous writings Hahnemann held that the disease "cause," inside the body but separate from it, was a mere figment of the imagination, impossible to isolate, and not treatable through application of a "contrary" remedy. His effort to elaborate a system of therapeutics that was not oriented toward a single "cause" inside the body represents the first systematic holistic therapeutics in the Western medical tradition.

The key to Hahneman's discovery of the homoeopathic system was provided by the principle of "similars" – in other words, that "likes are cured by likes." He wondered why malaria – characterized by chills and fever coming on with a certain periodicity – was often cured by the bark of the cinchona tree (containing quinine). As an experiment he took a quantity of this medicine over several days and found that under its influence he manifested chills and fever with the same periodicity as in malaria. This led him to the idea that quinine is curative in malaria through its "similarity" – meaning that, when administered to a healthy person, quinine gives rise to the typical symptom pattern of malaria.[2]

If this principle was correct, Hahnemann had found a direct relationship between medicines and the diseased conditions in which they act curatively. If a medicinal drug (or, as it later appeared, any substance from the animal, vegetable, or mineral worlds) is suitably prepared and administered systematically to healthy persons, it will give rise to a typical symptom pattern, one peculiar to that substance and differing from the symptom patterns of all other substances in the world. This symptom pattern is the guide to the disease conditions in which this substance has a curative effect. Even though Hahnemann did not call his approach "holistic," it can readily be seen to have been precisely that – a matching of the "whole" symptom pattern of the curative substance with the "whole" symptom pattern of the sick person.

In his lifetime Hahnemann investigated the effects of ninety-nine different substances on himself, the members of his family, and his followers. Since that time more than one thousand different substances have been investigated in this way by members of the homoeopathic school, and the records of these "provings" (from the German *Pruefung,* a trial or test) constitute the basic literature of homoeopathy.

A point of considerable interest to persons desiring to introduce holistic ways of thinking into medicine is the homoeopathic emphasis on the "strange, rare, and peculiar symptom." These physicians have found the unusual and unique symptoms, both in the symptomatic description of the patient and in that of the "proving," to be more useful characterizations of the remedy then the common symptoms that are encountered in many different diseased conditions and many different remedies. Homoeopathy holds that the key to the "wholeness" of the patient and of the remedy is found in their peculiarities or idiosyncrasies—in other words, in the factors that distinguish *this* patient and *this* remedy from other patients and other remedies that are similar but not the same as *this* one. Homoeopathy thereby incorporates into its method and, in fact, regards as invaluable those data that are usually discarded in conventional medical practice as representing the fleeting play of symptoms or the idiosyncratic peculiarities of the patient—such symptoms as "chilliness even during high fever" or "prostrating headache at the base of the brain, sometimes relieved by profuse urination."

Hahnemann thus aligned homoeopathic doctrine with an idea current in Western medicine since ancient times—symptoms can be divided into common (Latin, *communia*) and peculiar (Latin, *propria*) categories, with the latter symptoms being more useful than the former for diagnosis and treatment. Hahnemann inherited this concept from his empirical forebears; however, he provided it with a firm basis in method through the "proving." In the course of a "proving," the symptoms recorded by most or all of the "provers" and that, moreover, resemble the symptoms recorded in the "provings" of other remedies, are considered to be "common." The symptoms recorded by only a few of the "provers" and that are not found in the "provings" of other substances, are considered "strange, rare, and peculiar" in homoeopathy.

The importance of this analysis of symptoms for the definition of a holistic method in medicine can hardly be overestimated. The holistic dimension of the patient—as with the remedy—is described by the *peculiar* symptoms, those that set *this* patient and *this* remedy apart from others, not by those symptoms that *this* patient has in common with others.

Another holistic feature of homoeopathy is its concept of the "constitutional remedy." For each person there is a remedy matching his constitutional type, a remedy that will be indicated in whatever illness that person may have. Homoeopathic experience demonstrates that a person will manifest somewhat the same set of peculiar and idiosyncratic symptoms from whatever "disease" he may have. Consequently, his "constitutional remedy" will figure among the remedies indicated as part of the treatment whenever this person falls ill and regardless of the name given to his "disease" by conventional medicine.

While the heart of the homoeopathic doctrine is the matching of the patient's symptom pattern with that of the remedy—known as "treatment by similars"—Hahnemann proposed two additional rules: (1) the single remedy, and (2) the minimum dose. Treatment is through matching the "whole" remedy with the patient's whole set of symptoms. It would be incorrect to prescribe two or more medicines simultaneously—each for a part of the patient's symptom syndrome. Every remedy affects the patient as a whole organism, even though it may seem to have a selective effect on only one organ or function. Hence, when two or more medicines are administered simultaneously, they will have a synergistic effect that is unknown to the prescriber and not described in the homoeopathic books. While such multiple preparations exist, they represent a dilution of homoeopathic practice and a movement toward conventional medical thinking.

Thus homoeopathic treatment is not "symptomatic." Medicines are prescribed not to "remove" symptoms but to stimulate the healing powers of the organism along the correct lines. As the healing process proceeds, the symptoms disappear. Symptom analysis is only a way to discover the one remedy whose wholeness most closely matches the wholeness of the sick person and that is thus capable of initiating and maintaining the healing process.

Hahnemann's third principle, the minimum dose, held that medicine should be prescribed in a dose just sufficient to bring about the desired effect. The rationale of this principle is clear enough. When medicines are given according to the principle of "similars," they initially arouse in the patient a set of symptoms similar to the ones he is already manifesting. In other words, they exacerbate his existing condition. If the dose is too large, the exacerbation may be prolonged and violent. The minimum dose is that which arouses the necessary reaction but does not exaggerate it (like finding a skin test of the correct strength in allergy diagnosis).

Homoeopathic physicians have discovered by experience that medicine can be diluted to levels that appear inconceivable and incomprehensible to others, while still retaining their capacity to influence the organism toward cure. This use of the "high dilutions" is, in the public eye, one hallmark of homoeopathy and has been one of the principal points of confusion about homoeopathic practice. Homoeopaths have not resorted to the "high dilutions" out of perversity or to distinguish themselves from other physicians, but only because the experience of generations of homoeopathic physicians has dictated the necessity and validity of using such "high dilutions" to avoid harm to the patient. It must be emphasized that the "high dilutions" were an empirical discovery of Hahnemann's and are not an integral part of the homoeopathic doctrine.

This whole question is made more complex by two associated findings: (1) that medicines can be diluted even beyond the Avogadro Limit[3] and still retain their ability to affect the organism, and (2) that the dilution process actually *increases* the power of the medicine – especially beyond the Avogadro Limit. The less diluted doses are thought to act exclusively upon the physical plane and for a relatively short time, while the higher dilutions are thought to affect the mind as well as the body and to act for a longer time, but the problem of dose size remains to be worked out in many of its details (Boyd, 1954; Stephenson, 1955).

While the principles of homoeopathy are relatively few and easily mastered in theory, homoeopathic practice is extremely difficult, requiring a considerable talent for observation and the ability to remember the salient features of many dozens of remedies. The faculty of observation is not highly developed in modern Western medicine, and the would-be homoeopath thus starts at a disadvantage. The ability to question the patient carefully and thoroughly is also a learned art. Since the physician is searching for the peculiar and idiosyncratic symptoms of the patient (while not neglecting the common ones), he cannot be content with a cursory history but must penetrate into the difference between *this* patient and all others. Hahnemann (1974) advised his followers: "Each case of disease that presents itself must be regarded (and treated) as an individual malady that never before occurred in the same manner and under the same circumstances as in the case before, and will never again happen in precisely the same way."

When the physician has a record of the patient's symptoms, he compares them with the data from the provings. These materials, which constitute the basic materials of homoeopathy, have been gathered together in two major compendiums: Constantine Hering's *Guiding Symptoms of Our Materia Medica* (ten volumes, 1879-1891) and Timothy Field Allen's *Encyclopedia of Pure Materia Medica* (eleven volumes, 1874-1880). Another essential aid to practice is James Tyler Kent's *Repertory of the Homoeopathic Materia Medica* (first published in the 1890s). While the Allen and Hering compendiums list the symptoms pertaining to the parts of the body and physiological functions under the remedy name as the principal heading, the Kent *Repertory* is structured according to the parts of the body and functions affected, with the remedy names secondary. Thus they complement each other and together permit the practitioner to take as his starting point either the remedy or the part of the body affected.

Although the practitioner will always have these and other works available, he must make an effort to learn the major symptoms of the one or two hundred most commonly used remedies. This labor of study and memorization has always been an obstacle in the path of those who want to practice homoeopathy. The reward and compensation, of course, lie in the therapeutic results–which, in skilled hands, are strikingly good and indeed are better than the practitioner will be able to achieve using any other type of therapy. It is this that has kept homoeopathy alive and vigorous in most countries of the world–even though a minority movement in medicine–for almost two centuries.

Since preventive medicine and health enhancement are important aspects of holistic health practices, the value of homoeopathy in these areas is worth noting. Implicit in the concept of the "constitutional remedy," discussed above, is the idea that the individual tends to be sick in much the same way, whatever the name of his "disease." By the same token, he will manifest much the same pattern of symptoms, although in a modified and less striking form, even in health. It follows that prescribing the "constitutional remedy" in health has a protective or prophylactic effect, and homoeopathic patients usually visit their physicians regularly even when in good health in order to be prescribed their constitutional remedy. Homoeopathic techniques can also be combined with such other methods of health enhancement as regulation of diet, exercise, and yoga.

From the above it is clear that homoeopathy is radically different from conventional medicine (known to homoeopaths as "allopathy") in its use of drugs for healing. These differences (which have been analyzed in the author's *Divided Legacy*) reflect the differences between a holistic and a reductionist medicine, between a medicine that seeks to keep the whole body in view at all times and one that pursues the hypothesized disease "cause" through the body's fluids, solids, and interstices.

Of particular importance to contemporary orthodox medicine is the homoeopathic doctrine that much chronic disease is due to the incorrect treatment of prior acute illness—leading to its suppression and eventual emergence in a chronic form. This topic is gradually coming to the fore in the allopathic medical literature, and homoeopathic experience could shed much light on it.

Notes

1. For an account of the empirical tradition in medicine prior to Hahnemann, see the author's *Divided Legacy: A History of the Schism in Medical Thought* (Volumes 1 and 2). Washington, D.C.: Wehawken, 1975 (vol. 1), 1977 (vol. 2).

2. Hahnemann's account of his experiment with quinine was accepted by nineteenth-century pharmacologists even though it has been rejected by some in the twentieth century. [See L. Lewin, *Die Nebenwirkungen der Arzneimittel* (3rd ed.). Berlin: August Hirschwald, 1899. 421–422.] Pharmacologists today complain that the mode of action of quinine remains unexplained.

3. The Avogadro Limit or Avogadro Constant is named after Amadeo Avogadro (1766–1856), who discovered that one gram mole of any substance contains about 6.06×10^{-23} molecules. Thus if a homoeopathic remedy is diluted to 10^{-24} or beyond (the 24x potency), there is little probability that a single molecule of the original medicinal substance will remain in the dilution.

References

Boyd, W. E. Biochemical and biological evidence of the activity of high potencies. *British Homoeopathic Journal*, 1954. **44** (1), 6–44. (Reprinted in *Journal of the American Institute of Homeopathy*, 1969. **62** (4), 199–251.)

Hahnemann, Samuel. *Organon of Medicine* (6th ed.) (William Boericke, Trans.). New Delhi: Harjeet, 1974.

Stephenson, James. A review of investigations into the action of substances in dilutions greater than 1×10^{-24} (microdilutions). *Journal of the American Institute of Homeopathy*, 1955. **48** (11), 327–335.

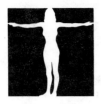 ANNOTATED BIBLIOGRAPHY

History and Philosophy for Physicians and Laymen

Coulter, Harris L. **Homoeopathic Medicine.** St. Louis: Formur, 1972.

> A concise account of homoeopathic philosophy and method, using the language of modern scientific method.

Coulter, Harris L. **Divided Legacy: A History of the Schism in Medical Thought.** Washington, D.C.: Wehawken Book Company. (Vol. 1, **The Patterns Emerge: from Hippocrates to Paracelsus,** 1975; Vol. 2, **Progress and Regress: J. B. VanHelmont to Claude Bernard,** 1977; Vol. 3, **Science and Ethics in American Medicine, 1800–1920,** 1973.)

> These books trace the history of the conflict between rationalist (reductionist) and empirical (holistic) medicine from ancient Greece to the early twentieth century. The history of medicine is presented as a history of ideas, using as materials the writings of the most eminent medical thinkers of the Western tradition. In Volume 2 homoeopathy is discussed as the most recent form of empirical (holistic) pharmacological medicine. Volume 3 is a history of nineteenth-century homoeopathy in the United States.

Hahnemann, Samuel. **Organon of Medicine** (6th ed.) (William Boericke, Trans.). New Delhi: Harjeet, 1974.

> The first and most comprehensive statement of homoeopathic philosophy, *Organon* was initially published in 1810 and since then has been translated into sixteen languages and published in eighteen countries in 115 editions. Several modern English translations are available. Although the language may at times seem a little old-fashioned, the concepts are entirely up-to-date. This work is as relevant today as the year it was first published. Harjeet and Co. is located at P.O. Box 5752, New Delhi, 110055, India.

Kent, James T. **Lectures on Homoeopathic Philosophy.** Calcutta: Sett Day, 1961.

> Thirty-seven lectures delivered to homoeopathic medical students by the man who

was one of the two greatest figures in U.S. homoeopathy. These lectures are in the form of comments on the sections of Hahnemann's *Organon* and are an elaboration of Hahnemann's teachings. Again, while the language may be a little out-of-date, the concepts retain their pristine freshness.

Roberts, Herbert A. **The Principles and Art of Cure by Homoeopathy.** London: Homoeopathic Publishing Co., 1936.

A somewhat pedestrian but comprehensive introduction – at the advanced level – to homoeopathic philosophy and practice by one of the United States's leading practitioners of the older generation. Important areas covered are the second prescription, suppression, the law of palliation, local applications, and the chronic diseases.

Materials for Beginning Students of Homoeopathy

Anderson, David; Buegel, Dale; and Chernin, Dennis. **Homoeopathic Remedies for Physicians, Laymen, and Therapists.** Honesdale, Pa.: Himalayan International Institute, 1978.

A recent publication by three young U.S. homoeopaths in three sections: (1) Principles of Homoeopathy, Remedy Selection, and Second Prescription; (2) Clinical Repertory (arranged according to allopathic disease categories); (3) Materia Medica (twenty-five homoeopathic remedies and eight biochemical remedies).

Clarke, John H. **The Prescriber** (9th ed.). Devon, England: Health Science Press, 1972.

About 500 remedies are discussed in this very handy pocket-sized guide. The subject matter is arranged according to the allopathic disease names, with the appropriate homoeopathic remedies given for the varieties and subvarieties of the allopathic "diseases." While this is not the best type of homoeopathy, it is easily understood by persons trained in the allopathic approach. Of particular value is the 69-page introduction discussing such topics as kinds and degrees of "similarity," the *genus epidemicus*, indications from heredity and history, differences among the principal homoeopathic repertories, etc.

Gibson, D. M. **First-Aid Homoeopathy in Accidents and Ailments.** London: British Homoeopathic Association, 1977.

A simple guide to the use of a limited number of remedies in emergency situations.

Shadman, Alonzo. **Who is Your Doctor and Why?** Boston: House of Edinboro, 1958.

This fire-breathing book by a physician who for many years conducted a homoeopathic hospital in the vicinity of Boston makes very exciting reading, as the author is unsparing in his criticism of almost all aspects of conventional medicine. The last 200 pages are reprints of a series of pamphlets published by the British Homoeopathic Association on the principal remedies and are a useful introduction to prescribing for the beginner.

Sharma, C. H. **A Manual of Homoeopathy and Natural Medicine.** New York: Dutton, 1976.

> An introductory guide to the use of forty-two remedies, this work also discusses the relations between homoeopathy, diet, ayurvedic medicine, and general hygiene.

Shepherd, Dorothy. **Homoeopathy for the First-Aider.** Surrey: Health Science Press, n.d.

> Discusses the use of forty-four remedies in emergency situations.

Shepherd, Dorothy. **The Magic of Minimum Dose.** London: Homoeopathic Publishing Co., 1938.

> An autobiographical account of the author's practice, this book is no less interesting than, and is similar in style to, the popular works by the British veterinarian, James Herriott (*All Creatures Great and Small,* etc.). Some chapters are on particular "diseases," others are on particular remedies.

Vithoulkas, George. **Homeopathy: Medicine of the New Man.** New York: Avon, 1972.

> This short work by a leading Greek practitioner is somewhat inspirational in tone but is very compelling reading nonetheless. It mixes philosophy, history, case histories from James Tyler Kent and others, and quotations from the leading homoeopaths of the past two centuries.

Materials for Advanced Students of Homoeopathy

Allen, Timothy Field. **The Encyclopedia of Pure Materia Medica** (11 vols.). New Delhi: Harjeet, n.d. (Originally published in 1874–1880.)

> The culmination of a lifetime's effort by the author, this work is too bulky and cumbersome to be useful in practice. However, as a compilation of all the symptoms from all the nineteenth-century provings, it is an indispensable reference work. Harjeet and Co. is located at P.O. Box 5752, New Delhi 110055, India.

Baker, Wyrth P., Young, W. W., and Neiswander, A. C. **Introduction to Homoeotherapeutics.** Washington, D.C.: American Institute of Homeopathy, 1974.

> This recent work by three American homoeopaths contains a materia medica of one hundred remedies, a sample repertorization chart, and a repertory. Simpler in format and presentation than other works of this nature, it is particularly suitable for use by the allopathic physician who is commencing the study of homoeopathy.

Blackie, Margery G. **The Patient, Not the Cure.** London: MacDonald and Jane's, 1976.

> A mixture of history, philosophy, and autobiography by the physician to Queen Elizabeth, this book contains much detail on the practical problems of prescribing not found in other similar works. The style and tone are similar to Dorothy Shepherd's *Magic of the Minimum Dose,* and this book makes equally absorbing reading.

Boericke, William. **Materia Medica with Repertory** (9th ed.). Philadelphia: Boericke and Tafel, 1927.

> Of all the short or pocket guides to homoeopathic remedies, this one best strikes the balance between conciseness and comprehensiveness. It is used by all professionals and by advanced laymen as well.

Boyd, W. E. **Biochemical and biological evidence of the activity of high potencies.** *British Homoeopathic Journal,* 1954. **44 (1),** 6–44. (Reprinted in *Journal of the American Institute of Homeopathy,* 1969. **62 (4),** 199–251.)

> This is an account of a six-year experiment to determine if an ultramolecular homoeopathic dilution could manifest a measurable effect under controlled laboratory conditions. The investigation was of the effect of a 61x (10^{-61}) dilution of mercuric chloride on the hydrolysis of soluble starch with malt diastase, and a statistically significant effect was found. Anyone in the future who wants to criticize homoeopathy because of the "high dilutions" must first cope with the results of this experiment.

Clarke, John Henry. **Dictionary of Practical Materia Medica with Clinical Repertory** (4 vols.). London: Homoeopathic Publishing Co., 1925.

> This monumental effort took the author fifteen years and gives information on more than 1,100 remedies. Presenting both the guiding symptoms for use of the remedies and the typical "diseases" in which the remedies are used, this work is especially useful to the allopathic physician commencing the study of homoeopathy.

Hering, Constantine. **The Guiding Symptoms of Our Materia Medica** (10 vols.). New Delhi: Harjeet, 1971. (Originally published in 1879–1891.)

> The life work of the "father of American homoeopathy," these volumes contain a critical selection of the symptoms also set forth in Allen's *Encyclopedia.* After the *Organon* itself and Kent's *Repertory* (see below) this is probably the greatest work produced by the homoeopathic movement. Indispensable for practice. Harjeet and Co. is located at P.O. Box 5752, New Delhi 110055, India.

Hubbard, Elizabeth Wright. **A Brief Study Course in Homoeopathy** (3rd ed.). Bombay: Roy and Co., 1959.

> Seventeen lectures by one of the most prominent modern U.S. practitioners. Concise and to the point, they reflect the character of their author. Very much for the advanced student, these lectures discuss, inter alia, the variable approaches taken by the authors and the differences among the standard repertories.

Kent, James Tyler. **Lectures on Homoeopathic Materia Medica.** New Delhi: Jain, 1971.

> The greatest figure in U.S. homoeopathy after Hering presents vivid, unforgettable symptom-pictures of about three hundred remedies. Kent's graphic style and penetration into the symptomatology of each remedy make this work one of the foundations of homoeopathic education. Available in a number of other editions.

Kent, James Tyler. **Repertory of the Homoeopathic Materia Medica.** New Delhi: Harjeet, 1977.

> One of the classics of world homoeopathy and used today in every country of the world, this volume indexes 630 remedies according to the parts of the body and functions affected. It is thus the indispensable complement to Hering's *Guiding Symptoms* and Allen's *Encyclopedia,* which group all information under the name of the remedy as the leading entry. First published in the 1890s, it has had several editions and numerous reprintings. Harjeet and Co. is located at P.O. Box 5752, New Delhi 110055, India.

Stephenson, James. **A review of investigations into the action of substances in dilutions greater than 1×10^{-24} (microdilutions).** *Journal of the American Institute of Homeopathy,* 1955. **48 (11),** 327–335.

> A valuable literature search of botanical, biological, physical, chemical, and zoological investigations into the action of the homoeopathic high dilutions. This article presents convincing evidence for the existence of a physico-chemical force in these ultramolecular dilutions.

Tyler, Margaret L. **Homoeopathic Drug Pictures.** Rustington, Sussex, England: Health Science Press, 1975.

> Similar to Kent's *Lectures on Homoeopathic Materia Medica* (above), this work is less systematic, more impressionistic, and perhaps more readable. It discusses 125 remedies on the basis of the author's own observations and case histories as well as materials from other sources. Indispensable for the advanced practitioner.

Vithoulkas, George. **The Science of Homeopathy, a Modern Text.** Athens, Greece: Athens School of Homoeopathic Medicine, 1978.

> This is the first of a projected three-volume work on homoeopathic theory and practice. The first section consists of nine chapters on homoeopathic philosophy; the second section contains twelve chapters on practice and is particularly valuable, giving precise data on the long-term management of patients, on the second and third prescriptions, etc., which are not available elsewhere in such a comprehensive form.

Many of the above materials may be purchased from the National Center for Homoeopathy, 6231 Leesburg Pike, Falls Church, Virginia 22044.

Editors' note: The word homeopathy/homoeopathy has been spelled according to the original reference.

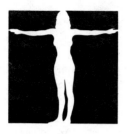

27

CHINESE MEDICINE AND HOLISTIC HEALTH

David E. Bresler, Ph.D.

Introduction

One of the earliest systems of holistic medicine was practiced by the ancient Chinese more than 5,000 years ago. Traditional Chinese medicine did not distinguish between mind and body but viewed physical and mental symptoms as manifestations of a unitary underlying energy imbalance that affected the entire organism. Thousands of years ago, Chinese physicians recognized the critical importance of environmental influences, diet and exercise, and preventive medicine. An ancient aphorism states "the superior physician cures before the illness is manifested. The inferior physician can only treat the illness he was unable to prevent."

Central to the practice of Chinese medicine is acupuncture, a technique that involves the stimulation of specific points on the body, usually by the insertion of tiny, solid needles. The acupuncture points may also be stimulated by using pressure, heat, cold, electricity, ultrasound, and even lasers to achieve therapeutic results. While acupuncture remains a controversial subject in contemporary U.S. medicine, it is routinely used to treat a wide variety of medical problems throughout the Far East, in Great Britain, Eastern and Western Europe, the Soviet Union, and Asia as well. As a medical system, it has endured over the centuries in spite of the tremendous cultural and political changes that have swept the Far East. Though considered "experimental" by many authorities, it has stood the test of time, and it is likely that more individuals have been treated by acupuncture in the course of human history than by all other known systems of medicine combined.

Origins of Chinese Medicine

The traditional Chinese concepts of health and disease are intimately tied to the philosophical constructs of classical Chinese thought. Man is a reflection of the universe, a microcosm in the macrocosm, and both are subject to the same universal, divine law – the law of the Tao. To live according to the Tao is to follow the "order of nature" and to live in harmony with the "ultimate principle." If one does not live according to the Tao, the resulting disharmony may be manifested as physical or psychological disease. Therapy must then be directed toward the re-establishment of balance and harmony if it is to have long-term effectiveness.

The terms yin and yang denote the twin polarities that were thought to regulate both man and the universe (see Table 27.1). Although Taoist philosophy describes yin as "negative" and "female" and yang as "positive" and "male," one should not consider this to be chauvinistic, as the terms "negative" and "positive" are used in the same sense that modern physics describes an electron as "negative"and a proton as "positive." A proton although positive is not superior to an electron! In the same manner, yin and yang refer to the opposing polarities, forces, or tendencies contained in all living entities.

Table 27.1
Polarities of Yang and Yin

Yang	Yin
Positive	Negative
Masculine	Feminine
Active	Passive
Sky	Earth
Sun	Moon
Splendorous	Plain
Hard	Soft
Left	Right
Black	White
Odd	Even
Light	Dark
Warm	Cold
Fullness	Emptiness

Yin and yang exist only in relation to each other, for, as the writings of the ancient Chinese state: "within each yang there exists yin, and within each yin must be yang." Nothing is pure yin or pure yang; there is always some yin and some yang in every living object. Thus, for example, no one is completely male or female; rather, masculinity and feminity are both present in each individual in varying degrees.

Yin and yang forces ebb and flow, and this undulatory nature affects not only individual health and character but all events in the universe. Their pulsation is found in the contraction and dilation of the heart (systole and diastole) and in the inhalation and expiration of the lungs.

Many sinologists have noted yin and yang relationships in the parasympathetic and sympathetic divisions of the autonomic nervous system. Overactivity of the sympathetic nervous system produces what the Chinese call "excess yang" ailments, whereas overactivity of the parasympathetic nervous system produces "excess yin" ailments. Yin and yang may also be reflected by the manner in which blood sugar is regulated by insulin and glycogen and by the way in which central nervous system activation and sleep are regulated by norepinephrine and serotonin.

The goal of Chinese medicine is to maintain or restore balance between yang and yin thus insuring proper health. In Western medicine, the term "homeostasis" refers to a similar concept in which a balance of opposite forces is maintained to insure proper functioning of physiological systems. Thus, it is intriguing to consider the possibility that many "incurable" ailments related to lack of homeostatic balance may someday be routinely treated by acupuncture therapy.

Traditional Theories of Acupuncture

The ancient Chinese discovered that certain loci on the skin, when pressed, punctured, or burned, could be used to alleviate pain, affect the course of certain ailments, and influence the functioning of internal organs. Of particular importance was the fact that widely separated loci affected the functioning of the same organ. These loci were connected and given the name "ching" or "meridian."

Originally, twelve double meridians were described with each pair placed symmetrically on either side of the body. Each meridian corresponded to one of twelve internal organs conceptualized by traditional Chinese medicine. In addition to these twelve paired meridians, two important nonpaired "control" meridians were postulated: the "Governing Vessel," which follows the spine and runs along the midline on the dorsal surface of the body, and the "Conception Vessel," which runs along the midline on the ventral surface of the body. These two plus six less important lines were called the eight "special" meridians. Later, "extra" meridians and "muscle" meridians were added, but in practice, the most commonly used acupuncture loci lie on the twelve main meridians and the two con-

Table 27.2
The Acupuncture Meridians

Yin	Yang
Lung	Large Intestine
Spleen	Stomach
Heart	Small Intestine
Kidney	Bladder
Liver	Gall Bladder
Circulation-Sex	Tri-Heater

trol meridians. The Chinese divided the twelve meridians into six yin-yang pairs representing the twelve traditional internal bodily functions (see Table 27.2). Two of these meridians are obscure to Western medicine: the "circulation-sex" (also called the "heart constrictor" or "pericardium") meridian probably relates to the endocrine system, while the "tri-heater" (also called the "triple warmer") meridian relates to the "heat" of respiration, digestion, and reproduction.

Unlike Western medicine, the ancient Chinese healing arts were not based on a knowledge of human anatomy. The Chinese worshiped their ancestors, so gross dissection of a cadaver was unthinkable. Instead, the Chinese system of medicine was based on an energetic concept of the body rather than a material one. In a sense, the early Chinese philosophers anticipated Einstein's theory of relativity, for they recognized that matter and energy were just two different manifestations of the same thing. Rather than focusing on the material aspects of the body (muscles, nerves, organs, bones, etc.), they concentrated on the vital life energy that creates and animates the physical body. This life energy, called *chi* (best translated as "breath"), is conceptually similar to the "orgone energy" described by Reich or *prana* in the Hindu theosophical tradition. Thus, all things that respirate have chi, including invertebrates and plants.

According to the classical Chinese theory, chi circulates through the body along the acupuncture meridians. Chi controls the blood, nerves, and all organs and must flow freely for good health to be maintained. When this energy flow becomes blocked or impaired—because of trauma, poor diet, excessive emotions, cold, stress, or any number of other factors—the individual becomes susceptible to illness. Consistent with this notion, pain is nothing more than an excess accumulation of energy that occurs when the flow of chi becomes blocked. Likewise, numbness or paralysis develops in areas of the body with insufficient chi flow. By selectively stimulating the acupuncture points that lie along the meridians, the ancient Chinese believed that the flow of chi in specific organ systems could be rebalanced, thus alleviating pain and strengthening the body's ability to combat disease. In addition to acupuncture, the Chinese utilized a variety of herbs, which were taken as broths, teas, or applied directly to the skin. Western medicine has not yet recognized the value of herbal therapy, but I believe that someday herbs will become an even more valuable therapeutic tool than acupuncture.

Before treating a patient, the traditional acupuncture practitioner first attempts to diagnose the nature of the imbalance of energy, utilizing a variety of diagnostic techniques. These techniques include a careful inspection of the general appearance of the patient, skin coloration, texture of the hair, color of the tongue's coating, and a general examination of the mouth, nose, eyes, and teeth. The rate and clarity of breathing, the patient's tone of voice and manner of speaking, and the determination of any foul or characteristic odors also provides important diagnostic information. The balance of the meridians is assessed by careful examination of the radial pulses. By palpation of these pulses, the traditional practitioner is reportedly able to discern which of the meridians is malfunctioning and whether this disturbance is due to increased or decreased chi flow. The link between philosophy and practice is demonstrated by the use of the yin-yang principle for arriving at a diagnosis. Yin is associated with cold, internal, and reduced functioning, while yang is related to overheating, external, and hyperactive functioning.

After a diagnosis has been made, the acupuncturist prescribes a course of acupuncture therapy. According to traditional Taoist philosophy, stimulation of appropriate acupuncture loci results in a restoration of balanced energy flow, which then permits the affected organ (and eventually the entire organism) to return to it's normal homeostatic state. Acupuncture loci may be stimulated by insertion of fine, solid needles, by intense heat (moxibustion), or by massage (acupressure), depending on the problem being treated. Modern technology has made available a variety of new techniques, including electrical stimulation of the needles (electroacupuncture), ultrasound stimulation (sonopuncture), and even laser beam stimulation (lasopuncture).

"Tonification-sedation," one of the fundamental principles of acupuncture therapy, is derived from the concept of yin and yang. In oversimplified terms, "tonification" techniques are utilized to replenish a deficiency of energy and "sedation" techniques are utilized to reduce an excess of energy. Either technique may be appropriate for restoring balance, depending upon the nature of a specific illness. For example, chronic fatigue in a thin, pale, asthenic individual may be related to a deficiency of yang energy, and tonification would be appropriate. On the other hand, sleep difficulties in a heavy, red-faced, plethoric individual may be related to an excess of yang energy, and sedation would be indicated.

This type of approach is representative of the holistic nature of acupuncture therapy. Rather than isolating and treating a specific medical symptom, the problem is seen as a single manifestation of the general condition of the individual. Acupuncture therapy involves the whole person, and the skilled acupuncturist treats the patient, not the disease. The rationale underlying the selection of other specific techniques and the loci used for treating a given illness involves a variety of rather complex theoretical relationships that are beyond the scope of this chapter. The interested reader is referred to the books by Palos (1971), Mann (1964, 1971, 1974), and Beau (1972).

Many people are unnecessarily frightened by the prospect of receiving acupuncture, for they incorrectly equate acupuncture needles with the type of needles used for hypodermic injections. Hypodermic needles are large and hollow with a razor-sharp beveled point for piercing through tissue. Acupuncture needles, on the other hand, are extremely thin—often no thicker than a human hair. They are made of solid stainless steel with a rounded pencil-tip point that pushes the tissue aside without cutting it. As a result, only a slight pin prick sensation is felt when they are inserted, and there is usually no bleeding during the entire treatment process. Once the needle is properly in place, a characteristic tingling or a heaviness is experienced. Although this sometimes may feel strange and unusual, most patients report that it is not painful.

After about twenty or thirty minutes, the needles are removed without discomfort. A brief rest will then be recommended after the treatment is completed because some patients experience light-headedness and even euphoria. Most patients describe a characteristic feeling of contentment and relaxation. The number of sessions required varies according to the individual and the problem being treated. For acute ailments, only a few treatments—sometimes just one—are necessary. Chronic problems usually require a greater number. Some people are fortunate, experiencing improvement in their condition immediately. However, others may instead feel even worse after the initial treatments and then begin making profound improvement later. If acupuncture is capable of helping, progress is usually noticeable by the tenth treatment. But for certain chronic ailments, fifteen to twenty treatments may be necessary. Typically, about two treatments are given per week.

Acupuncture facilitates the organism's own tendency toward homeostasis and health, and results are accomplished through the body's natural mechanisms of recovery and regeneration. This differs from Western medicine, which generally relies upon the introduction of some external substance to modify events within the body. Consequently, acupuncture seems to be most effective in those situations where the body's own life support and regenerative capacities are not too severely compromised.

Modern Concepts of Acupuncture

Although the terminology of traditional Chinese medicine often appears strange and unfamiliar to Western physicians, scientists have now begun to document the physiological, electrical, and chemical characteristics of the traditional acupuncture system. Many acupuncture points are anatomically identical to motor points of muscles, well known in electromyography, while others are identical to common trigger points, independently described by several Western investigators (Liu, 1975; Melzack et al., 1977; Vanderschot, 1976). Still others lie along major nerve trunks (Shanghai Medical College, 1972; Matsumoto and Lyu, 1975). Most interestingly, it has been found that the electrical resistance of the skin overlying acupuncture points is considerably lower than that of the surrounding area (Reichmanis et al., 1975, 1976; Becker et al., 1976), although the significance of this observation has yet to be explained. Basic research on acupuncture in the West has not been extensive, but it has been shown that stimulation of various acupuncture points can affect a great variety of physiological parameters. These include changes in red and white blood cell count, immunoglobulin levels, EEG and EKG recordings, bronchodilation, and vasodilation of the microcirculation, among others (see special reference section, Research in Acupuncture).

Most theories of acupuncture have focused on the nervous system, and it seems clear that the phenomena of acupuncture are at least in part mediated through the nervous system, through mechanisms that are not as yet well understood. Neurophysiological investigations of acupuncture have concentrated upon its analgesic effects, and various theories have been developed in an attempt to explain it. The existence of visceral-cutaneous reflexes and characteristic patterns of referred pain are well known, and it is possible that acupuncture may involve in part a complex manipulation of such reflexes (see special reference section on Reflexes and Neurophysiological Theories). Melzack and Wall (1965) have advanced the well known "gate theory" and others have amplified this with "multiple gate" theories (Man and Chen, 1972; Melzack, 1973). Basically, these theories propose that needle insertion at acupuncture points stimulates large diameter fibers in peripheral nerves, whose activity interferes at some level of the nervous system with the transmission of painful impulses mediated by small diameter fibers. The impulses produced by acupuncture thus close the "gate" to impulses mediating painful stimuli and prevent them from reaching the brain.

No single explanation of the phenomena has been generally accepted, and it is quite possible that a number of different factors may be involved, including peripheral neural stimulation, immune-inflammatory response to the needle insertion, and psychological factors (Bresler and Kroening, 1976). Quite recently, the discovery of endogenous polypeptides (endorphins) that bind to opiate receptors (Hughes et al., 1975; Terenius and Walhstrom, 1975; Cox et al., 1975) in the central nervous system has raised the intriguing possibility that release of these polypeptides may also be involved in mediating the analgesic effect of acupuncture (Pomeranz, 1977; Sjohund et al., 1977).

Endorphins are naturally occurring substances with opiate-like properties, whose analgesic actions can be reversed by opiate antagonists, such as naloxone. Preliminary investigations indicate that the analgesic effects of acupuncture may also be blocked by naloxone (Pomeranz and Chiu, 1976; Mayer et al., 1977), which suggests the existence of a similar mechanism.

Do all of these scientific findings mean that the traditional theory of energy flow has no practical validity? The answer to this depends upon the perspective of the questioner. Modern physics has shown that matter and energy are not distinct but represent two aspects of the same thing. In some situations, it is easier to explain a given phenomenon in terms of matter; in others, in terms of energy. Likewise, all events in the organism, whether psychological or physiological, involve both matter and energy. Thus, it does not seem at all contradictory to think both in terms of energy flow and of physiological mechanisms in order to explain what is happening when acupuncture is performed.

Clinical Applications of Acupuncture

Acupuncture is employed in China and elsewhere in the world for treatment of a great variety of medical problems. It is also considered a sophisticated form of preventive medicine, which may be utilized for the maintenance of health as well as for the treatment of disease. In light of its strong emphasis on nutritional, environmental, and psychological factors as well as physical symptoms, acupuncture may also be considered one of the earliest systems of holistic or integral medicine.

At present, the widest application of acupuncture in the United States has been for treatment of patients with chronic pain (Bresler, 1979 and in preparation). Certainly, it is no panacea. But often, when other types of therapy have failed, acupuncture can help. On the basis of my experience with it over the last eight years, I have found it to be astoundingly effective in treating a variety of chronic pain problems. They include:

- Musculoskeletal pain (e.g., low back, neck and shoulder, hip, and knee pain). As a rough guideline, areas close to the trunk seem to respond better than those in the extremities.
- Osteoarthritis localized in specific joints (Rheumatoid arthritis, a systemic illness affecting the entire body, does not appear to respond as well).
- Muscle contraction and migraine headaches. (There is no conclusive data yet available as to its effectiveness in treating allergic headaches.)
- Various neuralgias (e.g., trigeminal neuralgia, postherpetic neuralgia, etc.) and pain related to nerve injury.

Acupuncture may also be effective in treating psychological as well as physical pain. I have cared for many patients suffering from anxiety and severe depression, some of whom have been helped by acupuncture when accompanied by appropriate psychotherapeutic care. Other types of medical problems may also respond to acupuncture, but unfortunately, very little research has been conducted in this country concerning acupuncture therapy for problems other than chronic pain.

Acupuncture is not without its limitations, however. First, it is not readily available in most parts of the country. Although there might be many people in your community sticking needles in people, very few may be formally trained and experienced in traditional acupunctures. Those who are just poking needles in the body may be doing physical therapy, but acupuncture involves much more. Second, acupuncture is an invasive technique. It involves inserting a foreign object into the body, and for that reason, the possibility of infection or nerve, vessel, or organ damage – though minimal – always exists. Third, acupuncture therapy can be expensive. Depending on the practitioner, fees can range from $25 to $75 per treatment. Thus, if you were to undergo a typical therapeutic sequence – a consultation and eight to twelve treatments – the cost would be from $200 to as much as $900. Although Medicare does not yet cover acupuncture expenses, many private insurance companies will reimburse their policyholders in part or in full for this therapy.

Despite these shortcomings, acupuncture is an extremely safe technique when administered by a skillful, trained professional. At UCLA, after tens of thousands of acupuncture treatments, there has not been a single case of infection, broken needle, or nerve or organ damage. However, it is essential to find a competent therapist. Until the American Medical Association reverses its opposition to acupuncture and begins encouraging medical schools to teach it, this may not be easy to do. It seems ludicrous to me that this therapeutic system, which has been in continuous use for thousands of years, is still viewed today with such disdain by the medical establishment. I hope this will change in time; perhaps within ten to fifteen years acupuncture will become as accepted and commonly utilized in the United States as it has throughout the rest of the world.

Chinese Medicine and Holistic Health

In this era of nuclear energy, trips to the moon, and miracle drugs, it is difficult to accept a technique that seems so primitive and bizarre. Contemporary Western physicians stare in disbelief when they see a needle inserted into the ear to treat knee pain. But ancient healers would certainly have been equally baffled by the modern doctor placing a compressed white powder tablet (aspirin) into their patient's mouths. We, of course, know that the aspirin dissolves in the stomach, enters the bloodstream and quickly reaches the area of the knee. As we learn more about acupuncture and the way it works, I believe it too will become as acceptable and ordinary as our most commonplace treatments.

Most of us tend to think that the West is much more scientifically sophisticated than the East and that, if acupuncture had any validity, it would have been incorporated into our medical system long ago. But we are now discovering that the ancient Chinese were far more advanced than we had ever assumed. Although we give them credit for discovering porcelain, paper silk, and gunpowder, their insights into the field of medicine are even more astounding.

In a book called *Nei Ching* . . . *[The yellow emperor's classic of internal medicine],* the world's oldest known medical treatise dating back to the second century B.C., there is an explanation of blood circulation in the body – centuries before the English physiologist Sir William Harvey "discovered" how blood circulates. In the same book, vaccination against smallpox is described in detail – long before the English physician Edward Jenner devised his own smallpox immunization in the eighteenth century. The Chinese would scrape the pox off an infected person, grind it into a powder, and blow it through a tiny tube into the nostrils of anyone who came into contact with the victim. Smallpox was virtually unknown in ancient China, while it had devastating effects on Western civilization.

The ancient Chinese distinguished five levels of the healing arts. The lowest was practiced by the veterinarian, or animal doctor. Next came the acupuncturist and herbalist who treated minor symptomatic problems. The third level was the surgeon who treated more serious, life-threatening injuries. Second highest was the nutritionist who taught people what to eat; his was the science of longevity and preventive medicine. But, highest of all was the philosopher-sage who taught the "laws of the universe." He was the only practitioner who could effect a genuine cure, for he went directly to the heart of the problem: the patient's inability to live harmoniously with nature.

In the Western world, it is generally accepted that one can practice medicine without an underlying philosophy or religion; even an atheist can be an accomplished surgeon. But in the medical world of traditional China, this is inconceivable. Without proper knowledge of cosmic relationships and intense study of the weather, seasons, stars, and planets, medical treatment is impossible. Anything that affects the planets, seasons, and climates is thought to also affect the organs, tissues, and emotions of man. Western scientists are now only beginning to appreciate the powerful influence of climate on disease. For example, it is now known that cases of coronary occlusion occur more often on cold, cloudy days than on warm, sunny days. Chinese observers described this phenomenon nearly 5,000 years ago.

Traditional Chinese health care practitioners considered diet to be one of the most important factors in health and disease. Foods were evaluated in terms of their relative yin and yang energy. Certain types of grains and meats were thought to be either harmful or beneficial, depending on the energetic status of a given individual. The flavor and color of foods were also considered to be extremely important. It is difficult to determine if these complex correspondences have therapeutic validity or are merely superstitious customs handed down across generations. Nevertheless, the underlying importance of these general principles remain valid. The individual cannot be isolated from the environment in which he lives and the food that he eats.

Environmental factors may be even more important for contemporary man than for the Chinese who lived centuries ago. Modern man must face unprecedented environmental pollution, processed foods that lack critical nutrients, and the stresses of a noisy, crowded technological society. These and other environmental factors that affect health and disease must be carefully considered by contemporary practitioners just as ancient acupuncturists considered the wind, the cold, and the dampness.

Acupuncture in the United States

Traditional Chinese medicine approaches the concepts of health and disease from a totally different perspective than Western medicine, thus its ideas and terminology often seem strange or unfamiliar to most Western physicians. In addition, Western medicine has become increasingly specialized and it has not been clear where acupuncture, which approaches the treatment of the patient as a whole, should fit into this system of specialization. Thus, many physicians, while interested in the potential applications of acupuncture, are not sure how it could be included in their own medical practice, and few have access to formal training programs.

The legal status of acupuncture continues to be quite confused, with different states enacting widely differing laws regulating its practice. Despite its long history and the overwhelming scientific evidence of its efficacy, the American Medical Association and the Food and Drug Administration continue to insist that acupuncture be considered an "experimental" form of treatment. Because of this position, the Medicare and Medicaid agencies as well as most health insurance carriers will not provide reimbursement for acupuncture therapy, thus limiting its availability to those people fortunate enough to be able to pay for it.

It is hoped that this situation will change as acupuncture is more thoroughly investigated in this country. Acupuncture research is now being conducted at a number of medical schools in the United States, and although there is still disagreement as to its mechanism of action, most physicians who have seriously investigated acupuncture agree that it is a safe and effective form of therapy. It seems strange that acupuncture has been less readily available in the United States – with its sophisticated health care system – than in most other countries in the world. However, as new state laws are enacted to set standards for practice, and more and more people are helped, acupuncture may soon find a home in the United States as well.

References

Beau, G. *Chinese Medicine*. New York: Avon Books, 1972.

Becker, R. O.; Reichmanis, M.; Marino, A. A.; and Spadaro, J. A. Electrophysiological correlates of acupuncture points and meridians. *Psychoenergetic Systems* 1976. 1, 105–112..

Bresler, D. E. *Free Yourself from Pain*. New York: Simon and Schuster, 1979.

Bresler, D. E. Acupuncture and chronic pain: a critical review. In preparation.

Bresler, D. E., and Kroening, R. J. Three essential factors in effective acupuncture therapy. *American Journal of Chinese Medicine*, 1976. **4** (1), 81–86.

Cox, B. M.; Opheim, K. E.; Techmacher, H.; and Goldstein, A. A peptide-like substance from the pituitary that acts like morphine. *Life Sciences*, 1975. **16**, 1777–1782.

Hughes, J.; Smith, T. W.; Kosterlitz, H. W.; Fothergill, L. A.; Morgan, B. A.; and Morris, H. R. Identification of two related pentapeptides from the brain with potent opiate agonist activity. *Nature*, 1975. **258**, 577–579.

Liu, Y. K. The correspondence between some motor points and acupuncture loci. *American Journal of Chinese Medicine*, 1975. **3**, 347–358.

Man, P. L., and Chen, C. H. Mechanisms of acupunctural anesthesia: two gate theory. *Diseases of the Nervous System*, 1972. **33**, 730.

Mann, Felix. *The Meridians of Acupuncture.* London: William Heinemann Medical Books, 1964.

Mann, Felix. *Acupuncture: Cure of Many Diseases.* London: William Heinemann Medical Books, 1971.

Mann, Felix. *The Treatment of Disease by Acupuncture* (3rd ed.). Philadelphia: International Ideas, 1974.

Matsumoto, T., and Lyu, B. S. Anatomical comparison between acupuncture and nerve block. *The American Surgeon*, January 1975. 11–16.

Mayer, D. J.; Price, D. D.; and Rafii, A. Antagonism of acupuncture analgesia in man by the narcotic antagonist naloxone. *Brain Research*, 1977. **121**, 368–372.

Melzack, R. How acupuncture can block pain. *Impact of Science on Society*, 1973. **23**, 65–75.

Melzack, R.; Stillwell, D. M.; and Fox, E. J. Trigger points and acupuncture points for pain: correlations and implications. *PAIN*, 1977. **3**, 3–23.

Melzack, R., and Wall, P. Pain mechanisms: a new theory. *Science*, 1965. **150**, 971.

Palos, Stephen. *The Chinese Art of Healing.* New York: McGraw-Hill, 1971.

Pomeranz, B. H. Brain opiates at work in acupuncture? *New Scientist*, January 6, 1977. **73**, 12–13.

Pomeranz, B. H., and Chiu, D. Naloxone blockade of acupunture analgesia causes hyperanalgesia: endorphin implicated. *Life Sciences*, 1976. **19**, 1757–1762.

Reichmanis, M.; Marino, A. A.; and Becker, R. O. Electrical correlates of acupuncture points. *IEEE Transactions on Biomedical Engineering*, November 1975. **22** (6), 533–535.

Reichmanis, M.; Marino, A. A.; and Becker, R. O. D.C. skin conductance variation at acupuncture loci. *American Journal of Chinese Medicine*, 1976. **4**, 69–72.

Shanghai Medical College Acupuncture Anesthesia Group. Study of relations between the acupuncture points and surrounding nervous structure by anatomical dissection. *Liberation Daily News*, January 5, 1972.

Sjohund, B.; Terenius, L.; and Eriksson, M. Increased cerebrospinal fluid levels of endorphins after electroacupuncture. *Acta Physiologica Scandinavia*, 1977. **100**, 382–384.

Terenius, L., and Walhstrom, A. Search for an endogenous ligand for the opiate receptor. *Acta Physiologica Scandinavia*, 1975. **94**, 74–81.

Vanderschot, L. Trigger points vs. acupuncture points. *American Journal of Acupuncture*, 1976. **4**, 233–238.

Research in Acupuncture

Bresler, D. E. Electrophysiological and behavioral correlates of acupuncture therapy. In Z. Reidak (Ed.), *Konference o Vyzkumu Psychotroniky.* Prague: Sbornik Referatu, 1973.

Calehr, H. Acupuncture treatment of the asthmatic patient. *American Journal of Acupuncture*, 1973. **1**, 41–51.

Chen, K. C. Effects of electroacupuncture on the immunological reactions of rabbits to goat plasma anticoagulant factor. *Sansi China Report No. 103*, Sansi Acupuncture Symposium, April 1959. Available from Dr. David E. Bresler.

Chen, K. C. Effects of acupuncture and electroacupuncture on immunological reactions. *Sansi China Report No. 102*, Sansi Acupuncture Symposium, April 1959. Available from Dr. David E. Bresler.

Chu, Y. M., and Affronti, L. F. Preliminary observations on the effect of acupuncture on immune responses in sensitized rabbits and guinea pigs. *American Journal of Chinese Medicine*, 1975. **3**, 151–163.

Cracium, T.; Toma, C.; and Turdeanu, V. Neurohumoral modifications after acupuncture. *American Journal of Acupuncture*, 1973. **1**, 67–70.

Hu. H. H. Therapeutic effects of acupuncture: a review. *American Journal of Acupuncture*, 1974. **2**, 8–14.

Lee, G.T.C. A study of electrical stimulation of acupuncture locus Tsusanli (ST-36) on mesenteric microcirculation. *American Journal of Chinese Medicine*, 1974. **2**, 1–27.

Lung, C. H.; Sun, A. C.; Tsao, C. J.; Chang, Y. L.; and Fan, L. An observation of the humoral factor in acupuncture analgesia in rats. *American Journal of Chinese Medicine*, 1974. **2**, 203–205.

Omura, Y. Effects of acupuncture on blood pressure, leukocytes and serum lipids and lipoproteins in essential hypertension. *Federation Proceedings*, 1974. **33**, 430.

Tashkin, D. P.; Bresler, D. E.; Kroening, R. J.; Kerschner, H.; Katz, R. L.; and Coulson, A. Comparison of real and simulated acupuncture and isoproterenol in methacholine-induced asthma. *Annals of Allergy*, 1977. **39**, 379–387.

Wen, H. L., and Chan, K. Status Asthmaticus treated by acupuncture and electrostimulation. *Asian Journal of Medicine*, 1973. **9**, 191–195.

Yang, K. C. et al. Relationship between acupuncture-moxibustion and infection and immunity. In H. Yu and S. W. Hsieh (Eds.), *Advances in Immunity*. Shanghai: Shanghai Science and Technology Press, 1962. 140.

Reflexes and Neurophysiological Theories

Chang, H. T. Integrative action of the thalamus in the process of acupuncture for analgesia. *American Journal of Chinese Medicine*, 1974. **2**, 1–39.

Ionescu-Tirgoviste, C. Theory of mechanism of action in acupuncture. *American Journal of Acupuncture*, 1973. **1**, 193–199.

Looney, G. L. Acupuncture study. *Journal of the American Medical Association*, 1974. **228**, 1522.

Mann, F. *Acupuncture—The Ancient Chinese Art of Healing and How It Works Scientifically*. New York: Random House, 1974.

Small, T. J. The neurophysiological basis for acupuncture. *American Journal of Acupuncture*, 1974. **2**, 77–87.

Tien, H. C. Acupuncture anesthesia: neurogenic interference theory. *World Journal of Psychosynthesis*, 1972. **4**, 36–41.

Tien, H. C. Neurogenic interference theory of acupuncture anesthesia. *American Journal of Chinese Medicine*, 1973. **1**, 105.

Wancera, I., and Konig, G. On the neurophysiological explanation of acupuncture analgesia. *American Journal of Chinese Medicine*, 1974. **2**. 193–198.

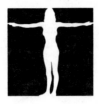 ANNOTATED BIBLIOGRAPHY

Academy of Traditional Chinese Medicine. **An Outline of Chinese Acupuncture.** Peking: Foreign Language Press, 1975.

> This is the most comprehensive English-language textbook yet published relating to the contemporary practice of acupuncture in the People's Republic of China. It includes thorough instructions in the use of acupuncture needles, moxibustion, and cupping techniques, as well as a description of several hundred acupuncture points. Full color charts are extremely helpful in visualizing the locations of these points. This text also contains chapters relating to other therapeutic methods, including auriculotherapy, point injection, and thread imbedding techniques.

American Journal of Acupuncture, 1973–. **1**–.

> This professional journal is an indispensible way for acupuncture practitioners to keep up with current developments. Most papers published are of general clinical interest and, although some lack scientific rigor, they are nevertheless relevant and informative. Particularly recommended are the "New Abstract" section, which summarizes research studies published in other journals, and the "Book Forum," which reviews new publications related to acupuncture and Chinese medicine. The address for this journal is 1400 Lost Acre Drive, Felton, California 95018.

American Journal of Chinese Medicine, 1973–. **1**–.

> This professional journal publishes wide-ranging research articles and essays relating to Chinese medicine. Translations of ancient and contemporary texts describing various aspects of the Chinese health care delivery system are included, as well as case reports. The address for this journal is P.O. Box 55, Garden City, New York 11530.

Beau, Georges. **Chinese Medicine.** New York: Avon Books, 1972.

> This fascinating book provides a general review of the subject of Chinese medicine. It includes a comprehensive section describing the principles of acupuncture and a brief review of the Chinese pharmacopoeia. It is not only rich in historical information but also surveys the status of traditional medicine in the People's Republic of China as of the early 1960s.

Bresler, David E., and Kroening, Richard J. **Three essential factors in effective acupuncture therapy.** *American Journal of Chinese Medicine,* 1976. **4** (1), 81–86.

Three essential factors for achieving effective therapeutic results utilizing acupuncture are described. First, immune/inflammatory reactions are mobilized when any area of the skin is sufficiently stimulated. Second, peripheral neural stimulation occurs when specific acupuncture loci are mechanically, electrically, chemically, or thermally activated. Precise stimulation of specific loci (i.e., peripheral neural receptors) may modulate central nervous system regulation of specific physiological functions in the body. And third, psychological support is well known as an important factor in all healing experiences, and that includes acupuncture therapy. The authors suggest that the most effective application of acupuncture involves sufficient stimulation of properly selected and precisely localized acupuncture loci combined with a dedicated concern for health that is clearly communicated to patients.

Bresler, David E.; Kroening, Richard J.; and Volen, Michael P. **Acupuncture – Can It Help?** Pacific Palisades, Calif.: Center for Integral Medicine, 1977.

This booklet provides answers to questions most commonly asked by individuals interested in receiving acupuncture therapy. These questions include: What is acupuncture? What advantages or disadvantages does it have compared to Western medicine? How does it work? Which medical conditions can it help? What is a typical treatment like? How many treatments are required? Are there any dangers associated with it? How can I find a competent acupuncturist?

    Single copies are available at no charge from the Center, c/o P.O. Box 967, Pacific Palisades, California 90272.

Carney, J. V. **Acupressure – Acupuncture Without Needles.** New York: Cornerstone Library, 1976.

The author presents his own enthusiastic, step-by-step approach to finger-pressure acupuncture. Although this book is directed to laypersons who wish to learn this self-management technique, it requires some diligence on the part of the reader to carefully follow all of the detailed recommendations. For those who are seriously interested in the subject, it contains an abundance of relevant information concerning the clinical indications of acupressure and is richly illustrated by the author.

Chaitow, Leon. **The Acupuncture Treatment of Pain.** New York: Arco, 1977.

This book is an excellent beginning text for medical practitioners interested in exploring the clinical effectiveness of acupuncture for the control and management of pain. The author, an osteopathic physician, briefly reviews his own experiences with acupuncture and then presents a "cookbook" approach that includes charts and descriptions of points used to treat pain in various parts of the body. Although severely limited in scope and perspective, this book is well organized and includes extensive charts that permit easy reference for those who are unfamiliar with the traditional anatomy of acupuncture.

Duke, Marc. **Acupuncture.** New York: Pyramid House, 1972.

This book is one of the best overall sources of information on acupuncture for both the serious student and interested laypersons. Written in a clear and concise manner, it provides a general overview of the development of acupuncture in the Far East and its introduction into Western civilization. It is fully illustrated and includes brief descriptions of the symptoms, illnesses, and diseases treated by stimulation of specific acupuncture points.

Huang, Helena L. (Trans.). **Ear Acupuncture.** Emmaus, Pa.: Rodale Press, 1974.

This translation of the training text written by the Nanking Army Ear Acupuncture Team is one of the most complete sources of information concerning the contemporary Chinese practice of auriculotherapy. It describes in detail the distribution and location of ear acupuncture points and contains tables of therapeutic indications. Techniques for examining and treating through the auricle are reviewed and the team's personal experiences using this approach are presented. This is an essential source book for those who wish to learn the practice of auriculotherapy.

Huard, Pierre, and Wong, Ming. **Chinese Medicine.** New York: McGraw-Hill, 1968.

The authors describe the general history of the growth and change of Far Eastern medical practices and the later Western influences that affected them. The traditional basis for various symptom complexes are explained, and a variety of therapeutic techniques and herbal remedies are reviewed. References to ancient Chinese medical sources are included.

Jenerick, Howard P. (Ed.). **Proceedings – NIH Acupuncture Research Conference.** Bethesda, Md.: National Institutes of Health, 1973. (Department of Health, Education, and Welfare Publication no. 74-165.)

This publication of the National Institute of General Medical Sciences contains summaries of research reports presented at a national conference sponsored by NIH in the spring of 1973. It represents the earliest attempts by contemporary U.S. scientists to evaluate the potential therapeutic value of acupuncture. This document also includes the names and addresses of fifty-nine participants, most of whom have continued to explore various aspects of traditional Chinese medicine.

John E. Fogarty International Center for Advanced Study in the Health Sciences (Trans.). **The Barefoot Doctor's Manual.** Bethesda, Md.: National Institutes of Health, 1974 (Department of Health, Education, and Welfare Publication no. 75-695). (Also published by Running Press, Philadelphia, 1977.)

This 960-page document is a translation of the well-known manual originally published by the Institute of Traditional Chinese Medicine of Hunan Province in September 1970. The focus of this book is on the improvement of medical and health care facilities in Chinese rural villages, and it represents a comprehensive attempt to integrate traditional and modern approaches to treatment and prevention of illness. The manual includes chapters on basic anatomy and physiology, hygiene, diagnostic and therapeutic techniques, birth control planning, and a thorough description of some 522 herbs (with 338 illustrations). Unfortunately, the manual was reproduced in limited quantities, so it may not be widely available. It has also been reprinted by commercial publishers in trade editions.

The Fogarty International Center has also published several other important documents relating to Chinese medicine.

Journal of Traditional Acupuncture. 1-.

This relatively new journal has two goals: (1) to educate lay persons about traditional acupuncture and the concepts of health inherent in this natural system of healing, and (2) to provide information and support for acupuncture practitioners so that they will continue to learn and grow in a nurturing environment. The address of this journal is Box 238, New York, N.Y. 10038.

Klide, Alan M., and King, Shiu H. **Veterinary Acupuncture.** Philadelphia: University of Pennsylvania Press, 1977.

In this text, the authors bring together diverse sources of information concerning veterinary acupuncture. The basic principles of traditional Chinese veterinary medicine are reviewed in a clear and concise manner, and the text is profusely illustrated with charts showing the locations of acupuncture points in both large and small animals. Various approaches to analgesia in veterinary surgery are included.

Kushi, Michio. **Oriental Diagnosis.** London: Red Moon Publications, 1976.

The author provides an absorbing introduction to the subject of traditional Far Eastern diagnosis. Edited and compiled from Kushi's lectures by his students, this book views the diagnostic process not as a method of classifying symptoms but as a way to understand the totality of an individual's health and life. Far Eastern diagnosis is based on the physiognomic principle that each person represents a walking history of his or her development. The strengths and weaknesses of parents, early environments, and general dietary habits profoundly influence all organs of the body and thus are reflected in the posture, color of skin, tone of voice, and other external traits. Kushi not only describes the diagnostic characteristics of the face, eyes, mouth, ears, hair, skin, and hands but also discusses pulse diagnosis and the diagnostic significance of the voice, handwriting, and various habits.

Lu, Henry C. **Tongue Diagnosis in Color.** Vancouver, B.C.: The Academy of Oriental Heritage, 1977.

This is a definitive text on Chinese tongue diagnosis. It includes a brief historical review and fifty-three color plates illustrating various conditions of the tongue that reflect illness. Diagnostic implications are discussed briefly in Western medical terms and more extensively in traditional Chinese terms (e.g., "disease of the bright Yang meridians"). Although this book would probably be of little interest to the casual reader, health professionals might find it to be a useful addition to their therapeutic armamentaria. It also contains more than sixty somewhat dated English language references concerning tongue diagnosis.

Mann, Felix. **The Meridians of Acupuncture.** London: William Heinemann Medical Books, 1964.

This book is intended for those who seek a more detailed understanding of the acupuncture system, its points, and their applications. It thoroughly describes the course of the fifty-six interconnecting meridians and includes a section in each of the twelve chapters devoted to "symptoms and signs." Although the important illustrations lack detail and clarity, this remains the best of the books on acupuncture written by Mann.

Mann, Felix. **The Treatment of Disease by Acupuncture.** (3rd ed.). Philadelphia: International Ideas, 1974.

This text is divided into two parts. The first contains a detailed listing of each acupuncture point, including its traditional Chinese name, English name, theoretical significance, and therapeutic indications. The second part, compiled by the Peking School of Chinese Medicine, consists of a general survey of common diseases, their symptoms and diagnostic features, and the principal acupuncture points utilized in their treatment. This book is one of the most detailed English-language sources of information concerning the individual acupuncture points and their use in the treatment of disease.

McGarey, William A. **Acupuncture and Body Energies.** Phoenix, Ariz.: Gabriel Press, 1974.

The author, a pioneering U.S. physician, presents a readable and balanced view of the principles of acupuncture with the hope that other doctors will become interested in utilizing it in their practices. Of particular interest are the chapters titled "A Western Approach to Therapy," which includes the author's personal experiences with acupuncture, and "Acupuncture in American Medicine," in which he synthesizes traditional Chinese theory with material from the readings of Edgar Cayce.

Nogier, Paul F. M. **Treatise of Auriculotherapy.** Moulins-les-Metz, France: Maisonneuve, 1972.

This is the classic text on the subject by the French physician who has been called the "father of auricular therapy." Thoroughly illustrated by R. J. Bourdiol, M.D., it reviews the anatomy, physiology, and theoretical significance of the external ear, presents methods and techniques of diagnosis and therapy, and discusses clinical indications in detail. Although later work by Chinese medical researchers has produced some discrepancies in the localization of certain auricular points, this text remains an invaluable source of information concerning the French school of auriculotherapy.

Palos, Stephan. **The Chinese Art of Healing.** New York: McGraw-Hill, 1971.

This book is one of the best sources of general information on various aspects of Chinese medicine, including massage, herbal medicines, physiotherapy, and respiratory therapy. Of special interest is Chapter 3, entitled The Human Body in Ancient Chinese Thought. Written from a scholarly point of view, it contains a fair and comprehensive treatment of the subject.

Porkert, Manfred. **The Theoretical Foundations of Chinese Medicine.** Cambridge, Mass.: Massachusetts Institute of Technology Press, 1974.

The author presents a detailed and systematic account of the theoretical notions that underlie traditional Chinese approaches to health care. The concepts of yin and yang and the law of five elements ("five evolutive phases," according to Porkert) are thoroughly discussed. Of particular interest is Chapter 2 on "phase energetics," in which the author reviews the interrelationship of meteorological, climatic, and immunological factors in health and disease. Unfortunately, Porkert utilizes his own unique system of Latin terminology throughout the book, which makes it an extremely difficult and often confusing book to read. However, it is rich in theoretical information and is recommended for serious students of ancient Chinese thought.

Serizawa, Katsusuke. **Massage – the Oriental Method.** San Francisco: Japan Publications, 1972.

This is a definitive work on Oriental massage, based on the author's amalgamation of traditional "amma" massage, shiatsu, and Western-style massage. It describes the major tsubo (acupuncture points) and provides instruction in practical massage techniques. Individual chapters review massage therapy, massage techniques for general well-being, and cosmetic massage procedures.

Veith, Ilza (Trans.). **The Yellow Emperor's Classic of Internal Medicine.** Berkeley, Calif.: University of California Press, 1972.

This book is a partial translation of one of the most ancient texts on traditional Chinese medicine. Compiled during the second century B.C., it is thought to be a collection of medical documents that were written several hundred years earlier. The text takes the form of a dialogue between the Yellow Emperor (the third legendary emperor of China, who ruled from 2697–2598 B.C.) and Ch'i Po, his court physician. They speak to each other about the causes and cures for illness and the relationship between man and nature. *The Yellow Emperor's Classic* provides a summary of the Chinese people's knowledge of anatomy, physiology, pathology, diagnosis, and treatment of various diseases as it existed at the time of its compilation. Covering a wide range of subjects, it laid the foundation of traditional Chinese medicine and is a "must" reading for the serious student.

Wallnofer, Heinrich, and von Rottauscher, Anna. **Chinese Folk Medicine.** New York: Bell, 1965.

This general but informative book reviews the fundamentals of traditional Chinese medicine and provides a historical summary of its evolution. In addition to brief reviews of Chinese anatomy, physiology, pathology, and various treatment approaches, the authors discuss medicinal herbs, drugs, "love medicines," traditional notions of aging and dying, and the use of various tortures to achieve "justice." This book also contains a fascinating chapter on tales, dreams, and their interpretations.

Wilhelm, Richard (Trans.). **The Secret of the Golden Flower.** New York: Causeway Books, 1975.

The Golden Flower is "that mysterious light in the human body which can be aroused by Taoist yoga and meditation practices, resulting in spiritual insights, wisdom and incomparable bliss." This translation by Richard Wilhelm is the definitive theoretical guide to traditional Chinese yoga. It also includes a fascinating commentary by C. G. Jung, which distinguishes and integrates the approaches of the East and West. In the introduction to this new edition, Charles San notes that certain ambiguities in the 1929 German translation can now be clarified, namely that "the key to the opening of the Golden Flower is the sexual energy of the individual, which must be aroused and converted into spiritual force." This is an amazing book in all respects.

Wu, Shui Wan. **The Chinese Pulse Diagnosis.** Los Angeles: Shui Wan Wu, 1972.

This pamphlet, published by the author, reviews various techniques used in conducting traditional Chinese pulse diagnosis. It also describes in some detail each of the twenty-eight unique qualities of the pulse and their implications from the point of view of traditional theory. It is one of the most thorough guides to the subject in English. This pamphlet is available from the author c/o P.O. Box 75023, Sanford Stations, Los Angeles, California, 90075.

Wu, Wei-F'ing. **Chinese Acupuncture.** Denington Estate, Wellingborough, Northamptonshire, England: Health Science Press, 1962.

This classic 1954 text was translated into French by Jacques Lavier and then into English by Philip Chancellor. For the student who wishes to learn the most basic fundamentals of traditional Chinese acupuncture, it is an invaluable reference source. Particularly useful are the detailed descriptions of the acupuncture points (although no anatomical charts are included) and the therapeutic repertory, which lists point combinations used to treat various illnesses.

28

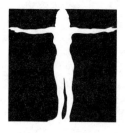

INDIGENOUS AND TRADITIONAL SYSTEMS OF HEALING

Arthur Kleinman, M.D.

Introduction

Over the past two decades, anthropologists and psychiatrists have extensively studied healing systems in non-Western societies and Western ethnic groups; such systems have been referred to as indigenous or traditional healing systems. My purpose is to alert health professionals in our own health care system about findings and concepts generated by these ethnographic and comparative cross-cultural studies that hold potential significance for them. I also sketch below a skeletal outline of what has been learned about universal and culture-specific structural processes mediating the healing process.

Besides early reviews by Sigerist (1951) and Ackerknecht (1971), relevant volumes have been edited by Kiev (1964), Kleinman et al. (1975, 1978a), Landy (1977), Lebra (1976), Leslie (1976), Middleton (1967), and Spicer (1977), among others. Monographs and journal articles that examine the healing systems of particular cultural groups are extremely numerous. Some of the best include: Crapanzano (1971), Fabrega and Silver (1973), Hallowell (1955), Harwood (1977), Horton (1967), G. Lewis (1975), I. M. Lewis (1971), Obeyesekere (1976), Reynolds (1976), Spiro (1967), Tambiah (1968), Turner (1967), and Young (1978). Several journals routinely publish studies of indigenous healing systems, including: *American Anthropologist, Culture, Medicine and Psychiatry, Ethnology,*

Medical Anthropology, Social Science and Medicine, Transcultural Psychiatry Research Review.

Jerome Frank's *Persuasion and Healing* (1974), however, still remains the most successful attempt to synthesize knowledge in this area to construct a comparative cross-cultural understanding of the healing process. Although it is an important synthesis, it, like most other comparative works by psychiatrists and psychologists, imposes a Western framework on the cross-cultural record by using psychotherapy as the guide to appreciate how healing systems work. In what follows, I shall try to provide a less ethnocentric and medicocentric account of indigenous healing, drawing on the groundbreaking work of Frank and the large body of data and concepts developed by the other scholars above. I will assess the present state-of-the-art and relate what we have learned to contemporary health care issues confronting health professionals in our society.

Indigenous Healing Systems: Structures and Processes

Anthropological and psychiatric studies of indigenous healing systems disclose that these systems perform two related functions: (1) the control of personal symptoms and socially disvalued behaviors, and (2) the provision of culturally approved meaning and social interventions for the experience of sickness (Kleinman, 1974). Although these core healing activities frequently occur together, they may be independent of each other. Healing, then, can be evaluated as change on any or all of four levels:

- physiological processes
- psychological processes
- social relationships
- cultural norms and meanings

Holistic healing, in one sense, might be taken to signify integrated change on each of these levels.

Turner (1967), for example, demonstrates how the community-wide healing rituals of a small-scale preliterate African society effect change on each level simultaneously, a finding supported by many other ethnographers (Douglas, 1970). In contrast, professional biomedical care has narrowed its therapeutic focus to technologically induced physiological responses (Reiser, 1978). It may be that professionalization and differentiation of allopathic healing in the West has fragmented the holistic approach characteristic of ancient Western, indigenous non-Western contemporary folk, and popular healing systems. Psychotherapy and the current renaissance of family care, from this perspective, might be regarded as attempts to reintegrate within professional biomedical care the core functions of traditional healing systems.

This increasingly accepted viewpoint requires qualification. In the first place, there is a tendency for field researchers to romanticize indigenous healing systems and, by the application of reverse ethnocentrism, to find in them what they criticize as missing from biomedical care. Recent studies suggest that indigenous healing may fall as far short of holistic practice as does biomedical care. That is to say, it may be chiefly oriented to providing "technological fixes." It may be equally if not more concerned with commercial profit, it may carry the added danger of uncontrolled hucksterism, and it may produce a full panoply of undesirable results (Snow, 1978). Moreover, few ethnographic and comparative studies of indigenous healing systems have actually determined that integrated healing does in fact occur on all four levels. Instead, this result has been inferred from the ideological commitment of field workers to the view that rituals in traditional societies *should* reaffirm threatened cultural values, reincorporate marginal individuals, and re-establish marginal relationships within the social group. This has been an article of faith in cross-cultural research much more frequently than it has been tested as a hypothesis. Field workers have spent even less time examining psychological and physiological change than these presumed social and cultural responses. Finally, more discriminating research in medical anthropology has shown that most indigenous healing systems are pluralistic. Therefore, statements about them need to be precisely related to the specific components, some of which can be very different (Kunstadter, 1975; Leslie, 1976). These cautions should be extended to historical studies as well. Frequently "holistic" healing seems to be more in the eye of the disaffected Western beholder than an attribute of the indigenous healing systems. Indeed indigenous people have repeatedly been shown to be utterly pragmatic in accepting what is most efficacious in Western medicine while retaining those instrumental and symbolic aspects of their healing traditions for which Western medicine has offered no acceptable substitute. Yet in the main it is probably correct to state that indigenous healing systems have more closely approximated the *ideal* of "holistic healing" than have modern professional systems of biomedical care.

One sign that this conclusion is justified is that no studies of biomedical health services that I am aware of use the term "healing," let alone "holistic." "Healing" has been relegated by biomedical researchers and clinicians to the dustbin of archaic and outmoded concepts. It is no longer seen to apply, and nothing has replaced it. Hence the core functions of traditional healing systems are no longer legitimated as a serious subject either for the discourse of medical science or for that of professional clinical care. Studies of indigenous healing systems highlight this strange development, and for this reason alone they deserve the attention of health professionals and the laity.

Indigenous healing systems have been categorized and compared chiefly from the standpoint of the healing role and, more recently, from that of the patient's role. My interest here is not to comment on these subjects, since they tend to be somewhat peripheral to the healing process itself. Instead I shall review what we presently know about indigenous therapeutic relationships and the universal and culture-specific healing activities they perform. Such a review should help the reader come to terms with the various healing approaches presented in this volume by providing an analytical framework for drawing comparisons and contrasts.

The relevant ethnomedical findings on therapeutic relationships (indigenous and biomedical) can be grouped under five headings (Kleinman, in press):

1. Institutional setting
2. Structure of the interpersonal interaction
3. Idiom of communication
4. Clinical construction of reality
5. Therapeutic stages

Though not exhaustive of the extensive information we possess on indigenous therapeutic relationships, these categories do cover the major dimensions of clinical praxis that are relevant to the practical interests of health professionals.

Institutional Setting

In most societies there are three distinguishable therapeutic arenas in which healing occurs. They are:

1. Popular nonspecialist care in the context of the family or social network
2. Professional bureaucratically organized orthodox healing specialists
3. Folk nonprofessionalized, nonorthodox, quasi-legal healing specialists

Professional and folk healing are further differentiated into specialized therapeutic roles and institutions. The institutional setting is a major determinant of differences in therapeutic relationships and treatment styles, as is well illustrated by the historical evolution of Western medical practice from the patient's home, to the doctor's private office (usually in his home), and finally to the bureaucratic setting (e.g., hospital or group practice clinic). The therapeutic relationship in the home includes certain of the affective ties, informality, and integration into everyday experience that characterizes *primary* role relationships. However, the therapeutic relationship in the bureaucratic setting is by definition a *tertiary* role relationship, characterized by emotional distance, formality, personal anonymity, and separation from day-to-day life transactions. Indigenous healing systems also function in distinctive social structural settings, such as community or kinship groups, private homes, traditional healers' shrines, and the like. One generalization that seems to hold across a variety of cultures is that indigenous healing tends to take place in more public settings than does professional health care, which is a private affair.

What is important for readers to recognize is that most traditional healing

health, and Chapter 14 discusses the uses of imagery in medicine – both good over-views.

Shealy, C. Norman, with Freese, Arthur S. **Occult Medicine Can Save Your Life: A Modern Doctor Looks at Unconventional Healing.** New York: Dial, 1975.

In this unfortunately titled book, Shealy, a neurosurgeon specializing in treating chronic pain, reports his investigation of unorthodox diagnostic and healing tech-niques. They include faith healing and psychic diagnosis (including a test in which selected psychics were 70–75 percent accurate in their diagnosis), acupuncture, biofeedback, electrical stimulation of the nervous system, autogenic training, graphology, and even astrology. (There are at least *astronomical* correlations with mental health and propensity to hemorrhage.) The author's examples and opinions reflect his belief in the potentials of some of these techniques, but he also points out precautions in using them and the need for orthodox medical diagnosis and treatment.

Vieth, Ilza (Trans.). **The Yellow Emperor's Classic of Internal Medicine.** Berkeley, Calif.: University of California Press, 1972.

This is a translation of the oldest known treatise on Chinese medicine, the *Nei Ching,* written about 1000 B.C. Pulse diagnosis and other diagnostic methods are described in detail. The book provides many poetic and precise examples of how the pulses feel: "When a man is tranquil and healthy the pulse of the spleen flows softly, coming together and falling apart like a chicken treading the earth" (p. 175); "When a man is sick the pulse of the spleen moves fully and is large and long and slightly tense, and there is a surplus of the number of pulse beats like a chicken raising its feet – and then one can speak of a sick spleen" (p. 175); "When the pulse is dense and coarse and large its content of Yin elements is insufficient, and there is a surplus of Yang elements which causes fevers within the body" (p. 167).

Chapters 17, 18, and 19 discuss examination by means of the pulse, colors, and vicera, and the differing effects of the seasons. The book is worth reading to ex-perience the mood and mode of the tradition.

Vithoulkas, George. **The Science of Homeopathy: A Modern Text Book** (Vol. 1). Athens, Greece: Athenian Society of Homeopathic Medicine, 1978.

This text, which organizes and explains the principles and practice of homoeopathy, contains three extensive chapters: case-taking (Chapter 12), evaluation of symptoms (Chapter 13), and case analysis and prescription (Chapter 14). The author draws on his experience for valuable details, discussing the process of case-taking, putting the patient at ease and eliciting a report of symptoms, weighting the symptoms, and ana-lyzing the case in terms of the repertory and materia medica. These chapters are espe-cially communicative of the open attitude of the homoeopath and the careful process of selecting a remedy to match the symptoms.

Wallnoffer, Heinrich, and von Rottauscher, Anna. **Chinese Folk Medicine.** New York: Mentor, 1965.

This book collects a vast amount of traditional Chinese medical information, though without evaluation as to its quality or efficacy. Chapter 5, "The Cause of Disease," reports some of the traditional diagnostic considerations based on land areas, climates, winds, colors, tongue, moods, and perspiration. A section on pulse diagnosis includes charts and descriptions of the various pulse characteristics and their related organs. It is useful in terms of information but disorganized and out of context.

Wexu, Mario. **The Ear: Gateway to Balancing the Body. A Modern Guide to Ear Acupuncture.** New York: ASI Publishers, 1975.

This is a thorough text on ear acupuncture and diagnosis, including discussions of 300 points on the ear, techniques of examination and selection, needling techniques, and case histories. Regarding diagnosis, the author explains general examination procedures of observation and questioning the patient and the special procedures for the ear examination of palpation, testing for heat and cold sensitivity, observation of skin changes, texture, electronic instruments, and comparative sensitivity between the two ears.

The book is especially good in discussing ear acupuncture within the larger context of traditional Chinese medicine – the meridians and their functions are explained, the relation of ear points to body points, and the role of colors in diagnosis. Included are chapters on anesthesia, drug addiction, obesity, deafness, special point locations developed by Nogier and Wexu, and historical traditions of auriculotherapy in India, Greece, Europe, the Mid-East, and China.

Part Six

SOCIAL AND POLITICAL IMPLICATIONS

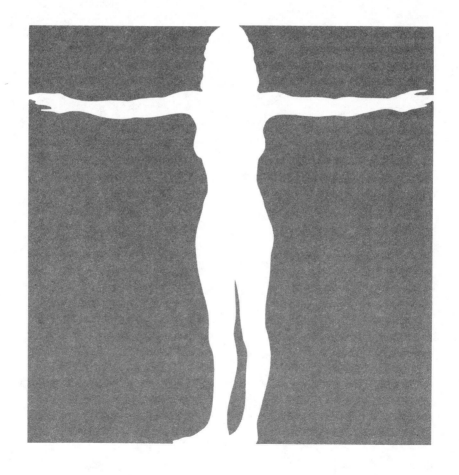

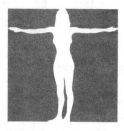

30

HOLISTIC HEALTH CENTERS

James S. Gordon, M.D.

Introduction

The future of holistic medicine will depend on the capacity of the holistic approach to cure the illnesses and improve the health of individuals, on the elaboration of its practice in centers specifically designed to accommodate it, and, ultimately, on its capacity to influence the larger health care system. In this chapter I want to deal particularly with the holistic health centers that have been established in the last several years, to place them in the context of a broader movement for creating humane and democratic alternatives to large impersonal and unresponsive services institutions, to describe their distinguishing characteristics, and to outline some of the ways they are affecting the larger system of health care.

Alternative Services

Alternative services began approximately twelve years ago. Most of the early ones were founded by indigenous helpers in direct response to the physical and emotional needs of the disaffected young people, who, in the mid- to late-1960s, had migrated to their communities. These services functioned as alternatives to health, mental health, and social service facilities that these young people found threatening, demeaning, or unresponsive.

The founders of the first alternative services resembled the earlier settlement-house workers in their idealism and humanitarianism. They differed in their commitment to the kind of participatory democracy that animated the civil rights, antiwar, youth, and women's movements of the 1960s. These activist workers believed that, given time, space, and encouragement, ordinary people could find the strength to help themselves and one another to deal with the vast majority of the problems that confronted them. They questioned the appropriateness of professional services that labeled or stigmatized those who came for help, and in their own work they blurred or obliterated boundaries between staff and clients. A teenager who was panicky one night might counsel another the next. Determined to remain responsive to their clients' needs, these early workers continually advocated the social changes that would make individual change more possible.

In 1967 a handful of switchboards, drop-in centers, free clinics and runaway houses served marginal young people in the "hip" neighborhoods of a few large cities. Today there are approximately 2,000 hot lines, more than 200 runaway houses, and some 400 free clinics. They have been organized by people of all ages, classes, and ideologies in small towns, suburbs, and rural areas as well as in the large cities. For example, in Prince George's County (a suburban and rural Maryland county), one of three hot lines receives 1,400 calls a month, one of two runaway houses gives shelter and intensive counseling to more than 350 young people each year, and a single one of the county's nine drop-in centers provides 600 hours of individual therapy each month.

In the early years alternative services were preoccupied with responding to the immediate needs of their young clients—for emergency medical care, a safe place during a bad drug trip, or short-term housing. More recently, they have expanded and diversified to offer longer-term and preventive services. Drop-in centers work with the families and teachers of the teenagers who come to them as well as with the young people themselves. Runaway houses have opened long-term residences and foster care programs for those who cannot return home or would otherwise be institutionalized. Free clinics and hot lines have helped initiate specialized counseling services for other and older groups—women, gays, the elderly, and so on.

During the 1970s, the alternative service model has been adopted and modified by people who have identified new community needs. They have created drug and alcohol counseling programs, rape crisis centers, shelters for battered women, peer counseling, street work projects, holistic health centers, home birthing services, and programs designed specifically for old people and particular ethnic minorities.

Free Clinics and Holistic Health Centers

In the late 1960s, while groups like the American Public Health Association and the Medical Committee for Human Rights struggled politically against the American Medical Association's position that health care was a "privilege not a right," free clinics (i.e., free at the point of delivery of care and relaxed in style) began to provide humane and easily accessible primary medical care to the young people who crowded into the centers of the counterculture.

The first free clinics—like the one in the Haight-Ashbury district of San Francisco—were inundated by young people looking for relief from a variety of physical, emotional, and drug-related problems. Physicians in emergency rooms gave intramuscular Thorazine to young people on bad drug trips and hospitalized them. At the Haight-Ashbury Free Clinic in San Francisco, street people—and mental health professionals willing to learn from them—were gently talking young trippers down in quiet, softly lit, pillow-filled rooms. In the medical part of the clinic, physicians and nurses carefully explained each aspect of their care to long-haired young people who had previously feared doctors and avoided treatment. It was as important at the free clinic not to condescend to patients, not to hurry them through procedures they feared or misunderstood and not to deny them information about preventing future illnesses as it was to prescribe the correct antibiotic. From the beginning these clinics readily included lay people in general, and patients in particular, on their staffs. They offered extensive paramedical training and education to their volunteers, emphasized collective decision making, and tried continually to respond to the community's changing needs.

Since the Haight-Ashbury Free Clinic opened in 1967 some 400 other free clinics have been created. Though some, like the Prince George's County Free Clinic and The Door in New York City, still focus on the physical problems (and their emotional sequelae) that particularly concern the young—birth control and prenatal care, minor urinary and respiratory ailments, venereal disease, and abortion—many others have become the primary health care resource for people of all ages in their area.

While the free-clinic movement was growing, health care professionals and their patients were becoming dissatisfied with the "best care that money can buy" and particularly with the care available to people who complained of feeling poorly but lacked organic pathology, the group that Sidney Garfield, creator of the Kaiser Permanente prepaid health program called the "worried well." This dissatisfaction was compounded by other aspects of medical practice: its focus on pathology and disease; its failure to prevent or adequately treat most chronic illness; its too rigid separation of physical, emotional, and spiritual problems; the iatrogenic illnesses that resulted from so many of its pharmaceutical and surgical remedies; and its failure to provide emotional satisfaction for either patients or practitioners.

Physicians, nurses, social workers, psychologists, and lay people who appreciated the interpersonal style and democratic policies of the free clinics but questioned the effectiveness of the conventional medicine practiced there began to study other approaches to health care and other traditions of healing. By the early 1970s they were stepping gingerly beyond the free-clinic model and away from their traditional training to create the services that would soon become holistic health centers.

Characteristics of Holistic Health Centers

There was, and is, no single model holistic health center. The programs that have evolved in the last decade are as varied as are the personalities and backgrounds, talents, and needs of their founders, the staffs they have attracted, and the clients who have made use of their services. There are, however, a number of characteristics that define and describe programs that are or might be called holistic health centers.

1. *Though they do so in a variety of ways, all holistic health centers are concerned with developing comprehensive programs that address the physical, psychological, and spiritual needs of those who come to them for help.* The Wholistic Health Centers, now a network of low-cost, primary care clinics in suburbs, cities, and rural areas on the East Coast and in the Midwest, began eight years ago with the establishment of a free clinic for low-income people in Springfield, Ohio, staffed by volunteers and operating out of a church basement. Its minister-founder, Granger Westberg, hoped to restore the Christian church's healing mission, to infuse medical practice with meaning, and to conserve resources by using the same building for two purposes. According to Westberg, these clinics, which stress "wholeness rather than piety," emphasize God's—and the clinic's—total acceptance of each person and a hope for the sick that is at once theologically sound and biologically useful. Teams of ministers, nurses, and physicians work jointly with clients in initial planning sessions to help them formulate health programs that address psychological and spiritual as well as physical needs. The treatment they offer is a synthesis of allopathic medical care, pastoral counseling, and biofeedback and is augmented by education in stress reduction, parent effectiveness training, yoga, meditation, and other physical and mental health practices.

At the Pain and Health Rehabilitation Center on a farm in LaCrosse, Wisconsin, Norman Shealy, a neurosurgeon who became disillusioned with the deleterious effects of drugs and the shortcomings of surgery, has created a program that addresses the bodies, minds, and spirits of sufferers from chronic pain. Shealy began eight years ago with a fairly mechanistic approach. Transcutaneous electrical nerve stimulation (TENS), facet rhizotomies, and behavior modification were his primary therapeutic modalities. Today he combines withdrawal from analgesics with diet, physical fitness, massage, biofeedback, TENS, and biogenics. The latter is a synthesis of progressive relaxation, autogenic training, Jungian therapy, and psychosynthesis, which is designed to help the practitioner to achieve the feeling of peace and acceptance that Shealy calls "spiritual attunement" as well as to relieve pain.

At the time that Westberg and Shealy were opening their clinics, Carl Simonton, a radiation oncologist in the U.S. Army, was beginning to study the therapeutic potential of the placebo response and of the faith and hope that are its constituents. After his discharge, he and his wife, Stephanie, opened the Cancer Counseling and Research Center in Fort Worth, Texas. Their program, which works primarily with people who have widely disseminated metastatic cancer, includes radiation therapy but relies to a large extent on procedures – visualization exercises, and individual, family, and group counseling in a supportive environment – that stimulate the person's will to live and with it, so far as they are able to tell, the body's immune response.

2. *Holistic health centers design health programs to meet the unique needs of each individual.* The lengthy meetings – "initial planning conferences" or "evaluations" – that are the first step in most programs generally produce a plan that includes ways to resolve the presenting problem, a summary of the client's long-term goals for health and well-being, and a strategy for achieving them.

A teenager with asthma who comes to a large and diverse program like the Wholistic Health and Nutrition Institute in Mill Valley, California, may get a shot of epinephrine for her acute attack, but her planning conference would probably develop a program to withdraw her from antihistamines and bronchodilators. It might include stress reduction through biofeedback, relaxation exercises, and a dietary change to eliminate foods that were allergenic for her. A longer-term strategy to help her achieve greater self-confidence and independence would perhaps involve counseling with her family to remove the interpersonal binds that precipitate and perpetuate this kind of psychophysiological condition and a jogging clinic to help her improve her vital capacity and her feelings about her own body. A second youngster with asthma with a different psychophysiologic make-up might be treated quite differently.

3. *All holistic health centers preferentially use therapeutic approaches that mobilize the individual's capacity for self-healing and independence rather than pharmacological or surgical remedies that have negative side effects and tend to promote further dependence.* In all centers there is an emphasis on techniques like biofeedback, progressive relaxation, acupressure, guided imagery, yoga, and tai chi, which enable people to experience and then alter physical and emotional states that they had always regarded as beyond their control. At the Pain and Health Rehabilitation Center and the UCLA Pain Control Unit, these modalities are used to help people who have been maintained on high doses of analgesics for years to quickly reduce or withdraw from them.

4. *Holistic health centers emphasize education and self-care rather than treatment and dependence.* Practitioners tend to believe that each person is his or her best source of care, that their job is to share rather than withhold and mystify their knowledge, to become "resources" rather than authorities. They tend to emphasize short-term problem-oriented psychotherapy and common-sense behavioral prescriptions rather than psychodynamic analysis.

Almost all centers provide extensive brochures and introductory talks about their approach to health care and the techniques they use. The vast majority present a variety of classes to increase the well-being and supplement the coping skills of those who come to them for help. Stress reduction, parent effectiveness, assertiveness training, communication skills, yoga, transcendental meditation, and jogging are staples. In programs like the Wholistic Health and Nutrition Institute and the Himalayan Institute (a network of primary-care clinics in which Western medicine, yogic practice, and psychotherapy are synthesized), the techniques used in the clinical services are also taught in programs specifically designed for lay people.

Other groups like the Berkeley Holistic Health Center; San Diego's Association for Holistic Health; the San Andreas Health Council, Palo Alto, California; and Interface in Brookline, Massachusetts, offer courses that are themselves a form of therapy. As one learns about visual retraining, massage, or meditation from a skilled teacher, one may indeed improve one's eyesight, relieve functional musculoskeletal problems, and reduce high blood pressure.

5. *Holistic health centers treat those who come to them for help as members of families and social systems.* This enables practitioners to view their clients' symptoms as reactions to and communications within their familial or social situation as well as biological phenomena. As part of their intake process most centers make extensive inquiries—both in person and through questionnaires—into job satisfaction, community involvement, and psychosocial stress. In some centers members of the family are interviewed together, and clinicians can observe the way they relate to one another.

Programs that work with people with chronic severe diseases (like the UCLA Pain Control Unit, the Pain and Health Rehabilitation Center in LaCrosse, Wisconsin, and the Cancer Counseling and Research Center) are particularly eager to mobilize the strengths of other family members to support the afflicted individual or, more often, to work together to resolve patterns that may encourage one of them to remain in a "sick role." In fact, several residential centers that recognize the therapeutic potential of this approach offer reduced rates to the symptomatic person's spouse. Programs for those who have relatively minor psychophysiological problems or for people who are concerned with health promotion also encourage family participation. Counselors work with couples to help them to stop smoking, lose weight, or to teach them how to massage one another.

6. *Holistic health centers view health as a positive state, not as the absence of disease, and emphasize health promotion and wellness.* This approach makes it possible for people who lack demonstrable organic pathology but feel poorly to enter holistic health programs, and encourages those who do have chronic organic disease to feel as well as they can within the limits set by the disease. Many centers offer courses to improve well-being by reducing stress and provide support groups for people who want to stop smoking, lose weight, become more physically fit, or improve their communication with others. In many cases, the techniques that are used to promote better health are identical with those that

are used to treat illness. At Oregon's Klamath Mental Health Center, for example, biofeedback is used to reduce stress and promote relaxation for those who simply want to feel better as well as those who have such conditions as migraine headache, back pain, and hypertension.

Since John Travis, a physician specializing in public health, first opened his Wellness Resource Center in Mill Valley, California, in 1974, "wellness" has become an influential concept, spurring the creation of programs like the Swedish Wellness Program at the Swedish Medical Center in Englewood, Colorado, and catalyzing an emphasis on wellness in holistic health centers. In wellness programs, individual counseling sessions and such standardized tests as health hazards appraisals, social readjustment rating scales, and wellness inventories are used to help clients understand the relationship between their behaviors and their health, to see that what and how much they eat, smoke, and exercise, how they drive, the way they work, and how they get along with their families all affect the way they feel physically and emotionally. Together staff and clients review the factors that are likely to make them ill or to shorten their lives and plan programs to eliminate or mitigate them.

7. *Though all holistic centers emphasize the preeminent importance of careful, sensitive history-taking and clinical examination, and most use such conventional diagnostic methods as X-rays, blood chemistry, urinalaysis, and psychological testing, some also include a variety of diagnostic techniques derived from other healing systems.* The Wholistic Health and Nutrition Institute, the Center for Traditional Acupuncture in Columbia, Maryland, and the UCLA Pain Control Unit, for example, all rely heavily on practitioners who have trained in both traditional Chinese and modern Western medicine and may compare and contrast findings obtained by pulse diagnosis and laboratory analysis. Some program directors, including Evarts Loomis at Meadowlark Center in Hemet, California; Norman Shealy of the Pain and Health Rehabilitation Center; and David Bresler of the UCLA Pain Control Unit have begun to bring scientific rigor to the study of such alternative diagnostic procedures as iridology, pulse diagnosis, ear diagnosis, and psychic diagnosis.

8. *Holistic health centers regard proper diet and exercise as cornerstones of healing.* Naturopathic physicians at the Clymer Clinic in Pennsylvania and at the Wholistic Health and Nutrition Institute use fasts, raw food diets, or increased amounts of particular foods therapeutically. The vast majority of centers simply advise their clients to cut down on processed, refined, and preserved foods as well as on sugar, artificial sweeteners, colorings, and flavorings; to increase the amount of fiber, complex carbohydrates, and raw food in the diet; and to eat somewhat less red meat and take stimulants like tea and coffee and depressants like alcohol in moderation. The meals they serve at parties or during workshops or residential sessions reflect these views.

Some programs emphasize the role that yoga, tai chi, or running may play in spiritual development as well as in improving physical and emotional health. Other centers are more concerned with the aerobic value of particular exercises.

Many centers have ongoing "clinics" devoted to particular physical disciplines, and running or doing yoga with a client is sometimes an integral part of the ongoing therapy.

9. *Holistic health centers maximize the therapeutic potential of the setting in which health care takes place.* The centers are generally both physically and interpersonally inviting and tend to inspire trust rather than fear or awe. The majority are free standing, but others like Westberg's and the UCLA Pain Control Unit occupy parts of such existing community institutions as churches and schools. The design leans heavily toward open spaces and attractively decorated, plant-filled rooms. Those who come for help are generally called clients rather than patients and are often encouraged to call staff members by their first names and to see the center as a place for education, volunteer work, and socializing as well as care in health and illness. Clients who do not have money often are able to barter services for health care.

10. *Holistic health centers rely on an active partnership between caregivers and consumers.* This connection is strongest in a program like the Eugene, Oregon, Community Health Education Center, which was started at the impetus of a broad-based neighborhood coalition supporting low-cost health care. This worker-managed collective of physicians, nurses, health aides, and social workers charges minimal fees (in 1979) for comprehensive primary care–$15.00 for the first visit and $8.50 for follow-ups–and is concerned with creating programs that respond directly to the felt needs of the community or for low-cost practical remedies to the problems that face them, such as child rearing, dietary management, physical fitness. Connections also exist with programs in more affluent areas. Community people are included on boards of directors, and their demands and needs shape the kinds of educational programs and health care techniques that are offered in the program.

11. *Holistic health centers include lay people and professionals with less prestigous degrees than M.D., Ph.D., and R.N. in the management of their centers.* A few programs have gone as far as the Community Health Education Center, a worker-managed collective in which all staff–from physicians to licensed practical nurses–are paid equally and participate equally in decision making, or the Mountain People's Clinic, whose physician makes $125 a week "sometimes when we've got it." However, virtually all centers make an active attempt to include nurses, massage therapists, receptionists, and health counselors in formulating policy and making day-to-day decisions about the center's operation.

12. *Holistic health centers provide an environment that is conducive to the personal growth of the staff as well as the clients.* Informality of staff relations, the relative absence of hierarchical distinctions, and the emphasis on cooperation and emotional sharing often make these centers feel more like a family than a physician's office or a clinic. A high value is placed on sharing feelings and on staff members' using their therapeutic talents and their emotional resources to help one another as well as their clients.

13. *Ongoing training of staff and of professionals in the community is an integral*

part of holistic health centers. Such training is one means by which nonprofessional staff can acquire skills and change their position within the center. It offers a way for practitioners to expand their knowledge and tends to catalyze changes in the therapeutic program.

Many centers also serve as resources for local professionals who are interested in incorporating a more holistic approach – or new techniques – in their practice. A number of programs (including the Pain and Rehabilitation Center, the Himalayan Institute, the San Francisco based East-West Academy of Healing Arts, and Los Angeles' Center for Integral Medicine have week- or month-long intensive courses and ongoing seminars for professionals. As they become more sophisticated, organizations are able to award continuing education credits for physicians and nurses.

Other groups like the Wholistic Health and Nutrition Institute, the Pain Control Unit, and San Francisco's Nurse Consultants and Health Counselors are actively involved in training students in the health care professions, and several programs, including the Pain and Health Rehabilitation Center, are looking forward to accredited rotations for interns and residents.

14. *Holistic health centers are concerned with incorporating healing systems and healers indigenous to their areas into their work.* This is an act of ecological faith as well as a matter of good clinical sense. Centers in western states have consulted with Native American healers and incorporated some of their rituals and herbs into their therapeutic programs. Centers in cities have made use of faith healers and *curanderos* (folk healers), and rural centers throughout the country have readily included indigenous plants in their pharmacopoeia.

15. *Holistic centers view illness as an opportunity for learning and change and are concerned with creating a context in which that kind of change can take place.* Even if it is not "natural" for Western-trained health professionals to regard illness as anything but an enemy, it is not difficult for them to realize that a flu or a bout of mononucleosis can be a sign of depression or that they can help a middle-aged executive to understand that a heart attack is a warning to slow down. It is far more difficult for centers that deal with people with chronic and often fatal illnesses to continue to help their clients wrest a sense of personal meaning from the illness that may soon kill them and for counselors and physicians to keep themselves from blame and self-doubt when their clients die. Work like this, which takes place at the Cancer Counseling and Research Center, requires a considerable amount of mutual support as well as extraordinary honesty.

16. *Though the absence of funds has handicapped research efforts, holistic health centers are beginning to study themselves and their work with clients.* An anthropological study of one Northern California center has already been completed and a second is under way at the Berkeley Psychosomatic Clinic. Most programs are keeping careful records and many are trying to move beyond anecdotal to systematic studies. The Pain and Health Rehabilitation Center, the UCLA Pain Control Unit, and the Cancer Counseling and Research Center have all been collecting follow-up data on their patients for some time. The results are

preliminary and in all cases the clients are their own controls. Still, all these programs have extremely high rates of success in reducing pain, amount of medication used, surgery, and cost of care. In the case of the Cancer Counseling and Research Center, the productive life of a number of patients with widely disseminated metastatic disease has been prolonged well beyond statistical probability and the expectations of their physicians.

The Future of Holistic Health Centers

As knowledge about a holistic approach to health and illness becomes more widespread, increased numbers of clients with a greater variety of problems are coming to the centers. Many centers are responding by changing to meet the needs of their clients. A program like the Holistic Rehabilitation and Health Center, which originally restricted itself to working with people with chronic pain, has now begun to apply its therapeutic approach to people who are simply stressed, and centers that initially worked with the "worried well" have begun to welcome the challenge of dealing with people who have serious illnesses.

The interest and the demand is widespread enough to stimulate Granger Westberg to plan for Wholistic Health Centers in a half dozen more cities, and intense enough—at least in northern California—to allow the staff of the Wholistic Health and Nutrition Institute to increase from six to twenty-three in the last two years.

Leslie Kaslof's 1978 volume *Wholistic Dimensions in Health* noted approximately fifty holistic health centers. Now, a year and a half after he compiled his listings, there may well be a hundred or more. In the Washington, D.C., area alone, three have opened in the last year.

At the same time that the model is being developed in holistic health centers it is also being applied in alternative services that confine their work to people at particular stages of the life cycle and in programs created by and for women. Comprehensive home birth programs, like Lewis Mehl's Berkeley Family Health Center, offer family counseling, prenatal care, and instruction in natural remedies as well as in natural childbirth. Runaway centers and group homes are beginning to pay more attention to the food they serve young people, to discuss exercise and health care as well as living places and schools, and to suggest meditation or relaxation exercises as well as family therapy. In Phoenix, physicians and psychologists who are disciples of Yogi Bhajan have created a comprehensive nondrug residential detoxification program for young addicts that combines Kundalini yoga, meditation, nutrition, and an intense group therapeutic experience. In Houston, Texas, plans are under way for a multimillion dollar holistic health and rehabilitation center, a city- and county-funded program for young people with psychosocial and drug-related problems. At the other end of the life cycle, programs for the elderly (like SAGE and the Institute for Creative

Aging) and projects for the dying (like SHANTI) have all adopted a holistic approach.

Women's programs (like the Berkeley Women's Health Collective and the Haight-Ashbury Women's Medical Clinic) combine general medical and gynecological care with an emphasis on prevention, natural remedies, and consciousness-raising groups. In Dorchester, Massachusetts, minority women who run the Columbia Point Alcoholism Program provide a comprehensive residential program for Hispanic and Black women and their children. The program uses fasts to detoxify alcoholics and combines instruction about natural foods and herbs, rhythmic breathing, physical exercise, and meditation with education, child care, rehabilitation counseling, and social services.

The model that has been created in holistic centers and applied in other alternative services is also being integrated into the mainstream of health care. Large corporations, alarmed by rising rates of absenteeism and alcoholism and by the increase in the cost of insuring their employees, have created wellness and health-promotion programs. Kimberly-Clark, a leader in this effort, is presently embarked upon a three-year experimental program that includes a comprehensive initial history and a physical, a screening battery of laboratory tests, consultation with a physician or nurse practitioner, and an orientation to physical fitness. A variety of educational experiences are available to enrollees free of charge, including courses in nutrition, cardiopulmonary resuscitation, smoking control, and stress management.

Donald Ardell, editor of the *American Journal of Health Planning*, notes that Health Systems Agencies, established under the Health Planning and Resource Development Act of 1974, are currently involved in providing technical assistance to health promotion and wellness programs in schools, the work place, hospitals, and neighborhood health centers. One of the most active of these, the Madison, Wisconsin, Health Planning Council, has helped a small hospital in Columbus, Wisconsin, to create a wellness program for employees that includes running, nutritional classes, yoga, transcendental meditation, cross-country skiing, and stress management.

Government bureaucracies, eager to practice some of what they preach, are also beginning to pay attention to improving their employees' health. At the Public Health Service's Center for Disease Control in Atlanta, 70 percent of the 2,200 employees are participating in health education programs that, like the Wellness Resource Center, begin by identifying physical and psychological risk factors in each person's life. And even the Department of Health, Education, and Welfare itself, which houses the newly created Office of Health Information and Health Promotion, is at work on its own internal health-promotion program.

Though there is little information so far on holistic health centers in the professional literature, they are being discussed in workshops at meetings of the newly created American Holistic Medical Association and the Congress of Nurse Healers. At public conferences across the country, groups like the San Diego

Association for Holistic Health, the Himalayan Institute, the Center for Integral Medicine, the East-West Academy of Healing Arts, and the Institute for the Study of Human Knowledge are presenting these programs and the techniques used in them to audiences that not uncommonly exceed one to two thousand professionals and lay people.

The effect of all this activity is now being felt in the schools of the health care professions. Departments of behavioral medicine, family practice, community medicine, and psychiatry and schools of nursing and public health are all sponsoring lecture series and elective courses in holistic approaches to health and medicine. Already at UCLA a joint effort of the Schools of Medicine, Public Health, and Nursing and the Department of Kinesiology has created the Center for Health Enhancement, Education, and Research (CHEER). This month-long residential program emphasizes exercise, diet, relaxation, stress reduction, education, and the development of mutual support groups for people who have frank cardiovascular disease as well as for the worried well. It will be carefully studied in the years to come.

Conclusion

As holistic health centers continue to grow and develop, their attitudes toward health and healing, the techniques they use, and the way they synthesize them will continue to be incorporated into the mainstream of medical care and of health promotion efforts. The holistic health centers themselves can serve as natural laboratories in which a variety of professionals (M.D.s, osteopaths, nurses, chiropractors, psychologists, massage therapists, and acupuncturists) and lay people will develop new therapeutic modalities and learn new ways to work together and with the clients who come to them for help.

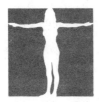

ANNOTATED BIBLIOGRAPHY

Ardell, Donald B. **From omnibus tinkering to high level wellness: the movement toward holistic health planning.** *American Journal of Health Planning,* October 1976. **1 (2)**, 15–34.

> In this essay Ardell, editor of the *American Journal of Health Planning* and author of *High Level Wellness,* shows how the attitudes and practices of the holistic health movement and the current emphasis on wellness rather than disease may be used to shape the work of health systems agencies and individual health planners.

Ardell, Donald B. **High level wellness in the HSAs: health planning success story.** *American Journal of Health Planning,* July 1978. **3 (3)**, 1–18.

> This article summarizes a survey of 198 Health Systems Agencies (HSAs). Ardell found that 20 of these local and regional planning agencies were actively involved in programs to promote wellness. Drawing heavily on the exemplary program of the Madison, Wisconsin, Health Planning Council, Ardell describes a paradigm for HSA involvement in wellness-related activity. He concludes by listing some of the factors that will be necessary to produce further interest in and awareness of wellness: increased support by the Department of Health, Education, and Welfare and the American Health Planning Association, information sharing among wellness promotion programs, training of wellness specialists, development of clear definitions for wellness and health promotion, and the creation of a local and national constituency for wellness.

Bloomfield, Harold H., and Kory, Robert B. **The Holistic Way to Health and Happiness.** New York: Simon and Schuster, 1978.

> A readable, popular volume that outlines the approach and programs of the Age of Enlightenment Center for Holistic Health in San Diego. At that center Dr. Bloomfield and his colleagues try to synthesize Western medicine with careful attention to diet, exercise, and the behavioral and environmental causes of illness. There is a particular emphasis at the center and in the book on the reduction of stress and the promotion of well-being through regular practice of transcendental meditation, which Bloomfield and Kory here describe as the "healing silence."

Fields, Suzanne. **Balm for the "worried well."** *Innovations,* Fall 1978, **5** (3), 3–10.

> This is a description of a pilot study that Kaiser Permanente, a comprehensive prepaid health program, has developed for "the worried well." Kaiser attempts to address the psychosocial problems of this group through counseling by its staff and educational programs stimulated by Kaiser and undertaken by a local community college.

Gordon, James S. **Final report of the special study on alternative services.** *Report to the President of the President's Commission on Mental Health.* Washington, D.C.: U.S. Government Printing Office, 1978.

> This comprehensive report places holistic health centers and health programs for specific groups—including women and elders—in the context of the larger movement to create systems of comprehensive community-based health and mental health care. It includes a historical section on the development of alternative mental health services, a summary of the characteristics of these services, and descriptions of the particular kinds of centers that have been developed to meet the needs of such diverse groups as runaway young people, battered women, and rape victims, as well as the elderly, the pregnant, and the ill. It concludes with recommendations for federal funding of alternative services.
>
> Available from Dr. Gordon at the Center for Studies of Child and Family Mental Health, National Institute of Mental Health, 5600 Fishers Lane, Rockville, Maryland 20857.

Gordon, James S.; Jaffe, Dennis T.; and Bresler, David E. (Eds.). **Mind, Body, and Health: Toward an Integral Medicine.** Rockville, Md.: National Institute of Mental Health, in press.

> This volume is a product of a 1977 conference titled New Directions in Health and Mental Health, sponsored jointly by the National Institute of Mental Health and the Los Angeles-based Center for Integral Medicine. The book's twenty essays provide the most comprehensive overview of the practical application of a holistic approach to health care presently available. The emphasis is on programs for the control of pain and chronic disease, including the Pain Control Unit at UCLA, the Pain and Health Rehabilitation Center in La Crosse, Wisconsin, and the Cancer Counseling and Research Center in Fort Worth, Texas. There are also chapters on holistic practice in alternative mental health centers, medical emergency rooms, private physicians' offices, birthing centers, and programs for the aged. The contributors, including C. Norman Shealy, Robert Rodale, Robert Swearingen, Richard Miles, Dolores Krieger, James Fadiman, and the editors, have long been active in the holistic health movement.

Kaslof, Leslie J. (Ed.). **Wholistic Dimensions in Healing.** New York: Doubleday, 1978.

> Though some of his listings are already out of date this volume still offers the most complete and comprehensive guide to groups and publications concerned with wholistic (or holistic) health. Listings for each holistic health center include name, address, phone number, director's name, a brief description of healing modalities employed, and date of founding. An exceedingly valuable reference for anyone interested in finding a local center or in surveying the holistic health movement.

Hayes-Bautista, David, and Harveston, Dominic S. **Holistic health care.** *Social Policy,* March/April, 1977. 7–13.

This paper presents a useful summary of what the authors call the "community clinic ideology," which suggests that "individual illness is a reflection of societal illness" with multiple causes, many of which lie outside of the individual's body or control. The authors suggest that multiple interventions, preventive care, health promotion, and social restructuring are all part of the therapeutic task.

Loomis, Evarts G., and Paulson, J. Sig. **Healing for Everyone.** New York: Hawthorne, 1975.

This is a personal account by a physician who has been practicing holistic medicine for more than twenty years, and his minister-colleague. It describes Dr. Loomis's Meadowlark Center and demonstrates how he and his staff have integrated pastoral counseling and Western medicine, diet, and exercise with such unorthodox modalities as megavitamin therapy and homoeopathy. Some of his techniques and his emphasis on the importance of spiritual factors in health and healing may seem alien to the medical profession, but Dr. Loomis's humane and sensitive approach to his patients will not.

Ng, Lorenz; Davis, Devra; and Manderscheid, Ronald. **The health promotion organization: a practical intervention designed to promote healthy living.** *Public Health Reports,* September/October 1978. **93 (5)**, 446–455.

In this paper three federal scientists propose the establishment of community-based health-promotion organizations that have as their function the creation of an active, healthy drug-free populace. Though the behaviorist emphasis seems a bit nightmarish (the authors suggest that rewards be given for "achieving certain desirable health norms"), the perspective and the proposal for integrating health promotion into the system of medical care is an interesting one.

Poesnecker, C. E. **It's Only Natural.** Hatfield, Pa.: Adventures Limited Press, 1978.

This account by the naturopath and chiropractor who is presently director of the Clymer Health Clinic is written for the lay person. Poesnecker details the clinic's diagnostic procedures from phonocardiography and thermography to reflexology and radiasthesia and describes a variety of natural, nonpharmacological therapies and their use at the clinic.

Some of Poesnecker's matter-of-fact and unsupported statements about pathological states and the therapies he uses to remedy them will undoubtedly make physicians bridle, but those who are curious about an unorthodox holistic practice will enjoy this chatty, opinionated book.

Simonton, O. Carl; Matthews-Simonton, Stephanie; and Creighton, James. **Getting Well Again.** Los Angeles: J. P. Tarcher, 1978.

The book presents accounts of some of the heroic therapeutic work the Simontons have been doing at the Cancer Counseling and Research Center in Fort Worth, Texas. It includes summaries of some of the scientific work that inspired their efforts, descriptions of visualization procedures and counseling sessions, frank discussions of the authors' reactions to the work they are doing, and preliminary statistics on the longer-than-average survival of some people who have come to them for help.

Though their therapeutic modalities are limited—they do not, for example, use the nutritional therapies that seem to be so useful to some people with cancer—this energetic, honest, and hopeful book still presents a fine model of holistic practice.

Travis, John W. **Wellness Workbook.** Mill Valley, Calif.: Wellness Resource Center, 1977.

Though it is a useful self-assessment tool for anyone who is concerned with improving his or her health, this attractive looseleaf workbook is particularly designed for clients coming to Travis's center. It includes numerous questions and questionnaires about health and health-related behaviors and provides practical suggestions for—among other things—relaxation, "ways to deal with anger," and "keeping a psychological journal."

The emphasis in the written material, as at the Wellness Resource Center, is on helping people to understand why they are not as well as they might be and encouraging them to "take charge of any areas [of their lives] which presently are not working well." Unfortunately, the *Wellness Workbook* costs $25 and a larger version for professionals still more. The Wellness Resource Center is located at 42 Miller Avenue, Mill Valley, California 94941.

Tubesing, Donald A. **The Wholistic Health Center.** New York: Human Sciences Press, 1979.

This book provides a comprehensive portrait of the philosophy and practice of the Wholistic Health Centers, a group of church-based primary-care facilities in Ohio and Illinois. In this account Tubesing, the former director of program development, sums up descriptive and statistical material earlier presented in a series of monographs. He emphasizes the Wholistic Health Centers' team approach—a physician, pastoral counselor, and nurse work together—its involvement of patients in their own care, and its emphasis on prevention and community education.

31

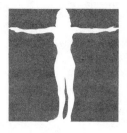

THE FUTURE OF HEALTH CARE IN THE UNITED STATES

Rick J. Carlson, J.D.

Speculation about the future is always problematic, and projecting the future for the institutions of health there is no exception. However, there is a central issue that can be used as an organizing principle. Simply, it is whether the human species is capable of adapting to the challenges of change, or if there are limitations to our adaptability – limits some think we have already reached. This issue is implicated in the many ideas, issues, and trends that will shape the future – many of which are discussed in this chapter. This question may not always be raised directly, but it is always present. It cannot be "answered"; it is as much a matter of belief as of proof. My task in this chapter is to present the ideas, issues, trends, and themes that will shape the future, and in turn, the future of the institutions of health *but* always with the cutting edge of adaptability in view.

A Trajectory of Ideas

It is possible to identify the key ideas that have characterized our society's thinking about its health and then to trace their interplay over time. Any historical examination will yield just a few central concepts – including such ideas as moderation, optimal performance, happiness, naturalness, social functioning, recovery and convalescence, equity, and wholeness. Ideas like these have always formed the foundation of the approaches the Western and Northern societies have

483

fashioned to improve their health. A historical examination is not possible in a chapter of this length, but a few summary comments can be made.

At the turn of this century, our society had some fundamental options before it. These choices can be characterized by this simple schematic:

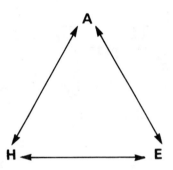

Letter "A" represents the *Agents* of disease. Much of current therapeutic medicine is based on counteracting the agents of disease and attempting to cure individuals who have become ill as a result of their action. "H" represents the *Human Host* and approaches to health that enhance the ability of the person to resist disease and to improve healing capacities of the body. Preventive medicine and health-enhancement programs illustrate these approaches. "E" represents the *Environment*, which includes social and ecological factors in health, such as sanitation, pollutant effects, and working conditions.

The evidence that identifies those factors associated with improvements in human health *prior* to the beginning of this century suggests that the principal gains were achieved through nontherapeutic methods (mainly public health measures affecting the environment) and through improvements both in the quality and in the amount of food (which strengthened the host). However, during this same period, therapeutic medicine was gaining ascendancy. Among the reasons for this seeming anomaly was the availability of the scientific method, which made it possible to draw causal relationships between a therapeutic intervention and the outcome of patient's disease. More importantly, medicine continued to gain political and economic strength as the number of its practitioners increased. For example, homoeopathic medicine, which focuses on the human host, was a major medical system of treatment at the turn of the century. As a result of the control gained by allopathic medicine and the Flexnor Report of 1910, homoeopathic medicine virtually went underground. For these reasons as well as a variety of others, society chose to emphasize the identification, management, and extirpation (in some cases) of the agents of disease as *against* equally plausible social choices that might have been made.

In my view, the choice to develop a medical-care delivery system through nearly exclusive allocation of resources for that purpose was made far more for political, social, and economic reasons than for therapeutic ones. A careful reading of the historical record at the turn of the century would have suggested a continuation and even an amplification of programs designed to improve the quality of the environment and to further strengthen the human host. The results of this choice have not been insignificant. We have gained considerable information about human biology, and human sickness, and we have discovered the means of curing and treating those sicknesses and diseases that lie beneath them.

The choice was not necessarily the wrong choice. Yet, it is my view that we are now poised for a fundamental change in perspective—a change that may restore social, environmental, and behavioral factors to a position of influence in public policy. Evidence is emerging that suggests that we will "rediscover" the critical importance of the determinants of health other than medical care. The "new" medicine will once again emphasize improvements in the quality of our environment and in the means and modes of strengthening the human host. If we change our perspective, it will not be a rejection of what we have learned and what we may continue to learn through the current system of medicine. Nonetheless future institutions of health will be quite different from what they are today.

Behind all of these options is a most fundamental question. Are we sufficiently adaptable (or do we believe ourselves to be) that we can continue to introduce new technologies in the service of growth and progress that have side effects that are neither so destructive to the species, nor so problematic as to create sicknesses and disease that our curative medicine cannot cope with? If we *are* sufficiently adaptable, the choice we have made about our health in the shank of this century—with continued investments in research and improvements in medical practice—should be sufficient for the foreseeable future. If we are *not* that adaptable, then either we will succumb to an increasingly toxic environment, or we will pioneer new approaches to health that will depend far less on after-the-fact medicine and far more on profound prevention and a population medicine. This choice will, in turn, shape the future institutions of health that must serve those ends.

Issues for the Future

The Philosophy of Limits: Appropriate Technology

As natural resources are now perceived to be finite and as the consequences of growth and development have become less tolerable, a movement (or a series of movements) has emerged proposing "limits" to growth. The work sponsored by the Club of Rome and authored by the Meadows et al., *The Limits to Growth* (1974), was one of the first books published concerning this issue. More recently, Lester Brown's *The Twenty-Ninth Day* (1978) updates the limits-to-growth debate in an excellent and comprehensive treatment of the arguments and issues. There is also literature on the "social" limits to growth, which examines the limits that have been imposed (or are likely to be imposed) on technological development for social reasons rather than – or in addition to – economic or technological ones. A good example of this literature is Fred Hirsch's (1976) book, *The Social Limits to Growth.*

The limits-to-growth rationale is closely related to, and in one sense pivotal to, another recent cultural trend: the "appropriate (or intermediate) technology" movement. Groups have sprung up throughout the world urging the development of more appropriate technologies to supplant those that are thought to be most damaging to our biology. The movement is most active in the United States and in the United Kingdom, where it had its classical origins with the work of E. F. Schumacher, principally in his seminal book *Small is Beautiful* (1976). The key premises of this movement are occasionally vague, but they center on technology that is "small, simple, capital saving, and nonviolent to people and to the environment." It is also often but not necessarily labor-intensive.

These companion movements influence future thinking about health. Medicine is so integral to our culture and so much a creature of society's technology that it cannot escape the analysis that these movements offer. This is true whether the analysis addresses each sector in our economy or is sweeping in its scope. In the health and medical sectors, the recent works that best apply the "limits" rationale to medicine are Illich's (1976) *Medical Nemesis,* Carlson's (1975) *The End of Medicine,* and Fuchs's (1975) *Who Shall Live?*

Holistic Thinking

One of the most overly used and abused words in our language is the term "holistic." First coined by Jan Smuts in 1926, the term has come to be applied to almost every aspect of human behavior. Smuts's original use of the word was epistemological; the word was a way of characterizing phenomena in a profoundly different way than the prevailing "reductionist" perspective. To Smuts – and to others – reductionist thinking resulted in an unrelenting analysis of the parts of systems without consideration of how those parts interacted and without consideration – or even acknowledgment – of phenomena that represented more than the sum of the parts. Hence, holistic thinking in its original and fullest sense is an antidote to the reductionist epistemology that underlies modern scientific thought.

In recent years the word "holistic" has applied perhaps more frequently in the health sector than in any other. This is not surprising. The practice of modern medicine is a case of reductionism run wild. While limiting, it is hardly an assault on human sensibility to examine the chemical constituents of a substance one at a time. But to many people it is not only limiting but impoverishing to assume that health is nothing more than the composite of "well-oiled" body parts. In this sense the application of the term "holism" to medicine is more than timely; it is profound. At the same time, the term is often glibly applied and frequently trivialized as well.

The power of holistic thinking lies in the perspective it brings to our perception of who we are as human beings. Reductionist thinking anywhere, medicine included, results in the compartmentalization of the human being and human experience into those aspects or parts that are amenable to detailed analysis or intervention. This is one of the basic premises that underlies the prevailing medical practice. Although it has its utility, it is a profoundly limited view of the human being.

This shift toward holism is really irreversible, not because it is being forced upon medicine so urgently and so successfully but rather because the shift is part of a much larger change in perspective about who and what the human being is. Its application to medicine is an aspect of a much more embracing paradigm shift. This is why the utility of the concept in a futures orientation has so much more power than could possibly be appreciated by attending a conference on "holistic" health in California, where the message is that carrot juice, massage, and running clinics represent the state-of-the-art.

The Placebo and the Self-Healing Patient

As medicine has evolved it has emphasized therapeutic interventions specific to the problems diagnosed: a drug, surgery, physical rehabilitation, and so on. Whenever possible, its mission has been to match a health problem with a specific treatment. The therapeutic results achieved have been believed to be associated with the specificity of the treatment—the more specific the treatment, the greater the likelihood of a good patient outcome. Any nonspecific aspect that appears to be related to patient outcome has either been ignored, given passing mention, or referred to as a placebo. This is the way most of medicine is practiced, but in the next few decades the real task of biomedical science should be to identify and learn to understand the dynamics of the placebo. It may be that most real healing is the consequence of nonspecific factors rather than the reverse. After all, if some percentage—say 40 percent—of any cure might be placebo, it suggests that at a minimum 40 percent of the disease experienced by the patient is a "placebo" as well.

The self-regulatory capacity of the human organism is imperfectly understood. The fast-growing biofeedback literature is evidence of the promise of self-regulation. Future biomedical research must place self-regulation high on the agenda; its potential is enormous. This does not mean that practitioners are unneeded. Far from it. As the "humanistic" medicine movement has valiantly sought to say, it is the quality of the person in the room with the patient that makes the difference, not the tool or the technique, however useful they may be.

The Larger Cultural Transformation

The institutions of health will not change in isolation. Many of the themes treated in this paper are drawn from change processes in larger cultural contexts. The largest of these contexts is the culture as a whole. In recent years, a substantial literature has emerged that focuses on the cultural transformation many believe is occurring. The issues and ideas raised by this literature are legion. Rather than deal with them individually, I would like to discuss the major thrust of the literature here. In the view of some (like George Leonard [1972] in his book, *The Transformation*, Jonas Salk [1973] in *The Survival of the Wisest*, and Theodore Roszak [1978] in *Person Planet*) we are living through the last stages—or gasps—of a materialistic world view. The values associated with material growth and technological progress are said to be yielding to more humanistic values and a less materialistic orientation. This is relevant because any medicine is rooted in its conception of the human being. Today's institutions of health are based on an approach to health that perceives the patient in materialistic and mechanistic terms. This is so in part because any medicine that would engage itself in the manifold aspects and realities of the patient would be paralyzed by information overload that would make an integrated delivery system very difficult to create. Still, the view of the human that animates medical practice is a very limited one. It is securely anchored in a mechanistic metaphor. The argument is that, as a materialistic reality dissolves and a more humanistic, spiritual reality takes its place, all human institutions will necessarily change—those dealing with health included.

A More Profound Ecology

One of the dominant intellectual disciplines in our society for the last few decades has been economics. As a result, public policy and our own perceptions of reality have been heavily shaped by the economist's perceptions, the tools economists use, and, for that matter, the indicators of our collective experience that economists offer as a way of characterizing that experience. Yet, these tools, concepts, and, indeed, the reality that economics forces upon us have compromised our capacity to devise a more profound ecological understanding of ourselves and our health in particular. There is a radical difference between cost-effectiveness analysis (and the measurement of the success of a society in terms of GNP) and the use of an ecological concept like "carrying capacity" to make judgments about growth, technological development, and progress. Moreover, we as human beings forget our animal origins and our continuing animal experience. We are a part of nature, not its subjugators. The notion, largely drawn from the Judeo-Christian tradition, that it is man's responsibility to exercise mastery over his environment has in many ways led us to the ecological and environmental pitfalls that we face today. Voices like Lester Brown's (1978) in *The Twenty-Ninth Day*, Kenneth Boulding's in much of his work, and even Barry Commoner's (though more polemical than the others) have urged upon us the essential need to understand our world ecologically rather than economically.

Health Promotion, Wellness, and the Super-Healthy

A little over thirty years ago, the National Institutes of Health (NIH) were conceived. In the decades that followed, the research conducted by and for NIH has resulted in an impressive body of knowledge about human biology and, in particular, states of disease in the human being. When the National Institutes of Health were created, as a society we had very little systematic information about disease and the sick person. Since the development of NIH, however, research has been done that has generated a systematic corpus of information. Much of the practice of a modern medicine is based upon the biomedical research conducted by NIH.

Yet neither the practice of medical care nor the research agendas of NIH have examined the healthy person. This is an anomaly because while we lack any systematic information about healthy people, interest in and enthusiasm for health promotion programs, wellness, well-being, and holistic approaches to health are rising fast. Any review of the literature over the last decade, either scholarly or popular, would quickly reveal that the programs related to health promotion and, indeed, the terms themselves were rarely found prior to the last few years. It is not surprising that interest in health promotion has increased. What is surprising is that this is happening without the existence of any kind of a theoretical base on which such programs can be grounded and without any systematic research effort to identify who healthy people are and why they are healthy.

There are already some small but significant changes. A branch for behavioral medicine has been created within the National Institutes of Health, an event that probably could not have occurred three or four years ago. Moreover, NIH appears to be more interested in the role of nutrition and human health than it has historically been. These are small changes, but they reflect the larger changes that are occurring.

If the new and quite fashionable interest in health promotion and wellness is to move beyond being a fad, more serious thought will have to be given to theory and research needs than has been given thus far. The National Institutes of Health will probably continue with their mandate to fund research to teach us more about disease and sickness even though there is no reason why we should know more. At the same time, research must be funded that tells us something about the healthy.

The Hypothesis of Biosocial Decline

During the years since World War II there has been an increase in chronic degenerative disease in the United States far greater than that accounted for by the aging of the population. We generally assume that increases in chronic degenerative disease are due principally to an increasingly aging population. There are some very impressive circumstantial data sources that do not agree. Commonweal, Inc., in Bolinas, California – a health and human ecology center whose staff has contributed to this volume – has collected most of this data, which can be found in journal articles published by Commonweal. These data were obtained through the examination of younger persons across a wide range of biological and social indicators, and it can be said that with no exception the quality of life or well-being reflected by those indicators has declined in the last twenty years. The indicators include chronic disease levels, serious crime rates, suicide rates, children with learning disabilities and behavioral disorders (such as hyperactivity), both quantitative and qualitative assessments of family life, illegitimacy rates, runaway rates for young people, accidental deaths, scores in scholastic aptitude testing, and so on. The cause of the "declines" is far from clear. The hypothesis generated at Commonweal is that these declines are associated with a wide range of environmental toxins which are in turn associated with a variety of technological and industrial processes and products. Many of these technologies and industrial products have been developed in the last twenty-five or thirty years to make our lives more comfortable and convenient. None of them was developed with the thought of high-level toxicity in mind. Nonetheless – and once again it must be stressed that it is only a hypothesis – the indicators suggest that the adaptability of our population, and in particular of young people, may be limited in the face of an increasingly toxic environment. There is much more work to be done on this hypothesis. It has only been propounded for the purpose of attracting attention and further work. But the data are chilling and highly suggestive nonetheless.

The Dialectics of Change
Countervailing Forces and Trends

The future is inherently contradictory. Some points in this chapter may contradict others. It would be impossible – or certainly foolish – to discuss the future as if all the trends and indicators were consistent, for of course, they are not. And yet most of the propositions offered thus far are of a piece. Taken together, they auger a certain kind of future, one characterized by deeper human values, a more humanistic perspective, the continuing ascendancy of holistic thinking, and less emphasis on specific therapeutics and excessive professionalism with a concomitant assumption of more responsibility by persons for their own health within a more sound ecological understanding of ourselves and our environment.

Taken together in an even larger sense, they argue for our frailty – our inability to adapt to the rigors of the industrial, technological society we have created. But there are cross-currents. Other trends and other ideas exist that project an alternative future – a future that is premised on our adaptability. These cross-currents deserve our full attention, but given the space limitations of the volume, they can only be mentioned here.

The Purpose of the Medical-Care Delivery System

It is generally assumed that modern medicine exists because it improves human health. Furthermore, it is also assumed that we have chosen to approach the improvement of our health for very reasonable, rational, and scientific reasons. But this is not the case. Modern medicine gestated for social, political and economic reasons, not therapeutic and scientific ones; it survives for the same reasons. There are many routes to improving health and there are many different medicines. The medicine that we have in our society is perhaps the only one that could have evolved, given the economic, social, and political conditions that prevailed at its birth and during its infancy. It is, however, conceivable that it could be based on a different theory of health and healing – some other system of medicine. There is nothing absolute about allopathic theory. But it is highly unlikely that the delivery system that has evolved, irrespective of the method of the medicine incorporated into it, could have been much different. Our medical-care delivery system is geared to the requirements of our political economy as much as is the steel industry. There is a product – medical-care services, the suppliers of the product; R&D to generate new products; financing mechanisms to insure adequate capital and sufficient cash flow; and marketing through insurance companies – and more than sufficient profits to keep things humming. The very penetration that the system has achieved into our economy, and its integral relationship with the viability of the economy as a whole, make it doubtful that it will yield any of its formidable power without the very nature of our economy first being transformed.

The Serviced Society

Recently, as industrial development has slowed and as new technologies and automation have steadily reduced the number of jobs available in manufacturing, the services sector has expanded. This expansion has been accompanied by the creation of jobs. Since our nation's economy and health is dependent upon a high rate of employment, the need for jobs has fueled a real search of growth in the services economy, an economy that by its nature is more job-creating and sustaining than manufacturing. As a result, for macro-economic reasons, our society "requires" a large and growing services sector of which medical care and the institutions of health are a large part.

As the population grows and automation continues to eliminate jobs, the demand for services will necessarily have to increase and this analysis applies to medical-care services perhaps better than to any of the other human services. The future may well belong to illness. As long as hospital beds have sheets on them, patients will be found to slip between them. A serviced society does not encourage self-responsibility or the development and implementation of programs designed to affect us all through improvements in the environment unless those initiatives guarantee at least as many jobs. In short, a serviced society demands illness, need, and dependence.

The Corporation and Human Services

Many employers have begun to perceive that one of their largest, if not the largest, outflows of capital is for medical care. At the same time, industry lacks the means to influence the level of that expenditure. Hence, corporations have recently become extremely interested in cost containment and have become further interested in health promotion programs ostensibly as a means of reducing their medical care costs. The fact that very little evidence exists that health promotion programs have that effect is proving to be no deterrent. Many companies have developed health promotion programs and still more are extremely interested in doing so. A good illustration is the lead article that appeared in the September 4, 1978, issue of *Business Week* describing the programs of many large corporations. Moreover, the office of Health Information and Health Promotion of the Department of Health, Education, and Welfare sponsored a conference in January 1979 bringing together a number of corporate executives to discuss corporate health promotion programs. This simply could not have occurred a few years ago.

Given the interest that corporations are now evincing in health and, further, given historical patterns of corporate interest in education and more generally in the welfare of employees and their families, within the next twenty years the corporation may become the prime deliverer of human services. The public is increasingly disenchanted with public solutions to critical human needs and it is unlikely that the other option – more individual responsibility – will be much accelerated even in the neoconservative mood of this country in the late 1970s. Under these circumstances the corporation – now directly influencing the lives of well over half of the members of our society – may be the only alternative left. This does not mean that government will step out of the picture; rather, it will continue to raise revenue and to pay for most, if not all, of the human services. But it may be that delivery units may soon come under corporate control.

Human Adaptability and the Future of Health

All that has been done in this chapter is to suggest some of the forces and trends that will "predispose" the future – a future that will ultimately depend on our adaptability to those varied forces and trends.

Prior to the industrial era, life was characterized by a simple diet; exposure to the outdoors and to the elements; hard but productive labor (often outdoors); more regularity of sleep, often more naturally wedded to night and day; little long-distance travel; and a set of interpersonal relationships that seldom varied and was nurtured by the extended family. Today all or most life functions have been altered for much of the population, particularly those living in the urbanized northeastern and western states. Diets are richer, more complex, and laced with a variety of chemicals to enhance both their appearance and their palatability; our lives are spent mostly indoors under artificial lighting conditions, in filtered air and controlled temperatures; people work hard but seldom with their bodies and often during hours least conducive to their own time clocks; work has been compartmentalized from the rest of life as something someone has to go somewhere else to do; many travel extensively, often crossing time zones, and even those who do not travel spend more and more time just getting to and from work – almost always by conveyance. Finally, high mobility and lack of the need for cooperative survival efforts have resulted in the diffusion, if not the elimination, of many traditional psychosocial supports. Whether these altered living conditions are conducive to ill health is impossible to prove except insofar as one or more of them can be associated with specific disease conditions that were greatly different.

Prior to 1900 the major killers were not chronic in nature; they were largely infectious and occasionally pandemic in nature. Today in the United States most infectious diseases (with the exception of some respiratory viral illnesses) are either under effective control or at least have been offset by biochemical means. But new health problems have arisen that may not be as amenable to the techniques currently available to medicine as those of the past. These include stress and illnesses that may be associated with stress; chronic conditions that result from multiple influences; accidental trauma and death due principally to the motor vehicle and acts of violence; degraded environmental conditions, including noise and other environmental contaminants; smoking; overindulgence in foods; and many other poor health habits that are related to the onset of disease. These new problems may be the result of rapidly changing ecological patterns – patterns that are foreign to those that nurtured the growth and development of the human species prior to the twentieth century.

So, again, the question remains. Will we or can we adapt to these changing conditions? The environments and cultures within which health and disease occur have changed and are changing. The health problems we experience today are clearly different than those of our past. But will we adapt to them with sufficient speed so as to keep them in check, or are they malaises so integral to the way in which we live our lives that they will eventually destroy the basis of life itself?

A Scenario for the Future

In the year 2000 there will still be a medical-care system, but it will be smaller than at present and will consume relatively fewer resources. The system will be organized around three types of facilities. The first is the neighborhood hospital and learning center, with fully staffed and equipped emergency-care facilities. The hospital will have emergency facilities, a large outpatient department for ambulatory care, and a resource center for general use by providers and consumers alike. The learning center will offer classes and seminars in health and provide outreach services as well. Up-to-date health information will be available as well as free consultations with trained personnel on health and treatment problems. All neighborhood hospitals will be community-owned and managed. The emphasis will be on patient learning. Further, admissions to the hospital will be made only on a voluntary basis and hospital privileges will not be limited to trained personnel.

The second key facility is the regional health center. More costly and sophisticated treatment will be provided here and only on an inpatient basis. Referrals will be made to the regional center from the neighborhood facilities. Residential complexes for the elderly, incorporating care, will be the third type of facility. These facilities will stress self-care and responsibility but will provide all necessary medical care on site.

Health care personnel in 2000 will no longer be rigidly stratified by training levels. Rather, health care teams will replace the solo physician. All teams will be hospital-based, although they will be deployed in emergency situations. There will be no independent office practice; all practitioners, however trained or with whatever skills, will practice in hospital or home settings.

The personnel engaged in health will differ greatly in social, education, and demographic terms from those now dominating the profession. Most will be trained in health or human ecology; few will be trained as physicians are now trained. Most training will be experiential, although the need for some didactic teaching will remain. No qualifications for training will be imposed, but the completion of training will not ensure placement with a hospital.

Astride the system will be the department of health affairs. The mission of this department will be to monitor the health environment and to intervene as appropriate. The department will work closely with agencies providing biomedical research support. Biomedical research will accordingly be refocused on social and environmental factors related to health. At the local level, citizens will control their own health care systems, featuring the neighborhood hospital and learning center. Each community will be given the necessary resources to design and implement health programs, subject only to broad specifications. Each citizen will have access to those drugs and tools of care necessary for treatment. Tools too costly to deploy at the local level or drugs for which citizens have not been given sufficient information will be available at the regional health center. Health care will be federally underwritten but largely on a bloc grant basis. In addition to grants to neighborhoods and regions, grants will also be made available for experimental projects on either a local or regional basis. Participation by healers and patients will be voluntary.

This may not sound very different, but given where medicine is today and the trajectory it is on, to accomplish this much by the year 2000 will be remarkable, even if it is only the first step toward health.

References

Brown, Lester. *The Twenty-Ninth Day.* New York: Norton, 1978.
Carlson, R. J. *The End of Medicine.* New York: John Wiley, 1975.

Fuchs, Victor. *Who Shall Live?* New York: Basic Books, 1975.

Hirsch, Fred. *The Social Limits to Growth.* Cambridge, Mass.: Harvard University Press, 1976.

Illich, Ivan. *Medical Nemesis.* New York: Pantheon, 1976.

Leonard, George. *The Transformation.* New York: Delacorte, 1972.

Meadows, Donella H., Meadows, D. L. et al. *The Limits to Growth* (2nd ed.). New York: University Books, 1974.

Roszack, Theodore. *Person Planet: The Creative Disintegration of Industrial Society.* New York: Doubleday, 1978.

Salk, Jonas. *The Survival of the Wisest.* New York: Harper and Row, 1973.

Schumacher, E. F. *Small is Beautiful.* New York: Harper and Row, 1976.

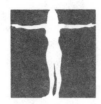 ANNOTATED BIBLIOGRAPHY

The literature on the future of the health field is very thin. The scattering of articles and essays are of generally poor quality, and most of them are focused on single aspects of the health scene – planning, for example. The annotated references that follow feature general futurist work that bears on the evolution of the institutions of health but with a few exceptions were not written with a health "futures orientation" as such.

Brown, Lester. **The Twenty-Ninth Day.** New York: Norton, 1978.

> Brown's book, though not centered on health and medical issues, supplies in my view the major blueprint for the institutions of health of the future, although this blueprint, like many others, lacks specific guidelines. It is the best contemporary statement of ecological thinking as applied to advanced cultures like the United States. To the extent that this is so, the very metaphors Brown uses are those that we, as a society, will need to completely understand and begin to use ourselves. If it is the case that the central metaphors of future health institutions will be ecological as opposed to economical in nature, then Brown's book is essential to an understanding of the transformation that might take place. Even though Brown offers no prescription to the institutions of health, the very fact that he sees the future direction as ecological supplies some guidelines for the health institutions of the future.

Carlson, Rick J. **The End of Medicine.** New York: John Wiley, 1975.

Carlson, Rick J. **The Frontiers of Science and Medicine.** Chicago: Henry Regnery, 1976.

> These books are reviewed in Chapter 1 of this volume, The Paradigm of Holistic Medicine, by James S. Gordon.

Dubos, René. **Man Adapting.** New Haven, Conn.: Yale University Press, 1965.

> The work of René Dubos is voluminous and profound. Rather than review any single

book—although *Man Adapting* is the best characterization of his work generally—it must be pointed out that Dubos has offered sage commentary on the state of our thinking about health for decades now, and his thoughts are as fresh and relevant today as they ever have been.

Dubos's central point has always been that an understanding of health requires an understanding of all factors relating to human health, most of which transcend the capacity of any medical-care system. He credits medicine with the contributions it has made and in many ways is less incisive in pointing out its limitations than other commentators. At the same time the breadth of his analysis makes it very clear that therapeutics in the form of modern medicine are distinctly limited in their capacity to improve the health of populations. In the *Mirage of Health* he makes these points most clearly, but in *Man Adapting* I find the real profundity of Dubos's contribution, particularly when he stresses the critical importance of the human being's adaptive capacities and the limitations of those capacities with respect to our health in the future. To Dubos, the ultimate question is the capacity of the human organism to adapt to social, biological, economic, technological, and cultural stresses imposed upon it.

Dubos points out that the human species' adaptive capacities have been little studied, but a determination of those capacities is absolutely critical in the crafting of the institutions of health for the future. Dubos is ultimately an optimist, as I am, but even while stressing man's adaptability, he is careful to point out that we are not infinitely adaptable and that it is critically important that we begin to understand the nature of our limitations as human organisms before it is too late.

Foucault, Michel. **Madness and Civilization.** New York: Pantheon, 1965.

Foucault's book is related to Rothman's but is far more complex and in many respects more erudite. Foucault examines the origins of the concepts of madness in the sixteenth- and seventeenth-century French society, and consequently, the context is less familiar to the American reader. I found it difficult going, although it was filled with insights and startling observations. Foucault's subtlety with concepts is almost unmatched in my own reading, but at times he seems to stretch points too thinly. Nonetheless, for someone interested in the future of the institutions of health in our society or anywhere, Foucault's book is essential.

In Foucault's examinations, concepts of madness cannot be understood outside of the widest possible context embracing a society's economical, political, social, and spiritual perspectives. To Foucault, definitions of the socially deviant (or again, by analogy, the diseased) are wholly dependent on the "needs" a given society has—those needs being best understood in social, political, and economic terms. He does not appear to go as far as Thomas Szasz in defining away mental illness—indeed, he is far more a historian than a polemicist like Szasz—but nonetheless, after reading him, it is hard to form a concrete impression of mental illness.

For me, the principal contribution of Foucault to an understanding of the future of the institutions of health in the United States is that he forces any analysis to take into consideration all of the contextual elements, including the economical, social, and political. It is often too easy to speculate on the future by simply examining the dynamics of the present. Foucault's analysis makes it clear that any such speculation, based on such a narrow scope, is bound to be incomplete.

Fuchs, Victor. **Who Shall Live?** New York: Basic Books, 1975.

There is a small handful of books on health and medical issues that might be categorized as "limits of medicine" books. Illich's *Medical Nemesis* and Carlson's *The End of Medicine* are in that category, and so is Fuchs's book. The fundamental difference in Fuchs's analysis and that of Carlson and Illich is that Fuchs has rooted his argument in more rational, economic terms. To Fuchs the question is not quite as fascinatingly cultural and need not be stated in such strident terms as those chosen by Illich and often by Carlson. In his analysis it becomes clear — at least to him and, I think, to many others — that hard choices about "who shall live" will force upon us the realization that we cannot continue to expend our human and social resources on medical care alone if we are interested in the improved health of our population in the future. In presenting this arguments, Fuchs examines what evidence there is available about the critical importance of life-style and of environmental variables versus therapeutic ones. He captures his argument in economic but easily understandable terms. In this sense, Fuchs's book is more approachable for many policy analysts than other books arguing the same case.

Illich, Ivan. **Medical Nemesis.** New York: Pantheon, 1976.

If the writings of Szasz are frustrating, then the writing of Illich may drive some readers to total distraction. This is largely, however, because people fail to penetrate his work to its clear juridical core. Illich, in *Medical Nemesis* and in his other work, stakes out rather unique ground. He argues simply that to the degree to which any society strips its members of participating equally in all decisions that affect their lives, that society will necessarily create institutions that are inherently undemocratic and that will serve the institutions' own interests to the derogation of the very people they were designed to serve. His analysis can be most clearly understood in a little known book called *Energy and Equity* in which he examines transportation policy. In that book he argues that any vehicle that exceeds the speed of eighteen miles per hour, or roughly that, necessarily creates inequities in a society because vehicular speed beyond that limit can only be "afforded by" those with more affluence and social power than others. (It should be noted that eighteen miles per hour is roughly the optimal speed for a bicycle or a very fast running donkey.) In all of his other books, *Medical Nemesis* included, Illich is striving to find the "eighteen-mile-an-hour-limit." Hence, in *Medical Nemesis* he argues that medicine and the institutions of medicine are undemocratic and actually socially destructive because they do not serve the interests of people generally but have come to serve only the professionals who organize and run them. And this is so because they have become so elaborate or — to put it another way — because they have so far exceeded the "eighteen-mile-an-hour limit."

Illich differs from someone like Szasz in that he is not fundamentally a libertarian in his political philosophy. He does not wish to abandon people to their fate but insists consistently, often to the frustration of the many who read him, that society must be constructed on juridical principles that offer equal opportunity for decision making to everyone. Once that is done, if a society chooses to exceed the "eighteen-mile-per-hour limit," so be it, even though Illich may not like it. In a libertarian society, although Szasz may not agree with this analysis, while people may be theoretically free to explore their own potential, more trust and reliance is placed on those institutions that congeal existing power relationships.

In the final analysis, Illich's insights are more than often staggering, but they are unrealistic benchmarks for the construction of future societies and to that extent equally doubtful as benchmarks for the construction of the future institutions of health.

Leonard, George. **The Transformation.** New York: Delacorte Press, 1972.

In recent years there have been a number of important books discussing the hope for transformation of human consciousness and, in turn, human institutions. Of these, George Leonard's *The Transformation,* while debated, is the most comprehensive. What Leonard has done in *The Transformation* is to examine historical roots and contemporary phenomena related to such a transformation to point out the rationale for its occurrence and to speculate on what life would be like should it occur. Since, in my view, the transformations of the institutions of health will depend on a larger cultural transformation, an examination of that larger cultural transformation is indispensable to an understanding of the future of the institutions of health. Leonard's book is unabashedly optimistic, even idealistic. He sees the transformation as inevitable if the human species is to survive and is positively lyrical about the possibilities. In this sense, the book is not an "analytical" one but more of a normative prescription for the best possible future. Nonetheless, for anybody interested in the future, the book is essential reading because the very sweep of his arguments and the power of his writing make a cogent case.

Levin, Lowell; Katz, Alfred; and Holst, Erik. **Self-Care: Lay Initiative in Health.** New York: Prodist, 1976.

Levin, Katz, and Holst have produced the single most comprehensive treatment of the self-care phenomenon. As they point out, self-care has always existed and, indeed, there is more self-care provided in the United States than professional care. Yet it has been rarely studied and little is known of its capacities and limitations. The reason for the almost sudden interest in self-care in recent years is due, at least in my view, to the general concern about the limitations of modern medicine as a means of improving our health. And, of course, it must also be related to the health promotion and self-improvement movements generally.

While there has been an interest in self-care for some time, that interest has risen fast in recent years, and terminological confusion has been rampant. What this book does is to clarify the fundamental principles upon which self-care is based and to pose a variety of questions that need to be investigated to fully understand the phenomenon. This book, then, represents a benchmark from which other work can proceed to further investigate self-care, and of particular importance in that examination should be the issue of how to encourage self-care without discouraging people from seeking curative aid when appropriate.

McKeown, Thomas. **The Role of Medicine: Dream, Mirage, or Nemesis.** London: Nuffield Provincial Hospitals Trust, 1976.

Thomas McKeown's book, *The Role of Medicine,* offers the most succinct synthesis of the current conceptual transformation in our thinking about health that is available today. McKeown, a professor of social medicine at the University of Birmingham, U.K., has long argued that any historical sense of our health and those things that have improved it would show unequivocally that therapeutics have always played a minor role and continue to do so today.

In his book, McKeown caps two decades of solid research and theoretical work on the potentials and limits of medicine. He points out the need for an imposition of limits. But in McKeown's case the imposition of limits arises less from political and economic reasons (as in the case of Illich or Carlson) but is based more on this historical record of what the determinants of health have always been and still remain. In his call for an increased emphasis on the behavioral and environmental determinants of health as against the therapeutic, he simply echoes arguments made by others, but he supplies what few others have been able to supply – a solid substantive base for the argument.

Rothman, David. **Discovery of the Asylum.** Boston: Little, Brown, 1971.

As a historian Rothman's task in this book is to examine the historical roots of the contemporary institutions of social control, principally the institutions that deal with mental illness and social and criminal deviance. Rather than a futuristic examination, Rothman's book is distinctly a history. Nonetheless, because of its analysis it offers clues to the future evolution of the institutions of health.

In Rothman's analysis, the fundamental model by which society approached social deviance prior to roughly the middle 1800s shifted dramatically at about that time, yielding a new model upon which contemporary institutions of social control have been based. Rothman traces the evolution of the institutions of social control (the asylum, poor house, alms house, and local jail and prison) in the seventeenth and eighteenth and into the nineteenth centuries. Most of those institutions were abandoned by society and replaced by the modern fortresslike institutions charaterized by the penitentiaries and mental hospitals located primarily in rural areas. He examines the propositions and assumptions that lay beneath the creation of those institutions and shows that society was capable of dramatic shifts in the nature of the institutions that it created to deal with social deviance. He postulates that it is equally possible for contemporary society to make such a dramatic shift, but as I have noted above his historical examinations stop short of a futurological speculation.

In my view, Rothman's book is salient in any examination of the future of the institutions of health because of the close relationship between those institutions and the institutions of social control.

Szasz, Thomas. **The Myth of Mental Illness.** New York: Hoeber-Harper, 1961.

Szasz is one of the most maddening contemporary analysts of the health and medical scene. This is primarily so because the argument found in all his books is seamless. What I mean is that, whether one agrees with him or not, his logic always hangs together. He attempts to understand and explain to others the workings of the mental health system based on assumptions that are so closely knit that you cannot break his argument at any point. All you can do if you wish to refute him is to deny all of his assumptions – or at least nearly all of them.

Szasz argues in *The Myth of Mental Illness,* as he does in many of his other books, that society has created deviance for "needs" of its own. In this sense, his analysis can be likened to that of Foucoult. He does not deny that people behave differently and that some people behave in a more socially destructive way than others. But he does argue—and this is essentially a political argument as opposed to a therapeutic one—that society has no business constraining the behavior of people through a system based on faulty premises, such as the mental health system, but should act instead through the criminal justice process. In other words, he allows that there are people who are antisocial and who, based upon their behavior, require some constraining by a truly effective criminal justice system. But to Szasz, mental illness as a separate category does not seem to exist.

Szasz fails to offer many useful futurological speculations, but it is clear from his writings what kind of society he would like to see. He is clearly, from a political point of view, a libertarian and consequently in his ideal future there would be no mental health institutions.

Torrey, E. Fuller. **The Death of Psychiatry.** Radmore, Pa.: Chilton, 1974.

In this book, Torrey argues that psychiatry as an approach to human problems has been based on the wrong model. He points out how often psychotherapeutic approaches, based on the model that he condemns, have failed to alter patients' lives. He feels that the fundamental proposition of contemporary psychiatry—that an individual's examination of his or her current behavior in terms of his past patterns—is at best heuristic and at worst destructive.

Torrey accumulates a substantial amount of evidence for the ineffectuality of psychotherapeutic intervention and argues for an abandonment of the psychiatric model and the development of an essentially educational model for psychiatric and psychological work. By an educational model, Torrey means a model that encourages the self-responsibility of the individual and a more collegial relationship between the professional and the patient as opposed to the dictatorial, at times autocratic, relationship that generally characterizes psychiatric interaction.

Torrey's analysis, although often compelling, offers little in the way of speculation as to the future of psychiatric work other than the wish he expresses that it turn to the educational model that he advocates.

NAME AND TITLE INDEX

Aaronson, B. S., 293, 294, 296a
Abbondanza, J., 126
Abu-Zeid, A.H.H., 197, 201
Achterberg, Jeanne, 110a, 448, 455, 458a
Ackerknecht, E., 427, 434, 436a
Acupressure – Acupuncture Without Needles, 421a
Acupressure Way of Health: Jin Shin Do, 244–245a
Acupuncture, 421a
Acupuncture and Body Energies, 424a
Acupuncture – Can It Help?, 421a
Acupuncture: Cure of Many Diseases, 418
Acupuncture – The Ancient Chinese Art of Healing and How It Works Scientifically, 419, 456, 462a
Acupuncture Treatment of Pain, The, 421a
Adulthood, 375a
Advanced Techniques of Hypnosis and Therapy: Selected Papers of Milton H. Erickson, 152, 155a

Advanced Treatise on Herbology, 273a
Advances in Immunity, 419
Advances in Parapsychological Research, xvii
Aerobics, 202
Aerobics Program at Oral Roberts University, The, 203
Aerobics Way, The, 110a
Affronti, L. F., 419
Aging in Mass Society: Myths and Realities, 372, 376a
Aikido in Daily Life, 245a
Airola, Paavo, 256a
Air Pollution, 82a
Aisenberg, Ruth, 390a
Ajaya, Swami (Allan Weinstock), 244a
Akroasis: The Theory of World Harmonics, 283a
Aleksandrowicz, M., 305, 315, 318a
Alexander, E. Russell, 434
Alexander, F. Mathias, 21, 23, 212–213, 216, 218–219a
Alexander, Franz, 10, 108, 357

Alexander Technique, The, 216
Alford, Robert R., 43, 46
Alike and Different: The Clinical and Educational Use of Orff-Schulwerk, 280
All Creatures Great and Small, 403
Allen, R. M., 291, 294
Allen, Timothy Field, 399, 403a, 404, 405
Allison, T., 129a
Almy, Thomas, 357
Altered States of Consciousness, xviii, 164, 456, 461a
Althabe, O., 305, 315, 318a
American Anthropologist, 427
American Health Empire, The: Power, Profits, and Politics, 24
American Indian Medicine, 269, 274–275a
American Journal of Acupuncture, 420a
American Journal of Chinese Medicine, 420a
American Journal of Health Planning, 477, 479
American Medicine and the Public

Interest, 48
American Way of Life Need Not Be Hazardous to Your Health, The, 111a
Amsterdam, E. A., 181, 183
Anand, B. K., 160, 164
Ancient Incubation and Modern Psychotherapy, 281
Anderson, Bob, 204a
Anderson, David, 402a
Anderson, Jean, 204
Anderson, Odin W., 44, 46
Andriese, P. C., 81a
Annas, George J., 319a, 330
Anthropology of Music, 281
Applied Kinesiology Notes, 234, 238a
Aramburu, G., 315, 318a
Archives, The: An Anthology of Literature Relative to the Science of Chiropractic, 236a
Ardell, Donald B., xv, 17, 20, 23, 24, 201, 202, 241, 477, 479a
Argumentation and Advocacy, Group Communication Through Computers, xvii
Arica Psychocalisthenics, 242a
Aristotle, 382
Arms, John, 315
Arms, Suzanne, 13, 24, 305, 309, 310, 311, 315, 319a, 327
Ashiba, M., 81a
Asian Medical Systems, 435, 439–440a
Assagioli, Roberto, 244, 449, 455, 456, 459a, 461a, 462a
Aston, S. M., 288, 290, 294, 296a
Atchley, Robert, 373a
Atteneave, Carolyn, 17, 27
Audiometric Changes under Specific Chiropractic, 235
August, Ralph, 153a
Aura, The. See Human Aura, The
Autogenic Therapy, 135, 136a
Avogadro, Amadeo, 400
Awareness of Dying, 390a
Awareness Through Movement, 24, 216, 220a
Away with All Pests: An English Surgeon in People's China, 1954–1969, 25, 31a

Bach, Edward, 267–268, 270a
Bach, Marcus, 236a

Bäckman, H., 181, 183
Back to Eden, 272a
Bagnall, Oscar, 453, 455
Baker, Elsworth, 214, 216, 219a
Baker, Lester, 26, 60, 62a
Baker, Wyrth P., 403a
Baldwin, H. S., 181, 183
Baldwin, T., 217
Balint, Michael, 56, 59
Ballentine, Rudolph, 244a
Banks, Jane, 257a
Banta, H. David, 305, 315, 319a
Barber, T. X., 125a, 128a
Barefoot Doctor's Manual, The, 274a, 422a
Barlow, Wilfred, 212, 216
Barry, Jean, 170, 171, 172a
Basic Chiropractic Procedural Manual, 234, 238a
Basmajian, J. V., 125a, 126, 128
Baum, Allyn Z., 236a
Be Alive As Long As You Live: Mobility Exercises for the Older Person, 205a
Beard, Toni Roberts, 94, 97
Beatty, J., 128a
Beau, Georges, 412, 417, 420a
Becker, Ernest, 389a
Becker, R. O., 413, 417, 418
Beecher, Henry K., 181, 183, 184, 186a, 187a
Behavioral Control and the Modification of Physiological Processes, 168a
Behavioral Toxicology, 85a
Behring, Emil von, 5
Beiman, I., 163, 164
Bellchambers, H. E., 288, 290, 294, 296a
Belleza, T., 217
Belloc, N. B., 196, 202
Benefits and Hazards of the New Obstetrics, 322a
Benefits of Chiropractic Inclusion in Your Health and Welfare Program, 234
Benjamin, B., 26
Benjamin, L. S., 356
Bennett, Hal, 34a, 448, 457
Benson, Herbert, xv, 11, 16, 24, 161, 162, 163, 164, 165, 166a, 168a
Benson, R. C., 322a
Bereavement, 391a

Berenson, B., 381, 388
Bergson, Henri, 18
Berkman, Lisa F., 45, 47, 49a
Bernard, Claude, 7
Bernheim, H., 139, 140, 151
Bertrand, F. R., 334, 339
Beyond Biofeedback, 25
Bhajan, Yogi, 476
Bibliography of Books and Journals Related to Marital and Family Therapy, 61a
Billy Jack (film), 195
Binstock, Robert H., 373a
Bioenergetics, 26, 216, 222–223a
Biofeedback and Self-Control, xvii, 128a
Biofeedback and Self Control Annual, 125a
Biofeedback and Self-Regulation, 126a
Biofeedback: A Survey of the Literature, 127a
Biofeedback Primer, A, 127a
Biofeedback—Principles and Practice for Clinicians, 125a
Biofeedback, Theory and Research, 128a
Biological Effects and Health Hazards of Microwave Radiation, 71a
Bird, Christopher, 273a
Birdwhistell, Ray L., 445, 446, 455
Birren, Faber, 296a
Birren, James E., 373a
Birth Book, 327a
Bitcon, C. H., 280
Blackie, Margery G., 403a, 458
Blanchard, E., 127a
Bloomfield, Harold H., 28a, 110a, 479a
Blum, Henrik L., 45, 47, 49a
Blumberger, S. R., 136
Boadella, David, 214, 216
Body and Mature Behavior: A Study of Anxiety, Sex, Gravitation and Learning, 216
Body Awareness in Action, 216, 222a
Body Fantasy, 217, 225a
Bodymind, xvi, 24, 375a, 456, 459–460a
Body Reveals, The, 456, 461a
Boericke, William, 400, 404a

Bogdanoff, M. D., 182, 183
Bogen, J. E., 279, 280
Bokert, E., 162, 165
Bonny, Helen Lindquist, xv, 278, 279, 280, 282a
Book of Ki, The: Coordinating Mind and Body in Daily Life, 245a
Book of Life, The, 243a
Book of the It, The, 25, 31a
Borchers, Jane, xv
Boudreau, Frank G., 255
Boulding, Kenneth, 488
Bourdiol, R. J., 424
Bourne, H. R., 180, 181, 183
Bowen, Murray, 59, 61
Bowerman, Charles E., 360a
Boyce, P. R., 290, 291, 294
Boyd, Doug, 14, 24
Boyd, W. E., 398, 400, 404a
Brackbill, Yvonne, 305, 315, 320a
Bradley, Robert A., 307, 315
Brain Mind Bulletin, 311, 315
Bramwell, S. T., 356
Brand, R. J., 197, 203
Brand, Stuart, 193
Brattnäs, Berit, 204a
Brazelton, T. B., 305, 315, 320a
Breakthrough to Creativity: Your Higher Sense Perception, 456, 460–461a
Breathe Away Your Tension, 375a
Brecher, Arlene, 252, 255, 256a
Brecher, Edward M., 9, 24
Breckinridge, Mary, 309
Brenner, Harvey, 10, 24
Brenner, Paul, 480
Bresler, David E., xv, 17, 18, 19, 24, 25, 26, 31a, 241, 413, 414, 417, 418, 419, 421a, 451, 455, 473, 480a
Breslow, Lester, 78, 196, 202
Brewer, G., 321a
Brewer, T., 321a
Breyer-Brandwijk, Maria Gerdina, 275a
Bricklin, Mark, 29a
Brief Study Course in Homoeopathy, A, 404a
Brier, Robert, 453, 456
Briggs, A. H., 181, 184
Bright, E., 280, 281
Brint, Armand Ian, 454, 455, 456, 459a

British Herbal Pharmacopoeia, 270a
British Homoeopathic Journal, 275a
Brodeur, Paul, 83
Brodmann, K., 131
Brody, Howard, 16, 24
Broman, Sarah, 305, 315, 320a
Brook, Robert H., 9, 24
Brooks, Charles, 213, 216, 219–220a
Bross, I.D.J., 356
Brown, B., 125
Brown, B. S., 193, 202
Brown, Lester, 485, 488, 494, 496a
Brown, Malcolm, 446, 456
Brown, Robert, 199
Brown, Walter A., 305, 315, 321a
Budzynski, T., 125, 126, 128, 129
Buegel, Dale, 402a
Bulletin of the Oregon State Health Division, 316
Burchell, R. C., 305, 315, 321a
Burmese Supernaturalism: A Study in the Explanation and Reduction of Suffering, 435, 441a
Burnet, Macfarlane, 78
Burney, S. W., 295, 298a, 336, 340
Burnout Prevention for Doctors, 92
Business Week, 492
Butler, Francine, 127a
Butler, Robert N., 364, 371, 374a

Caldeyro-Barcia, Roberto, 305, 315, 318a, 321a, 331
Calehr, H., 419
Camerino, M., 10, 19, 27
Cannon, Walter B., 9, 20, 24, 108
Canter, A., 181, 184
Cantwell, J. D., 192, 197, 198, 202
Capra, Fritjof, 11, 24
Cardon, P. V., 354
Caring for Your Unborn Child, 324a
Caring for Youth: Essays on Alternative Services, xvii
Carolson, J., 126
Carlson, M. L., 162, 165
Carlson, Rick, J., xvi, 9, 17, 24,

29a, 50, 486, 494, 496a, 498, 500
Carkhuff, R., 381, 388
Carney, J. V., 421a
Carpenter, W. A., 339
Carrie, L., 316, 326a
Carson, Rachel, 76
Casarett, Louis J., 70a
Case of Nora, The: Body-Awareness as Healing Therapy, 216, 221a
Castelli, W. P., 197, 202
Cayce, Edgar, 424
Chaitow, Leon, 421a
Challenge Without Competition, 207a
Chalmers, Ian, 322
Chan, K., 419
Chancellor, Philip, 426
Chang, H. T., 419
Chang, Y. L., 419
Change, Principles of Problem Formation and Problem Resolution, 63a
Changing Families: A Family Therapy Reader, 61a
Changing Images of Man, xvii
Chapman, L. F., 153a, 156
Character Analysis, 217, 223
Charcot, J. M., 108
Chard, T., 322a
Chase, T. N., 25
Cheek, David B., xvi, 141, 144, 145, 146, 147, 148, 149, 150, 151, 154a
Chemical and Pharmaceutical Bulletin, 275a
Chen, C. H., 413, 418
Chen, K. C., 419
Cheng, Man-ch'ing, 241a
Cheraskin, E., 251, 252, 255, 256a, 257a, 338, 339
Chernin, Dennis, 402a
Chessick, R. D., 182, 183
Chhina, E. S., 160, 164
Childbearing: Its Social and Psychological Aspects, 328a
Childbirth Without Fear, 307, 315, 322a
Childhood and Society, 375
Child Is Born, A, 329a
Chinese Acupuncture, 426a
Chinese Art of Healing, The, 418, 424a

Chinese Folk Medicine, 425a, 457, 463–464a
Chinese Herbs, 274a
Chinese Medicine (Beau), 417, 420a
Chinese Medicine (Huard and Wong), 422a
Chinese Pulse Diagnosis, The, 426a
Chiropractic: A Modern Way to Health, 234, 236a
Chiropractic: An International Bibliography, 237a
Chiropractic Story, The, 236a
Chiropractic Textbook, 235
Chiu, D., 413, 418
Chopra, I. C., 274a
Chopra, R. N., 274a
Chopra's Indigenous Drugs of India, 274a
Christensen, A., 195, 202
Christenson, W. W., 356
Christianson, Alice, 374a
Christopher, John R., 270a
Chu, Y. M., 419
Churchman, C. West, 39, 47, 49a
Clark, J. W., 251, 255, 257a
Clark, R. K., 182, 183
Clarke, Edmund R., 355, 360a
Clarke, John Henry, 402a, 404a, 459
Cleve, T. L., 257a
Cleveland, G. S., 232, 234
Clinical and Experimental Hypnosis, 156a
Clinical Ecology, 24
Clinical Feedback: A Procedural Manual, 127a
Clinical Hypnosis: Principles and Applications, 152, 154a
Clinical Hypnotherapy, xvi, 152, 154a
Clymer, R. Swineburn, 271a
Clynes, Manfred, 282a
Coffin, David L., 82
Cole, Warren H., 11, 24, 109
Collen, F. Bobbie, 97
Collins, John S., 287, 294
Collins, U. B., 322a
Color Psychology and Therapy, 296a
Comfort, Alex, 374a
Coming of Age, The, 374–375a
Commoner, Barry, 488

Common Knowledge, xv, xvii, xviii
Commonsense Psychiatry of Dr. Adolf Meyer, The, 353
Complete Book of Running, The, 205a
Complete Book of Vitamins, The, 255, 258a
Complete Family Guide to Dental Health, The, 340, 341–342a
Complete Illustrated Book of Yoga, The, 246a
Conference on Future Directions in Health Care: The Dimensions of Medicine, 49–50a
Conger, G. B., 355
Conner, Dan, 47
Conrad, C. C., 193, 202
Consciousness and Self-Regulation, 128a
Consciousness: East and West, xviii
Cooper, Kenneth H., 20, 24, 110a, 192, 196, 199, 202, 204a
Copernicus, Nicolaus, 33
Corey, Laurence, 47, 50a
Correlative Chiropractic Techniques, 235
Corrigan, A. B., 196, 202
Cost and Quality of Health Care: Unnecessary Surgery, 27
Coulson, A., 419
Coulter, Harris Livermore, xvi, 401a, 447, 456
Cousins, Norman, 30a, 110a
Cox, B. M., 413, 418
Cracium, T., 419
Crapanzano, V., 427, 434, 436a
Crasilneck, Harold B., 142, 152, 154a
Creativity—Road to Self Discovery, xvi
Creighton, James, 12, 17, 21, 27, 113a, 448, 457, 481a
Crile, George, 145, 152
Critchley, M., 279, 281, 282a
Crocker, Lucy H., 42, 47, 51a
Cultural Warping of Childbirth, The, xvii, 324–325a
Culture, 427
Culture and Experience, 434, 437a
Culture and Healing in Asian Societies: Anthropological, Psychiatric, and Public Health Studies, 434, 438–439a
Culture-Bound Syndromes, Ethnopsychiatry, and Alternative Therapies, 435, 439a
Culture, Disease and Healing, 435, 439a
Culver, D., 126
Cundiff, David, 196, 202
Cunningham, D. A., 196, 202, 340, 342a
Cunningham, L., 288, 295
Cunningham, Robert, 29a
Cureton, T. K., 291, 294
Current Obstetric and Gynecological Diagnosis and Treatment, 322a
Curtin, Sharon R., 366, 371, 374a
Curtis, W. D., 163, 164
Cutright, D. E., 338, 339
Czerski, P., 71a, 82

Danaher, Kate, 87, 88, 90, 91, 95, 96, 99
Dangott, Lillian, 366, 372, 374a
Daniels, J., 230, 234
Dantsig, N. M., 292, 294
Darwin, Charles, 57
David, J., 326a
Davidson, J., 161, 164, 167a
Davidson, R., 161, 163, 164, 165, 168a
Davis, Devra, 481a
Davis, T.R.A., 294, 298a, 340
Death Does Not Exist, 28
Death of Psychiatry, The, 501a
Deaths of Man, 391a
DeBakey, Michael, 111a
de Beauvoir, Simone, 374a, 389a
Deikman, A., 162, 164
DeJarnette, J., 229, 234
Delassio, Donald J., 358a
DeLee, Joseph, 304, 315
DeLeo, J., 161, 165
Den Boer, James, 47, 50a
Denial of Death, The, 389a
Descartes, René, 4
Design of Inquiring Systems, Basic Concepts in Systems Analysis, 47, 49a
Desoille, R., 449, 456, 461
Des Pres, Terrence, 390
Devloo, R. A., 181, 184
Dewey, John, 212, 218, 222

Diamond, S., 126
DiCara, L., 125a, 128a
Dickey, Lawrence D., 20, 24, 72a, 79
Dick-Read, Grantly, 147, 307, 315, 322a
Dickson, W. J., 182, 184
Dictionary of Practical Materia Medica with Clinical Repertory, 440a
DiCyan, Erwin, xvi
Die Nebenwirkungen der Arzneimittel, 400
Diet and Disease, 255, 257a
Dietary Goals for the United States, 27, 35a, 250, 255, 260a
Dietrich, John, 197-198
Differential Effects of Colored Lights on Psychophysiological Functions, 294, 297a
Differential Mortality in the United States: A Study in Socioeconomic Epidemiology, 47
Digest of Chiropractic Economics, 238a
Dilemmas of Punishment, The, xvi
Dilfer, Carol, 204a
Dinnerstein, Albert J., 187a
Dintenfass, Julius, 233, 234, 236a
Directed Daydream, The, 456
Discovery of the Asylum, 500a
Diserens, C. M., 279, 281
Divided Consciousness, 152
Divided Legacy: A History of the Schism in Medical Thought, xvi, 400, 401a
Dixon, Norman P., 452, 456
Dlin, B. M., 182, 184
Doctor, His Patient, and Illness, The, 59
Doctors in Hospitals: Medical Staff Organizations and Hospital Performance, 48
Doering, S., 322a
Doing Better and Feeling Worse: Health in the United States, 25, 32a, 50a, 112a
Donaldson, Rory, 205a
Dong, Collin H., 257a
Doongaji, D. R., 161, 165
Dorland's Illustrated Medical Dictionary, 180, 183
Dorpat, T. L., 356

Douglas, M., 428, 434, 436a
Doull, John, 70a
Downing, George, 210, 216, 220a
Doyle, J. T., 197, 202
Dr. Airola's Handbook of Natural Healing, 256a
Dream Telepathy, xvii
Drinking Water and Health, 79a
Dubin, L. L., 165
Dubos, René, 6, 7, 8, 12, 24, 30a, 35, 78, 238, 496-497a
Dudley, Donald L., 360a
Duffy, D., 233, 234, 236a
Duke, Marc, 421a
Dunbar, Helen Flanders, 10, 108, 148, 152
Duncan, C. H., 353, 354
Duhl, Leonard J., xvi, 40, 41, 44, 46, 47, 50a
Duszynski, K. R., 10, 27
Dychtwald, Ken, xvi, 19, 24, 375a, 446, 455, 456, 459a

Eagle, C. T., 278, 279, 281
Ear Acupuncture, 422a, 456, 460a
Ear Acupuncture Diagnosis in Musculoskeletal Pain: Final Report of Preliminary Investigation, 24, 455
Ear, The: Gateway to Balancing the Body. A Modern Guide to Ear Acupuncture, 457, 464a
East/West Exercise Book, The, 208a
Easy Does It Yoga for Older People (originally Easy Does It Yoga for People Over Sixty), 202, 374a
Eckholm, Erik, 72a
Economic Botany, 275a
Ecstatic Religion: An Anthropological Study of Spirit Possession and Shamanism, 435, 440a
Edgar Cayce and the Palma Christi, 269
Edwards, C. J., 355
Effects of Noise on Man, The, 281
Ehrenreich, Barbara, 12, 24
Ehrenreich, John, 12, 24
Ehrlich, Anne, 72a
Ehrlich, Paul, 5

Ehrlich, Paul R., 72a
Einstein, Albert, 11, 33, 410
Eisenberg, Leon, 10, 14, 24, 25, 30a, 60, 94, 99, 102a, 432, 434, 439a
Electrocardiograph Changes under Specific Chiropractic, 235
Elementary Treatise in Herbology, 273
Eleven Lourdes Miracles, 171, 177a
Ellingwood, Finley, 271a
Ellis, William R., 41, 47
Ellison, Jerome, 366, 372, 375a
Ellman, G., 217
Elman, David, 145, 152
Elmfeldt, D., 196, 203
Elvin-Lewis, Memory P. F., 268, 269, 272a
Emergency Childbirth, 332a
Emmons, Patty, 203
Emotions and Bodily Changes, 152
Encyclopedia of Pure Materia Medica, The, 399, 403a, 404, 405
End of Medicine, The, xvi, 24, 29a, 486, 494, 496a, 498
Energy and Equity, 498
Engel, George L., 10, 24, 30-31a, 111a, 125, 354
Engelhardt, D. M., 181, 182, 184, 187a
Enkin, M., 323a
Entwisle, D., 322a
Environmental Psychology: People and Their Physical Settings, 47, 52a
Epstein, L., 127a
Epstein, Mark D., xvi, 11, 24
Estein, Samuel M., 73-74a
Erh Chen, 460a
Eric, 391a
Erickson, Elizabeth M., 155a
Erickson, Erik H., 375a
Erickson, Milton H., 61-62a, 142, 145, 147, 152, 154a, 155a, 156a, 158
Eriksson, M., 418
Ernest, Eunice K. N., 307, 316, 328a
Esdaile, James, 139, 144, 152
ESP: A Scientific Evaluation, 456
Essays in Humanistic Medicine, 26

Essential Guide to Prescription Drugs, The, 102a
Estabrooks, G. H., 139, 140, 152
Estimating the Social Costs of National Economic Policy: Implications for Mental and Physical Health, and Criminal Aggression, 24
Ethnic Medicine in the Southwest, 435, 441a
Ethnology, 427
Ethno Medicine, 275a
Evaluation of Caesarian Section in the United States of America, An, 316, 328a
Evaluation of Health Aspects of GRAS Food Ingredients: Lessons Learned and Questions Unanswered, 80a
Evans, F. M., 355
Evans, W., 181, 183
Everson, Tilden C., 11, 24, 109
Exercise and Coronary Heart Disease, 202
Exerciser's Handbook, The, 202
Exercise Testing and Training of Apparently Healthy Individuals, 202
Expanding Health Care Horizons, 47, 49a
Experimental and Clinical Hypnosis, 342–343a
Exploring Madness, xvi

Fabrega, H., 427, 434, 437a
Facilitating GIM Sessions, xv, 280
Facts and Myths About Aging, 372
Fadiman, James, xiii, xvi, 24, 480
Family Networks, 27
Family Process, 61
Fan, L., 419
Farnsworth, Norman R., 264, 269
Farnsworth, Paul R., 278, 279, 281
Farquhar, John W., 111a
Feifel, Herman, 379, 388, 389a
Feingold, Ben F., 67, 74a
Feldenkrais, Moshe, 20, 24, 213, 216, 220–221a
Feller, R. P., 295, 298a, 336, 340
Fentem, P., 197, 202
Ferguson, M., 279, 281
Ferguson, Tom, xvi, 13, 19, 25,

89, 94, 95, 96, 98, 100a, 102, 103
Fernando, C. K., 125, 126
Field of Family Therapy, The, 53, 60
Fields, Suzanne, 480a
Finch, Caleb E., 373a
Fine, H., 279, 281
Fink, Donald, 98
Finkelman, A., 340
Finley, W. W., 126, 129a
Firestein, S. K., 336, 339, 341a
First-Aid Homoeopathy in Accidents and Ailments, 402a
Fisch, Richard, 63a
Fischer, H. K., 182, 184
Fist of Fury (film), 195
Fitch, K. D., 196, 202
Fit for Fun: A Swedish Message, 204a
Fitzgerald, Dorothy, 323a
Fitzgerald, R. G., 26
Fitzherbert, Joan, 170, 171, 173a
Fixx, James F., 205a
Fleming, Alexander, 5
Fletcher, G. F., 197, 198, 202
Florey, Howard Walter, 5
Fluegelman, Andrew, 205a
Flynn, A., 305, 315, 323a
Fonder, A. C., 335, 339, 341a
Food Additives and Federal Policy: The Mirage of Safety, 76a
Forest of Symbols, The, 435, 441–442a
Forward Plan for Health— 1977–1981, 197, 203
Fosshage, James L., 172, 173a, 175
Fothergill, L. A., 418
Fotopoulos, S., 126
Foucault, Michel, 497a, 500
Fowler, C. Ray, 61
Fox, E. J., 418
Fox, Renée, 51
Frager, Robert, xvi
Framo, James L., 61a
Frank, Cyril, 168a
Frank, Jerome D., 10, 11, 25, 31a, 50, 109, 170, 171, 172, 173–174a, 181, 184, 428, 433, 434, 437a
Frankel, Laurence J., 205a, 376a
Frederking, Walter, 461
Fredricks, Carlton, 252

Freedman, N., 181, 182, 184, 187a
Freedom from Pain, 24
Freese, Arthur S., 457, 463a
Free Yourself from Pain, xvi, 417
Freud, Sigmund, 18, 21, 31, 108, 199, 214, 244
Friberg, Lars T., 82
Friedman, Jay, 43, 48
Friedman, Meyer, 10, 25, 108, 109, 111a, 357, 445, 456
Fritsch, Albert J., 74a
From the Inside Out: A Self-Teaching and Laboratory Manual for Biofeedback and Self-Regulation, xviii
Frontiers of Science and Medicine, The, xvi, 29a, 496a
Fuchs, Victor R., 50, 75a, 486, 495, 498a
Fulton, C. D., 193, 202
Function of the Orgasm, The, 217
Fundamental Basis of Iridiagnosis, 456
Funderburk, James, 242a
Furst, M. L., 165
Fusco, Paul, 221
Future Directions in Health Care: A New Public Policy, xvi, 29a

Gaardner, K., 126, 127a
Gajdusek, D. C., 10, 25
Gale, James L., 434
Gantt, W. H., 182
Garfield, Charles A., xvi, 386, 388, 389a, 390a
Garfield, Sidney, 469
Gartner, Alan, 95, 98, 100a
Gaskin, Ina May, 307, 310, 315, 324a, 327
Gaskin, Stephen, 324
Gaston, E. Thayer, 278, 281
Gatewood, T. Schley, 309, 315
Geannette, Gloria, 191, 202
Geba, Bruno, 375a, 376a
Geiger, H. Jack, 40, 47, 50a
Gellman, D. D., 191, 202
Generalov, A. A., 294
Genes, Dreams, and Reality, 78
George Crile, An Autobiography, 152
Gerard, R. M., 293, 294, 297a
Gerras, Charles, 253, 255, 258a

Getting Well Again, 27, 110, 113a, 457, 481a
Gibbs, C. J., 10, 25
Giber, D., 161, 165, 167a
Gibson, D. M., 402a
Gindler, Elsa, 214
Ginn, D. L., 75a
Ginsburg, Eli, 51
Giotto, Antonio, 111a
Glaser, Barney, 390a
Glasser, William, 205a
Gliedman, L. H., 181, 182, 184
Glover, Bob, 199, 202
Gluck, L., 315, 321a
Glueck, D. C., 161, 164
Goddard, K., 316, 327a
Gold, Edwin, 324a
Goldberg, George, xvi
Golding, K., 193, 203
Goldsmith, John R., 82
Goldstein, A., 418
Goldstein, Murray, 232, 234
Goleman, Daniel, 161, 162, 163, 164, 165, 166a, 167a, 168a, 385, 388
Good Age, A, 374a
Good, Byron, 14, 25, 60, 432, 434, 439a
Goode, R. C., 340, 342a
Goodell, Helen, 153a, 156, 358a
Goodhardt, Robert, 253, 255, 258a, 340, 343a
Goodheart, G., 228, 229, 234
Goodrich, Joyce, 173
Gordon, James S., xiii, xvii, 3, 13, 18, 24, 25, 26, 31a, 311, 315, 316, 480a
Gordon, T., 197, 202
Gorlin, R., 181, 183
Gorton, Bernard E., 155
Gots, B., 324a
Gots, R., 324a
Gould, D., 197, 202
Grace, William J., 349, 354, 359-360a, 361a
Grad, Bernard, 11, 25, 170, 171, 172a, 173a
Graettinger, John, 13, 25
Graham, David T., 346, 349, 354, 355, 356, 357, 361a
Graham, F. K., 349, 356
Graham, Frank, Jr., 76a
Graham, L. E., 164
Grant, Richard H., 96, 98, 101a

Gravenstein, J. S., 181, 184
Green, Alyce, 18, 25, 125
Green, Elmer E., 18, 25, 125, 134, 135
Green, Lawrence W., 96, 98
Green Medicine, 269, 272a
Grenfell, R. F., 181, 184
Grief Observed, A, 391a
Grieve, Maude, 265, 269, 271a
Griffin, R., 217
Grinker, Roy, 357
Groddeck, Georg, 21, 25, 31a
Grodin, Jay, 321a
Gross, Leonard, 207a
Groswald, Douglas, 231, 234
Guidelines for Successful Jogging, 205a
Guide to Fitness After 50, 376a
Guiding Systems of Our Materia Medica, 399, 404a, 405
Gullers, K. W., 204a
Gunderson, E. K. Eric, 111a
Gunther, Bernard, 214, 216, 221a
Guttmacher, Alan, 328a
Gutwirth, S. W., 338, 339

Hahnemann, Samuel, 395-399, 400, 401a, 402, 458
Haire, Doris B., xvii, 13, 25, 324a, 331
Hale, W. E., 197, 198, 203
Haley, Jay, 61-62a, 142, 152, 154, 155a, 156a
Hall, James A., 142, 152, 154a
Hallowell, A. I., 427, 434, 437a
Halm, Jerome, 187a
Halpern, S., 279, 281
Hamadsha, The: A Study in Moroccan Ethnopsychiatry, 424, 436a
Hamilton, D., 163, 165
Hammer, D. C., 193, 202
Handa, K. L., 274a
Handbook of Aging and the Social Sciences, 373a
Handbook of Parapsychology, 457
Handbook of Physiology, 77a
Handbook of the Biology of Aging, 373a
Hankoff, L. D., 181, 182, 184, 187a
Hansel, C.E.M., 453, 456
Happich, Carl, 448, 449, 461
Haraldsson, Erlender, 385, 388

Hardy, A. C., 287, 294
Hare, Clarence C., 353, 357a
Harper-Shove, F., 271a
Harrington, Janette, xiii
Harris, Raymond, 376a
Harveston, Dominic S., 481a
Harvey, William, 4, 416
Harwood, A., 427, 433, 434, 437a
Hassett, J. A., 127a
Hastings, Arthur, xiii, xvii, 24, 241, 338, 340
Hauser, Philip, 39, 40, 47
Haverkamp, Albert, 305, 316, 325a, 331
Hawkins, Norman G., 360a
Hayes-Bautista, David, 481a
Hayflick, Leonard, 373a
Hazell, Lester D., 325a
Headache and Other Pain, 358a
Healing Factor, The: Vitamin C Against Disease, 255, 260-261a
Healing for Everyone, 481a
Healing: Implications for Psychotherapy, 173a
Health Activation for Senior Citizens, 98, 101a
Health Activation News, The, 94
Health and Light, 298a
Health Care in Transition: Directions for the Future, 48
Health Care Politics, 46
Health Department Data Shows Danger of Home Births, 315
Health Education Monographs, 95
Health Effects of Environmental Pollutants, The, 84a
Health of the Individual, of the Family, of Society, 47
Healthwise Handbook, 97
Heal Thyself, 270a
Healthy State, A: An International Perspective on the Crisis in the United States Medical Care, 81a
Heilpflanzenkunde Der Mensch Und Die Heilpflanzen, 273a
Heisenberg, Werner, 11, 25
Help Yourself, 96, 98, 102a
Hematological Changes under Specific Chiropractic, 235
Hendricks, C. Davis, 363, 364, 372, 376a
Hendricks, Jon, 363, 364, 372, 376a
Henson, R. A., 279, 281, 282a

Herbal Pharmacology in the People's Republic of China, 269, 274a

Herb and Ailment Cross-Reference Chart, xvii, 272a

Herbs, 272a

Herbs for Health, 272a

Hering, Constantine, 399, 404a, 405

Hernandez-Peon, R., 140, 152

Herrigel, Eugen, 206a

Herriott, James, 403

Hessel, Dieter, 364, 372, 377a

Hicks, J., 326a

High Level Wellness: An Alternative to Doctors, Drugs, and Disease, xv, 23, 202, 479

High Level Wellness for Young People or Anyone Under the Influence of an Adult, xv

Hilgard, Ernest, R., 128, 142, 144, 152, 156a, 337, 340, 341a

Hilgard, Josephine R., 156a, 337, 340, 341a

Himber, Jacob, 335, 340, 341a

Himmelfarb, P., 297a

Hinkle, Lawrence E., Jr., 346, 351, 354, 355, 356, 357a

Hintze, Naomi, 169, 171, 175a

Hippocrates, 9, 18, 20

Hirai, T., 160, 164

Hirsch, Fred, 486, 495

History of Medicine, A, 435, 441a

Hoebel, F. C., 17, 25

Hoffman, Dietrich, 82

Hoffman, Lloyd E., 101a

Hoffman, Lynn, 61

Holism and Evolution, 27

Holistic Health Handbook, The, 28a, 203, 456, 459a

Holistic Health in Perspective, 26, 33a

Holistic Medicine: From Stress to Optimum Health, xviii

Holistic Way to Health and Happiness, The, 28a, 110a, 479a

Holland, W. C., 181, 184

Hollins, C., 315, 323a

Holmes, Thomas H., xvii, 10, 18, 25, 45, 47, 50a, 349, 351, 355, 356, 357, 358a, 360a, 361a, 362a

Holst, Erik, 87, 88, 95, 96, 98,

101a, 499a

Home Birth Book, The, 331a

Home Oriented Maternity Experience: A Comprehensive Guide to Home Births, 323a

Homeopathic Digest, The, 275a

Homeopathy: Medicine of the New Man, 403a

Homeotheraphy, 275a

Homewood, A. E., 233, 234

Homoeopathic Drug Pictures, 405a

Homoeopathic Medicine, xvi, 456

Homoeopathic Remedies for Physicians, Laymen, and Therapists, 402a

Homoeopathy for the First-Aider, 403a

Hopkins, H. K., 217

Horn, Joshua, S., 14, 25, 31a

Horney, Karen, 201

Horton, R., 427, 434, 437–438a

Horwitz, Ten, 242a

Hoult, I., 305, 316, 326a

Household Pollutants Guide, The, 74a

Houston, Jean, 448, 456, 462a

Houston, W. R., 182, 184, 188a

Howard, J. H., 338, 340, 342a

How Business Can Promote Good Health for Employees and Their Families, 99

How Could I Not Be Among You?, 391a

How to Be Your Own Doctor (Sometimes), 26, 94, 98, 99, 102a

How Your Body Works, 95, 98

Hoyle, C., 181, 183

Hsieh, S. W., 419

Hu, H. H., 419

Huang, Helena L., 422a, 450, 451, 456, 460a

Huard, Pierre, 422a

Hubbard, Elizabeth Wright, 404a

Hubbard, R., 217

Huffman, B. Leslie, Jr., 87

Hughes, J., 413, 418

Hughes, Philip C., xvii, 297a

Human Atmosphere, The. See Human Aura, The

Human Aura, The (Kilner) (originally *The Human Atmosphere*), 456, 461a

Human Aura, The (Regush), 457

Human Colon, The, 359–360a

Human Ecology, 72a

Human Ecology and Susceptibility to the Chemical Environment, 79a

Human Gastric Function: An Experimental Study of a Man and His Stomach, 359a

Humanist, The, 376a

Human Potential: Glimpses into the 21st Century, xvi

Humphrey, B., 281, 283a

Hunt, Valerie, 211, 216

Hunter, Beatrice Trum, 76a

Husband-Coached Childbirth, 307, 315

Hutchens, Alma R., 271a

Huxley, Aldous, 212, 222

Hyde, R. T., 197, 198, 203

Hypnosis, 152, 157a

Hypnosis in Marriage and Divorce, xviii

Hypnosis in Medicine and Surgery (originally *Mesmerism in India*), 152, 155a

Hypnosis in Obstetrics, 153a

Hypnosis in the Relief of Pain, 156a, 340, 341a

Hypnosis of Man and Animals, 157a

Hypnotic Susceptibility, 152

Hypnotism, 152

Ichazo, Oscar, 242a

Ikegami, R., 163, 164

Illich, Ivan, 9, 25, 32a, 78–79, 486, 495, 498a, 500

Illness and Shamanistic Curing in Zinacantan: An Ethnomedical Analysis, 434, 437a

Imagery and Daydream Methods in Psychotherapy, 457

Imagery of Cancer: IMAGE-CA, 110a, 455, 458–459a

Imber, S. D., 181, 184

Immaculate Deception: A New Look at Women and Childbirth in America, 24, 315, 319a

Independent Studies of Industrial Back Injuries, 234

Indian Herbology of North America, 271a

Ingram, K. G., 196, 202

Inman, O., 229, 234

Inner and Other Space:

Introduction to a Theory of Social Psychiatry, xviii, 62a
Inner Game of Tennis, The, 207
Instructions for Nursing Your Baby, 324a
Interactional View, The, 25
International Chiropractic Association Manual, 234
International Review of Chiropractic, 238a
Introduction to Homoeotherapeutics, 403a
Introduction to the Methods of Autogenic Therapy, 135
Introductory Musical Accoustics, 281
Ion Effect, The, 81a
Ionesco-Tirgoviste, C., 419
Isayeva, E. A., 294
It's Only Natural, 481a
Ivey, H. F., 288, 294
Iyengar, B.K.S., 242-243a

Jääskeläimen, A., 196, 203
Jackson, Don, 61
Jackson, Ian, 206a
Jacobson, Nils, 454, 456
Jacoby, Heinrich, 214
Jacoby, James D., 342a
Jaffe, Aniela, 376a
Jaffe, Dennis, 18, 25, 26, 31a, 480
Jaffe, R., 161, 165
James, Dorothy, 43, 47
Jayson, J. K., 291, 294, 298a
Jefferson, Thomas, 93
Jenerick, Howard P., 422a
Jenner, William, 5, 416
Jennings, Charles, 195, 203
Jensen, Bernard, 454, 456, 460a
Jerome, C. W., 288, 294
Jeste, D. V., 161, 165
Jevening, R., 163, 164
Johnson, S. A., 164
Jiyu-Kennett, Roshi P.T.N.H., 243a
Joffe, Joy R., 360a
Jogger, The, 203
Johnson, Karen, 94, 98
Johnson, S. A., 164
Johnson, Virginia, 149
Jones, Franklin, 212, 216, 222a
Journal of American Insurance, 196, 202
Journal of Chiropractic, 239a
Journal of Ethnopharmacology,

275a
Journal of Music Therapy, 278, 281
Journal of Parapsychology, 172
Journal of Pharmaceutical Sciences, 275a
Journal of Psychosomatic Research, 351
Journal of the American Institute for Homeopathy, 275a
Journal of the American Medical Association, 154, 179, 352
Journal of the American Society for Psychical Research, 172
Journal of the American Society of Psychosomatic Dentistry and Medicine, The, xviii
Journal of Traditional Acupuncture, 423a
Jouvet, M., 152
Joy, 217
Joy of Running, The, 25, 199, 202, 206a
Judd, D. B., 288, 294
Jung, Carl Gustav, 18, 199, 244, 376a, 425

Kabler, J. D., 354, 356
Kaleidoscope of Childbearing, 315, 321a, 325a
Kalish, Richard A., 366, 372, 374a, 377a
Kalita, Dwight, 253, 255, 262a
Kalliola, H., 181, 183
Kamiya, Joanne Gardiner, xvii
Kamiya, Joe, xvii, 125a, 128a
Kane, F. D., 356
Kantor, H., 305, 316, 326a
Kanzler, M., 181, 184
Kapur, L. D., 274a
Karagulla, Shafica, 452, 453, 456, 460a
Karmel, Marjorie, 307, 316, 326a
Kasamatsu, A., 160, 164
Kaslof, Leslie J., xvii, 32a, 269, 272a, 456, 476, 480a
Kast, E. C., 182, 184
Kastenbaum, Robert, 387, 388, 390a
Kattus, A. A., 196, 202
Katz, Alfred H., 87, 88, 95, 96, 98, 101a, 499a
Katz, R. L., 419
Kayser, H., 283a

Kelling, George, 199, 202
Kelly, J., 315, 323a
Kemper, Donald W., 94, 97
Kennedy, Edward M., ix-x
Kennedy, John F., 192
Kennell, John, 20, 25, 305-306, 316, 327a
Kent, C., 229, 230, 234
Kent, James Tyler, 399, 401a, 403, 404a, 405a
Kerr, Michael E., 58, 60
Kerschner, H., 419
Keyes, Ancel, 197
Keyes, John D., 274
Kiev, A., 427, 434, 438a
Kilner, Walter J., 453, 456, 461a
Kimmelman, Susan, 242a
Kimura, S., 81a
Kinesics and Context: Essays on Body Motion Communication, 455
Kinesiology, 235
King, Shiu H., 423a
Kinsman, R., 126
Kirkpatrick, T., 192, 202
Kitigawa, Evelyn, 39, 40, 47
Kitzinger, S., 326a
Klaus, Marshall, 20, 25, 305-306, 316, 327a
Kleiber, D. A., 291, 294, 298a
Klein, Judith, 170, 171, 172, 177a
Klein, Lawrence, 237a
Klein, R. F., 182, 183
Kleinman, Arthur, xvii, 10, 14, 17, 25, 56, 60, 427, 428, 430, 431, 432, 434, 435, 438a, 439a
Klerman, G. L., 182, 184
Klide, Alan M., 423a
Kling, R., 217
Kloosterman, G. J., 327
Kloss, Jethro, 272a
Klumbies, Gerhard, 157a
Klumpp, Theodore G., 196
Knapp, Mark L., 445, 456
Knapp, P. H., 277, 281
Knowledge of Illness in a Sepik Society, 435, 440a
Knowles, John, 7, 8, 12, 25, 32a, 50a, 51a, 112a
Koch, Robert, 5, 346
Kohr, R., 162, 164
Kolomiytseva, M. G., 292, 294
Konference o Vyzkumu Psychotroniky, 418

Konig, G., 419
Korr, I. M., 230, 232, 234
Kory, Robert B., 28a, 110a, 479a
Koski, S., 294, 298a, 340
Kosterlitz, H. W., 418
Kostrubala, Thaddeus, 20, 25, 199, 202, 206a
Kostuk, W. J., 196, 203
Kotaka, S., 81a
Kotin, Paul, 78a
Kretschmer, W., 446, 448, 449, 456, 459, 461a
Krieg, Margaret B., 268, 269, 272a
Kriege, Theodore, 454, 456
Krieger, Dolores, 12, 19, 20, 25, 170, 171, 172, 175a, 480
Krippner, Stanley, xvii, 170, 171, 172, 173, 175a
Kristein, Marvin M., 95, 98
Krivitskaya, E. I., 291, 292, 295
Kroening, Richard J., 24, 413, 418, 419, 421a, 451, 455
Kroger, William S., 156a, 342a
Kron, R., 305, 316, 327a
Krueger, Albert P., 81
Kryter, K. D., 279, 281
Kübler-Ross, Elisabeth, 28, 382, 386, 388, 390a
Kuhlman, W. H., 129a
Kuhn, Maggie, 364, 372, 377a
Kuhn, Thomas S., 33a
Kum Nye Relaxation, 245–246a
Kundalini: Yoga for the West, 243–244a
Kunish, N. O., 356
Kunstadter, Peter, 429, 434, 435, 439a
Kuntzleman, Charles T., 192, 202, 206a
Kurtz, Ron, 446, 456, 461a
Kushi, Michio, 423a, 458

Lachaine, R., 191, 202
LaLonde, Marc, 14, 26, 33a, 47, 51a, 112
LaLonde Report. See New Perspective on the Health of Canadians, A
Lamaze, Fernand, 307
Landy, D., 427, 435, 439a
Lang, Raven, 327a
Langer, S., 278, 281

Language of the Body, The, 216
Laqueur, Peter, 61
Larson, Daniel, 203
Lasagna, L., 181, 184
Laskin, Daniel M., 335, 340
Later Life: Applying Social Gerontology, 377a
Lavely, R., 161, 165
Lavier, Jacques, 426
Lavoisier, Antoine Laurent, 33
Law, M. M., 191, 202
Lawlis, G. Frank, 110a, 448, 455, 458a
Lawrence, Ron, 199
Lazarev, D. N., 294
Leaf, A., 191, 202
Leavitt, Judith Walzer, 98
Leboyer, Frederick, 147, 306
Lebra, W. O., 427, 435, 439a
LeCron, Leslie M., 143, 144, 145, 150, 152, 154a, 158a
Lectures on Homoeopathic Materia Medica, 404a, 405
Lectures on Homoeopathic Philosophy, 401–402a
Lee, Bruce, 193, 195
Lee, Douglas H. K., 77–78a
Lee, G.T.C., 419
Lee, Philip R., 50, 101a, 260a
Leeuwenhoek, Anton van, 4
Leger, J. P., 450, 456
Lemaigre-Voreaux, P., 288, 291, 294
Lemons, T. M., 290, 294
Leonard, George, 195, 207a, 488, 495, 499a
Lerner, Michael, xvii
Lerner, Stephen, xviii, 83
Lesh, T., 161, 164
LeShan, Lawrence, 10, 11, 12, 26, 108, 109, 170, 171, 172, 173, 175a
Leslie, C., 427, 429, 434, 435, 439–440a
Lesse, S., 179, 181, 182, 184
Lester, B. A., 315, 320a
Leuner, Hans Carl, 448, 449, 456, 459, 461, 462a
Leung, P., 161, 164
Levenson, G., 326a
Levin, Arthur, 101a
Levin, Lowell S., 87, 88, 95, 96, 98, 101a, 499a

Levinson, Bernard, 145, 152, 157a
Levi-Strauss, Claude, 436
Levy, B., 309, 316, 327a
Lewin, L., 400
Lewis, Charles E., 95, 98
Lewis, C. S., 387, 388, 391a
Lewis, G., 427, 435, 440a
Lewis, Mary Ann, 95
Lewis, Thomas, 358
Lewis, Walter H., 268, 269, 272a
Lewis, W. C., 356
Liberman, R., 181, 184
Licit and Illicit Drugs: The Consumer's Union Report on Narcotics, Stimulants, Depressants, Inhalants, Hallucinogens, and Marijuana, Including Caffeine, Nicotine, and Alcohol, 24
Lidz, Theodore, 357
Liebeault, 139
Lief, A., 353
Liegner, L., 383, 388
Life, 375
Life After Life, 385
Life Before Birth, 328a
Life Crisis and Disease Onset: A Prospective Study of Life Crises and Health Changes, 47
Lifelong Health and Well-being, xvi
Life's Second Half: The Pleasures of Aging, 372, 375a
Life Stress and Bodily Disease, 345, 353
Life Stress and Essential Hypertension: A Study of Circulatory Adjustments in Man, 354
Life Stress and Illness, 111a
Life Style, 196, 202
Light on Yoga, 242a
Lillard, Harvey, 228
Limits to Growth, The, 285, 495
Lindemann, Hannes, 136a
Lipnack, Jessica, 327a
Lister, Joseph, 155
Little Red Book of Acupuncture, The, 456, 461–462a
Liu Y. K., 413, 418
Lives of a Cell, The, 78
Living Heart, The, 111a
Lloydia: The Journal of Natural

Products, 276a
Lockey, 72
Loesch, J. A., 182, 184
Long, James, 102a
*Look at Chiropractic Spinal
   Correction, A,* 235
Loomis, Evarts, 473, 481a
Loomis, W. F., 287, 288, 294,
   297a
Looney, G. L., 419
Lorenz, T. H., 355
Loughlin, Tom, 195
Louis XIV, 305
Lowen, Alexander, 21, 26, 210,
   215, 216, 222-223a
Lowen, Leslie, 216, 223a
Lu, Henry C., 423a, 450, 456, 458
Lubar, J. F., 129a
Lubic, Ruth Watson, 307, 316,
   328a
Lucas, O. N., 337, 340
Luce, Gay, 377a
Lucey, Jerold F., 293, 294
Lui, H. H., 242
Lund, Doris, 391a
Lundy, R. M., 356
Lung, C. H., 419
Lunsford, L., 354
Luthe, Wolfgang, 131, 132, 133,
   134, 135, 136a
Luther, Martin, 94
Luttges, Marvin, 231, 234, 235
*Lying In: A History of Childbirth
   in America,* 317, 331a
Lynch, P., 315, 323a
Lyon, T. C., 339
Lyu, B. S., 413, 418

Maas, J. B., 291, 294, 298a
MacAdam, D. L., 288, 294
McAdam, D. W., 281, 283a
McFarland, R. L., 182, 183
MacFarlane, A., 305, 317, 331a
McGarey, William A., 267, 269
*McGovern Report. See Dietary
   Goals for the United States*
MacGraegor, R. J., 235
McGuigan, F. G., 339, 341a
McGuire, Thomas, 335, 340, 342
McKee, G., 279, 281, 283a
McKeown, Thomas, 7-8, 26, 30,
   33a, 50, 78a, 499-500a
Mackler, D., 355

MacLennon, A., 316, 326a
McNerney, Walter J., 50
MacPhillamy, Rev. Daizui, 243a
Madness and Civilization, 497a
Maggie Kuhn on Aging, 372, 377a
Magic, Faith and Healing, 434,
   438a
Magic of the Minimum Dose, The,
   273, 403
Magic, Witchcraft and Curing,
   435, 440a
Magoun, H. W., 140, 152
Maigne, Robert, 227, 234
Majestic, H., 164
Major Medicinal Plants, 273a
Mäkäräinen, M., 196, 203
*Making Whole: Health for a New
   Epoch,* xvi, 47, 50a
Malec, J., 163, 164
Malitz, S., 181, 184
Man, P. L., 413, 418
Man Adapting, 496-497a
Management and the Worker, 184
Manber, Malcolm, 232, 234
Mandell, 72
Manderscheid, Ronald, 481a
*Man in the Trap: The Causes of
   Blocked Sexual Energy,* 216,
   219a
Mann, Felix, 412, 418, 419,
   423-424a, 450, 452, 456, 458,
   462a
Manning, Tracey, 321a
*Manual of Homoeopathy and
   Natural Medicine, A,* 403a
Marathon, The, 203
Marieskind, Helen, 305, 316,
   328a
Marine, W., 316, 327a
Marino, A. A., 417, 418
Marllatt, Allen, 163, 164
Marti-Ibanez, Felix, 7, 26
Martin, C. J., 360a
Martin, J. S., 165
Martin, R. A., 232, 234
Maslow, Abraham, 42, 44, 201,
   244
Massage Book, The, 216, 220a
Massage—the Oriental Method,
   425a
Massey, Wayne, 211, 216
Mass Psychology of Fascism, The,
   26, 34a

Masters, Robert, 448, 456, 462a
Masters, William, 149
Masuda, Minoru, 10, 45, 47, 50a,
   356, 360a, 362a
Materia Medica and Therapeutics,
   271a
Materia Medica with Repertory,
   404a
Maternal and Infant Bonding, 316,
   327a
Maternal-Infant Bonding, 25
Mather, H. G., 9, 26
Matsumoto, T., 413, 418
Matsushima, L., 81a
Matthews-Simonton, Stephanie,
   12, 17, 21, 27, 28, 29, 31, 113a
   448, 457, 471, 481a
Mattson, Phyllis, 23, 26, 33a
Maupin, E., 162, 164
Mausert, Otto, 272a
Mauz, Friedrich, 461
Maximum Performance, 207a
Mayer, D. J., 413, 418
Mayron, L. W., 336, 340
Mead, M., 328a
Meadows, Donella H., 485, 495
Meadows, D. L., 485, 495
Meaning of Death, The, 389
Medical Anthropology, 428
*Medical Botany: Plants Affecting
   Man's Health,* 269, 272a
*Medical Discoveries of Edward
   Bach, Physician: What the
   Flowers Do for the Human Body,*
   269
Medical Nemesis, 25, 32a, 78, 486,
   495, 498a
*Medical Self-Care: Access to
   Medical Tools,* xvi, 25, 96, 98,
   99, 100a, 102, 103
Medical Self-Care Magazine, 88,
   94, 96, 98, 100a, 103
Medical Tribune, 311
Medical World News, 87
*Medicinal and Poisonous Plants of
   Southern and Eastern Africa,*
   275a
Medicina Traditional, 276a
Medicine and Ethnology, 434, 436a
Medicine and Psychiatry, 427
*Medicine and the Reign of
   Technology,* 79a, 440a
Medicine in a Changing Society, 47,

Medicine in America: Life, Death, and Dollars (television special), 47

Medicine in Chinese Cultures, 434–435, 438a, 439a

Medicine Without Doctors, 96, 98

Meditation: Self-Regulation Strategy and Altered States of Consciousness, xviii, 164, 165, 166a

Medium, the Mystic and the Physicist, The, 26, 171, 175a

Mehl, Lewis E., 310, 316, 330, 476

Meier, C. A., 278, 281

Melzack, R., 413, 418

Memories, Dreams and Reflections, 376a

Mendelsohn, Robert, 310, 316

Mental and Elemental Nutrients: A Physician's Guide to Nutrition and Health Care, 255, 259a

Mental Health and Chiropractic, 235, 238a

Meridians of Acupuncture, The, 418, 423–424a

Merriam, A. P., 278, 281

Mesmer, Franz, 139

Mesmerism in India. See Hypnosis in Medicine and Surgery

Meyer, Adolf, 346

Meyer, Sharon, 237a

Michael, Donald N., 51a

Michel, D. E., 280, 281

Middleton, J., 427, 435, 440a

Milechnin, Anatol, 140, 152, 154, 157a

Miles, Richard, 480

Miller, Eddie, 96, 98, 102a

Miller, Emmett, 31

Miller, N., 125a, 128a

Miller, Stuart, 14, 26

Mills, Nancy, 330

Milo, Nancy, 96, 98, 102a

Minard, David, 78a

Mind as Healer, Mind as Slayer: A Holistic Approach to Preventing Stress Disorders, xviii, 26, 34a, 112a, 377–378a

Mind, Body, and Health: Toward an Integral Medicine, xvi, xvii, 25, 27, 31a, 480a

Mind-Body Effect, The, xv, 24

Mind/Body Integration: Essential

Readings in Biofeedback, xviii

Mind Games: The Guide to Inner Space, 456, 462

Minuchin, Salvador, 11, 16, 17, 26, 59, 60, 61, 62a

Mirage of Health, 6, 24, 30a, 78, 497

Mitchell, Edgar D., xiii, 453, 456

Mittleman, B., 354

Modern Developments in the Principles and Practice of Chiropractic, 234, 236a

Modern Herbal, A, 269, 271a

Modern Nutrition in Health and Disease, 255, 258a, 340, 343a

Modern Perinatal Medicine, 315, 321a

Molière (Jean Baptiste Poquelin), 55

Monkerud, D., 197, 203

Montagu, Ashley, 209, 217, 328a

Montgomery, Penelope, 127a

Moody, Raymond, 385, 386, 388

Morehouse, Laurence E., 207a

More Magic of the Minimum Dose, 273

Morgan, B. A., 418

Morgan, William P., 199

Morita Psychotherapy, 435, 440a

Morris, H. R., 418

Morris, J. D., 171, 176a, 456

Morris, R. L., 171, 176a

Morse, R., 163, 165

Moss, Aaron A., 158, 337, 340, 342a

Mostofsky, D. I., 168a

Motoyama, Hiroshi, 19, 26

Multiple Factors in the Causation of Environmentally Induced Diseases, 78a

Murai, Juro, 245

Murphy, F. A., 108, 109

Murphy, Michael, 199, 203

Musical Experience of Composer, Performer, and Listener, The, 281

Music and the Brain: Studies in the Neurology of Music, 281a, 282–283a

Music and the Language of Emotion, 281

Music and Your Mind: Listening with a New Consciousness, xv, 281, 282a

Music in Developmental Therapy, 281

Music in Geriatric Care, 281

Music in Therapy, 281, 283a

Music Therapy, 281

Music Therapy as a Career, 280, 281

Music Therapy for Handicapped Children, 284

Music Therapy in Action, 284a

Music Therapy Index, 281, 283a

Music Therapy in Special Education, 284a

Myers, C. R., 193, 203

Myers, R., 305, 316, 329a

Myers, S., 305, 316, 329a

Myth of Mental Illness, The, 500–501a

Namikoshi, Tokujiro, 211, 217, 223a

NAPPSAC Directory of Alternative Birth Services and Consumers' Guide, 311, 316, 330a

Naranjo, C., 166a

Nash, E. H., 181, 184

National Formulary, 263

Nature's Healing Agents, 271a

Needleman, Jacob, 23, 26

Neer, R. M., 287, 292, 294, 297a, 298a, 336, 340

Nei Ching. See Yellow Emperor's Classic of Internal Medicine, The

Neiswander, A. C., 403a

Nervous System, The, 25

Neurodynamics of the Vertebral Subluxation, 234

Neustadt, J. O., 181, 184

New Aerobics, The, 24, 202, 204a

New Age Journal, 327, 377a

New Age Politics: Healing Self and Society, 48, 52a

New American Materia Medica Therapeutics and Pharmacognosy, 271a

New England Journal of Medicine, 30a

New Games Book, The, 205a

New Hope for the Arthritic, 257a

New Meanings of Death, 389a

New Perspective on the Health of Canadians, A (LaLonde Report), 14, 15, 26, 33a, 43, 47, 51a, 112

Newsweek, 379
Newton, N., 328a
New Yorker, The, 62
New York State Health Code, 329a
Ng, Lorenz, 481a
Nichols, C. R., 182, 183
Nickerson, D., 288, 294
Nilsson, Lennart, 329a
Ninety Days to Self-Health, 137a
Nobody Ever Died of Old Age, 371, 374a
Nogier, Paul F. M., 424a, 450, 456, 464,
Nolewajka, G., 196, 203
Nonverbal Communication in Human Interaction, 456
Nordoff, Paul, 284a
Norton, Julia F., 273a
Nose, The: An Experimental Study of Reactions Within the Nose in Human Subjects During Varying Life Experiences, xvii, 358-359a
Nouwen, Henri, 380, 388
Numbers, Ronald A., 98
Nutrition Against Disease, 113a, 255, 261a
Nutrition Almanac, 255, 258a
Nutrition in a Nutshell, 261a

Obeyesekere, G., 427, 435, 440a
Obstetrical Medication and Development in the First Year of Life, 315, 320a
Occult Medicine Can Save Your Life: A Modern Doctor Looks at Unconventional Healing, 457, 463a
Ogden, Horace G., 96, 98
O'Halloran, D., 164
Oleson, Terrance D., 24, 451, 455
Olson, Paul, 172, 173a, 175
Omura, V., 419
On Death and Denying, 391a
On Death and Dying, 390a
One Surgeon's Experience with Hypnosis, 158a
On Learning to Plan—and Planning to Learn, 51a
Ophiem, K. E., 418
Opportunities in a Chiropractic Career, 236a
O'Regan, Brendan, 17, 24
Organon of Medicine, 401a, 402,

404, 458
Oriental Diagnosis, 423a
Origin and Properties of the Human Aura, 455,
Orleans, Peter, 41, 47
Orlick, Terry, 207a
Orme-Johnson, D., 161, 165
Ornstein, R., 166a
Orthopedic Medicine, 234
Osis, Karliss, 162, 165, 385, 386, 388
Osler, William, 3, 9
Ostfield, A., 356
Östling, G., 181, 183
Otis, L., 163, 165
Ott, John, 262, 298a
Our Bodies, Ourselves, 24, 28-29a, 100a
Outline of Chinese Acupuncture, An, 420a, 455, 458a
Over Easy (television show), 371

Paffenbarger, R. S., Jr., 197, 198, 203
Pahnke, W. N., 278, 280
Pain Game, The, 27
Palmer, B. J., 229, 231, 235
Palmer, D. D., 228, 233, 235, 237a
Palos, Stephen, 412, 418, 424a
Paperte, F., 278, 281
Paracelsus, Philippus, 268
Parascandola, L., 288, 295
Parkes, Colin Murray, 391a
Parkes, C. N., 16, 18, 26
Parsons, Talcott, 22, 26
Passarelli, E. W., 181, 184
Passwater, Richard A., 249, 253, 255, 258-259a
Pasteur, Louis, 7, 107
Patel, C. H., 161, 165
Patient Brochure and Self-Help Manual, 91, 99, 102a
Patient, Not the Cure, The, 403a
Patients and healers in the Contest of Culture: An Exploration of the Borderland between Anthropology, Medicine, and Psychiatry, xvii, 434, 438a
Pauling, Linus, 238, 253, 255, 259a, 260, 334, 340
Paulson, J. Sig, 481a
Pavlov, I., 108, 157, 326
Pearse, Innis H., 42-43, 47, 48,

51a
Peckham Experiment, The: A Study of the Living Structure of Society, 47, 51a
Pediatrics, 318, 320
Pelikan, Wilhelm, 273a
Pelletier, Kenneth R., xviii, 10, 19, 26, 34a, 112a, 377a, 386, 388
Pender, Nola J., 102a
Peper, Erik R., xviii, 126, 133, 135
Perinatal Factors Affecting Human Development, 315, 318a
Perry, J., 126
Personality and Personal Growth, xvi
Person Planet: The Creative Disintegration of Industrial Society, 488, 495
Perspectives on Health Promotion and Disease Prevention in the United States, 202
Persuasion and Healing: A Comparative Study of Psychotherapy, 25, 31a, 109, 171, 173a, 428, 434, 437a
Pesticide Conspiracy, The, 83a
Pesticides and Human Welfare, 75a
Pfeiffer, Carl, 251, 255, 259a
Pharmacopoeia of the United States, 263
Philosophy in a New Key, 281
Physician's Handbook on Orthomolecular Medicine, A, 255, 262a
Physician's Posy, A, 273a
Physics and Philosophy, 25
Physiology, Environment, and Man, 78a
Picture of Health, The: Environmental Sources of Disease, 72a
Pills, Profits, and Politics, 260a
Pinsky, R. H., 355, 356
Place of Birth, The, 326-327a
Plack, J. J., 292, 294, 295
Planning for Health: Development and Application of Social Change Theory, 47, 49a
Planta Medica, 276a
Plantes Medicinales et Phytotherapy, 276a
Plato, 382

Plummer, Norman, 356, 357a
Po, Ch'i, 425
Poesnecker, C. E., 481a
Poley, Jane, 95, 98
Politics of Cancer, The, 73–74a
Pomeranz, B. H., 413, 418
Pope, Alexander, 346
Popenoe, Cris, 34a
Population, Resources,
    Environment, 72–73
Porkert, Manfred, 424–425a
Positive Addiction, 205a
Poverty, Politics, and Change, 47
Powles, John , 35
Practical Encyclopedia of Natural
    Healing, The, 29a
Pratt, C. C., 278, 281
Pratt, J. G., 169, 171, 175a
Pratt, Lois, 96, 98
Precise, Posture Constant
    Spinograph Comparative Graphs,
    235
Precision Nirvana, xviii, 165,
    166a, 168a
Pregnant Patient's Bill of Rights,
    The, 325a
Prescriber, The, 402a, 459a
Prescriber and Clinical Repertory
    of Medicinal Herbs, 271a
Prestera, Hector, 446, 456, 461a
Prevention Magazine, 29, 255, 258
Prevention of Embryonic Fetal and
    Perinatal Disease, xvii
Preventive Medicine U.S.A., 51a
Pribram, Karl, 128
Price, D. D., 418
Priestly, Mary, 284a
Primer of Psychophysiology, A,
    127a
Principles and Art of Cure by
    Homoeopathy, The, 402a
Problem Solving Therapy: New
    Strategies for Effective Family
    Therapy, 62a
Proceedings–NIH Acupuncture
    Research Conference, 422a
Proceedings of the Hearings on
    Obstetrical Practices in the
    United States, 331a
Proceedings of the Third World
    Congress of Psychiatry, 135
Promotion and Maintenance of
    Health: Myth and Reality, 50a
Proshansky, Harold M., 39, 41,

47, 52a
Prugh, Dane, 357
Psychic Exploration, 456
Psychic Realm, The: What Can We
    Believe?, 171, 175a
Psychic Side of Sports, The, 203
Psychodietetics, 255, 256–257a
Psychological Care for the Dying
    Patient, 389a
Psychology of Color and Design,
    The, 299a
Psychology of Death, The, 390a
Psychology of Meditation, The,
    166a
Psychology of Music, A, 281
Psychology Today, 168
Psychophysiology, 128a
Psychophysiology of Respiration in
    Health and Disease, 360a
Psychosocial Care of the Dying
    Patient, xvi
Psychosomatic Families: Anorexia
    Nervosa in Context, 26, 60, 62
Psychosomatic Medicine: Its
    Clinical Applications, 136
Psychosynthesis: A Manual of
    Principles and Techniques, 455,
    456, 461a, 462a
Puente, A., 164
Purvis, J. P., 280, 281

Quarterly Journal of Crude Drug
    Research, 276a
Queen Elizabeth, 403
Quigley, W. H., 233, 235

R., Karen, 251, 255, 259–260a
Rabkin, Richard, xviii, 62a, 63a
Race, Change, and Urban Society,
    47
Radha, Swami Sivananda,
    243–244a
Rafii, A., 418
Rahe, Richard H., 18, 25, 45, 47,
    111a, 351, 361a
Ralston, D., 305, 316, 329a
Rama, Swami, 244a
Randolph, Theron G., 67, 72a,
    79a
Rank, Otto, 389
Rankin, David, 374a
Rappaport, M., 217
Rashkis, H. A., 182, 184
Raskin, D., 195, 202

Rating the Exercises, 206a
Reader's Digest, 375
Reading Disabilities and
    International Perspective,
    330–331a
Realms of Healing, The, xvii, 171,
    175a
Rechnitzer, P. A., 196, 202, 203,
    340, 342a
Rechung, Jampal Kunzang
    Rinpoche, 451, 456
Redmont, R., 356
Reed, E. J., 81a
Regush, Nicholas M., 453, 457
Reich, Wilhelm, 10, 19, 21, 26,
    34a, 210, 214–215, 217, 219,
    222, 223–224a, 244, 410
Reichmanis, M., 417, 418
Reichsman, F., 354
Reidak, Z., 418
Reiser, Morton, 357
Reiser, Stanley Joel, 79a, 428,
    435, 440a
Relaxation: A Bibliography, xviii
Relaxation Response, The, xv, 24,
    164, 166a, 168a
Relieve Tension the Autogenic
    Way, 136a
Relman, Arnold S., 455, 457
Renewal in Psychiatry, xvii
Repertory of the Homoeopathic
    Materia Medica, 399, 404, 405a
Report of the Secretary's
    Commission, 80a
Report on Smoking and Health
    (U.S. Surgeon General), 6, 27
Report to the President's
    Commission on Mental Health,
    25, 26, 315–316, 480a
Research in Parapsychology, 1972,
    171
Research in Parapsychology, 1973,
    456, 457
Research in Parapsychology, 1975,
    456
Research Status of Spinal
    Manipulative Therapy, The,
    234, 237a
Responsibilities of the Health Team
    in Maternity Care, The, 315
Resurrection of the Body, The, 23,
    216, 218a
Reynolds, D. K., 427, 433, 435,
    440a

Richard, Betty Byed, 205a
Richards, Martin, 322a
Richardson, S., 328a
Riessman, Frank, 95, 98, 100a
Rights of Hospital Patients, The: The Basic ACLU Guide to a Hospital Patient's Rights, 319a
Rindfuss, Ronald R., 331
Ringler, Norma E., 306, 316
Ringsdorf, W. M., Jr., 251, 252, 255, 256a, 257a, 338
Ripley, Herbert S., 352, 353, 354, 356, 357, 360a, 362a
Rise of Music in the Ancient World, East and West, The, 281
Risse, Guenter B., 96, 98
Robbins, Clive, 284a
Roberts, Herbert, 402a
Robinson, A. V., 290, 294
Rodale, Robert, 248, 480
Roemer, Milton J., 43, 48
Roethlisberger, F. J., 182, 184
Rogers, Carl, 201
Role of Medicine, The: Dream, Mirage, or Nemesis?, 26, 33a, 78–79a, 499–500a
Role of Taped Music Programs in the Guided Imagery and Music Process, The, xv
Rolf, Ida P., 20, 26, 211, 217, 224–225a, 446, 457, 462a
Rolfing: The Integration of Human Structures, 26, 217, 224–225a, 462a
Roll, W. G., 171, 176a, 456, 457
Rolling Thunder, 24
Rosa, K. R., 132, 135, 137a
Rosenman, Ray, 10, 25, 108, 109, 111a, 445, 456
Rosenthal, D., 181, 184
Rosenthal, Ted, 391a
Rosenzweig, Sandra, 87, 98
Rosman, Bernice, 26, 60, 62a
Roszack, Theodore, 488, 495
Rothman, David, 497, 500a
Rousseau, Jean Jacques, 12
Runner's Handbook, The, 199, 202
Runners' World, 203, 207
Running and Being: The Total Experience, 207a

Sab-feng, Cheng, 242
Saccharine Disease, The, 257a

Sachs, C., 278, 281
Sacro-Occipital Technique Notes, 234
Safe Alternatives in Childbirth, 316, 331a
Saint Augustine, 55
Salk, Jonas, 488, 495
Samet, S., 280, 281
Samuels, Michael, 34a, 112a, 378a, 448, 449, 457, 462a
Samuels, Nancy, 112a, 378a, 449, 457, 462a
San, Charles, 426
Sandweiss, J., 126
Sanne, H., 196, 203
Sargent, J. D., 134, 135
Satin, Mark, 43, 48, 52a
Satir, Virginia, 61
Savary, L. M., 278, 281, 282a
Savits, Barry, 453, 456
Saward, Ernest, 112a
Schafer, R. C., 238a
Schaie, K. Warner, 373a
Schapis, P., 294, 298a, 340
Scherrer, H., 152
Schiavi, R. C., 10, 19, 27
Schick, J., 292, 294, 295
Schmale, A. H., 16, 26
Schmeidler, Gertrude, 453, 456
Schneider, J. M., 183, 185
Schneider, Nina, 95, 98
Schneider, R. A., 354
Schneiderman, Marvin A., 8, 26
School of Natural Healing, 270a
Schottstaedt, W. W., 354, 355
Schultz, J. H., 131, 132, 133, 135, 136a
Schultz, Karen, 328
Schumacher, E. F., 486, 495
Schutz, Will, 211, 214, 217, 225a
Schwarcz, R., 315, 318a
Schwartz, Gary E., 125, 128a, 161, 163, 164, 165, 168a
Schwartz, Herman S., 233, 235, 238a
Science, 30a
Science and Practice of Iridology, The, 456, 460a
Science and the Evolution of Consciousness, 26
Science, Art, and Philosophy of Chiropractic, The, 235, 237a
Science of Homoeopathy, a Modern Text, The, 405a, 457, 463a

Science Studies Yoga: A Review of Physiological Data, 242a
Science, Synthesis, and Sanity, 48
Scott, A., 297a
Scott, J. P., 47, 50a, 362a
Season to Be Born, A, 315
Secret Life of Plants, The, 273a
Secret of the Golden Flower, The, 425–426a
Seeing with the Mind's Eye, 112a, 378a, 457, 462–463a
Segal, H. L., 354
Sehnert, Keith S., 19, 26, 87, 88, 90, 93, 94, 95, 96, 98, 99, 101a, 102a
Selected Writings: An Introduction to Orgonomy, 26, 34a, 217, 223a
Self-Care Information Sheet, 98
Self-Care in Health, 95, 96, 99, 103a
Self-Care: Lay Initiatives in Health, 96, 98, 101a, 499a
Self-Help in the Human Services, 95, 98, 100a
Self Hypnotism, 152
Selver, Charlotte, 210, 214
Selye, Hans, 9, 10, 26, 108, 357a
Senay, E. C., 47, 50a, 362
Sense Relaxation, 214, 216, 221a
Sensory Awareness, 216, 219a
Sentics: The Touch of the Emotions, 282a
Separation and Depression: Clinical and Research Aspects, xvii, 47
Serizawa, Katsusuke, 425a
Serve the People: Observations on Medicine in the People's Republic of China, 27
Sessions, R., 278, 281
Shadman, Alonzo, 402a
Shafii, M., 161, 165
Shanas, Ethel, 373a
Shapiro, Arthur K., 11, 26, 179, 180, 181, 182, 184, 188a
Shapiro, Deane H., Jr., xviii, 125a, 128a, 161, 162, 163, 164, 165, 166a, 167a, 168a
Sharma, C. H., 403a
Sharon, I. M., 292, 295, 298a, 336, 340
Sharpe, Deborah T., 299a
Sharpless, S. K., 231, 235
Shaw, George Bernard, 212, 222

Shaw, James H., 334, 336, 340, 343a
Shealy, C. Norman, 17, 18, 27, 31, 126, 137a, 453, 457, 463a, 470, 471, 473, 480
Sheehan, George, 207–208a
Sheldon, William, 446
Shepard, E. J., 354
Shepard, Leslie, 461a
Sheperd, Jack, 199, 202
Sheperd, Dorothy, 273a, 403
Sher, 268
Sherrington, Charles, 108, 222
Shiatsu: Japanese Finger-Pressure Therapy, 217, 223a
Shils, Maurice, 253, 255, 258a, 340, 343a
Shireson, S., 340
Shneidman, Edwin, 391a
Shnider, S., 305, 316, 326a, 329a
Shook, Edward E., 273a
Shore, M. L., 71a
Shore, Nathan A., 335
Shorter, Frank, 192
Sidel, Ruth, 14, 27, 81a
Sidel, Victor, 14, 27, 81a
Sigerest, H., 427, 435, 441a
Silent Spring, 76
Silver, D. B., 427, 434, 437a
Silverman, J., 212, 217
Silverman, Milton, 260a
Simkin, P., 311, 312, 315, 316, 321a, 325a, 330a
Simons, Victoria, xviii, 229, 234
Simonton, O. Carl, 12, 17, 21, 27, 28, 29, 31, 110, 113a, 448, 457, 471, 481a
Since Silent Spring, 76a
Singer, Jerome L., 449, 457
Singh, B., 160, 164
Sinning, W., 193, 203
Sipprelle, C., 163, 164
Sivananda, 244
Sjohund, B., 413, 418
Skibbe, R., 229, 234
Slome, C., 309, 316
Small, T. J., 419
Small Is Beautiful, 486, 495
Smarr, E. R., 182, 184
Smith, David, 208a
Smith, J., 163, 165, 167a
Smith, M. J., 11, 27, 170, 171, 176a

Smith, R. F., 81a
Smith, Robert W., 241a
Smith, T. W., 418
Smuts, Jan Christian, 3, 27, 486
Snow, L. F., 429, 435, 441a
Snyder, Solomon H., 109
Sobel, David, 16, 24, 35a
Social Forces in Later Life, The: An Introduction to Social Gerontology, 373a
Social Limits to Growth, The, 486, 495
Social Psychology of Music, The, 281, 283a
Social Science and Medicine, 428
Social Structure and Personality, 26
Soghikian, Krikor, 97
So Human An Animal, 24
Sokolov, M. V., 294
Solovey, Galena, 157a
Somers, Anne R., 40, 48
Song of the Siren, xvii
Sound and Symbol: Music and the External World, 281, 284a
Soyka, Fred, 81a
Spadaro, J. A., 417
Special Study of Alternative Services: Report to the President's Commission on Mental Health, xvii
Specific Relations of Attitude to Physiological Change, 349
Speck, Ross V., 17, 27, 61
Spetz, M., 57, 60
Spicer, E. H., 427, 435, 441a
Spiegel, Herbert, 155
Spiegelford, Morton B., 343a
Spiritual Midwifery, 315, 324a
Spiro, M., 427, 435, 437, 441a
Spontaneous Regression of Cancer, 24, 109
Standards for Obstetric-Gynecologic Services, 319, 325
Statistical Abstract of the United States, 1977, 24
Strategic Psychotherapy, xviii, 63a
Stein, M., 10, 19, 27, 316, 327a
Steiner, Rudolf, 273
Stent, Gunther, 445, 457
Stephenson, James, 398, 400, 405a
Stephenson, R. W., 228, 235

Sterman, M. B., 128, 129a
Stern, Arthur C., 82a
Stern, J. A., 356
Stevens, J.G.R., 75a
Stevens, Rosemary, 43, 48
Stevenson, Ian P., 353, 354, 357
Stewart, David, 311, 316, 330a
Stewart, Lee, 316, 330a
Stewart, Richard B., 309, 315
Stickl, 268
Still, Andrew, 227
Stillwell, D. M., 418
Stirman, 154
St. Martin, Alexis, 359
Stokinger, Herbert, 82
Stoll, Walt W., 91, 99, 102a
Stone, Irwin, 253, 255, 260a
Stone, R. A., 161, 165
Stoyva, J., 125a, 127, 128a
Strauss, Anselm, 390a
Street, G., 229, 235
Stress and Survival: The Emotional Realities of Life-Threatening Illnesses, xvi, 390a
Stress of Life, The, 26
Stretching, 204a
Stroebel, C. F., 126, 161, 164
Structure of Scientific Revolutions, The, 33a
Study and Analysis of the Treatment of Sprain and Strain Injuries in Industrial Cases, A, 234
Subliminal Perception: The Nature of a Controversy, 456
Suggestive Therapeutics, 151
Suh, Chung Ha, 231, 235
Sullivan, H. S., 244
Sun, A. C., 419
Sun, Patricia, 28
Superhealthy, The, 24
Supernutrition, 255, 258–259a
Surgical Performance: Necessity and Quality, 27
Survival of the Wisest, The, 488, 495
Survivor, The, 390
Swanson, Susan, xiii
Swearingen, Robert, 20, 27, 31, 480
Sweeney, Edward A., 334, 336, 340, 343a
Syme, Leonard F., 45, 47

Szasz, Thomas, 497, 500–501a

Tager, Mark, 195, 203
Tai Chi, 241a
Tai Chi Chuan, 242a
Tai Chi Chuan: A Simplified Method of Calisthenics for Health and Self Defense, 241a
Talk Back to Your Doctor: How to Demand and Recognize High Quality Health Care, 101a
Tambiah, S. J., 427, 433, 435, 441a
Tandy, B., 126
Tao of Physics, The, 24
Tarnopol, L., 330a
Tarnopol, M., 330a
Tart, Charles T., 164, 453, 456, 457, 461a
Tashkin, D. P., 419
Taub, E., 126, 128
Taylor, I., 294, 298a, 340
Taylor, I. A., 278, 281
Techmacher, H., 418
Techniques of Hypnotherapy, 152, 154
Teeguarden, Iona, 244–245a
Teitelbaum, H. A., 182
Tension Control: Proceedings of the Second Meeting of the American Association for the Advancement of Tension Control, 339, 341a
Terenius, L., 413, 418
Testimony before the Subcommittee on Health and Scientific Research, 26
Thacker, Stephen, 305, 315, 319–320a
Thank You Dr. Lamaze: A Mother's Experience in Painless Childbirth, 316, 326a
That First Bite: Journal of a Compulsive Overeater, 251, 255, 259a
Thayer, P. S., 297a
Theoretical Foundations of Chinese Medicine, The, 424–425a
Thetford, W. N., 356
Thie, John, 238a
Thiede, Henry A., 309, 317
Thomas, Caroline B., 10, 27, 108, 109
Thomas, Lewis, 50, 78

Thomas, L. J., 335, 340
Thompson, J., 229, 235
Thompson, K. F., 337, 340
Thompson, Samuel, 263
Thompson Technique, 235
Thorington, L., 288, 294, 295, 298a, 340
Thurber, James, 253
Tiber, N., 340
Tibetan Medicine, 456
Tien, H. C., 419
Time to Enjoy, A: The Pleasures of Aging, 372, 374a
Tinbergen, Nikolaas, 35a, 212, 217
Tinker, Kathleen McIntosh, 94, 97
Tocantius, L. M., 340
Todd, Malcolm C., 196, 203
Toftness, I. N., 229, 235
Tohei, Koichi, 245a
Toma, C., 419
Tompkins, Peter, 273a
Tongue Diagnosis in Color, 423a, 456
Tooth Trip, The, 335, 340, 342a
Torrey, E. Fuller, 501a
Total Fitness in 30 Minutes A Week, 207
Touch for Health, 238a
Touching, 209, 217
Toward a Science of Consciousness, xviii
Toxicological Evaluations of Some Food Additives Including Anticaking Agents, Antimicrobials, Antioxidants, Emulsifiers and Thickening Agents, 76–77a
Toxicology: The Basic Science of Poisons, 70–71a
Training Workshop for Professionals, A: Introduction to the Methods of Autogenic Therapy, 136a
Transcultural Psychiatry Research Review, 428
Transformation, The, 488, 495, 499a
Traut, E. F., 181, 184
Travis, John, 17, 27, 28, 87, 88, 92, 99, 473, 482a
Treatise of Auriculotherapy, 424a, 456

Treatment of Disease by Acupuncture, The, 418, 424a
Troiani, J., 126
Trotter, Robert J., 306, 317
Trubo, Richard, 17, 18, 24
Tryphonopoulou, Y., 315, 320a
Tsaknis, P. G., 339
Tsao, C. J., 419
Tubesing, Donald A., 19, 27, 482a
Tulku, Tarthang, 245–246a
Tuning the Human Instrument, 281
Turdeanu, V., 419
Turner, Evelyn, 212, 217, 225a
Turner, S., 81a, 305, 317, 331a
Turner, Victor, 427, 428, 435, 436, 441a
Turshen, Meredith, 12, 27
Twelve Healers and Other Remedies, The, 270
Twenty-Ninth Day, The, 485, 488, 494, 496a
Tyler, Margaret L., 405a
Tyler, Paul, 82a
Type A Behavior and Your Heart, 25, 109, 111a, 456

Uhlenhuth, E. H., 181, 184
Ullyot, Joan, 208
Ultimate Athlete, The, 207a
Uncommon Therapy: The Psychiatric Techniques of Milton Erickson, 61a, 156a
Uneasy Equilibrium, The: Private and Public Financing of Health Services in the United States, 1875–1965, 46
United States Dispensatory, 273–274a
Urban Condition, The: People and Policy in the Metropolis, 47, 50a

Vahia, N. S., 161, 165
Van Den Bosch, Robert, 83–84a
Vanderschot, L., 413, 418
Varieties of the Meditative Experience, The, 166a
Vaughan, Alan, 454, 457
Veith, Ilza, 425a, 450, 457, 463a
Very Easy Death, A, 389a
Vesalius, Andreas, 4
Veterinary Acupuncture, 423a
Villforth, J. C., 71

Villoldo, Alberto, 170, 171, 172, 175a
Virchow, Rudolph, 7, 107
Vishnudevananda, Swami, 246a
Vitality Training for Older Adults, 376a
Vitamin C, the Common Cold and the Flu, 255, 259a, 340
Vitamin E and Aging, xvi
Vitamins in Your Life, xvi
Vithoulkas, George, 403a, 405a, 447, 457, 463a
Vogel, Marcel, 29
Vogel, Richard, 334, 340
Vogel, Virgil J., 263, 269, 274a
Vogl, A. J., 238a
Vogt, O., 131
Volen, Michael P., 421a
Volgyesi, Ferenc András, 154, 157a
Volkman, Janice, 47, 50a
Volkova, N. V., 292, 295
von Felsinger, J. M., 181, 184
von Rottauscher, Anna, 425a, 450, 457, 463a
Voznesenskaya, E. A., 294
Vuori, I., 196, 203

Wagner, M. J., 277, 281
Wagner, N. N., 356
Walcott, A., 294, 298a
Waldbott, George L., 84a
Walhstrom, A., 413, 418
Walker, E. H., 175
Wall, P., 413, 418
Wallace, R. K., 161, 164, 165, 437
Wallnofer, Heinrich, 425a, 450, 457, 463a
Walrath, L., 163, 165
Walsh, R., 164, 165, 166a, 167
Walters, David, 238a
Walters, E. D., 134, 135
Wancera, I., 419
Ward, Charlotte, 331a
Ward, Fred, 331a
Warnes, H., 136
Warren, Frank, 460
Waterman, D., 126
Watkins, Anita M., 170, 171, 172, 176-177a
Watt, E. W., 198, 202
Watt, John Mitchell, 275a
Watzlawick, Paul, 25, 63a

Ways of Health: Holistic Approaches to Ancient and Contemporary Medicine, 24, 35a
Way to Vibrant Health, The: A Manual of Bioenergetic Exercises, 216, 223a
Weakland, John, 25, 63a
Weeks, Nora, 268, 269
Weinstock, Allan (Swami Ajaya), 244a
Weisel, J., 287, 292, 295
Weisman, Avery, 391a
Weiss, Bernard, 85a
Weitzenhoffer, André M., 155
Well Body Book, The, 34a, 448, 457
Wellness, 34a
Wellness Inventory, 27
Wellness Workbook, 99, 482a
Wells, K., 229, 235
Wells, Roger A., 170, 171, 172, 176a, 177a
Wen, H. L., 419
Werbel, Ernest W., 158a
Werner, A., 183, 185
Werner, David, 97, 99
Wertz, Dorothy C., 304, 317, 331a
Wertz, Richard W., 304, 317, 331a
Wessberg, H. W., 163, 164
West, D. J., 169, 171, 177a
Westberg, Granger, 470, 471, 474, 476
Wexu, Mario, 450, 457, 464a
What Every Woman Should Know: The Truth About Diets and Drugs in Pregnancy, 321a
Wheatley, D., 182, 185
Where There Is No Doctor, 99
Whitaker, Carl, 61
White, G., 332a
White, Kerr, 30
White, Rhea, 199, 203
Whitehead, W., 126
Who Is Your Doctor and Why?, 402a
Whole Earth Catalog, 193
Whole Person Health, 203
Wholistic Dimensions in Healing, xv, xvii, 32a, 269, 272a, 456, 476, 480a
Wholistic Health: A Whole Person

Approach to Primary Health Care, 27
Wholistic Health Center, The, 482a
Who Shall Live? Health Economics and Social Choice, 75a, 486, 495, 498a
Why Survive? Being Old In America, 371, 374a
Why Your Child Is Hyperactive, 74a
Wiklund, Nils, 454, 456
Wilhelm Reich: The Evolution of His Work, 216
Wilhelm, Richard, 425a
Wilhelmsen, L., 196, 203
Wilkinson, F., 316, 327a
Williams, Elizabeth Ann, xviii
Williams, Roger J., 20, 27, 113a, 251, 252, 253, 255, 261a, 262a
Williamson, G. S., 42-43, 48, 51a
Williamson, John D., 87, 88, 90, 91, 95, 96, 99, 103a
Wilson, A. F., 161, 165
Wing, A. L., 198, 203
Winikoff, Beverly, 30
Winokur, G., 356
Wirth, Victoria, 198, 203
Wisdom of the Body, The, 24
Without Prescription, xvi
Wittkower, E. D., 136
Wolf, Stewart G., Jr., 352, 353, 354, 355, 357a, 358a, 359-360a, 362a
Wolf, S., 181, 183, 185
Wolff, Harold G., 153a, 155, 156, 345, 352, 353, 354, 355, 356, 357a, 358a, 359-360a, 362a
Wolfson, S., 181, 183
Wolman, Benjamin, 453, 457
Wollman, Leo, xviii
Women Running, 208a
Wonderful World Within You, The: Your Inner Nutritional Environment, 255, 261a
Wong, Ming, 422a
Woodyat, R. T., 57, 60
Woolfolk, R., 161, 165, 167a
Working Papers (newsletter), xviii, 83
World of Light, The, 294
Worthington, R. E., 10, 26
Wright, C., 126
Write Yourself Slim, xviii

Wurtman, R. J., 286, 287, 292, 294, 295, 298a, 340
Wu, Shui Wan, 426a, 458
Wu, Wei-F'ing, 426a
Wyler, A. R., 129a, 356
Wynder, Ernst L., 82
Wynne, Lyman, 61
Wyszecki, G., 288, 294

Yang, K. C., 419
Yannacone, Victor J., Jr., 76
Yeager, Robert C., 87, 99, 103a
Yellow Emperor, The, 425
Yellow Emperor's Classic of Internal Medicine, The (Nei Ching), 415, 425a, 457, 463a
Yoga and Psychotherapy: The Evolution of Consciousness, 244a
Yoga and the Athlete, 206a
You and AT, 135, 137a
Young, A., 427, 433, 435, 442a
Young, W. W., 403a
Your Baby, Your Body, 204a
Your Second Life, 377a
Y's Way to Physical Fitness, The, 203
Yu, H., 419

Zahn, D. W., 355
Zamkova, M. A., 291, 292, 295
Zapping of America, The, 83
Zaret, Milton, 71a
Zeiger, David J., xviii
Zeldow, Leonard L., 335, 340
Zen and the Art of Archery, 206
Zifferblatt, A., 168a
Zuckerkandl, Victor, 278, 281, 284a

SUBJECT INDEX

Acupressure, 243–245, 411, 421, 471
Acupuncture, 4, 19, 407–426, 450–452, 458, 460, 461–462, 463, 473
  clinical applications, 414–415
  and the ear. *See* Auriculotherapy
  moxibustion, 411
  theories of, 412–414
  and veterinary medicine, 423
  See also Acupressure
Additives. *See* Food additives
Aerobics, 110, 192, 196, 199, 204
Aerobics Center (Dallas, Tex.), 199
Age of Enlightenment Center for Holistic Health, 479
Aging, 101, 195, 205, 363–378
  attitudes toward, 364–365, 377
  and exercise, 195, 205, 376
  population statistics, 363–364
  programs for the elderly, 367–371, 375, 377
  and self-care, 101
  and yoga, 195, 374
Aikido, 192, 195, 245
Air pollution. *See* Pollution, air

Alcoholism, 8, 134, 477
Alexander technique, 21, 35, 212–213, 216, 218–219, 222
Allopathic medicine, 395–396, 400. *See also* Biomedicine
Almega Institute, 241
American College of Obstetricians and Gynecologists (ACOG), 309, 310, 312, 325
American Dental Association (ADA), 337
American Health Foundation, 95
American Health Planning Association, 479
American Herbal Pharmacology Delegation, 265, 269, 274
American Holistic Medical Association, 23, 477
American Indian medicine. *See* Native American medicine
American Institute of Homoeopathy, 395
American Medical Association (AMA), 151, 196, 260, 395, 415, 417, 469
American Public Health Association, 468

American Society of Clinical Hypnosis, 151
Anesthesia
  and childbirth, 326, 329
  and hypnosis, 156–157
  and hypnotic awareness, 145, 154, 157
Anorexia nervosa, 17, 62
Anthrax, 268
Antibiotics, 5, 6, 8, 85
Apgar scores, 310. *See also* Childbirth
Arica psychocalisthenics. *See* Psychocalisthenics
Arthritis, 18, 134, 257, 364
Asbestos, 41, 73
Aspirin, 7, 187
Association for Holistic Health (San Diego, Calif.), 23, 472, 477–478
Association for Humanistic Gerontology (AHG), 370
Asthma, 16, 17, 55, 57, 134, 348
Astrology, 463
Attitudes and disease, 9–10, 108–109, 113, 346–349, 361, 481

Aura, 453, 461
Auriculotherapy, 422, 424, 450–
451, 458, 460, 464, 473
Autism, 35
Autogenic therapy, 18, 108,
131–137, 463
exercises, 132–133
history, 131
research and theory, 134–135
Autogenic training. See
Autogenic therapy
Avogadro limit, 398, 400, 404

Bach Flower Remedies, 267–
268, 270
Berkeley Family Health Center,
307, 311, 476
Berkeley Holistic Health Center,
28, 456, 459, 472
Berkeley Psychosomatic Clinic,
475
Berkeley Women's Health
Collective, 477
Bioenergetics, 21, 210, 215,
222–223, 446, 459. See also
Touch
Biofeedback, 4, 17, 18, 19, 115–
129, 463, 471, 487
clinical applications, 116–117,
127
definition, 116
evaluation of, 121–124
and non-stress disorders, 120–
121
and stress disorders, 117–120
Biofeedback Society of America,
126
Biomedicine
background, 4–6
challenge to, 6–7, 30–31, 111
consumer critique, 13
contextual critique, 10
cross-cultural critique, 14–15,
433, 437–438
ecological critique, 12–13
general critique, 7–15, 29, 30,
32, 33, 498–499, 500
historical reevaluation, 7–8
humanistic critique, 13–14
political critique, 12
psychosomatic critique, 9–10
spiritual critique, 11–12
task of, 487
See also Allopathic medicine

Birth. See Childbirth
Bloodroot, 268
Blue Cross Association, 96, 102
Body therapies. See Touch
Bodywork. See Touch
Boston Women's Health Book
Collective, 13
Breathing exercises, 218, 375,
376
Bridge Project (Bellingham,
Wash.), 367

Cancer, 8, 17, 72, 108, 109, 110,
113, 268, 364, 458–459, 471,
481
politics of, 73–74
Cancer Counseling and Reseach
Center, 471, 472, 475, 476,
480, 481
Cardiovascular disease, 8, 21,
108, 111, 120, 197, 364
Center for Continuing Health
Education, 93
Center for Disease Control, 477
Center for Health Enhancement,
Education, and Research
(CHEER), 478
Center for Integral Medicine
(Los Angeles, Calif.), 475,
478, 480
Center for Traditional
Acupuncture (Columbia,
Md.), 473
Cerebrovascular disease, 8
Chevreul pendulum, 143, 147
Chi energy, 10, 18, 245, 410
Childbirth, 5, 13, 21, 303–332,
476
alternative birth movement,
306–309, 314, 319, 323, 324,
325, 327–328, 330, 476
and anesthesia, 326, 329
electronic fetal monitoring
(EFM) 147, 305, 319–320
home births, 303, 307, 309–
311, 313, 323, 324, 325,
326–327, 331
and hypnosis, 146–148, 153
Lamaze method, 146, 307, 326
Leboyer method, 147, 306, 323
midwifery, 5, 13, 303, 307,
309–310, 324, 327
and physical exercise, 198,
204–205

Chinese medicine, 14, 19, 31–
32, 211, 266, 407–426, 431,
432, 438, 439, 440, 449–452,
458, 462, 463–464
and herbs, 265, 274, 422
and holistic health, 415–417
origins of, 407–409
theory of, 408–409, 424–425
yin and yang, 408–409, 410,
411, 416, 449–450, 463
See also Acupressure;
Acupuncture; Diagnosis,
traditional Chinese
Chiropractic, 5, 227–239
cost effectiveness, 232–233
diagnosis in, 229–231, 238
history, 227–228, 236, 237–238
kinesiology, 228, 238
and mental health, 238
research, 231–232, 237
subluxation, 228–231
Chloramphenicol, 7
Clairvoyant diagnosis. See
Diagnosis, psychic
Clinical ecology. See
Environment, clinical ecology
Club of Rome, 485
Clymer Health Clinic, 473, 481
Color and health, 292–293, 296,
297, 299. See also Light and
health
Columbia Point Alcoholism
Program (Dorchester,
Mass.), 477
Committees for the Defense of
the Revolution (Cuba), 313
Commonweal, Inc., 83, 489–490
Community Health Education
Center (Eugene, Oreg.), 474
Congress of Nurse Healers, 23,
477
Corporate health programs, 196,
477, 491–492
Cost of medical care. See
Medical care, cost

Death
emotional reaction to, 387–388,
389–391
near-death experiences, 384–
387
social concern with, 379–380,
390
See also Dying

Demographics and health, 41–42
Dentistry, 333–343
  holistic dentistry, 338–339
  and hypnosis, 337, 341, 342–
    343
  and mental health, 334–335,
    343
  and nutrition, 334, 343
  and patient anxiety, 336–337,
    341
  preventive oral health, 335–
    336
Dentists, health of, 337–338,
  342
Denver Birthing Center, 307,
  311
Depression, 181, 193, 198–199
Diabetes, 17, 57–58, 59, 134,
  349, 459
Diagnosis
  alternative forms of, 19, 423,
    443–464, 473
  in clinical ecology, 67
  ear. See Auriculotherapy
  in homoeopathy, 398–399,
    447–448, 459, 463
  imagery in, 448–449, 458–459,
    461, 462–463
  mind control programs and,
    453–454
  observation in, 19, 224–225,
    398–399, 445–447, 449,
    451–452, 459–460, 461, 462
  psychic (clairvoyant), 452–454,
    460, 473
  pulse, 411, 426, 449, 450,
    462, 463, 473
  Tibetan, 451
  tongue, 411, 423, 449, 450
  traditional Chinese, 411, 449–
    452, 463
  validity of alternative systems,
    444–445
Diet. See Nutrition
Dieting, 250–252, 256–257,
  259–260. See also Nutrition;
  Overweight
Digitalis, 263–264
Disease. See Illness
Door, The, 469
Drugs, 102, 260, 268, 471. See
  also Antibiotics; Food and
  Drug Administration; Plants,
  drugs derived from

Dying, 5, 22, 379–391, 477
  and care of the dying, 243,
    380–383, 389–390, 477
  emotional issues, 381–383, 390
  hospice and counseling
    programs, 383–384
  and life-threatening illness, 390
  See also Death

East-West Academy of Healing
  Arts (San Francisco, Calif.),
  475, 478
Ecology. See Environment
Economic conditions and health,
  10, 40. See also Medical
  care, costs
Education and health, 40, 42
Élan vital, 18
Elderly. See Aging
Elmhurst Hospital (Queens,
  N.Y.), 55
Elvirita Lewis Foundation (Santa
  Cruz, Calif.), 369
Endorphins, 109, 413
Environment, 8, 12, 30, 33, 43,
  50, 52, 53, 65–85, 488, 496–
  497
  carcinogens in, 73–74, 78, 84
  clinical ecology, 66–67, 72, 79
  effects of environmental
    toxins, 65, 490
  See also Food additives;
    Pesticides; Pollution;
    Radiation; Toxicology
Epilepsy, 121, 129
Ethnic background and health,
  41
Exercise. See Physical
  exercise
Extrasensory perception, 453–
  454, 456, 460

Faith healing. See Psychic
  healing
Family therapy, 17, 53–63
  definition, 53
  effect of illness on family, 58–
    59
  and physical illness, 56–58
  school of, 53–56, 62
Farm, the, 307, 310, 324
FDA. See Food and Drug
  Administration
Feldenkrais exercises, 213, 216,

220, 221
Flexnor Report of 1910, 484
Food. See Food additives;
  Nutrition
Food additives, 67, 74, 76–77,
  80–81, 248–249, 490. See
  also Food and Drug
  Administration
Food and Drug Administration
  (FDA), 249, 250, 324–325,
  332, 417
Foot reflexology, 444, 459
Free clinics, 468–470
Frontier Nursing Service, 309
Future health care, 49–50, 200–
  201, 493–494. See also
  Health policy

Garden of Eden, 55, 272
Georgetown Family Center, 58
Gerontology, 370, 373, 377. See
  also Aging
Gestalt therapy, 18
Gray Panthers, 370–371, 377
Guided fantasy, 225, 448–449,
  461, 462. See also
  Guided Imagery and
  Music; Visualization
Guided imagery. See Guided
  fantasy; Guide Imagery
  and Music
Guided Imagery and Music
  (GIM), 278–279, 280
Gynecology
  hypnosis in, 148–150.
  See also Childbirth

Haight-Ashbury Free Medical
  Clinic, 94, 469
Haight-Ashbury Women's
  Medical Clinic, 477
Hawthorne effect, 182
Headaches, 8, 118, 181, 358
  migraine, 118, 134, 348, 358
Health, definition, 17. See also
  High level wellness
Health centers, holistic, 22,
  467–482
  characteristics of, 470–476
  future of, 476–478
  See also Free clinics
Health education, 95
Health planning, 14, 49, 51,
  200–201, 479, 498. See also

Health policy
Health Planning and Resource Development Act of 1974, 477
Health Planning Council (Madison, Wisc.), 477, 479
Health policy, 12, 22, 29–30, 39, 44, 51, 204, 483–501
  in China, 14, 31
  future, 493–494
  human adaptability, 492–493, 496–497
  issues in health care, 485–490
  and trends in health care, 490–492
  See also Future health care; Health planning
Health promotion, 17–18, 50, 66, 196, 200–201, 472–473, 488–489, 492. See also High level wellness
Health Skills Associates (Dayton, Ohio), 95
Health Systems Agencies, 477
Healthwise (Boise, Idaho), 94
Heart disease. See Cardiovascular disease
Herbs. See Plants
High level wellness, 17, 193, 201, 479. See also Health promotion
Holistic health. See Health centers, holistic; Holistic medicine
Holistic medicine
  definition of, xi, 3, 89–90, 338–339, 433–434, 486
  paradigm of, 15–23, 115
Holistic thinking, 486–487
Home births. See Childbirth, home births
Home Oriented Maternity Experience (HOME), 323
Homoeopathy, 5, 174, 273, 275, 395–405
  diagnosis in, 398–399, 447–448, 459, 463
  history of, 395, 401, 484
  and holistic principles, 397, 399
  practice, 398–399, 403–405
  principles of, 396–398, 401
Hospitals, 5, 9, 304–306, 307,

309–310, 311, 493–494. See also Health centers, holistic
Household pollutants, 74
Humanistic medicine, 13. See also Holistic medicine
Humor in healing, 110
Hunza, 364
Hyperactivity, 67, 74
Hypertension, 10, 17, 18, 118–119, 134, 161, 166, 167, 197, 268, 347, 472. See also Cardiovascular disease; Stress
Hypnosis, 18, 108–109, 139–158, 167–168, 173
  autohypnosis and autogenic therapy, 131
  and childbirth, 146–148, 153
  concepts of, 139–140
  and dentistry, 337, 341, 342–343
  and gynecology, 148–150
  and meditation, 167–168
  and pain, 144, 156, 337, 341
  and paranormal healing, 173
  and surgery, 145, 155, 158
  theories of, 140
  use in emergencies, 145–146
Hypnotherapy, 154

Iatrogenic illness, 9, 19
Ideomotor questioning, 149, 150–151, 154
Illness
  definition, 55, 56, 68
  distribution, 43, 57, 96, 346–351
  See also Cardiovascular disease; Depression; Iatrogenic illness; Mental health; Psychosomatic illness; and names of other specific illnesses
Image-CA, 110, 448, 458–459
Imagery. See Guided fantasy; Guided Imagery and Music; Visualization
Immune system, 18, 19, 458, 471
Indigenous healing, 14–15, 17, 23, 263, 265–266, 268, 271–272, 274–275, 427–442, 475
  and holistic care, 433–434
  institutions, 430–431
  levels, 428–430

therapeutic stages, 433
  See also Chinese medicine; Native American medicine; Tibetan medicine
Insomnia, 119
Institute of Consciousness and Music, 279, 282
Institute for Creative Aging, 476–477
Institute for the Study of Humanistic Medicine, 14
Institute of Noetic Sciences, xiii
Integral medicine, 31. See also Holistic medicine
Integrated Pest Management (IPM), 83
Interface (Brookline, Mass.), 472
Intergenerational Child Care Center (Santa Cruz, Calif.), 369
International Center for Autogenic Therapy, 137
International Childbirth Education Association, 321, 324, 325
International Chiropractic Association (ICA), 231, 237, 238
International Committee on Autogenic Therapy (ICAT), 134
International Society of Clinical and Experimental Hypnosis, 151
Iridiagnosis. See Iridology
Iridology, 444, 454–455, 459, 460, 473

Jin Shin Do, 244–245. See also Acupresssure
Jogging. See Running and jogging

Kaiser Permanente medical care program, 92, 469, 480
Ki energy. See Chi energy
Kinesiology. See Chiropractic, kinesiology
Klamath Mental Health Center, 473
Kum nye, 245–246
Kundalini. See Yoga, Kundalini

Lamaze method. See Childbirth, Lamaze method
Laying-on-of-hands, 19–20, 169,

170, 174, 175–176. *See also*
Psychic healing; Touch
Leboyer method. *See* Childbirth,
Leboyer method
Lifestyle and health, 17, 33, 43,
72, 75, 111, 112–113, 191–
208
Light and health
color rendering index (CRI),
286, 288–291
indoor illumination, 286–287
spectral power distribution
(SPD), 288–290
sunlight, 285–286
therapeutic uses, 293, 297–298
See also Color and health
Lourdes, 169, 174, 177

Malnutrition, 72
Martial arts, 192, 193, 195, 241,
242, 245
Maryland Psychiatric Research
Center, 278
Massage, 20, 210–211, 216, 220,
446, 472
Esalen, 230
Japanese, 223
Oriental, 425
shiatsu, 211, 216, 223
Maternity Center Associates
(New York, N.Y.), 307
Maternity Center Association,
307, 328
Meadowlark Center (Hemet,
Calif.), 473, 481
Medical botany. *See* Plants
Medical care
cost, ix, 7, 9, 12, 15, 97, 232–
233, 474
See also Biomedicine
Medical Committee for Human
Rights, 12, 22, 469
Medicare and Medicaid, 7, 233,
417
Meditation, 4, 16, 18, 28, 159–
168, 242, 244–246, 425, 461,
472, 476, 479
as altered state of
consciousness, 161–162, 166
clinical applications, 161–167
and hypnosis, 167–168
as self-regulation strategy, 159,
161, 163, 165, 166
Mental health, 5, 8, 30, 31, 52,

53–63, 162, 188–189, 243–
244, 256–257, 259, 267–268,
439, 448–449, 497, 500–501
and chiropractic, 238
and oral health, 334–335
and physical exercise, 198–
299, 200
Menninger Foundation, 244
Meyer life chart, 346
Midwifery. *See* Childbirth,
midwifery
Midwifery Program (the Farm),
307
Mountain People's Clinic, 474
Multiple sclerosis, 268, 348
Music and Health, 277–284
music therapy, 278–284
and physiological effects, 279
sound, 279
Myasthenia gravis, 268

Naloxone, 109, 413
National Association of Parents
and Professionals for Safe
Alternatives in Childbirth
(NAPPSAC), 311, 312
National Center for
Homoeopathy, 405
National Health and Resources
Development Act (1974), 233
National Hospice Organization,
384
National Institute of Mental
Health (NIMH), x, xiii, xiv
National Institutes of Health,
488–489
Native American medicine, 14,
31–32, 139, 263, 268, 271–
272, 274–275, 437, 441. *See
also* Indigenous healing
Natura system. *See* Thomsonian
system
Naturopathy, 5
Networking, 44–46, 49
Neuromuscular dysfunctions,
120
New Games, 193, 205
Nurse Consultants and Health
Counselors (San Francisco,
Calif.), 475
Nursing Home Residents'
Advisory Council (NHRAC),
369–370
Nursing Home Residents

Advocates, 370
Nutrition, 8, 16, 19, 20, 33, 35,
65, 72, 113, 199, 247–262,
334, 400, 471, 473, 476
critique of American diet, 35,
249–250, 257, 259, 260
diet and disease, 249–251,
256, 257, 258, 261, 334
food processing, 248–249
See also Dieting; Overweight;
Vitamins and minerals

Obesity. *See* Overweight
Observation. *See* Diagnosis,
observation in
Obstetrics
hypnosis in, 146–148, 153,
154, 157
See also Childbirth
Occupation and health, 40–41,
42, 72
Office of Health Information
and Health Promotion, 477,
492
Office of Technology Assessment
(OTA), 305, 319–320
Oral health. *See* Dentistry
Oral Roberts University, 194
Orgone research, 34, 224. *See
also* Reichian therapy
Orthomolecular medicine, 262
Osteopathy, 5, 174, 227–228
Overeaters Anonymous, 252, 260
Overweight, 8, 20, 251–252,
259–260, 459. *See also*
Dieting

Pain, 143–144, 154, 155, 156,
181, 186, 187, 336–337, 341,
383–384, 386, 413, 414, 421,
470, 471, 472
Pain and Health Rehabilitation
Center (La Crosse, Wisc.),
453, 470, 471, 472, 473, 475,
476, 480
Pain Control Unit (UCLA), 451,
471, 472, 473, 474, 475–480
Palmer Research Clinic, 231
Pastoral counseling, 11, 470
Patient education. *See* Self-care
Patients' rights, 319
Peckham experiment, 42–43, 51
Pellagra, 251
Pesticides, 73, 75–76, 79–80,

83–84. *See also* Environment
Phoenix Society, 375
Physical exercise, 16, 20, 191–
    208, 374, 376, 400, 472, 473
    and aging, 205, 374, 376
    and health, 196–199
    and mental health, 198–199,
        200
    Swedish approach, 204
    See also Aikido; Kum nye;
        Psychocalesthenics; Running
        and jogging; Taì chi chuan;
        Yoga
Physicians for Social
    Responsibility, 22
Physics, 11
Pioneer Health Center, 42, 47,
    51
Placebo effect, 11, 109, 110,
    121–123, 179–189, 487
    definition, 181
    and schizophrenia, 187–188
    and stress, 186–187
Plants, 263–276
    administration, 267
    drugs derived from, 264, 268–
        269
    early uses, 263
    herbal and plant remedies,
        270–275
    preparation, 266–267
    subtle energies, 267–268, 270
    variability, 265–266
Pollution
    air, 72, 82, 84
    environmental, 73–74, 78, 84
    household pollutants, 74
    water, 79
    See also Environment;
        Pesticides; Radiation;
        Toxicology
Population growth, 72–73
Preventive medicine, 17–18,
    488–489. *See also* Dentistry,
    preventive oral health;
    Health promotion; High level
    wellness
Prince George's County Free
    Clinic, 469
Psi, 453
Psychiatry. *See* Psychotherapy
Psychic diagnosis. *See* Diagnosis,
    psychic

Psychic healing, 11, 169–177,
    463. *See also* Laying-on-of-
    hands
Psychocalisthenics, 208, 242
Psychokinesis, 172, 176, 453
Psychophysiology, 115, 127, 128
Psychosomatic illness, 9–10, 62,
    107–113, 345
Psychosynthesis, 459
Psychotherapy, 16, 30, 31, 161,
    166–168, 181, 182, 187,
    188–189, 214–215, 219, 222,
    223, 225, 352, 362, 440, 500,
    501. *See also* Gestalt
    therapy; Mental health
Pulse diagnosis. *See* Diagnosis,
    pulse

Radiation
    ionizing, 77, 81
    microwave and non-ionizing,
        68, 71–72, 77–78, 82–83
Raynaud's disease, 119, 347
RDA. *See* Recommended Dietary
    Allowance
Recommended Dietary
    Allowance (RDA), 253, 338
Reichian therapy, 34, 214–215,
    219, 223–224, 446. *See also*
    Touch
Reston-Herndon Medical Center
    (Herndon, Va.), 93
Retired Senior Volunteer
    Program (RSVP), 371
Rickets, 251, 297–298
Rolfing, 211–212, 216, 224–225,
    446, 459, 462. *See also*
    Touch
Royal Air Force exercise
    program, 110
Running and jogging, 192, 199,
    204–208, 472, 473. *See also*
    Physical exercise

SAGE. *See* Senior Actualization
    and Growth Explorations
San Andreas Health Council
    (Palo Alto, Calif.), 472
Santa Cruz Birth Center, 310
Santa Cruz Midwives, 307, 311
Schistosomiasis, 72
Schizophrenia, 181, 187–188
Scurvy, 250–251

Self-care, 18, 19, 34, 87–103,
    471, 487, 499
    classes, 93–94, 101
    clinics, 90–92
    definition, 88
    health education, 95
    and holistic health, 89–90
    issues in, 97
    publications, 95–96, 100, 102
Self-regulation. *See* Autogenic
    therapy; Biofeedback;
    Meditation, as self-regulation
    strategy
Senior Acutalization and Growth
    Explorations (SAGE), 368,
    377, 476
Senior citizens. *See* Aging
Senior Companion Program
    (Santa Cruz, Calif.), 369
Senior Health Source (SHS)
    (Albuquerque, N.M.), 369
Seniors Health Program
    (Chicago, Ill.), 368
Sensory awareness, 213–214,
    219–220, 221–222
Sentics, 282
Sexuality and health, 20–21,
    149, 194–195
SHANTI Project, 383, 384, 390,
    477
Shiatsu massage, 211, 216, 223
Sinus tachycardia, 119, 134. *See
    also* Cardiovascular disease
Social and Athletic Readjustment
    Rating Scale (SARRS), 356
Social context of health, 17, 39–
    52, 472, 474
    demographic changes, 41–42
    networks, 44–46
    Peckham experiment, 43–44
    statistical approach, 40
Social Readjustment Rating Scale
    (SRSS), 18, 45, 350, 351,
    353, 361–362
Sound. *See* Music and health
Spiritual healing, 11, 16, 243,
    245–246. *See also* Psychic
    healing
Spontaneous remission, 11, 109,
    169
Sports, 193–195. *See also*
    Physical exercise
Sports medicine, 196

Stress, 8, 10, 18, 34, 45, 59, 108, 110, 111–112, 186–187, 345–362, 375, 376, 377–378, 472, 479, 493
    biofeedback treatment, 117–120
    and breathing, 375–376
    and the colon, 359–360
    and disease, 108, 345–353, 357
    and the nose, 358–359
    Schedule of Recent Experience (SRE), 362
    and the stomach, 359
    treatment techniques, 108–109
    See also Cardiovascular disease; Hypertension
Structural integration. *See* Rolfing
Students International Meditation Society (SIMS), 162
Subluxation. *See* Chiropractic, subluxation
Sugar, 35, 257
Superhealth. *See* High level wellness
Surgery, 4, 9, 145, 155, 158
Swedish Medical Center, 473
Swedish Wellness Program, 473

Tai chi chuan, 22, 192, 195, 241, 242, 471
Technology, medical, 79
Telekinesis. *See* Psychokinesis
Television, 42, 65, 68
Tension. *See* Hypertension; Stress
Thematic Apperception Test, 462
Thermonuclear war, 73
Thomsonian system, 5, 271
Tibetan medicine, 245–246, 451
Touch, 11, 19–20, 21, 34, 35, 175, 209–225, 425, 446, 459, 472. *See also* Alexander technique; Bioenergetics; Feldenkrais exercises; Kum nye; Laying-on-of-hands; Massage; Reichian therapy; Rolfing; Sensory awareness; Shiatsu massage
Toxicology, 70–71, 76–77, 85. *See also* Pesticides; Pollution; Radiation

Traditional healing and medicine. *See* Indigenous healing
Tuberculosis, 57, 349, 360–361
Type A behavior, 10, 108, 111

UCLA Pain Control Unit. *See* Pain Control Unit
Urban condition and health, 50, 102

Vaccines, 5
Visualization, 18, 19, 34, 110, 112, 113, 378, 448–449, 458–459, 461, 462–463, 471, 482. *See also* Diagnosis, imagery in; Guided fantasy; Guided Imagery and Music
Vitamins and minerals, 110, 248, 251, 252–253, 254, 258, 259, 260–261, 264. *See also* Nutrition
    vitamin C, 258, 259, 260–261

Weight Watchers, 252
Wellness Resource Center (Mill Valley, Calif.), 92, 473, 477, 482
Wholistic Health and Nutrition Institute, 471, 472, 473, 475, 476
Wholistic Health Centers, 470, 476, 482
Wolf-Parkinson-White disease, 120
Women's health, 13, 28–29, 100, 208, 477
World Health Organization, 17, 313

Yan and yang, 408–409, 410, 411, 416, 449–450, 463
Yoga, 22, 159, 160, 192, 195, 206, 208, 242–243, 244, 246, 374, 400, 425, 459, 471, 472, 473–474
    hatha, 195, 206, 242, 246, 374
    Kundalini, 243–244, 476

Zen Buddhism, 206, 243